Lymph Node Biopsy Interpretation

To the memory of
the late Dr Iris Hamlin
who first began writing this book

Lymph Node Biopsy Interpretation

EDITED BY

A G Stansfeld
Department of Histopathology,
St Bartholomew's Hospital, London

CHURCHILL LIVINGSTONE
EDINBURGH LONDON MELBOURNE AND NEW YORK 1985

CHURCHILL LIVINGSTONE
Medical Division of Longman Group Limited

Distributed in the United States of America by Churchill Livingstone Inc., 1560 Broadway, New York, N.Y. 10036, and by associated companies, branches and representatives throughout the world.

First published 1985

ISBN 0-443-03291-2

British Library Cataloguing in Publication Data
Lymph node biopsy interpretation.
1. Lymphatics — Biopsy
I. Stansfeld, A.G.
616.4'207583 RC646

Library of Congress Cataloging in Publication Data
Main entry under title:
Lymph node biopsy interpretation.
1. Lymph nodes — Biopsy. 2. Lymph nodes — Diseases — Diagnosis. 3. Histology, Pathological. I. Stansfeld, A.G. [DNLM: 1. Biopsy — methods. 2. Lymph Nodes — pathology. 3. Lympatic Diseases — pathology. WH 700 L986]
RC646.L93 1985 616.4'207'58 85-12731

Printed and bound in Great Britain by
William Clowes Limited, Beccles and London

Preface

The primary aim of this book is to assist the general hospital histopathologist in the interpretation of lymph node biopsy sections and most of the chapters have been written with this objective directly in view. A prime necessity is to realise that the static picture seen down the microscope represents only a moment in time and that the cells of the lymphoreticular system are normally in a constant state of dynamic activity. This aspect is emphasised in the introductory chapter, which relates the structural features of the lymph node to its functional characteristics.

Secondly, whilst morphology, as revealed by the light microscope, has been the mainstay of diagnosis and is likely to remain so in the foreseeable future, the pathologist can no longer afford to neglect the impact which other methods of investigation are making on lymph node biopsy interpretation. In particular, immunostaining and the increasing development and use of monoclonal antibodies are refining the diagnosis of malignant lymphomas, as of many other neoplasms. It is not to be expected that every hospital laboratory will have either the time or the facilities to use such techniques to the full, but it is important that histopathologists should be aware of the scope of such methods of study.

There have been such rapid advances in immunopathology in recent years that one may not doubt that some of our present concepts are likely to be out of date almost before the ink is dry on the page, but whatever their precise interpretation, the morphological appearances will remain the same.

I am indebted to my fellow authors who have contributed individual chapters to this book and to a number of histopathologists, both in Britain and abroad, who have kindly contributed material from which illustrations have been made. In particular I wish to thank Drs K L Agarwal, M A Ahmed, K J Arulambalam, S J Beales, W L Brander, C M Chabrel, K W Chan, F W Chandler, I Chorlton, R M Cross, P Davies, J Diebold, F E Dische, J L Dyson, M D E Evans, R Finlayson, N E France, C V Harrison, W J Harrison, E H Hemsted, W M R Henerson, K A Jasim, B S Jones, M Kikuchi, G Krasznai, I Lampert, P W Leedham, J J Lucey, A MacFarlane, L E McGee, J B MacGillivray, F McGinty, I M Magrath, O Mioduszewska, J A K Missen, E E Peters, D M Pryce, J I Pugh, D B Rimmer, E Sato, R M Seal, S G Subbuswamy, T Suchi, A C Thackray, K A D Turk, K Valteris, L Vogel and I G Williams.

I owe much to the expert technical assistance of Miss Gillian Latham and other members of the technical staff of the histopathology department at St Bartholomew's Hospital. I would like to thank Mr Peter Crocker and his staff and also the department of medical illustration for photographic assistance. I have benefited greatly from collaboration with Dr John Habeshaw in understanding the immunological aspects of malignant lymphomas and have enjoyed close cooperation with my clinical colleagues on the staff of the ICRF Medical Oncology Unit at St Bartholomew's Hospital. Of the many people from whom I have learned, I am particularly grateful to Professor Karl Lennert, both for his instruction and for his friendship.

Finally, I wish to thank Miss Jill Grimsey for typing the entire manuscript and the publishers for their tolerance and patience over the long gestation period which this book has had.

London, 1985 A.G.S.

List of contributors

Dr J. A. L. Amess
Department of Haematology, St Bartholomew's Hospital, London

Dr A. J. Blackshaw
Department of Pathology, St Bartholomew's Hospital, London

Dr T. J. Chambers
Department of Experimental Pathology, St Bartholomew's Hospital, London

Dr J. D. Davies
University Department of Pathology, Bristol Royal Infirmary, Bristol

Dr J. A. Habeshaw
Medical Oncology Unit, St Bartholomew's Hospital, London

Dr J. G. Hall
Chester Beatty Institute, Royal Marsden Hospital, Sutton, Surrey

Miss Gillian Latham
Department of Histopathology, St Bartholomew's Hospital, London

Dr F. Paradinas
Department of Histopathology, Charing Cross Hospital, London

Dr A. G. Stansfeld
Department of Histopathology, St Bartholomew's Hospital, London

Dr G. T. Williams
Department of Pathology, University Hospital of Wales, Cardiff

Contents

1

J.G. Hall

The functional anatomy of lymph nodes

INTRODUCTION

The lymph nodes of mammals are aggregates of precisely structured lympho-reticular tissue which are placed at intervals along the lymphatic vessels that return excess tissue fluid to the blood. The main function of lymph nodes is to arrest, neutralise and eliminate antigenic materials and micro-organisms that have gained entry to the tissue fluids and have been conveyed to the nodes by their afferent lymph. The initial arrest of such immunogens is brought about usually by phagocytic macrophages. Many macrophages simply degrade the foreign material that they have engulfed but others, probably rather specialised 'dendritic' cells, present the antigen in an easily recognisable form to the T and B lymphocytes which respond to the proffered antigens by transforming into blast cells and undergoing mitotic division. Some of these blast cells become plasma cells and migrate to the medulla of the node where they make the antibodies which opsonise bacteria and neutralise viruses and toxins: some migrate to the primary lymphoid follicles in the cortical regions and participate in the formation of germinal centres; others produce lymphokines or become cells which mediate 'cellular' immunity and delayed-type hypersensitivity so that some of them can kill allograft cells or cells infected with viruses. None of these lymphoid cells is confined to the node which produced them. They are carried first by the lymph, and then by the blood, and become disseminated throughout the lymphoid tissue of the body to produce a state of systemic immunity which will deal effectively with the next onslaught of the particular pathogen which elicited their generation.

In other words, the cells which have passed through a lymph node are quantitatively and qualitatively as important to an understanding of what is going on inside it as the numbers and types of cells that happen to be present when the node is dropped into fixative and prepared for microscopical examination. Even under basal conditions a lymph node will transmit its own weight of recirculating lymphocytes from blood to lymph in about 12 days, and the extent of this traffic will double or treble when the node reacts to an antigenic stimulus. This is made possible by a rich supply of blood which flows through the node at a rate of at least 1 ml per minute per gram node weight. Similarly, there is a significant flow of tissue fluid, or lymph, through the node which is of the order of 10 ml per hour per gram node weight. These figures relate to basal conditions and they are liable to substantial increases when the cardiovascular system is in a hyperdynamic state.

When a node is biopsied all these processes are brought to a halt and, perhaps inevitably, attention becomes focused on the more static elements of the node. Because of this it is necessary to make a conscious effort while at the microscope to remember the vigorous and abundant traffic of cells and fluid which constitute the real 'raison d'être' for the histological features of a lymph node. The biological function of this traffic of cells has always been something of a puzzle. No one really knows why, or even if, it is essential for immunological reactivity. It is believed at the moment that the modulation of immune responses is brought about by the critical but large scale interactions of B cells and subsets of T cells. Presumably, these interactions only can be brought about under properly controlled and regulated conditions in organised lymphoid tissues such as lymph nodes where the continual reassortment of lymphocyte subsets is possible. Unfortunately, there is no way of describing these events in the micro-anatomical terms derived from our rather simple ideas about the structure of lymph nodes. The truth of the matter is that we know very little indeed about how lymph nodes really work, and this makes writing about them, in ways which will help a pathologist, very difficult. The other difficulty is the lack of a common and comprehensive terminology. Experimentalists have to employ a simple terminology that can be applied to all experimental animals and they cannot always use easily the detailed nomenclature of cell types which pathologists apply, quite properly, to human material. Those concerned with basic research on cytological aspects of immuno-biology are prepared to recognise fibrocytes and fibroblasts, the endothelial cells of blood and lymphatic vessels, blood leucocytes, macrophages, small lymphocytes and large lymphocytes (i.e. immunoblasts which are either of T- or B- cell lineage) and plasma cells. Terms like centrocyte, centroblast, histiocyte and reticulum cell have little general currency. This does not mean necessarily that the existence of such cells is denied but merely that the terms are either too restrictive or imprecise to be used in general immunobiological discussions. Today, the classification of subsets of the major cell types is carried out by immuno-histological or automated electronic cell-sorting techniques that depend on the recognition of type specific membrane antigens by monoclonal antibodies. These special techniques are discussed further in chapter 4.

GENERAL ORGANISATION OF LYMPH NODES AND LYMPHATICS

Lymph nodes, like the lymphocytes, are heterogeneous and it is necessary to be aware both of the differences between them and the terminology that describes them.

Lymph nodes made a fairly late appearance on the evolutionary scene and fully organised nodes are restricted to mammals. However, lymphatic vessels make a much earlier appearance for they are, after all, an integral part of any high-pressure, circulatory system. The lymphatics exist to collect the proteinaceous tissue fluid formed in the capillary beds by the excess of filtration over reabsorption, and return it to the blood vascular compartment. This fluid, or lymph, which is formed in the peripheral tissues, is known as 'peripheral lymph'; it is lymph that has not passed through a lymph node, and it contains very few cells. The lymph vessels which collect it join together to form larger peripheral lymphatic vessels which in mammals, convey it to peripheral lymph nodes like the popliteal or epitrochlear lymph nodes of man. Such nodes are characterised by having their entire supply of afferent lymph made up of peripheral lymph. The efferent ducts from such nodes are of course 'afferent' to the next nodes up the chain (e.g. the inguinal or axillary nodes in man). The lymph in ducts between lymph nodes is known as 'intermediate' lymph; the composition of the actual lymph plasma is similar to that of the peripheral lymph from which it is derived but, of course, it does contain many more cells. These are recirculating lymphocytes which entered the lymph stream from the blood, as it passed through the peripheral lymph nodes. Intermediate lymph nodes, like the inguinal or axillary nodes, will thus have two sorts of afferent lymph supply. One will be true, peripheral, hypocellular afferent lymph formed in the local tissues which they drain, the other will be the highly cellular efferent from more peripheral nodes. The efferent ducts from the first set of intermediate nodes go to deeper, internal nodes and the efferents from these ultimately join together to form the main lymph trunks (i.e. the lumbar, intestinal, cervical and thoracic ducts) the contents of which are referred to as 'central' lymph, i.e. lymph which will not pass through any more lymph nodes before it reaches the blood. Thus, lymph formed, say, in the foot will traverse many groups of lymph nodes before it reaches the thoracic duct but this is not an invariable pattern. In the gut, for example, things are organised a bit differently. The gut itself is a major lymphoid organ; there is much lymphoid tissue scattered in the *lamina propria* of the intestine and in addition there are macroscopic aggregates of organised lymphoid tissue — the Peyer's patches. The effect of this is to endow the peripheral lymph formed in the gut with an unusually large population of lymphocytes so the mesenteric nodes, which technically could be considered peripheral nodes, have a supply of unusually cellular afferent lymph. Also, this lymph has only to traverse one set of nodes, the mesenteric lymph nodes, before it becomes 'central lymph' in the intestinal duct. These peculiarities are reflected to some extent in the structure and function of the mesenteric nodes and will be mentioned later. Similar considerations apply to some of the cervical lymph nodes which drain 'Waldeyer's ring' (i.e. the lymphoid tissue of the pharynx — tonsils, adenoids etc.) and whose efferent ducts discharge directly into the deep cervical lymph duct.

Lymph nodes have many more afferent ducts, which convey lymph to them, than efferent ducts that carry the lymph away. Commonly, lymph nodes have only two or three efferent ducts but there are usually at least half a dozen afferent ducts and sometimes over a score.

All lymph ducts from the most peripheral afferents to the central thoracic duct contain smooth muscle in their walls. The active contractions of these muscle fibres, together with the numerous bicuspid valves which prevent retrograde flow, are responsible for forcing the lymph powerfully in a central direction (Hall et al, 1965).

These features are shown in the accompanying schematic diagram of a lymph node (Fig. 1.1), but before discussing the detailed structure of lymph nodes it will be convenient to consider the cells travelling in the lymph stream.

CELLULAR COMPOSITION OF LYMPH

Peripheral lymph

By constructing chronic lymphatic fistulae in experimental animals peripheral lymph has been collected under physiological conditions from the soft tissues of the limbs and torso, from the testis,

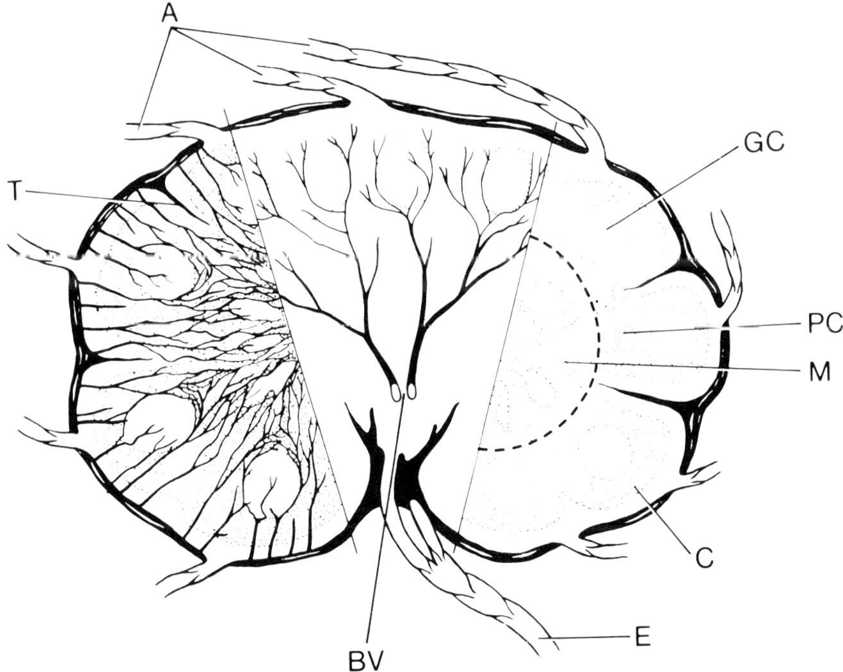

Fig. 1.1 Schematic diagram of a lymph node. A, afferent lymphatics. BV, blood vessels. C, cortex. E, efferent lymphatic. GC, germinal centre. M, medulla. PC, paracortex. The left hand portion of the diagram shows the capsule and trabeculae and suggests the network of reticulin fibres, which is relatively sparse in actual germinal centres. The middle portion shows the blood vessels; again, these do not penetrate the germinal centres to any great extent but enfold them in a 'goblet-like' configuration. The right hand portion shows the main areas of the lymphoid component and the broken line arbitrarily demarcates the medulla from the cortex. Immediately above the medulla, and beneath the germinal centres and the true cortex, is the paracortex — an area which can expand greatly during the inductive phase of an immune response and which is the site of much lymphocyte traffic and T cell proliferation.

ovary, thyroid, liver, kidney and intestine. Also, peripheral lymph has been collected from the limbs of man.

Intestinal lymph apart, the cellular composition of peripheral lymph from these various sources is rather similar. The cell count is low, usually about 200 per mm^3 and rarely more than 1000. Under normal conditions the cells are virtually all mononuclear, though occasional eosinophil granulocytes may be present. Up to 15% are cells of the macrophage-monocyte series and the rest are recirculating lymphocytes. These lymphocytes can only have come from extravasation from the blood and their presence in peripheral lymph is important evidence that ordinary capillary beds, which lack any specialised cuboidal endothelium at their venular end, are perfectly capable of at once transmitting lymphocytes into the tissue spaces and preventing the escape of other formed elements from the blood. Most of the lymphocytes in peripheral lymph are T cells as only 10% of them bear surface Ig, compared with 25% or so in the blood or intermediate lymph, and this indicates that their extravasation from the blood cannot have been an entirely random event.

Many of the macrophage-like cells in the peripheral lymph have all the cytological and histochemical features of conventional macrophages and monocytes and most people are content to accept them as such. A minority of the macrophage-like cells is characterised by a very active membrane which gives the living cells a spectacular 'veiled' or 'frilly' appearance when they are observed with phase-contrast optics (Fig. 1.2). There is some argument about the nature of these veiled cells. Some believe they are not true macrophages

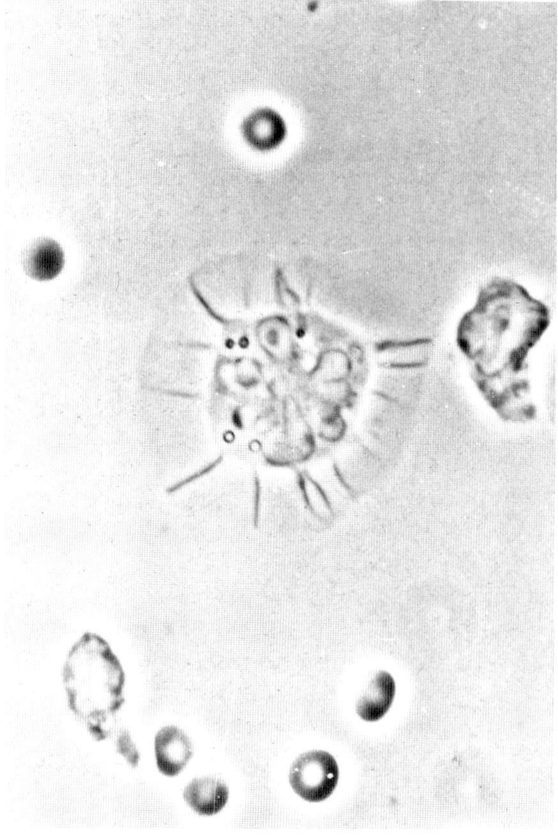

A

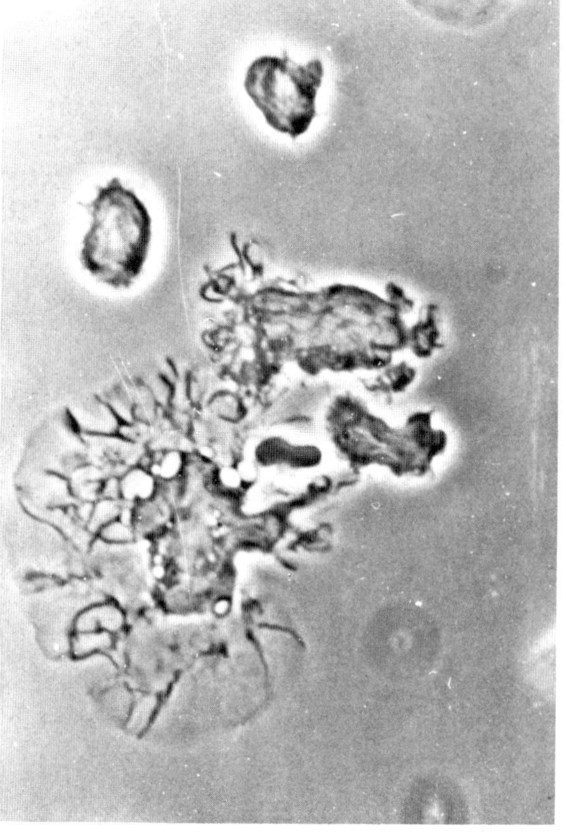

B

Fig. 1.2 Phase contrast photomicrographs of peripheral leg lymph of sheep (approx. × 1700) to show living, dendritic macrophages; small lymphocytes and red cells are present as well. A shows a 'classical' dendritic cell, while the two in B are more pleomorphic.

and are related to or derived from the dendritic Langerhans cells which are found (e.g.) at the base of the epidermis. Such cells (either in skin or in lymph) are believed to be important in the induction of cutaneous hypersensitivity reactions and they are supposed to have a crucial, UV-sensitive role in this specialised type of antigen presentation. The matter is controversial. For the sake of simplicity, it is easier to think of all the macrophage-like cells in lymph as being macrophages for, as the accompanying illustrations show, even the most dendritic cells are capable of phagocytosing immune complexes (Fig. 1.3). One of the difficulties in investigating the properties of these cell types is that they tend to perform badly in in vitro systems. In vivo they take up particulate material like carbon or immune complexes quite avidly but tend not to do so to nearly the same extent in vitro. However, whatever rôle one attributes to these cells one must remember that in absolute terms their numbers are very, very small. For example, if one injects even sterile saline subcutaneously the traumatic inflammation is sufficient to elicit a flood of neutrophil granulocytes in the regional peripheral lymph. If immune complexes (which can activate complement) are injected instead of saline, even more acute inflammatory granulocytes are called forth, and most of the injected antigen is conveyed to the regional node either free in the lymph plasma or inside polymorphonuclear neutrophil granulocytes. That moiety of the antigen that reaches the regional node on or in dendritic macrophages is a very small part of the total, though this need not mean that such cells have no importance. It is likely though that their rôle in inducing immune responses relates to cellular antigens like transplantation antigens or chemical haptens that have become fixed to (e.g.) epidermal cells. Such antigens cannot gain direct entry into the lymph but they can, conceivably, be 'sampled' by wandering dendritic macrophages which then enter the peripheral lymph and carry the 'antigenic message' to the regional node. As a group the macrophages of peripheral lymph express abundant Ia antigens on their surfaces and this is believed to facilitate the presentation of antigen to T lymphocytes. These macrophages are perhaps most abundant in peripheral lymph from the liver and it is easy to show, by a prior intravenous injection of indian ink, which labels the phagocytic Kupffer cells of the hepatic sinusoids with carbon, that many of the dendritic macrophages in peripheral lymph become labelled and must have been derived from the phagocytic cells in the tissue in which the lymph was formed.

The cell types in peripheral lymph from the intestine are similar to those described above: the main difference is a quantitative one, the cell count being up to 100 times higher than in peripheral lymph from other organs. Also, a few of the macrophage-like cells are replete with fat droplets which derive, presumably, from the products of digestion.

Intermediate and central lymph

The cell count of intermediate and central lymph varies widely between species, between individuals and between different anatomical locations and may range from 5000 to 50 000 white cells per mm^3. Under normal circumstances lymph of this description is populated almost entirely by normal small lymphocytes which have been derived from the blood by extravasation in the paracortices of lymph nodes and which comprise the 'recirculating pool'. About 25% of them bear surface Ig and are thus B lymphocytes, the remainder is made up of the various subsets of T cells. Occasional neutrophil and eosinophil granulocytes are present but macrophage-like cells are hardly ever seen. Apparently the dendritic macrophages from peripheral lymph are almost quantitatively retained by the first lymph nodes they reach but their ultimate fate and function are uncertain.

The rather uniform appearance of the lymphocytes in intermediate and central lymph changes dramatically after antigens have impinged on the lymph nodes. This subject will be dealt with in detail later but one or two points should be made right away. The salient observation is that within about 100 hours of the antigenic stimulus large numbers of lymphoid blast cells start to appear in the lymph (Fig. 1.4). These immunoblasts may account for nearly half the cells in the efferent lymph from a stimulated node and they display frequent mitotic figures. It is important to stress that, neoplasia apart, the presence of such cells is indicative of the fact that an immune response is

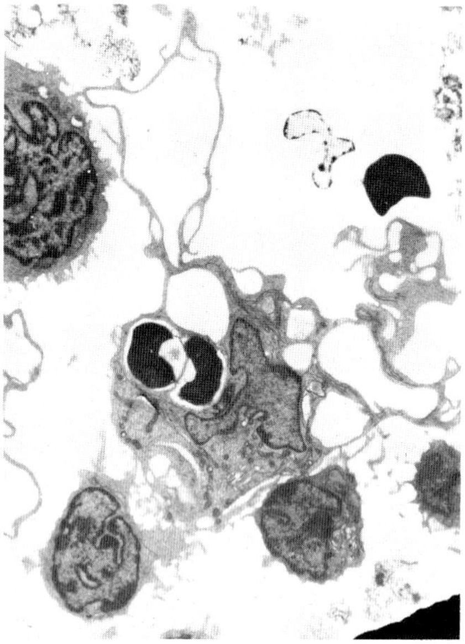

A

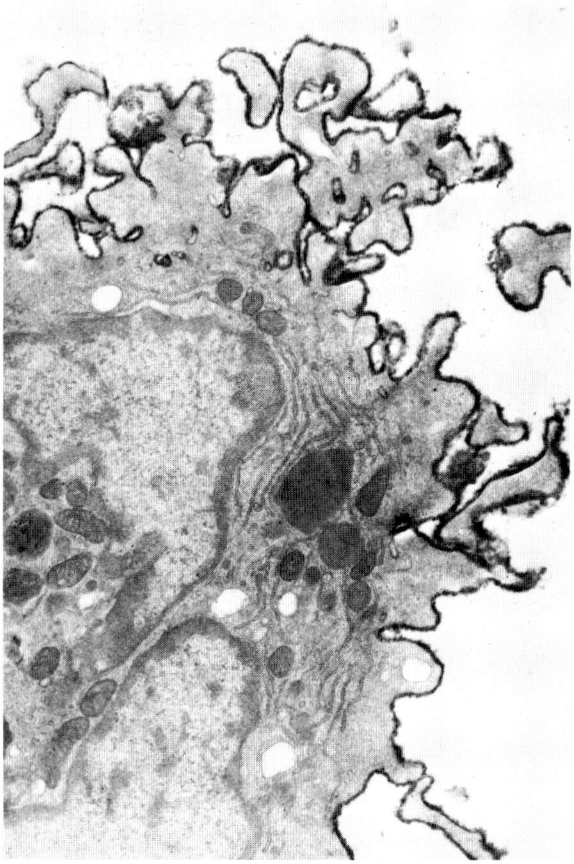

B

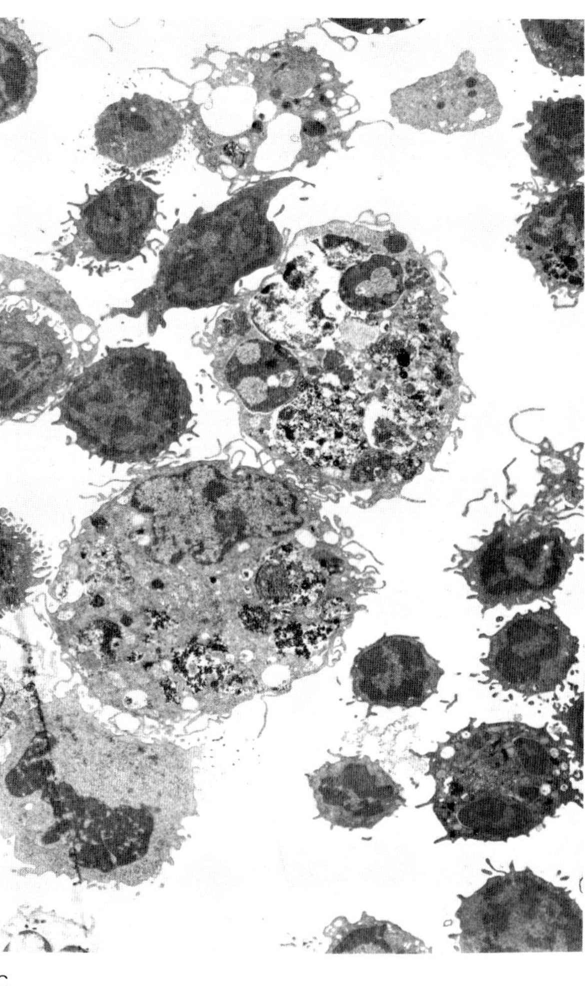

C

Fig. 1.3 Transmission electron micrographs of peripheral lymph. A. Dendritic macrophage, containing phagocytosed red cells and closely applied to two lymphocytes, from the peripheral intestinal lymph of a sheep (approx. × 3000). B. Dendritic macrophage from the peripheral intestinal lymph of a rat. The membrane has been stained with immuno-peroxidase reagents, the primary antibody being a mouse monoclonal directed against rat Ia-like antigens. Many cells of this type have abundant Ia antigens on their surfaces. (approx. × 16 500). C. Macrophages in peripheral lymph from the leg of a sheep. The dark staining material in their phago-lysosomes is horseradish peroxidase which they had engulfed in vivo in the form of immune complexes (approx. × 4 400). N.B. Figure A is reproduced from *Blood Cells*, 5, 479–492 (1979) by permission of the Editors.

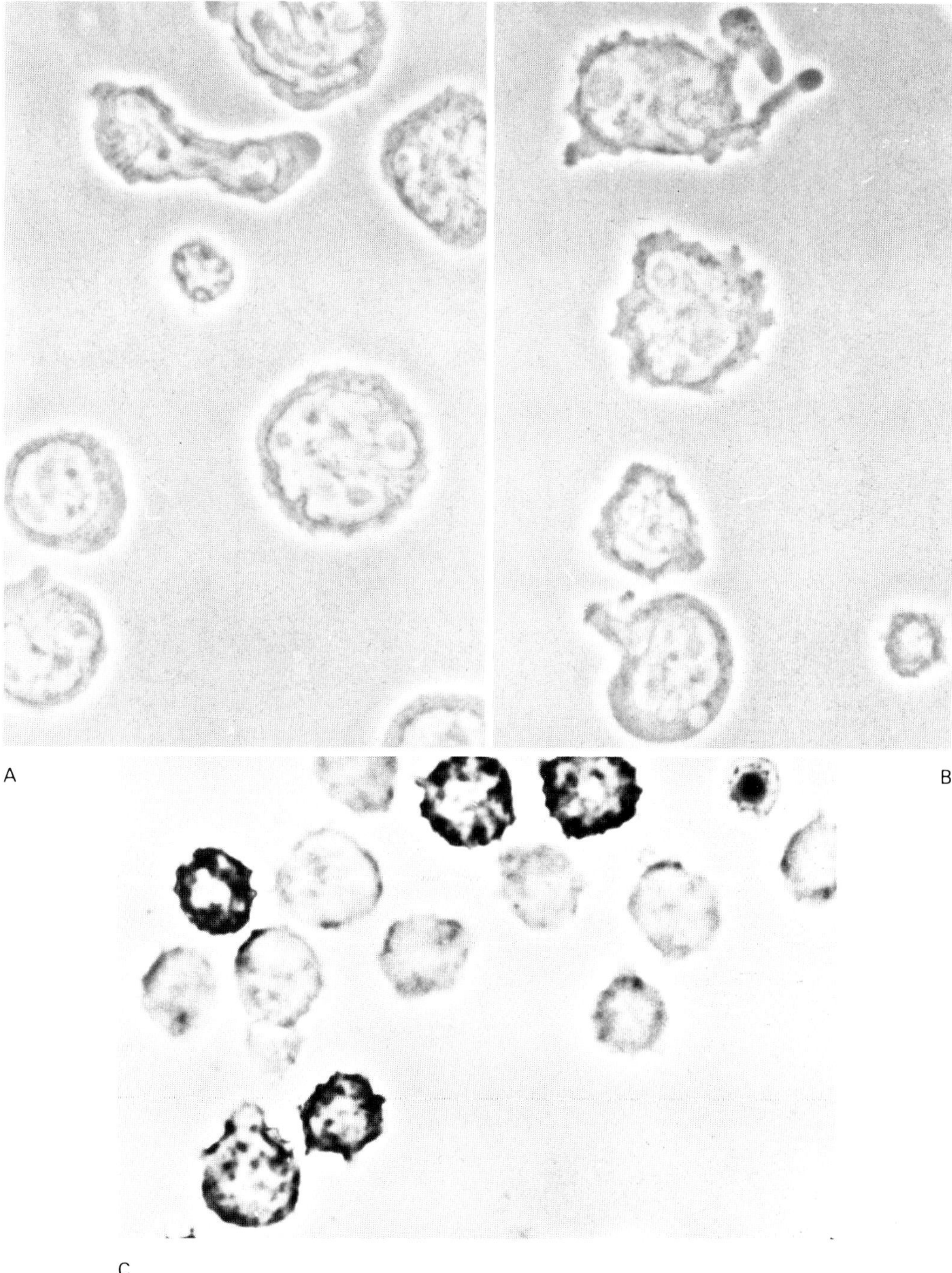

Fig. 1.4 Phase contrast photomicrographs of cells in efferent lymph. A and B, live preparations (approx. × 1200) showing numerous immunoblasts, with a small lymphocyte for comparison, at the height of an immune response, about 100 h after primary antigenic stimulation. C, fixed preparation (approx. × 2000) showing small lymphocytes. The Ig-bearing, 'B' lymphocytes have been stained with anti-immunoglobulin immunoperoxidase reagents.

in progress. It follows that lymph from nodes which receive chronic stimuli should always contain some immunoblasts. This, in fact, is the case and intestinal lymph from all healthy, normal animals contains always a few percent of immunoblasts. These are generated in response to the dietary and microbial antigens from the gut which impinge continually on the intestinal lymphoid tissue and mesenteric lymph nodes.

THE STRUCTURE OF LYMPH NODES

A schematic diagram of a lymph node is shown in Figure 1.1 (p. 3). Many textbooks of histology start to describe lymph nodes by showing a sketch of an idealised lymph node, crowded with primary follicles, germinal centres, a proliferating paracortex and a well demarcated medulla. It is certainly true that one can find lymph nodes, like the mesenteric nodes which receive continual antigenic stimulation from the gut, which really do show all these features but one can also find many that do not.

The appearance of a lymph node in an adult individual is, like that of the individual, the product of the interaction between the environment and a basic, genetically determined structure. In the case of the lymphoid system the important environmental influence is the continual onslaught of immunogens, usually in the form of bacteria and their toxins, viruses and dietary antigens. Many animals, particularly the usual laboratory rodents, are born before the lymphoid system is properly developed and so its normal growth and development occur side by side with the reactive proliferation caused by exogenous stimuli. Indeed, some would go as far as to say that in these species continual antigenic stimulation is essential for the proper morphogenesis of lymphoid tissue. In any event, it is not easy always to decide whether the changes that take place in the lymph nodes of young rats and mice are caused by antigens, by normal growth and development, or by both. However, some animals have lymphoid systems that are well developed, both anatomically and functionally, well before birth exposes them to an antigenic environment. This applies particularly to ruminants and it is a happy circumstance for the experimenter. A study of the lymph nodes of fetuses of such animals shows what they look like before they have been exposed to any antigen and shows which types of cellular activity take place spontaneously, as opposed to those which occur only in response to antigenic challenge. In this way it is possible to discern more easily the true structure of a lymph node and how its later experiences lead it to acquire the appearances of the so-called 'normal' node of traditional histological texts.

The reticular structure and phagocytic functions

As has been implied already, most of the lymphocytes, and perhaps even some of the macrophages in a lymph node are really only temporary visitors to lymph nodes, the basic structure of which consists of a meshwork or 'reticulum' of fibres, the cells which secrete them and the macrophages which cover them (Greek: rete = meshwork, or net). There is some argument about the nature of the cells and fibres that make up the reticulum of the node. Hard-line cell biologists take the view that all the non-contractile, extracellular fibres in the reticulum are composed of variants of the collagen molecule, and that the cells which secrete them are therefore fibrocytes or fibroblasts. In active lymph nodes the reticular meshwork is not uniform, it is distorted and modified by the presence of the lymphoid component, especially when the latter is in a phase of ebullient activity or proliferation, but these are essentially secondary effects. Perhaps the most striking demonstration of the primary structure of lymph nodes is seen shortly after high doses of whole body irradiation or cytotoxic drugs have eradicated the lymphocytes. In such circumstances the lymph nodes do not disappear, they are still perfectly tangible structures only marginally smaller to casual inspection than their normal counterparts. Microscopical examination reveals that, although there are few lymphocytes, there is surprisingly little empty space, instead there are sheets of fibrocytes and macrophages. The lymph nodes from patients with Swiss-type agammaglobulinaemia present a similar appearance (see Fig. 8.5). The only easy way to demonstrate the basic structure of normal nodes is to employ silver impregnation methods which show up the agyrophilic extracellular fibres of the reticulum.

Like any organ the lymph node requires some sort of structural scaffolding to give it enough mechanical strength to maintain its generally reniform shape. This is provided by a capsule and internal trabeculae composed of dense collagenous fibres and smooth muscle fibres. The capsule is penetrated by numerous afferent lymphatics which discharge their lymph into the subcapsular sinus. After flowing through the node parenchyma, via the lymph sinuses, the lymph leaves the node via one or two efferent lymphatics which leave the node where the blood vessels enter, in the hilus. It is to this capsule and trabeculae of dense collagenous tissue that the meshwork of more delicate fibres is attached. The fixed macrophages of the lymph node are attached, in their turn, to the meshwork of fibres so that the basic reticulum of the node is covered with macrophages which thus present an enormous area of phagocytic surface to the lymph stream which percolates through the node. From a functional point of view the reticulum of the node is made up therefore of the fibres and fibre-forming cells on which is superimposed a layer of phagocytic, macrophage-like cells. Most of these seem to be fixed phagocytic cells which line the lymph sinuses; more specialised 'dendritic' cells, whose functions and lineages are matters of hot debate, are associated with the afferent lymph and germinal centres. Any or all of these cell types could thus be termed a 'reticulum' cell but it is better to use a more precise terminology whenever possible. However, it is the basic structure that is important and if this is kept in mind there is little difficulty in appreciating the anatomical basis for the filtering function of lymph nodes. In spite of this it is sometimes stated that lymph nodes are poor filters (Humphrey & White, 1970). In any general sense this statement is wrong. It is true that when soluble materials such as heterologous plasma proteins are present in the lymph stream the lymph node retains only a small proportion of the foreign material (Hall & Morris, 1963), but filters of any sort are not designed usually to retain soluble substances. Where particulate materials are concerned the filtering capacity of a lymph node can be impressive. Dead bacteria are removed almost quantitatively from the lymph stream (Hall et al, 1967). Living bacteria too, are usually cleared very efficiently when specific opsonising antibody is present though virulent, pathogenic bacteria may sometimes escape phagocytosis (Yoffey & Courtice, 1970). However, the fact that occasional pathogens with special surface properties, like certain strains of virulent pneumococci, are able to evade the phagocytic defence mechanisms (Humphrey & White, 1970) is no reason to deny the general filtering efficiency of lymph nodes. After all, pathogens are, by definition, organisms that possess special properties which allow them to elude the defences of the host for sufficient time to produce obvious disease.

The above observations refer to situations in which relatively large amounts of particulate antigens were given as single doses. In real life the amount of antigen, in absolute terms, may be much smaller but may impinge on the node for several days or weeks or months. Under these conditions the macrophages lining the lymph sinuses hypertrophy, presumably in response to chronic stimulation, and because of their abundant eosinophilic cytoplasm they become much more obvious in standard histological preparations. This tends to delineate the lymph sinuses more effectively and gives rise to an appearance known as 'sinus histiocytosis' (see p. 345).

The lymphoid component

Like the kidney and adrenal gland a lymph node has cortical and medullary regions which are sufficiently demarcated to be discerned by the naked eye in fresh material. Under the microscope the transition is less clear cut and there is an intervening no-man's land which is sometimes referred to as the paracortex. The cortex is composed of more or less densely packed lymphocytes and is bounded by the subcapsular sinus above and separated from the trabeculae by the lymph sinuses that penetrate into the node. The lymphocytes in the cortex tend to be grouped into large spherical masses called primary nodules (follicles). When, in post-natal life, these primary lymphatic nodules become the site of focal cellular proliferation, i.e. when germinal centres are formed, the nodular pattern becomes even more apparent. The cortical tissue gradually merges into the medullary region where the lymphoid tissue is arranged in interlacing finger-like processes, the 'medullary cords'. In post-natal life these cords are the principal habitat of plasma cells and thus of large scale antibody production. In appropriately stained sections it can be seen that the reticular meshwork is more open in the cortex than in the medulla, indeed in some areas of the cortex, where germinal centres are present (q.v.) it disappears altogether. It may be that the looser arrangement in the cortex permits a greater degree of cellular movement than in the more straight-laced, slit-like reticulum of the medulla.

Although it is customary to talk of lymph 'sinuses' it should be remembered that these are merely the main channels that are obvious to standard methods of examination. The lymph fluid is not really confined to a few sinuses but is free to percolate through most of the cortical tissue before it is collected into the medullary sinuses and discharged into the efferent ducts.

This, then, is the basic arrangement of the lymphoid tissue within a node. It can be seen best by studying the nodes of fetuses, like those of sheep, where in the terminal third of gestation the fetus is fully immunocompetent and possesses a full complement of lymphocytes but is as yet unaltered by contact with antigen. It cannot be stressed too often that until post-natal life exposes a lymph node to the onslaught of antigens, there are no germinal centres in the cortex, no immunoblasts in the paracortex, no plasma cells in the medulla and no immunoglobulins in the plasma of blood or lymph (Cole & Morris, 1973). Nonetheless, in spite of the absence of antigenic stimuli, the recirculation of small lymphocytes (i.e. the entry into the node of lymphocytes by transmigration across venular endothelium) is in vigorous progress in the paracortical areas (Pearson et al, 1976). It is thus quite clear that the continual migration and redistribution of circulating lymphocytes is something that happens quite independently of antigens and soluble mediators released as a consequence of antigen–antibody interactions.

The blood supply of lymph nodes; the wherewithal for lymphocyte recirculation

A good, modern account of the blood vasculature of lymph nodes is available (Herman, 1980). The arterial blood supply approaches the node at the hilus, usually as one major vessel, the branches of which may form an arcade just before they disappear into the parenchyma of the node. Branching arterioles course from the hilus and follow the trabeculae and some supply the capillary beds of the medulla. Most reach the cortex where they supply a rich capillary network and the post-capillary venules which drain from it pass downwards and supply the deeper regions of the cortex and paracortex before coalescing into collecting veins which leave the hilus of the node as one or two major vessels.

The post-capillary venules in the paracortical regions are an important feature of the microvasculature of lymph nodes because they have a special function. The walls of these vessels seem to be selectively 'permeable' to small lymphocytes so that they are able to transmit these cells from the blood to the lymph stream, while, at the same time, they exclude the other formed elements of the blood from the lymph node. Whether the active partner in this process is the lymphocyte or the endothelial cell, or both, is unknown and the biochemical basis is obscure. In rodents, many of these venules have a high, cuboidal endothelium and in Gowans' original description of the phenomenon of lymphocyte recirculation it seemed that not only were cuboidal endothelial cells an essential structural requirement for this function, but also that the lymphocytes actually passed through the cytoplasm of the endothelial cells during the process of extravasation (Gowans & Knight, 1964). However, more recent studies (Schoefl, 1972) have shown that the lymphocytes probably pass between, and not through, the endothelial cells. There are some grounds for doubting whether the high, almost cuboidal type of endothelium that characterises some of the post-capillary venules in the lymph nodes of rats and mice, is essential for the transmigration of lymphocytes. For example, in the lymph nodes of sheep, where lymphocyte recirculation occurs on a substantial scale it has not been possible to find post-capillary venules with high endothelium. Similarly, some selective extravasation of lymphocytes goes on in peripheral tissues generally where no specialised post-capillary venules have been described. However, although the details of the mechanism by which small lymphocytes extravasate into lymph nodes are uncertain, and may vary between species, there is general agreement that it occurs mainly through post-capillary venules in the paracortical regions. Because the majority of recirculating lymphocytes are of thymic derivation it follows that much of the traffic of lymphocytes in the paracortex of the node is composed of T cells. For this reason the paracortex is often spoken of as being a 'thymus dependent' area (c.f. Parrott & de Sousa, 1971). Thus, when a mammal suffers either an experimental or naturally occurring deficit in circulating T cells the paracortices of the lymph node undergo a type of disuse atrophy and become collapsed and relatively sparsely populated, even though the true cortex, primarily a B cell area, may be unaffected.

Obviously, the exact route taken by a lymphocyte that has extravasated into a lymph node will depend to some extent on whether the lymphocyte is a B cell or a T cell. The former is more likely to move into the cortex before gaining the main lymph stream while the latter will perhaps merely traverse the paracortex. The truth is that we really know very little about the subject; three main migratory pathways have been proposed, viz. the perifollicular route, the paracortical sinus route and the paracortical cord route (Kelly, 1975), but they are easier to imagine than to demonstrate.

While the blood flows through the vascular system of the node something between 10% and 20% of the available blood lymphocytes are extracted from it and conveyed to the lymph compartment. The mechanisms which regulate the blood flow through the node are difficult to investigate and few data are available. Numerous arterio-venous communications and venous sphincters, innervated by unmyelinated nerve fibres, are said to exist in the cortical vascular bed (Anderson & Anderson, 1975) and such structures may play a role in regulating the blood flow through the post-capillary venules in the paracortex. Again, the time lymphocytes take to pass through the vascular endothelium, wander through the parenchyma of the node and emerge in the efferent lymph has not yet proved susceptible to precise measurement but a figure of about 5 hours has been proposed; lymphocytes which extravasate in non-lymphoid tissue appear to take a similar amount of time to regain the lymph stream (Hall et al, 1976).

Lymphocyte recirculation through nodes at different sites: somatic versus visceral recirculation

Until recently it was supposed generally that the lymphocytes in the blood and lymph recirculated more or less randomly through all the major lymphoid organs, i.e. the lymph nodes, the Peyer's patches and the spleen. However, about 10 years ago it was discovered that this is not so; small lymphocytes collected from intestinal lymph of sheep showed a predilection for recirculating through the gut-associated lymphoid tissues (GALT) (i.e. the mesenteric nodes, Peyer's patches and lamina propria), whereas those collected from intermediate somatic lymph recirculated preferentially through the peripheral somatic lymph nodes (PSLNs). This was an unexpected finding and at first it was suggested that this recirculatory bias might be a property of B lymphocytes, reflecting variations in the nature of their surface immunoglobulins (Igs). It seems now that this explanation was wrong. Further work in a similar experimental system indicated that recirculating T lymphocytes show the same bias. It must be concluded now that both T and B lymphocytes can be further categorised as to whether they have gut-associated or somatic-associated proclivities. The possibility that these properties may also be manifested by malignant lymphocytes has been mooted already (Hall et al, 1977). It is not impossible that each major organ may have its own 'standing army' of lymphocytes that migrate preferentially through the regional lymph nodes, particularly during phases of cyclical activity (e.g. the lactating mammary gland). At the moment, though, such speculations are without an experimental foundation and they are mentioned only to show the direction and preoccupations of some current research.

THE EFFECT OF ANTIGENIC STIMULI ON THE STRUCTURE AND FUNCTION OF LYMPH NODES

This subject is large and controversial and anything written about it is going to be considered inadequate, misleading or offensive by someone. This has been the case for nearly a century. Part of the trouble lies in the fact that any two immune responses are rarely identical. Even when equal doses of the same antigen are administered in the same way to animals of the same breed, age, weight and sex the resulting immune responses often yield specific antibody molecules with obvious structural and biological differences. When one considers the antigenic complexity of the environment, and biological variation of outbred individuals, both in terms of genetics and previous experiences, it is hardly surprising that different investigators of the histology of the immune response have published descriptions which differ a good deal. The mistake has been to assume that one finding is 'right' and another 'wrong' and that the histology and cytology of every immune response can be categorised meaningfully according to the prejudices of contemporary fashion. By varying the dose, route and timing of the administration of a given antigen the experimentalist can arrange matters to give a wide range of results. It is as well to bear this in mind when reading accounts of experiments which are limited, as experiments must be, to a particular set of conditions.

Nature of the antigen

A large number of factors are important in shaping the reaction of lymphoid tissue to foreign, antigenic macromolecules. Some molecules, for no very obvious reason, seem to be intrinsically more immunogenic than others. For example, some soluble serum proteins, or linear polysaccharide dextrans, are only feebly immunogenic in their native form. They are not trapped by the RES and they circulate freely for considerable periods. If they are aggregated by mild denaturation, or mixed with adjuvants before being injected, they become much more immunogenic. As mentioned above, these differences can be explained partly on the susceptibility of the antigen to rapid phagocytosis but this is not the whole story. Other antigens, e.g. synthetic polypeptides or pneumococcal polysaccharide (Humphrey, 1976), tend to be localised in the macrophages of the medullary regions but are only degraded and processed very slowly.

Antigens like ficoll or branched-chain dextrans become localised in the macrophages lining the subcapsular sinus and, again, they remain present for considerable periods (Humphrey, 1976). Most antigens however are degraded fairly quickly and, if retained at all, seem to be taken up by the macrophages in both cortical and medullary regions. Some soluble antigens with special biological properties like the lectins or bacterial endotoxins bind to specific receptors on the surfaces of most cells and perhaps because of this are often potent immunogens.

However it happens, though, the decisive events in the genesis of an immune reaction in a lymph node are the retention of some antigen by the macrophages and its subsequent recognition by the lymphocytes. The exact site, or sites, in the node where antigen is first 'presented' by macrophages to the lymphocytes is uncertain, as is the exact nature of the macrophages or reticulum cells concerned. Reference has been made already to specialized dendritic cells that are to be found in the afferent lymph and cortical regions; these are not the only candidates, some suggest that 'interdigitating' cells in the paracortex may be involved. These cells are characterised by long villous processes which, in organised lymphoid tissue, are responsible for interdigitating with their fellows. Are these cells related to the dendritic cells of the cortex? Are they involved in antigen presentation? At the moment, no one seems to know what these cells really are but it is as well to be aware of their existence. They certainly increase markedly in some pathological conditions (Wright, 1982) but their immunological rôle remains to be defined, though they are believed to encourage the extravasation of T cells and thus to maintain the T cell microenvironment.

Early events; the induction of primary immune responses

The arrival of antigenic material at a lymph node causes an immediate perturbation of lymphocyte recirculation so that the number of lymphocytes leaving the node in the efferent lymph falls dramatically. At first it was thought that during this phase of 'shutdown' lymphocytes no longer entered the node from the blood. More recently, it has become apparent that lymphocytes continue to enter the node (Hall, 1974) and that something prevents them from leaving. The mechanism is, as usual, obscure; perhaps the engagement of antigen with cellular or humoral receptors leads somehow to the release of pharmacologically active products from lymphocytes or macrophages which have the effect of sticking lymphocytes together, so causing 'sinus plugging' (Kelly, 1970) which prevents the lymphocytes from leaving the node in the efferent lymph fluid which, it should be noted, continues to flow without impediment. However, although 'shutdown' can be a dramatic phenomenon it lasts usually only a few hours and its biological significance is unknown. Its importance, to us, is that it shows that the lymph node is a functional unit that is capable of responding virtually instantaneously to the presence of antigenic material.

After the transient 'shutdown' phase, lymphocyte re-circulation through the node increases several fold (Hall, 1971). Probably, this is brought about by an increase in blood flow through the node and hence an increased total supply of blood-borne lymphocytes, rather than an increase in the proportion of blood-borne lymphocytes that actually extravasate in the node. Again, the details of the mechanism are obscure but there can be little doubt that during the first 3 days that follow an antigenic stimulus a lymph node is supplied with a 'throughput' of recirculating cells that is even larger than the substantial numbers available under basal conditions. This situation seemed to accord excellently with the clonal selection theory of acquired immunity (Burnet, 1959) and to give it a simple, objective physiological basis. In this way, so it seemed to many, the node was presented with vast numbers of lymphocytes from which those with appropriate genetic potential could be selected and retained in the node to react with the antigen that had been sequestered by the macrophages. This phase of increased lymphocyte recirculation was thus referred to as a phase of 'recruitment' (Hall, 1967) and apparent experimental validation of the concept was presented in due course, but in spite of the attractions of logic and simplicity, these ideas cannot yet be accepted wholeheartedly and although they are helpful in envisaging what goes on, the true situation is probably a good deal more complicated (Hay & Morris, 1976). Nonetheless, few would quarrel with the notion that a characteristic feature of the induction of a primary immune response in a lymph node is an increased traffic of lymphocytes through an expanded and hyperaemic paracortical region. As detailed above many of these incoming cells will be T cells and it is these that are the first lymphocytes to recognise the antigen and go into mitosis (Davies et al, 1969) and populate the paracortex with large, pyroninophilic blast cells. The trophic, 'helper' action of the dividing T cells stimulates the appropriate B lymphocytes to become producers of the required immunoglobulin, first as blast cells in the paracortex and as free blast cells in the efferent lymph and, later, as true plasma cells in the medullary cords of both the regional and distant lymph nodes. Thus, the peak of T cell mitosis in the paracortex is reached on day 4, while the maximal proliferation of B cells may be as late as day 8 (Davies et al. 1969). Nonetheless, it is important to remember that we are talking about 'peaks' and the overlap of their bases is considerable. Consequently, it is possible to detect cells forming specific antibody, as well as humoral antibody, in the efferent lymph by fairly simple methods as early as day 4 or 5.

Many primary immune responses are almost absolutely dependent for their proper development on the participation of T cells, secondary responses to the same antigen may be less so (Davies, 1969). However, most animals possess traces of antibody to traditional immunogens such as heterologous red cells or vaccines of the common bacterial or viral pathogens. The responses to these antigens are thus rarely 'primary' in the strict sense of the word, they are usually modified to some extent by the presence of trace amounts of pre-existing antibody, however that antibody may have been acquired. On the other hand, when an animal is presented with an immunogen that does not occur commonly in nature, such as a synthetic aromatic organic compound like dinitrophenol or oxazolone, the response is more likely to be truly primary and unmodified by the effects of previous experience. Because some chemicals of this nature bind to the skin and elicit ultimately delayed hypersensitivity reactions rather than obvious antibody formation it is assumed sometimes that the exuberant reactions they provoke in the paracortices of the regional nodes are concerned exclusively with the genesis of T cell mediated phenomena. Such a view is too extreme and the original descriptions make it clear that the paracortical response was followed always by some degree of medullary plasmacytosis and antibody formation. It is now accepted generally that the majority of primary antibody responses depend on the participation of the T cells and thus of enlargement and hyperplasia of the paracortices of the involved lymph nodes. After repeated stimuli with the same antigen (as in the mesenteric nodes) the need for T cell participation is less crucial; the paracortical responses to successive stimuli become less dramatic, and the medullae expand as sheets of plasma cells are formed. This shift of histological emphasis is mediated to some extent by two interdependent systems, one cellular, the other humoral; the germinal centres and the immunoglobulins.

GERMINAL CENTRES, ANTIBODIES AND SECONDARY RESPONSES

It is just about 100 years since Flemming's original descriptions of germinal centres were published (e.g. Flemming, 1885). Since then an enormous amount of literature on the subject has accumulated. One reason for this is that even with fairly primitive techniques germinal centres appeared as obvious and dramatic structures which were implicated in the reactive changes associated with immunity to those infectious diseases which, until the arrival of antibiotics, formed the main business of many pathologists and clinicians. Most of this literature is now only of historical interest and it seems best to proceed by listing the few important facts about germinal centres that are accepted today:

1. In spite of their name, germinal centres are not a primary source of new, uncommitted lymphocytes and they have nothing to do with lymphopoiesis in any general sense. They represent a focal proliferative reaction to antigen and for this reason they are never seen in antigen-free fetuses *in utero*.
2. They are part of the B cell system and can remain present and active after depletion of the T cell pool.
3. Although they are composed of B cells which have surface, and sometimes intracytoplasmic, immunoglobulin they are not quantitatively important in mammals in the actual bulk manufacture of specific antibody immunoglobulin. That is the business of the plasma cells in the medullary cords.
4. Although they arise most often in primary lymphoid follicles in the cortices of lymph nodes they are by no means confined to lymphoid organs. They can be found beneath many healthy mucosae and also in pathological tissue such as the synovia of joints afflicted with rheumatoid arthritis.
5. Their essential structure is comprised of a central group of dendritic cells which display trapped antigen or antigen-antibody complexes on their cytoplasmic processes. Around these cells lymphocytes cluster, undergoing blastogenesis and mitotic division. The cells in the germinal centre need not have come from the node itself, cells coming from the blood or, in particular, from the afferent lymph, may make a very substantial contribution.
6. The timing of the appearance of germinal centres in relation to the antigenic stimuli which provoke them is very variable but, in general, they appear *after* antibody production is well established. Thus their function appears to be in mediating the production of 'memory cells' so that the cellular basis of secondary responsiveness becomes established. In addition they may 'fine tune' the spectrum of antibody isotypes which are produced.

Some of the above statements require qualification and expansion and the actual structure of germinal centres must first be considered in more detail.

Structure of germinal centres

After antigenic stimulation some of the dendritic reticular cells in the cortex become coated with antigen–antibody complexes and, if C_3 is present (Humphrey, 1976), they aggregate and become associated with dividing lymphoid blast cells. In conventional histological preparations the area occupied by these large mitosing cells stands out as a paler area in the primary nodules of cortical regions which stain darkly because of the dense masses of small lymphocytes of which they are composed. In human material the smaller lymphocytes in germinal centres are spoken of as 'centrocytes' and tend to display a markedly irregular, 'cleaved' nucleus but this feature is not conspicuous in experimental animals. The larger, blast cells in the germinal centres in humans are spoken of as 'centroblasts'. Here, again, experimentalists tend to regard such cells as common or garden immunoblasts. Indeed many immunoblasts in intermediate lymph can be shown to enter into the germinal centres in the first node to which the lymph carries them (Morris et al, 1980). In other words, a cell which is first observed as a large pyroninophilic cell in the paracortex of a node can, after a few seconds of lymph-borne travel, become a so-called 'centroblast' in the next node up the chain.

During the expansion of the focus of proliferating blast cells, which characterise a germinal centre, the surrounding small lymphocytes become compressed into concentric cuffs of cells which have the effect of delineating the germinal centre and so emphasising its presence. At the same time, the reticulin of the cortex is also pushed aside and in sections prepared by silver impregnation methods the presence of active germinal centres can be deduced from the corresponding holes in the agyrophilic reticulin network. Similarly, the blood vessels are displaced so that the middle of the germinal centre often becomes almost avascular; the more peripheral parts have a rich blood supply, the arteries and veins being arranged in a goblet-like configuration which surrounds and enfolds the developing tissue (Herman, 1980).Associated with the proliferating lymphoid cells are variable numbers of macrophages. These were called 'tingible-korper' cells by Flemming (1885) because they contained intracellular objects that took up histological stains. Many of these 'stainable-bodies' are pieces of nuclear debris from dead cells. Some of these may come from the apparently premature death of the proliferating lymphoid cells themselves, perhaps the result of lethal or inappropriate mutations. The life span of germinal centres is very variable and estimates vary from days to weeks (Yoffey & Courtice, 1970). Some merely seem to fade away; in others the proliferating cells seem to be replaced by more and more macrophages, and yet others become replaced partly with fibrinoid or amyloid-like material and thus leave a semi-permanent scar in the cortex. Direct evidence about the fate and function of the cells formed in the centres is hard to come by; we do not know whether they become plasma cells elsewhere or contribute directly to the pool of circulating lymphocytes, as B memory cells, or whether their effects are mediated more indirectly by humoral factors. Although germinal centres are part of the B cell system they may be absent when the development of the lymphoid system has been blighted from the outset by congenital thymic aplasia (de Sousa & Pritchard, 1974) but remain intact after depletion of the pool of T cells (Parrott et al, 1966). As has been emphasised already this does not mean that all the proliferating blasts in germinal centres are busy making antibody. Early immunofluorescence studies detected Igs in germinal centres because antibody had become compounded with the antigen and C_3 on the dendritic cells, rather than because of its local production. Some genuine antibody forming cells do occur in germinal centres, especially in fowls (Humphrey & White, 1970) but this is not an essential feature of germinal centres. Even so, if the ability to form some antibody is absent germinal centres do not develop, and if germinal centres do not develop then neither does the ability to mount a rapid secondary antibody response to a later challenge with the same antigen. These observations are clear and compelling but it is not easy to explain them simply in terms of cytology and morphology. A possible sequence of events for the genesis of germinal centres during a primary immune response is as follows:

1. Antigen is deposited in a subcutaneous or submucosal site. If there is no pre-existing antibody and if it is not inflammatory in its own right the mere presence of the antigen will not elicit much cellular reaction and some of it will be absorbed into the peripheral lymph and conveyed to the regional node, the rest will remain at the site of original deposition.
2. When the antigen arrives at the node it will

be phagocytosed; efficiently if it is particulate in form or denatured, inefficiently if it is soluble.

3. Some of the paracortical T and B cells will recognise the antigen presented by the macrophages and a phase of paracortical blastogenesis and cell division will ensue. The population of B plasmablasts will expand under the influence of trophic lymphokines from 'helper' T blasts. The histological picture at this stage may be rather unimpressive. The paracortex will be hyperaemic and the site of an increased traffic of cells and will contain increased numbers of blast cells. However, since these changes are diffuse and there is no convenient yardstick with which to compare them, they may easily escape detection in all but the most vigorous responses. Some of the plasmablasts will move to the medulla and some will pass via the lymph to other nodes. In either situation they will secrete specific immunoglobulins so that humoral antibody will appear in the blood and lymph plasma.

4. Much of the early humoral antibody will be IgM, an efficient opsonin and binder of complement. When antibody penetrates to the site of original antigen deposition, immune complexes, perhaps involving complement, will be formed locally. These may become phagocytosed or otherwise associated with the dendritic macrophages which are ever present in peripheral tissues, and conveyed in this cell-associated form via the afferent lymph to the subcapsular sinus of the regional node.

5. The afferent macrophages bearing the antigen may enter the cortex and initiate the formation of a germinal centre which will start to produce memory lymphocytes and perhaps mediate the switch of immunoglobulin production from IgM to IgG.

This is, no doubt, a rather fanciful scheme but it goes some way to explain the 'chicken and egg' relationship of germinal centres and antibody. Although I have deliberately stressed the role of migrant cells I do not mean to suggest that it is the only way things may come about; many other scenarios are equally feasible. It is a fact though, that lymph nodes whose afferent lymph contains an abundance of dendritic cells and immunoblasts do in fact tend to contain a great many active germinal centres. This situation occurs most obviously in the case of the mesenteric nodes in which active germinal centres can always be found. This finding led Yoffey (Yoffey & Courtice, 1970) to denote such nodes as 'polysynthetic', in contrast to the more 'oligosynthetic' peripheral nodes like the popliteal.

Incidentally, there is another feature of mesenteric nodes which should be noted. In these nodes many plasma cells can sometimes be found lining lymph sinuses in the cortex and even in the subcapsular sinus itself. Such findings are particularly striking in immuno-histochemical preparations for the demonstration of intracellular IgA. This unusual appearance does not mean that mesenteric nodes are intrinsically different from others; it shows merely that the diffuse lymphoid tissue in the wall of the gut is capable of producing IgA (and other) plasmablasts and plasma cells; some of these gain entry to the lymph and are swept up into the mesenteric nodes where they lodge in the cortical sinuses.

THE DISCHARGE OF CELLS INTO THE CIRCULATION BY ANTIGENICALLY STIMULATED LYMPH NODES

Although a lymph node may retain quantitatively a particulate immunogen and thus prevent the antigenic or pathogenic entity as such from reaching its fellows it can none the less communicate to them the specification of the antigenic structure by means of immunologically-activated, lymph-borne cells. These cells can colonise lymphoid tissue remote from the site of the actual localisation of antigen so that lymph nodes higher up the chain may be regarded as 'slave stations' which both carry out and transmit the instructions for immunological activity contained in the cells discharged by the node which received the original stimulus. Morris (1972) has prepared an illustrated review of the subject.

Numbers and types of cells involved

Within 100 hours of a primary antigenic stimulus, and as little as 50 hours of a secondary stimulus,

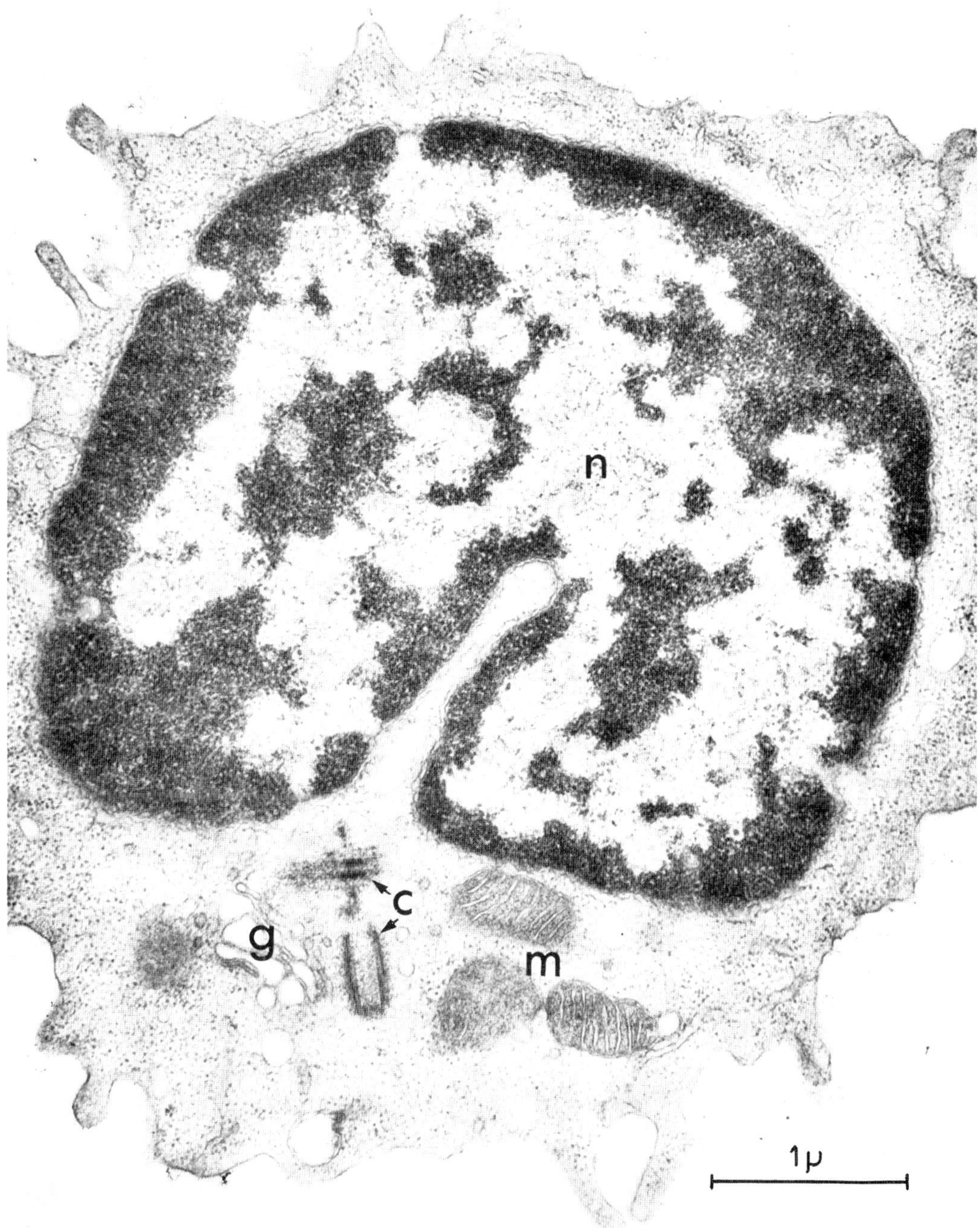

Fig. 1.5 Transmission electron micrograph of a typical small lymphocyte. The scanty cytoplasm which surrounds an indented nucleus (n), is sparsely populated with ribosomes and displays a few mitochondria (m), centriole (c) and Golgi membranes (g). Reproduced from the *Journal of Experimental Medicine*, 125, 91 (Hall, Morris, Moreno and Bessis, 1967) by permission of the Editors.

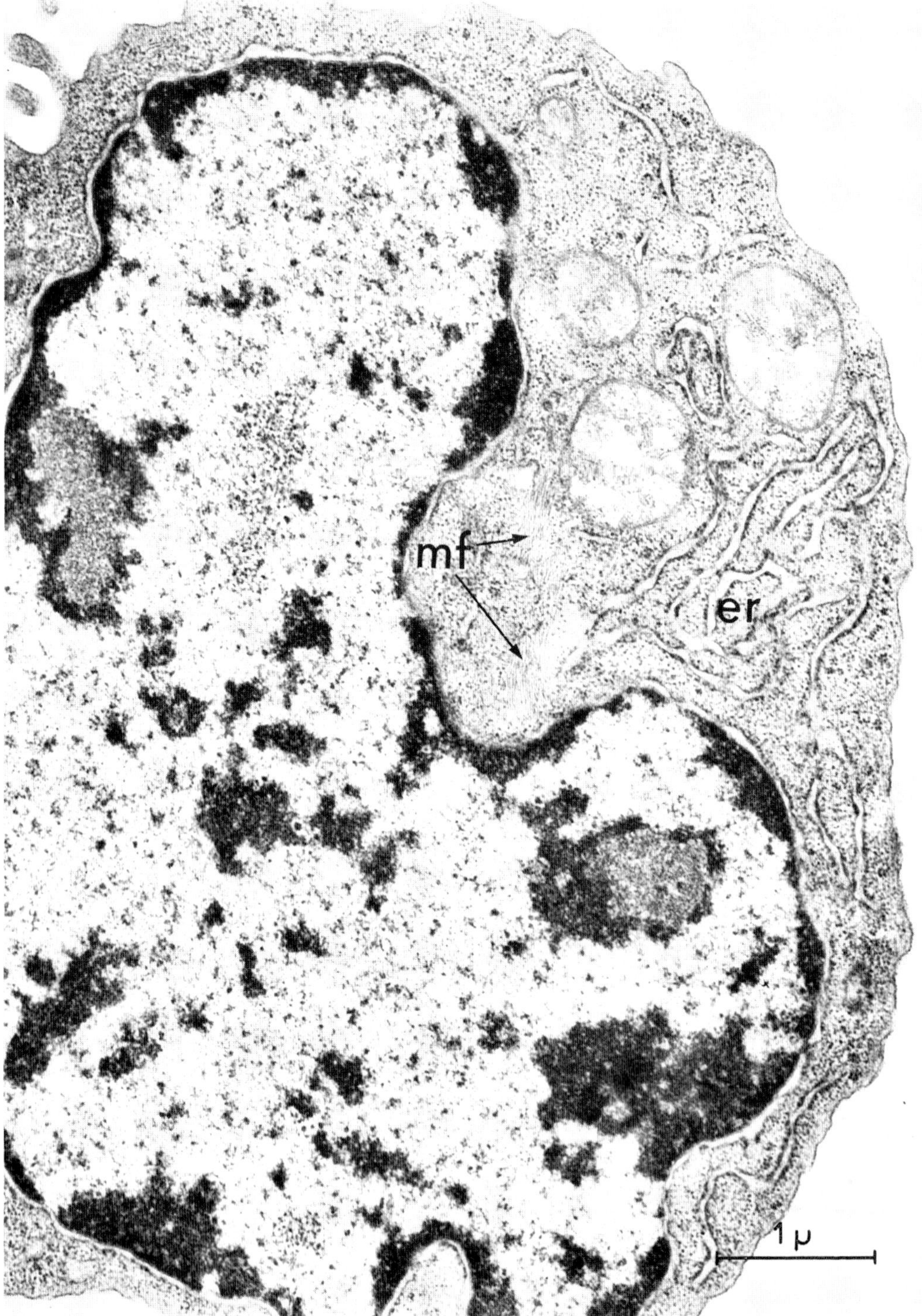

Fig. 1.6 Transmission electron micrograph of a lymph-borne immunoblast from the efferent lymph of an antigenically stimulated lymph node. The cytoplasm is replete with ribosomes some of them arranged as polyribosomes in rosettes or spirals; microfilaments (mf) have developed as has endoplasmic reticulum (er). The latter feature is indicative of protein (Ig) synthesis and suggests that this cell arose by transformation of a 'B' small lymphocyte. Reproduced from the *Journal of Experimental Medicine*, 125, 91 (Hall, Morris, Moreno and Bessis, 1967) by permission of the Editors.

large lymphoid 'immunoblasts' start to appear in the efferent lymph of the stimulated node (Hall & Morris, 1963). Although lymphoid blast cells are functionally heterogeneous they are structurally fairly similar and their salient properties are as follows. In the first place it should be remembered that they are actively motile cells whose true configuration is anything but the inert spherical blob of conventional representation. They divide rapidly and at the same time engage in protein synthesis both for self-renewal and for secretion. Accordingly, they have basophilic and pyroninophilic cytoplasm and incorporate avidly radioactive precursors of DNA such as ^{3}H-thymidine and ^{125}Iodo-deoxyuridine; genuine small lymphocytes do not have these characteristics. Also, the large cells incorporate amino-acids and precursors of RNA at 10 to 100 times the rate at which small lymphocytes do so. The real test of the difference between a large lymphoid blast cell and an ordinary small lymphocyte is thus a biochemical one, and since such tests cannot be performed on fixed tissue one often has to make do with inferences drawn from ultrastructural or histochemical studies.

A comparison of the ultrastructure of small lymphocytes with that of the large lymphocytes into which they metamorphose reveals the structural basis for these biochemical differences (Figs. 1.5–1.7). The cytoplasm of the small lymphocyte is meagre and contains a centriole, some Golgi bodies and a few mitochondria; the content of RNA is low, as shown by the sparse distribution of monoribosomes (Fig. 1.5). The large lymphoid blast cells have a more abundant cytoplasm which, in addition to the mitochondria, Golgi bodies, etc. is replete with polyribosomes which are often arranged in rosettes and spirals (Fig. 1.6). It has been claimed that the T blasts have ribosomes which are sparser and arranged in smaller clusters than in the corresponding B cell. This may be so but is difficult to substantiate and helps little with the classification of an individual cell. These cells are relatively large and each one can be cut into several ultrathin sections; in some equatorial sections the cytoplasm may appear to be rather sparsely populated, yet examination of sections towards the 'tail' of the cell may reveal many more ribosomes and even some identifiable endoplasmic reticulum (ER). The presence of ER in large lymphocytes can be taken usually as evidence of Ig synthesis and thus of B cell status. Although while in the blast phase large B lymphocytes do not display the abundant, concentric lamellae of ER that characterise the mature plasma cell, they do have some ER that contains easily demonstrable amounts of both specific antibody activity and immunoglobulin (Fig. 1.7). In vivo, some of the large B lymphocytes transform fairly rapidly (24–48 hours) into the classical plasma cells that populate the medullary cords of lymph nodes (Birbeck & Hall, 1967). Appropriate treatment of the large B lymphocytes shows that like small B lymphocytes they have Ig on their surfaces but although an Ig positive blast can be assumed to be a B cell one should hesitate before assigning T cell status to Ig negative blasts. When B lymphocytes enlarge as they transform into blasts the Ig on their surfaces becomes sometimes too sparse for easy detection. Also, a very immature B blast may lack endoplasmic reticulum and intracytoplasmic Ig. When working with large lymphocytes from species where direct serological detection of T-associated antigens is not practicable it is wise not to be too ready to identify T blasts solely on the basis of negative attributes.

Methyl green-pyronin stains polymerised ribonucleoprotein red and hence can be used to assess the amount of cytoplasmic RNA. It is best used on formalin fixed sections; in cell films and imprints the cells are too spread out for their cytoplasm to stain really intensely with pyronin and the degree of cytoplasmic basophilia, as revealed by conventional Romanowsky stains, is often just as informative. However, because of the identification of large pyroninophilic cells in the paracortices of lymph nodes regional to skin allografts or the sites of application of sensitising chemicals it is sometimes assumed that large pyroninophilic cells (LPC) have some particular association with cell mediated immunity and delayed type hypersensitivity, and are thus likely to be T cells. This is not so. In so far as large B cells may have more RNA than large T cells it might be expected that LPC would be particularly evident in B cell responses. In fact, no such distinction is possible and LPC are detectable in lymphoid tissue at some stage of all types of immune responses.

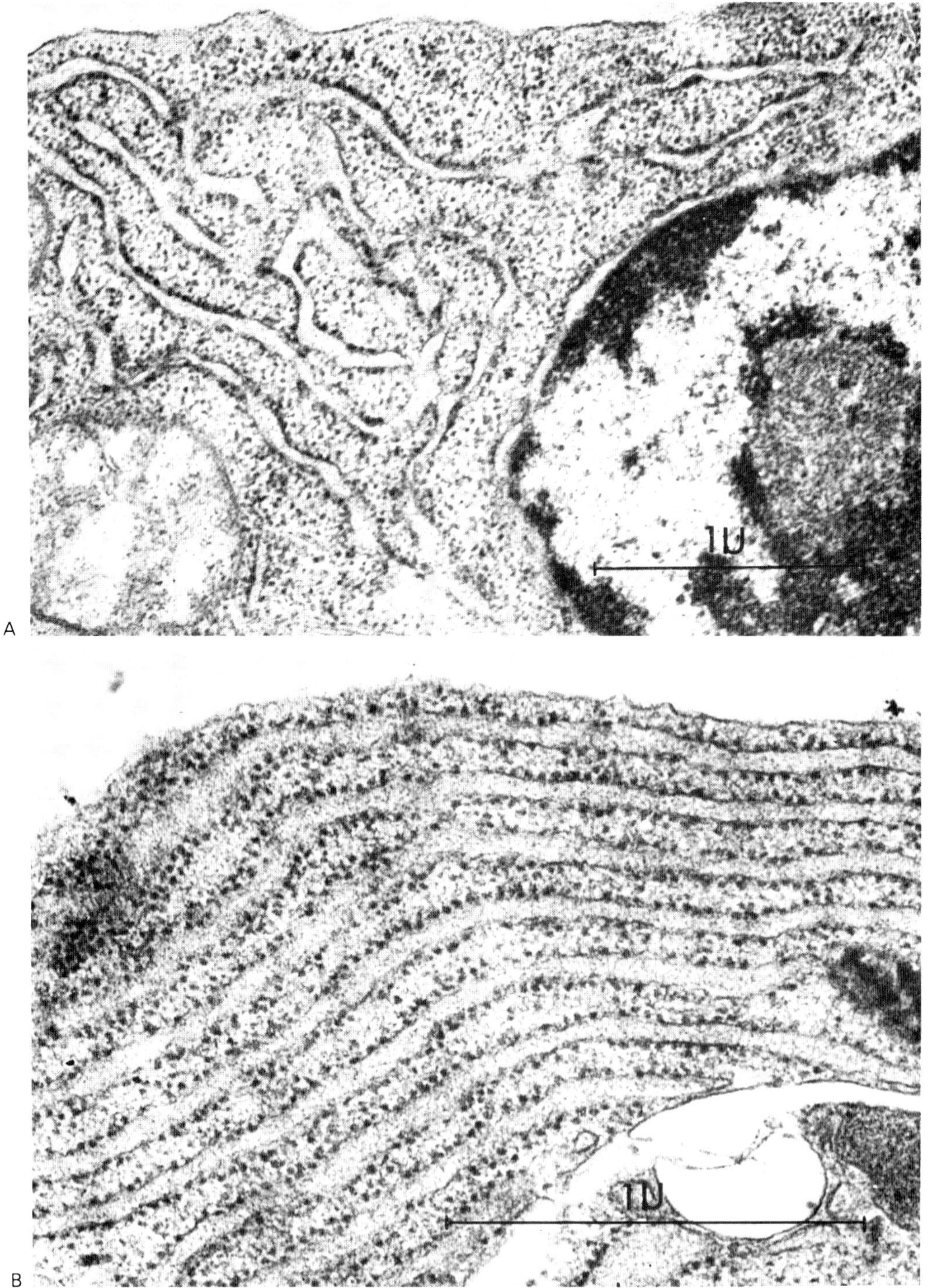

Fig. 1.7 Transmission electron micrographs. The somewhat disorganised endoplasmic reticulum of a lymph-borne immunoblast (A) contrasts with the concentric, lamellar endoplasmic reticulum of a fully fledged plasma cell (B) in the medulla of the lymph node. In spite of this difference it takes no more than 24 h for the immunoblast to become a plasma cell once the lymph conveys it to another node, or the blood conveys it to the spleen or the bone marrow. Reproduced from the *Journal of Experimental Medicine*, 125, 91 (Hall, Morris, Moreno and Bessis, 1967) by permission of the Editors.

The problem of what to call large lymphoid cells has no generally acceptable solution. Terms like 'large lymphocyte' or 'plasmablast' carry the implication that the later fate, function and progeny of lymphoid cells can be predicted reliably on the basis of their appearance. Terms like 'large basophilic lymph cell' or LPC can refer only to particular situations where particular stains have been used and, together with ultrastructural terms, are unsuitable for general use. The term 'immunoblast' (Dameshek, 1963) is here preferred for the large lymphoid blast cells that occur in lymphoid tissue and lymph as a result of an antigenic stimulus. This term can be used without prejudice as to the cell's T/B status or later fate and function. The numbers of these immunoblasts released during immune responses is considerable, and during vigorous responses a single node may release gramme (10^{10} lymphoid cells have a wet weight of approximately 1 g) quantities of such cells. Such large quantities of cells are unlikely to represent nothing more than an inadvertent and unimportant overflow from the pool of proliferating cells within the node. Indeed, there is quite good evidence that one function of these lymph-borne cells is to establish systemic humoral (Hall et al, 1967) and cell mediated immunity. The B immunoblasts do this by turning into plasma cells after reaching other lymph nodes or after extravasation in the tissue spaces generally. The cells efferent from a node depend absolutely on the lymphatic system for their transport to the blood and thus to their final destination; occasionally lymphatic-venous anastamoses within the nodes permit their direct entry into the blood but this is not usually the case. In all responses, even those to skin-sensitising chemicals (Hall et al, 1980), some of these blasts contain and secrete immunoglobulin and specific antibody and are thus, presumptively, B cells (Fig. 1.8). The precise ratios of T to B blasts has not been investigated in detail; probably, in primary T-dependent responses T cells may be in the majority. The site in the node from which the lymph-borne immunoblasts originate is not easy to determine but the timing of their appearance in the lymph seems to correspond with the paracortical hypertrophy and hyperplasia and it is presumably from this region that most of them are launched into the lymph.

Fate and distribution of lymph-borne immunoblasts

Mention has been made already of the fact that the migratory route of all circulating lymphoid cells depends on whether they come from the GALT or from the PSLNs. This difference is most striking in the case of lymph-borne immunoblasts. It has been demonstrated often that many of the immunoblasts present in rat thoracic duct lymph enter the blood stream and then extravasate in the lamina propria of the small gut (Gowans & Knight, 1964; Hall et al 1972). This property is shared by immunoblasts teased from mesenteric nodes, whereas similar cells from PSLNs show no such propensity. This striking 'gut-seeking' property of immunoblasts from the GALT does not seem to be mediated primarily by an affinity for dietary or microbial antigens within the lumen of the gut for it occurs just as obtrusively in situations where the influence of antigens can be excluded (Halstead & Hall, 1972; Moore & Hall, 1972). This work relates to laboratory rodents but experiments on sheep, where precise surgery is easier, have made it clear that the immunoblasts from the GALT of large mammals behave in the same way irrespective of whether they are generated in the mesenteric nodes or the wall of the gut as such (Hall et al, 1977).

Many of the B immunoblasts in thoracic duct and intestinal duct lymph can be shown to be making IgA and, after entering the blood circulation, many extravasate in the lamina propria of the gut where they become plasma cells. These plasma cells that lie beneath the epithelium of the gut and in lesser numbers beneath most mucous membranes, are concerned particularly with furnishing the secretory immunoglobulins (usually of the IgA class) that probably play a major role in protecting these vital surfaces both by inactivating pathogenic micro-organisms and by modulating the absorption e.g. of dietary antigens (see review by Lamm, 1976). Much of the IgA produced by these submucosal plasma cells is swept into the regional lymphatics and conveyed to the blood. However, IgA is rapidly cleared from the blood by hepatocytes, which secrete it into bile, so that the biliary system is a major route by which secretory immunoglobulins reach the gut (Hall & Andrew,

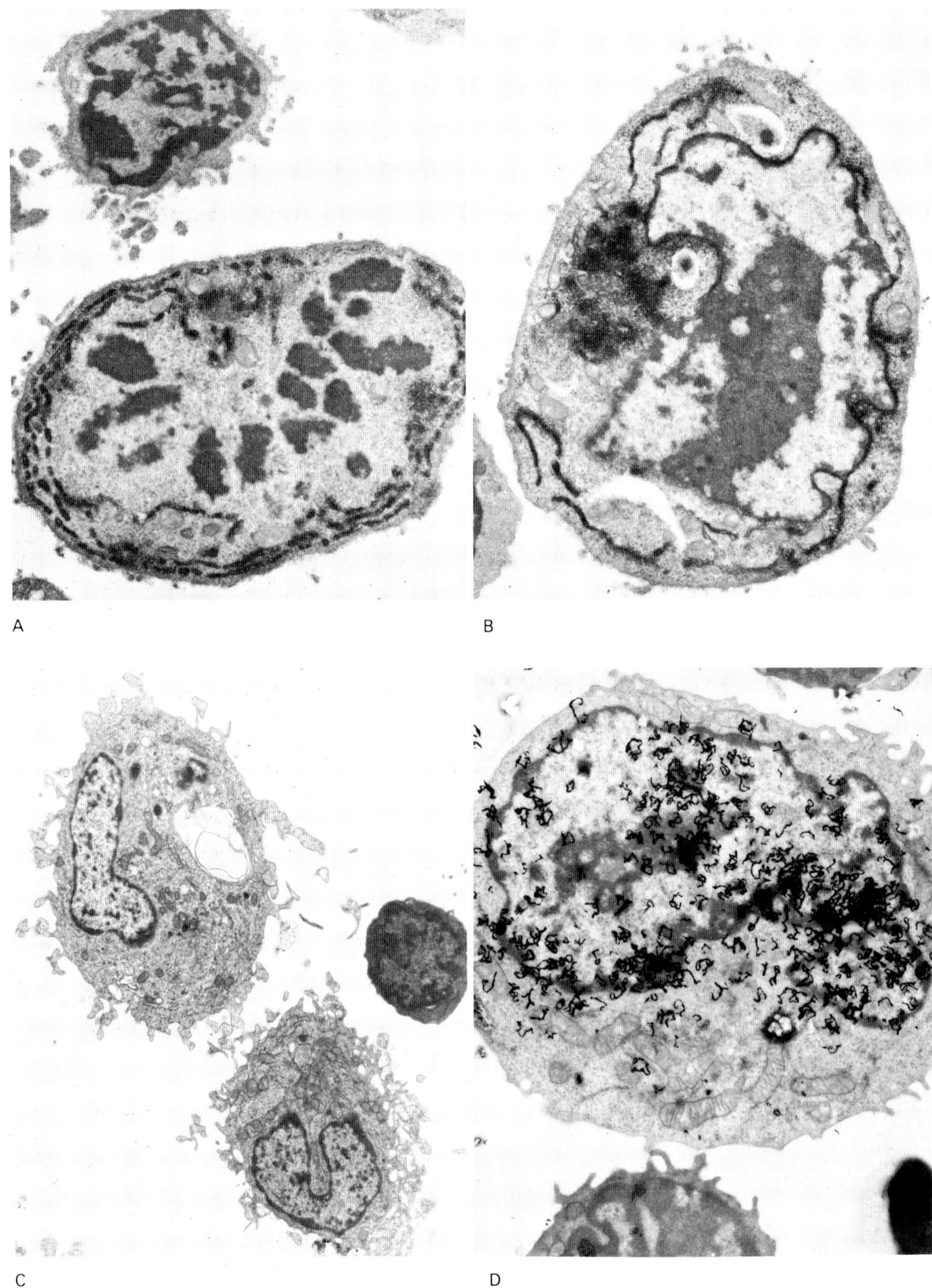

A
B
C
D

Fig. 1.8 Transmission electron micrographs of cells from the lymph of a node draining an area of skin that had been painted with contact-sensitizing agent, oxazolone, 5 days previously. A. Immunoblast from efferent lymph (approx. × 7 000) to show mitotic figure and endoplasmic reticulum full of immunoglobulin. The latter has been revealed by treating the fixed cell with detergents to allow the penetration of an anti-F(ab')$_2$-peroxidase conjugate. B. Another, similarly treated immunoblast from efferent lymph. Immunoglobulin is present in the Golgi region and around the nuclear membrane as well as in fragments of endoplasmic reticulum (approx. × 7000). C. An autoradiograph of an immunoblast from efferent lymph that had been incubated with ^{125}I-iododeoxyuridine before fixation. The nucleus of the cell is heavily labelled; the cytoplasm contains little endoplasmic reticulum, and the cell may be a 'T' blast (approx. × 8 500). D. Macrophages from afferent (peripheral) lymph, showing curved or 'horseshoe' nuclei and characteristic ruffled cytoplasmic membranes (approx. × 4 500). A and C illustrate the capacity of immunoblasts for rapid cell division. A and B show that immunoglobulin producing cells are an inevitable feature of all immune responses, even those that may be associated obviously with 'cell-mediated' phenomena. Reproduced from *Immunology*, 39, 141 (1980) by permission of the editors.

1980). After a few days of antibody production these plasma cells die off and so make room for the newcomers that are arriving continually. However, on general grounds it would be predicted that some of the immunoblasts that 'home' to the gut would be T cells and, indeed, this has been demonstrated directly. The function of such cells is less easy to understand. They extravasate mainly in the inter-follicular regions of the Peyer's patches rather than throughout the lamina propria; presumably, they have some trophic effect on local B cells and it has been suggested that they may develop into intra-epithelial lymphoid cells.

After receiving an appropriate stimulus with soluble antigens or bacteria, viruses, allografts, skin sensitising chemicals or local antigenic, neoplastic lesions even a single PSLN will discharge a large cohort of immunoblasts. These cells, however, do not usually find their way to the gut but go for the most part to other PSLNs, the spleen and the alveolar parenchyma of the lung. Those of them that are B cells make IgM or IgG antibodies but not IgA (Hall et al, 1977).

It might be imagined that since these cells are carried by the blood throughout the body they would have the ability to 'home' into lesions that contained the same antigen(s) that had initiated their discharge into the circulation. Unhappily, this simple and apparently logical arrangement has not yet been provided with a firm experimental basis. Immunoblasts from PSLNs seem just as obtusely indifferent to the call of specific antigens as the immunoblasts from the GALT. Many attempts have been made to demonstrate the selective extravasation of specifically activated lymphoid cells into the sites e.g. of allograft rejection. Usually these attempts failed (Hall et al, 1980); more recently some success has been claimed but the phenomenon is far from impressive and similar equivocal results have rewarded attempts to show the specific homing of immunoblasts to intradermal foci of antigens.

Long-term fate of lymph-borne immunoblasts

Some of the B immunoblasts obviously turn into plasma cells, which are end cells with a relatively short life span. Some, as we have seen, participate in the formation of germinal centres and it would seem reasonable if some of them reverted to the form of recirculating small lymphocytes which are known to help mediate immunological 'memory' and secondary responsiveness (Gowans & Uhr, 1966). Such cells are often referred to as 'B-memory cells' and a similar category of sensitised or 'educated' T cells must also be presumed to exist. However, although the reversion of lymphoid blast cells to small lymphocytes in vitro has been well documented (Hayry, 1976) it has proved harder to demonstrate in vivo in any experimental animal.

CONCLUSION

In the above account of the functional anatomy of lymph nodes the most overworked phrase is 'the mechanism is obscure', or words to that effect. Thirty years ago we did not know what lymphocytes did or what they were for. Now we know that they are a varied and mobile population made up of co-operating sub-groups which interact with endothelial cells and macrophages and which modify each other's activities in bringing about the various effects of specific, immunological reactions. What we do not know is exactly why and how they do it. The answers lie in biochemistry, somatic cell genetics, and the physio-pharmacology of cell membranes and it may be years before they are all found, recognised and comprehended. In the meantime we have to cope with a dismaying barrage of phenomenology. The discoveries of recondite functions and surface markers for lymphoid cells in in vitro systems burgeon faster than the number of elementary particles in physics, but their biological significance is not always immediately apparent. In spite of all this activity it is still impossible to manipulate the immune response so as to prevent the rejection of a renal allograft or to promote the destruction of an antigenic tumour. This may be annoying to those who have spent their careers trying to achieve such goals but younger people who have embarked more recently on the study of lymphoid tissue have grounds for mild exhilaration. The best is yet to come.

REFERENCES

Anderson A O, Anderson N D 1975 Studies on the structure and permeability of the microvasculature in normal rat lymph nodes. American Journal of Pathology 80: 387–412

Birbeck M S C, Hall J G 1967 Transformation in vivo of basophilic lymph cells into plasma cells. Nature 214: 183–184

Burnet F M 1959 The clonal selection theory of acquired immunity. The University Press, Cambridge

Cole G J, Morris B 1973 The lymphoid apparatus of sheep: Its growth, development and significance in Immunologic Reactions. Advances in Veterinary Science and Comparative Medicine 17: 225–263

Dameshek W 1963 Immunoblasts and immunocytes — An attempt at a functional nomenclature. Blood 21: 243–245

Davies A J S 1969 The thymus and the cellular basis of immunity. Transplantation Review 1: 43–91

Davies A J S, Carter R L, Leuchars E, Wallis V 1969 The morphology of immune reactions in normal, thymectomized and reconstituted mice. II. The Response to Oxazolone. Immunology 17: 111–126

de Sousa M A B, Pritchard H 1974 The cellular basis of immunological recovery in nude mice after thymus grafting. Immunology 26: 769–776

Fahy V A, Gerber H A, Morris B, Trevella W, Zukoski C F 1980 The function of lymph nodes in the formulation of lymph. Monographs in Allergy (Karger/Basel) 16: 82–99

Flemming W 1885 Studien uber regeneration der Gewebe. Archiv fur Mikroskopische Anatomie und Entwicklungsmechanik 24: 50–97

Gowans J L, Knight E J 1964 The route of recirculation of lymphocytes in the rat. Proceedings of the Royal Society. Series B. 159: 257–282

Hall J G 1967 Quantitative aspects of the recirculation of lymphocytes. An analysis of data from experiments on sheep. Quarterly Journal of Experimental Physiology and Cognate Medical Science 52: 76–85

Hall J G 1971 The lymph-borne cells of the immune response: A review. In: Gilliland I, Francis J (eds) The Scientific Basis of Medicine. Annual Reviews. University of London, Athlone Press, p 39–57

Hall J G 1974 Observations on the migration and localization of lymphoid cells. Progress in Immunology 3: 15–24

Hall J G, Andrew E 1980 Biliglobulin: a new look at IgA. Immunology Today 1: 100–103

Hall J G, Hopkins J, Orlans E 1977 Studies on the lymphocytes of sheep. III. Destination of lymph-borne immunoblasts in relation to their tissue of origin. European Journal of Immunology 7: 30–37

Hall J G, Hopkins J, Reynolds J 1980 Studies of efferent lymph cells from nodes stimulated with oxazolone. Immunology 39: 141–149

Hall J G, Morris B 1963 The lymph-borne cells of the immune response. Quarterly Journal of Experimental Physiology and Cognate Medical Sciences 48: 235–247

Hall J G, Morris B, Moreno G D, Bessis M C 1967 The ultrastructure and function of cells in lymph following antigenic stimulation. Journal of Experimental Medicine 125: 91–108

Hall J G, Morris B, Woolley G 1965 Intrinsic rhythmic propulsion of lymph in the unanaesthetised sheep. Journal of Physiology, London 180: 336–349

Hall J G, Parry D M, Smith M E 1972 The distribution and differentiation of lymph-borne immunoblasts after intravenous injection into syngeneic recipients. Cell and Tissue Kinetics 5: 269–281

Hall J G, Scollay R G, Smith M E 1976 Studies on the lymphocytes of sheep. I. Recirculation of lymphocytes through peripheral nodes and tissues. European Journal of Immunology 6: 117–120

Halstead T E, Hall J G 1972 The homing of lymph-borne immunoblasts to the small gut of neonatal rats. Transplantation 14: 339–346

Hay J B, Morris B 1976 Generation and selection of specific reactive cells by antigen. British Medical Bulletin 32: 135–140

Hayry P 1976 Anamnestic responses in mixed lymphocyte culture induced cytolysis (MLC-CML) reaction. Immunogenetics 3: 417–453

Herman P G 1980 Microcirculation of organised lymphoid tissues. Monographs in Allergy (Karger, Basel) 16: 126–142

Humphrey J H 1976 The still unsolved germinal centre mystery. In: Feldman M, Globerson A (eds) Immune, Reactivity of Lymphocytes. Plenum Press, New York, p 711–723

Humphrey J H, White R G 1970 The fate of antigen and the process of antibody production. Chapter 7 in: Immunology for Students of Medicine. 3rd edn. Blackwell Scientific Publications, Oxford, p 238–305

Kelly R H 1970 Localization of afferent lymph cells within the draining node during a primary immune response. Nature 227: 510–511

Kelly R H 1975 Functional anatomy of lymph nodes. 1. The paracortical cords. International Archives of Allergy and Applied Immunology 48: 836–849

Lamm M E 1976 Cellular aspects of immunoglobulin A. Advances in Immunology 22: 223–290
Marchesi V T, Gowans J L 1964 The migration of lymphocytes through the endothelium of venules in lymph nodes: an electron microscope study. Proceedings of the Royal Society. Series B. 159: 283–290
Moore A R, Hall J G 1972 Evidence for a primary association between immunoblasts and the small gut. Nature 239: 161–162
Morris B 1972 The cells of lymph and their role in immunological reactions in: Handbuch der Allgemeinen Pathologie Springer-Verlag, Berlin, p 405–420
Parrott D M V, de Sousa M A B 1971 Thymus-dependent and thymus independent populations: Origins migratory patterns and life span. Clinical and Experimental Immunology 8: 663–684
Parrott D M V, de Sousa M A B, East J 1966 Thymus dependent areas in the lymphoid organs of neonatally thymectomised mice. Journal of Experimental Medicine 123: 191–204
Pearson L D, Simpson-Morgan M W, Morris B 1976 Lymphopoeisis and lymphocyte recirculation in the sheep foetus. Journal of Experimental Medicine 143: 167–186
Schoefl G I 1972 The migration of lymphocytes across vascular endothelium in lymphoid tissue. A re-examination. Journal of Experimental Medicine 136: 568–584
Wright D H 1982 Immunological aspects of diagnostic histopathology. In: Lachmann P J, Peters D K (eds) Clinical Aspects of Immunology Blackwell Scientific Publications, Oxford, p 443–461
Yoffey J M, Courtice F C 1970 Lymphatics, Lymph and the Lymphomyeloid Complex. Academic Press, New York

2

A.G. Stansfeld

Indications, technique and applications for lymph node biopsy

Lymph node biopsy, like any other surgical operation, is not to be lightly undertaken. A careful history of the patient's present and past illnesses and family history may throw light on the nature of the lymphadenopathy and, of course, a thorough examination is mandatory. Less invasive investigations, such as a complete blood count and examination of a blood film, may obviate the need for lymph node biopsy. It should not be uncritically assumed, however, just because the patient is known to have a particular disease which may cause lymphadenopathy, that the lymph node enlargement in his or her case is necessarily due to that cause.

Some guidelines to the taking of lymph node biopsies and the investigations which may be carried out on excised nodes are given in this chapter.

INDICATIONS FOR LYMPH NODE BIOPSY

There are five main reasons for performing a lymph node biopsy which are:

1. To make a diagnosis in a case of persistent, unexplained lymph node enlargement

The lymphadenopathy may be localised or generalised and the approach to the problem will differ depending upon this, as upon other considerations, such as the patient's age, general state of health, and other findings on physical examination. The presence of localised lymphadenopathy, especially in a superficial node or group of nodes, will arouse suspicion of a focus of infection within the lymph drainage area and such should always be sought with great care before embarking on lymph node biopsy. How long should one observe an unexplained enlarged lymph node before removing it for biopsy? It is impossible to give a generally applicable answer to this question. So much will depend upon the circumstances of the case. A rubbery or hard node demands immediate exploration, regardless of the length of history. Conversely, soft and moderately enlarged nodes, especially in children, should seldom be removed at all unless there are other indications (see below).

2. To make a diagnosis or assist in the investigation of a patient who has unexplained symptoms, such as fever or loss of weight, accompanied by lymphadenopathy

The lymph node enlargement may be relatively insignificant in cases of this kind and obviously lymph node biopsy is only indicated where other investigations have failed to establish a diagnosis. Examination of a node may then be made to *exclude* the possibility of malignant lymphoma being responsible for the patient's symptoms. The findings, on the other hand, may lead to a suspicion of systemic lupus erythematosus or a diagnosis of tuberculosis or other infection.

3. To confirm a diagnosis already suspected on other grounds

The clinical history or findings on physical examination may be highly suggestive of malignant disease, but even where the primary tumour is obvious, removal of an involved lymph node may be indicated, for example, to discover the histological type of a bronchial carcinoma, as a necessary basis for planning treatment. In the same way, the presence of multiple nodes in different groups may suggest a malignant lymphoma, but lymph node biopsy is necessary to confirm and elaborate on this diagnosis.

Other examples in this category might include the confirmation of a diagnosis of dermatopathic lymphadenitis in a patient with chronic skin disorder accompanied by grossly enlarged superficial nodes, or the exclusion of other disease in the enlarged nodes of a patient with chronic rheumatoid arthritis.

Again it should be stressed that lymph node biopsy should never be performed merely to satisfy the curiosity of the attendant physician, but only where reasonable doubt exists about the diagnosis.

4. *To assess the extent of spread of known malignant disease*

The removal of lymph nodes in a radical operation for carcinoma or the excision of individual nodes as part of a staging procedure come under this heading. In both these circumstances, histological examination of the excised nodes will help to determine the extent of spread of the disease which, in turn, may influence prognosis and treatment.

5. *To monitor the progress of disease in patients with malignant lymphomas*

Today, when physicians and radiotherapists are aiming at a curative treatment in these diseases, it is no longer sufficient merely to establish the primary diagnosis with a lymph node biopsy. Further node biopsies are often taken in Hodgkin's disease, in the course of a staging laparotomy operation, as mentioned above. In addition, excision of other nodes may be indicated during the course of the disease. Two specific indications for biopsy are: (a) enlarged nodes persisting after therapy which would normally be effective in that particular disease and situation; (b) enlarged nodes which appear in a patient previously in remission after effective therapy.

Nodes which continue to be palpable and to feel abnormal after treatment may show one of three changes on biopsy — (a) destruction of the lymphoma with fibrosis and hyalinisation of the node, (b) persistence of the original disease or (c) the presence of a different disease. The last is most likely to be a lymphoma of a higher grade of malignancy, as a result of blastic transformation in the original neoplasm. More rarely, it is a different disease altogether, such as tuberculosis or a fungal infection. Obviously it is important for the future management of the patient to know the precise cause of such persistent lymphadenopathy.

The appearance of newly enlarged nodes in a patient previously in complete remission of malignant lymphoma/leukaemia is equally an indication for repeat biopsy. It is important for the radiotherapist to know whether such nodes have appeared within or outside previously treated areas. In Hodgkin's disease, it is not uncommon for the repeat biopsy to show simple reactive hyperplasia in the enlarged node, especially if the patient is under 30, and it should therefore never be assumed, without biopsy, that the fresh appearance of enlarged nodes means relapse of the disease. In the malignant lymphomas other than Hodgkin's disease, it is again important for the rational planning of treatment to know whether such newly appearing nodes show the same features as the original biopsy or indicate progression to a higher grade of malignancy (see Ch. 10).

TECHNIQUE OF LYMPH NODE BIOPSY

A detailed description of surgical techniques would be out of place in this book, but certain general principles are worthy of attention. The first point to make is that this is not an easy operation than can safely be left to the surgical tyro. It may be easy enough to remove a normal lymph node, but it often requires great skill to remove intact an enlarged and diseased node. For the interpretation of a difficult lymph node biopsy, it is important not only that the node should be intact, if possible, but that it should be subjected to the minimum of trauma in the process of removal — indeed until the tissue is fixed. Trauma, whether caused by pinching or pulling on the tissue, not only tears the capsule and disrupts the architecture of the node, but also severely distorts the lymphoid cells, producing the so-called 'stringy artefact' of the nuclei. A badly traumatised biopsy may be completely uninterpretable. If the node capsule is still intact it is unlikely that the cells inside will have been severely damaged, even though the internal architecture may be disrupted (see p. 73–74).

The second point concerns the choice of node for biopsy. If there is only a single enlarged node, then clearly that node is the one to remove. If, on the other hand, there is widespread lymphadenopathy, then other considerations apply. Inguinal nodes should be avoided where possible in adults, because they so often show scarring or other evidence of past lymphadenitis which may complicate interpretation. Axillary nodes not infrequently show fatty involution of their centres, so that from the histopathologist's point of view, cervical nodes are generally to be preferred. (For the patient, cosmetic considerations may be paramount!) The most accessible node is not always the best one to remove and, generally speaking, the best node from the point of view of the pathologist is the largest one available. All too often the surgeon is tempted to remove a smaller, more accessible node, but this may not be representative and the diagnosis may consequently be missed. If there are multiple enlarged nodes, the removal of several nodes may be easily achieved and may give more information than can be obtained from a single node, for even two adjacent nodes do not always look alike.

These remarks apply chiefly to biopsy of superficial lymph node groups. However, there are occasions when it is necessary to obtain material from thoracic or abdominal nodes. Mediastinal nodes may be biopsied on mediastinoscopy, but it is often difficult to get a satisfactory (i.e. untraumatised) biopsy by this means and it may be necessary to resort to open operation to make a diagnosis. Scalene node biopsy often provides useful information about the nature of underlying lung disease, e.g. sarcoidosis or carcinoma. Abdominal nodes are now commonly removed in the course of staging laparotomy operations and the sites of removal of such nodes may be indicated by small metal clips to enable subsequent abdominal X-ray films to be compared with preoperative lymphangiograms. Routine biopsy of mesenteric lymph nodes in the staging laparotomy procedure for Hodgkin's disease is not advisable, for mesenteric nodes are rarely involved, except in very advanced Hodgkin's disease, and there is a significant risk of adhesions with attendant complications developing after mesenteric node biopsy. It may, of course, be necessary to take biopsies of mesenteric nodes in other circumstances, e.g. when enlarged mesenteric nodes are the presenting feature at laparotomy in a patient explored for appendicitis or in suspected malignant disease of the intestine.

In this account of technique, no mention has been made of drill or needle biopsy of lymph nodes. Drill biopsy may, of course, provide adequate material for the diagnosis of metastatic carcinoma in selected cases, but its applicability is strictly limited in an area where the pathologist generally needs as much tissue as he can get to arrive at a diagnosis. The same applies to needle aspiration of lymph nodes, but this technique has been less practised in Britain than elsewhere in Europe, and it is almost certainly true that diagnostic skill in this, as in other fields, increases with increasing experience of the technique.

APPLICATIONS OF LYMPH NODE BIOPSY

Whilst in many cases a single routine-stained section of paraffin embedded tissue is all that is required to make a diagnosis, a great deal more information can often by elicited from the biopsy tissue by the use of additional techniques (see Fig. 2.1). The particular circumstances of the case may dictate whether any additional investigations are likely to be required. These are generally not indicated, for example, in a patient who has obvious metastatic carcinoma. If there is any doubt, it is a wise precaution to examine the node before it is put into fixative, especially in cases of suspected infection or lymphoma. Indeed, it is an ideal practice for the pathologist to examine every excised lymph node fresh, soon after its removal from the body, but this necessitates close cooperation between the pathologist and the surgical team.

On receipt, the fresh node should be cleanly sliced in half with a new scalpel blade. If the history or the appearance of the node suggest infection, one half of the node should be immediately placed in a dry sterile container for the appropriate

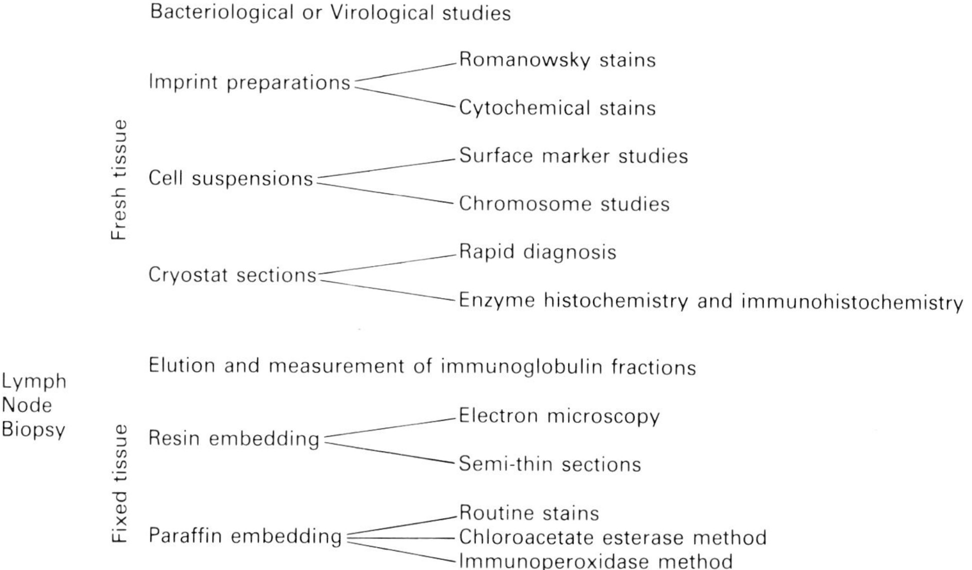

Fig. 2.1

bacteriological (or virological) investigations. These will not be detailed here but, obviously, tuberculous nodes demand that precautions should be taken to prevent the spread of infection and cultures should be set up on an appropriate medium. The other half of the node may then be placed in fixative.

If infection is unlikely, imprint preparations may be made with one half of the freshly sliced node as detailed in Chapter 3. If facilities are available for cell marker studies, cell suspensions may be prepared from the same half of the fresh node, as set out in Chapter 4. Immunoglobulin extraction is a technique requiring special research facilities and is not generally applicable. This investigation demands that sufficient fresh tissue is available for the accurate measurement of the various immunoglobulin fractions. Any reserve tissue required for this or any other purpose may be snap frozen in isopentane and stored in liquid nitrogen.

Imprints are valuable, not only for showing the appearance of the cells in a cytological preparation stained by a Romanowsky method (and thus for comparison with blood or bone marrow smears), but also for cytochemical studies. Enzyme histochemical tests can also be performed on cryostat sections of the fresh node (see Ch. 3). In general, the use of rapid frozen sections to provide a quick diagnosis is not to be encouraged in the case of lymph node biopsies, for diagnostic difficulties are magnified by the thicker and often less clear sections obtained by freezing. There are, however, occasions when a confident diagnosis can be made on a rapid cryostat section of a lymph node. Furthermore, the immunofluorescent or peroxidase antiperoxidase (PAP) methods, for the detection of immunoglobulins or other antigenic determinants in tissue, are much more sensitive when carried out on frozen sections of fresh tissue, rather than paraffin sections of fixed tissue.

It is a useful practice in research centres, if sufficient tissue is available from the biopsy, to retain a block of the fresh tissue, deep frozen in a −70° C freezer or stored in liquid nitrogen, in case it is required for future studies (see above). The block already used for frozen sections may serve this purpose.

Having taken all that is required of the fresh tissue and cells, the remaining lymph node tissue (generally not less than half the node if it is a small one) is put into fixative solutions. Cubes of tissue not more than 2 mm in diameter should be put into glutaraldehyde for subsequent resin embedding and electron microscopy and this should be done soon after the fresh node is bisected, before any autolysis has taken place. Larger, but still thin, blocks may be fixed in glutaraldehyde for resin embedding and semi-thin (1–2 μm) sections. Finally, a block or blocks (if the node is a large one) should be taken across the equator of the node and placed in formol-saline or other suitable fixative solution for subsequent processing and paraffin embedding. Details of recommended methods and techniques are given in the next chapter.

3

G.R. Latham

Routine laboratory methods

In this chapter the methods of handling and staining biopsy material of lymphoreticular tissue are mainly those methods which have been tried and found successful in the Histopathology Department of St Bartholomew's Hospital, London. Most of the staining methods have been published elsewhere and in such cases the source of the method is acknowledged. In cases where modifications to the original method have been found to be an improvement, attention is drawn to the modifications. In the few instances where we have not had practical experience of a particular method, this is stated. Only those methods which seem to us to be of real value have been included and the uses of each method are briefly indicated, after details have been given of the technique in question.

The order in which methods are dealt with is not in order of preference but is governed by the chronological order of events, from the moment of receipt of a fresh lymph node biopsy specimen. Thus the technique of making imprints is dealt with first. Then methods for which frozen sections are required. Thirdly, methods employed on sections of paraffin or resin embedded fixed tissue.

The vital importance of careful handling and prompt fixation of specimens has been emphasised in the previous chapter. It cannot be overstressed that faults in dealing with the specimen at this critical stage will lead to artefacts which cannot later be corrected, no matter how impeccable the subsequent technique.

IMPRINT PREPARATIONS (TOUCH PREPARATIONS, 'DABS')

One of the many advantages of receiving lymph node biopsies fresh from the operating theatre, rather than in fixative, is that imprint preparations can be made. To prepare these imprints, the freshly cut surface of the node is lightly blotted with soft absorbent paper, to remove excess blood and fluid. The cut surface is then lightly touched on to a clean, grease-free glass slide. Some operators prefer to hold the back of the lymph node with forceps and dab the cut surface of the node on to glass slides placed flat on the bench. Others place the cut lymph node on the bench and bring the glass slide down into contact with it. The important point is that only the lightest pressure should be applied and any lateral movement should be avoided as this will cause 'streaking' or 'tailing' of the cells. With a small lymph node several imprints can be made on one slide and it is useful to prepare several slides (4–6), not only because the first prints taken may prove too thick, but in order that different staining methods may be applied.

Staining imprints

Two or more imprint slides should be stained by the May-Grünwald Giemsa (Pappenheim) method (or whatever Romanowsky method is in use in the laboratory). Study of these slides will enable the pathologist to get a general idea of the proportions of different types of lymphoid and other cells represented in the node, for comparison with the biopsy section in due course. A cytological diagnosis of Hodgkin's disease, other malignant lymphoma, or metastatic carcinoma may be possible. In cases of malignant lymphoma, it is particularly valuable to have Romanowsky stained imprints of the node for comparison with similarly stained marrow preparations, for it may enable lymphoma cells to be identified in the marrow at a stage when very few are present. Other methods of value for staining imprints are:

PAS (Periodic Acid-Schiff) — for glycogen granules in cells, (positive staining abolished by prior diastase digestion), immunoglobulin in cells of plasma cell lineage, or mucin in identifying signet-ring cell carcinoma.
Oil Red O for intracytoplasmic lipid (in Burkitt's and other high grade lymphomas).
Enzyme methods, especially:
Acid Phosphatase for histiocytes, T-cells and 'hairy cells' (in which the enzyme is tartrate resistant).
Non-specific Esterase for histiocytes.
Acid Esterase (α-naphthyl acetate esterase) for T-lymphocytes.
Chloroacetate Esterase for neutrophil granulocytes and their precursors and for mast cells.

These methods, which are the same as those employed for frozen sections, are given in the following pages.

Other enzyme methods for lymphoid cells (not given here), include those methods for β-glucuronidase, adenosine triphosphatase, 5-nucleotidase, and diaminopeptidase IV (Feller & 1981).

FROZEN SECTIONS

Demands for rapid frozen cryostat sections for the diagnosis of lymph node biopsies should, wherever possible, be resisted. The interpretation of top quality paraffin sections may be difficult enough and there is no doubt that the interpretation of frozen sections is even more difficult, for the sections are often thicker and the cells less distinct. Where there is any suspicion that a lymph node is tuberculous, a frozen section of unfixed tissue should be refused. Frozen sections are necessary for certain histochemical and immunohistochemical studies and for the demonstration of lipids. Sections are cut on the cryostat at 5 μm, either from a snap-frozen block of the fresh, unfixed lymph node, or from the reserve tissue stored in liquid nitrogen.

Methods applicable to frozen sections

For topographical study of a node a standard haematoxylin and eosin procedure is all that is required. On the few occasions when it is necessary to demonstrate lipids in lymph node sections, the Oil Red O method for neutral fats (Lillie, 1963) will be found to be satisfactory.

ENZYME HISTOCHEMICAL METHODS

The activity of most enzymes is destroyed or severely diminished by the standard fixation and processing required to produce paraffin section. For this reason, imprints or cryostat sections are required for these methods. The outstanding exception is the Naphthol ASD Chloroacetate Esterase method (p. 35) which works perfectly satisfactorily on fixed, paraffin sections. The method is included at the end of this section for completeness' sake.

Naphthol AS-B1 phosphate for acid phosphatase

(Barka & Anderson, 1962)

Hexazotized pararosanilin (HPR)

A. Dissolve 1.g pararosanilin hydrochloride in 20 ml distilled water, add 5 ml conc. (concentrated) HCl. Warm gently, cool and filter. Store in the dark.
B. Freshly prepared 4% sodium nitrite.

For use, mix equal quantities of A and B solutions and refrigerate at 4°C for 5 minutes for hexazotization to take place.

Solutions

1. HPR working solution.
2. Dissolve 10 mg naphthol AS-B1 phosphate (sodium salt) in 1.0 ml dimethyl formamide.
3. Stock 0.2 M sodium acetate/glacial acetic acid buffer pH 5.2.

Incubating solution

1. Stock sodium acetate/acetic acid buffer — 5 ml
2. Distilled water — 12 ml

3. Naphthol AS-B1 phosphate/dimethyl formamide 1 ml
4. HPR 1.6 ml

Adjust to pH 5.2 with either N/NaOH or N/HCl

Method

1. Fix smears, imprints or cryostat sections in formol calcium fixative at 4°C for 10 minutes.
2. Wash well in distilled water.
3. Place in the filtered incubating solution ½–1½ hours at room temperature. Check microscopically at intervals. The end point is reached when the macrophages are a deep red colour.
4. Wash well in distilled water.
5. Counterstain the nuclei with Mayer's haematoxylin — 30 seconds.
6. Blue in running tap water.
7. Dry sections or smears.
8. Clear in xylene and mount in DPX.

Results

Sites of acid phosphatase activity	red
Nuclei	blue

Uses

Monocytes and histiocytes show abundant red granules throughout their cytoplasm, as do neutrophil polymorphs. Some T-cell subsets and T-cell precursors show focal spot-like activity in the Golgi zone. Other T-cells show more diffuse activity. 60% of the neoplastic cells (Catovsky et al, 1974) in cases of hairy cell leukaemia show moderate amounts of diffuse acid phosphatase activity which is not destroyed by tartrate treatment. This is therefore a very useful confirmatory test for the diagnosis of hairy cell leukaemia, especially in imprint preparations.

Tartrate resistant acid phosphatase

The method is identical to the above, except that sodium acetate tartrate buffer is used in place of stock acetate buffer. To prepare, add 75 mg of tartaric acid to 10 ml of stock buffer solution.

Notes

1. Smears and imprints can be stored unfixed at room temperature for at least 2 weeks prior to staining, without any appreciable loss of enzyme activity. When smears are stored in the refrigerator they should be fixed first, as very often moisture condenses on the slides causing haemolysis.

2. Acid phosphatases are usually demonstrated between pH 4.8–6.0. Above pH 6.0 and below pH 3.0 complete inhibition occurs. At pH 5.5 and above, some background staining occurs, therefore a compromise pH 5.2 is used. (Janckila et al, 1978).

3. Hexazonium pararosanilin is said to give a final reaction product (FRP) which is insoluble in alcohol and xylene. However, personal experience has shown that there is some loss of the product in dilute alcohol and the sections or imprints are therefore dried prior to clearing in xylene.

A modified coupling azo dye method for alkaline phosphatase

(Pearse, 1972)

Solution

Dissolve 20 mg of sodium α-naphthyl phosphate in 20 ml of stock 0.2 M tris buffer (pH 10), add 20 mg fast red TR (5-chloro-O-toluidine). Mix well.

Method

1. Cut cryostat sections 5 μm thick.
2. Fix in buffered neutral formalin or formal calcium for 10 minutes at 4°C.
3. Wash in running tap water, rinse in distilled water.
4. Filter on the staining solution and incubate for 10–60 minutes at room temperature.
5. Wash in distilled water.
6. Counterstain in Mayer's haematoxylin — 30 seconds.
7. Blue in running tap water, mount in glycerin jelly.

Results

Sites of alkaline phosphatase activity	reddish brown
Nuclei	blue

The demonstration of alkaline phosphatase activity is of limited value in the distinction of different types of lymphoma. The T-cell regions are weakly positive for alkaline phosphatase and others have shown positive staining in cells of the mantle zone of follicles (Lennert, 1978).

Non-specific esterase

(Nachlas & Seligman, 1949; use of hexazonium — Davis & Ornstein, 1959)

Solutions

A. 10% formol calcium

Analar formaldehyde	11 ml
M calcium chloride	9 ml

Distilled water to 100 ml
Calcium carbonate approximately 0.5 g to pH 7.0

B. 0.2 M phosphate buffer
(a) Monobasic sodium phosphate (NaH_2PO_4 $2H_2O$) 2.76 g/100 ml
(b) Dibasic sodium phosphate (Na_2HPO_4 $12H_2O$) 7.16 g/100 ml
19 ml (a) + 81 ml (b) = pH 7.4

C. Hexazotized Pararosanilin
Solution (a)
Dissolve 1 g of pararosanilin hydrochloride in 20 ml distilled water and add 5 ml conc. HCl. Warm gently, cool and filter. Store in the dark.
Solution (b)
Freshly prepared 4% sodium nitrite.
For use, mix equal parts of (a) and (b) and leave in the refrigerator for 5 minutes.

Substrate

Freshly prepare as follows:
Dissolve 5 mg of l-naphthyl acetate in a few drops of acetone. Add 5 ml 0.2 M phosphate buffer pH 7.4 and 2 drops of hexazotized pararosanilin. Mix well, avoiding contact with the skin.

Method

1. Fix cryostat sections of fresh tissue in 10% formol calcium for 10 minutes at 4°C. Rinse in distilled water.
2. Filter freshly prepared substrate on to the sections and incubate at room temperature for 10 minutes. Do not use substrate which has turned brown, otherwise a precipitate forms.
3. Wash in water.
4. Counterstain in 0.1% light green — 10 seconds.
5. Wash in tap water.
6. Dehydrate rapidly in alcohol.
7. Clear in xylene and mount.

Results

Non-specific esterase activity	reddish brown
Nuclei	green

This technique has in the past been very useful for the demonstration of histiocytic reticulum cells, which contain a large amount of non-specific esterase. However, since like all monocyte-derived macrophages they contain an abundance of lysozyme (muramidase), this method has now been largely superseded by the more specific immunoperoxidase technique using an antibody to human muramidase.

Acid esterase (α-naphthyl acetate esterase — ANAE)

(Kulenkampff et al, 1976)

The incubating solution is identical to that for non-specific esterase except that an acid medium, pH 5.8–6.4 is used.

Method

1. Fix cryostat sections or smears in formol calcium or neutral buffered formalin at 4°C for 10 minutes.
2. Wash well in distilled water.
3. Hexazotized pararosanilin solution 2–4 ml
0.7 M phosphate buffer pH 5.0 40 ml
adjust to pH 5.8 with N/NaOH
Add 10 mg of α-naphthyl acetate (dissolved in a few drops of acetone)
Filter into a Coplin jar
Incubate sections in a covered Coplin jar at 37°C for 3 hours.
4. Wash well in distilled water.
5. Counterstain in 0.5% light green — 30 seconds
6. Rinse in distilled water.
7. Dehydrate rapidly in alcohol, clear in xylene, mount in DPX.

Results

Sites of acid esterase activity red-brown
Nuclei light green
The acid esterase method is a useful one for mature T-lymphocytes; the vast majority show a lo-localised dot reaction product in the Golgi region of the cytoplasm.

Notes

1. The pH of the solution varies according to the species cell to be demonstrated, e.g. for mouse T-cells use pH 6.4, for human T-cells pH 5.8 (Müller et al, 1975).
2. Three hours at room temperature will normally show the full activity of T-lymphocytes, if longer incubation times are used some activity in B-cells is also seen.
3. Monocytes show a diffuse cytoplasmic red-brown reaction product, T-lymphocytes a solitary intense cytoplasmic dot, or a few scattered granules at one pole.

There is some discrepancy in the staining of thymic lymphocytes, which contain little or no α-naphthyl acetate esterase (Pinkus et al, 1979), suggesting that T-cells must reach a certain stage of maturity to acquire ANAE activity.

Naphthol AS-D chloroacetate esterase
(Leder, 1964)

The naphthol AS-D chloroacetate esterase method is applicable to frozen sections, imprints and formalin fixed paraffin sections. There is marked impairment of the reaction on bone marrow trephine sections after decalcification in formic acid, but the enzyme is still active and can be demonstrated after the use of a chelating agent, e.g. ethylenediaminetetracetic acid (EDTA) for decalcification.

Preparation of solutions

1. Prepare hexazotized pararosanilin (HPR) (see page 34)
2. Buffer: Michaelis' Veronal Acetate
   A. N/10 HCl
   B. Veronal acetate solution
      Sodium acetate 19.4 g
      Sodium diethyl barbiturate 29.4 g
      Dissolve in 1 litre of distilled water.

For use, 10 ml A + 10 ml B, distilled water 30 ml.

Working solution

1. To 30 ml of veronal acetate/HCl buffer add 0.5 ml of HPR, adjust to pH 6.3.
2. Dissolve 10 mg naphthol AS-D chloroacetate in 1 ml dimethyl formamide.

Mix 1 and 2, shake well (milky, pink flaky deposit formed), filter.

Method

1. Deparaffinize sections and take to distilled water. Smears, imprints and blood films: fix in 1 part methanol, 9 parts 4% formalin, or formol calcium at 4°C for 10 minutes.
2. Wash well in distilled water.
3. Incubate for 20 minutes in working solution at room temperature.
4. Wash in running tap water.
5. Counterstain lightly with Mayer's haematoxylin — 30 seconds.
6. Blue in running tap water.
7. Air-dry sections.
8. Clear in xylene.
9. Mount in synthetic resin.

Results

Sites of chloroacetate esterase activity red
Nuclei blue
The chloroacetate esterase method is very useful for the demonstration of mast cells, granulocytes (except eosinophils), and their precursors.

IMMUNOHISTOCHEMISTRY

Immunofluorescence methods

The immunofluorescence technique is useful for specifically localising antigens in cells or tissues. The method involves the use of antibodies conjugated to fluorochromes (fluorescein or rhodamine B isothiocyanates), which fluoresce when excited by ultraviolet light. The antigen–antibody complexes are visualised using a U-V microscope.

Direct method

1. Cut thin 4–5 μm cryostat sections and dry in a stream of warm air for 1 hour.
2. Cover the section with appropriate fluorescein conjugated antiserum at optimal dilution. Leave in a moist chamber for 30 minutes.
3. Wash well with phosphate buffered saline (PBS), (3 changes of 20 minutes each), using a mechanical agitator to remove excess fluorescent antibody.
4. Mount in buffered glycerol.
5. View using a U-V microscope.

Notes

1. The specificity and avidity of each batch of fluorescent antibody should be checked before it is brought into routine use.
2. Adequate controls should be taken through in parallel with each batch of test sections. These should include both known positive and negative sections.
3. Tissue autofluorescence and the fluorescent labelling of non-specific antibodies are difficult to prevent.

This *direct* method is used for the examination of renal biopsies, skin, gut and lymphoid tissue.

In the *indirect* immunofluorescence technique, the tissue is first treated with a non-conjugated antibody raised to the specific antigen which it is desired to demonstrate. Visualisation is brought about by the use of a second, fluorescein-conjugated, anti-immunoglobulin serum. The second antibody is raised in an animal of different species to that of the non-conjugated antibody. The fluorescein-conjugated antibody attaches to the first antibody, now fixed to the tissue antigen. The indirect method produces an amplified fluorescence, since several fluorescein-anti-immunoglobulin molecules will bind to each molecule of the first antibody. It also has the advantage that a single fluorescent reagent can be used to detect a wide range of unconjugated antibodies. The indirect immunofluorescence technique is widely used for the detection of autoantibodies in the sera of patients suffering from autoimmune diseases. Each patient's serum is tested against a composite block of appropriate tissues. After thorough washing in PBS the second conjugated antibody is applied; the section is then once more thoroughly washed in PBS, mounted in buffered glycerol and examined under the U-V microscope.

Immunoperoxidase techniques

Fluorescein-conjugated antibody methods have several inherent disadvantages:

1. Frozen sections are required (unless special processing methods have been used) and therefore retrospective studies are not usually possible.
2. Cell morphology is relatively poor.
3. The preparations are not permanent.
4. A U-V microscope and darkroom are necessary to view the preparations.

Labelling antibodies with either horseradish peroxidase or alkaline phosphatase overcomes many of these disadvantages since the enzyme-labelling methods are often applicable to paraffin sections of fixed tissue.

There are, however, pitfalls in the performance and interpretation of immunoperoxidase methods which may be briefly mentioned here:

1. *Endogenous peroxidases.* Naturally occurring enzymes of this type are found in many cells, e.g. erythrocytes and leucocytes. These must be blocked or inhibited to prevent a false positive reaction when the diaminobenzidine reagent (DAB) is applied. Inhibition is achieved by pretreatment of the section with a 0.3% solution of hydrogen peroxide in absolute methanol (see below) (Streefkerk, 1972).
2. *Irregular staining.* Sometimes sections show heavy and unselective brown staining around the edges or in an irregular fashion. On occasions this artefact can be attributed to faulty fixation, but the explanation is not always clear.
3. *Backgound staining.* This problem is discussed on pages 38–39.
4. *Non-specific absorption of immunoglobulin by cells.* Positive staining of a cell for Ig does not necessarily imply that it is of B lymphocyte lineage, or has synthesised the immunoglobulin in question, for it is now known that many cells besides macrophages may absorb plasma pro-

teins from their surroundings and give positive results. The phenomenon may be suspected when positive cells are: (a) in a minority, (b) mainly the largest cells present, and (c) very variable in depth of staining. Demonstration of both types of light chain in a single cell by double labelling (Mason & Sammons, 1978) is proof of non-specific absorption.

The 'DAB' Reaction

Antigenic sites, localised by peroxidase conjugated antisera are usually visualised by the diaminobenzidine (DAB) reaction (Graham & Karnovsky, 1966). The peroxidase catalyses the transfer of oxygen from hydrogen peroxide in the presence of a chromogenic hydrogen donor (e.g. diaminobenzidine) to form an insoluble stable brown coloured product at the site of antigen activity (Drury & Wallington, 1980). Ethyl carbazole may be used as a substitute for DAB. Since this reaction product is soluble in alcohol, the sections should be mounted in glycerin jelly.

The direct method

In the direct method an antiserum to the tissue antigen to be demonstrated is labelled with horseradish peroxidase and applied to sections of the tissue (Heyderman, 1979). Antigen sites are visualised by the DAB reaction.

The method is now seldom used because of its relative insensitivity, and also because it is only suitable when large amounts of antisera are available for labelling.

The indirect method

In the indirect method a primary *unlabelled* antiserum, directed against the specific antigen which it is desired to demonstrate, is applied to the tissue sections. After thorough washing, this is followed by a peroxidase conjugated antiserum, raised in a different species and directed against the IgG of the primary antiserum (Taylor, 1978). Visualisation for light microscopy is again achieved by the use of a peroxidase-specific chromogen, e.g. hydrogen peroxide/diaminobenzidine, to produce a stable coloured product.

Method

1. Paraffin sections are cut at 4 μm thick, mounted on clean grease-free slides and dried in the oven at 45°C for 1 hour.
2. Dewax sections in xylene, hydrate in alcohol and wash briefly in methanol.
3. Block endogenous peroxidase activity in 0.3% hydrogen peroxide in absolute methanol — 30 minutes.
4. Wash well in 0.5 M tris buffer pH 7.6 diluted 1:10 with normal physiological saline. Three washes of 3 minutes each. Agitate continuously. Wipe off excess fluid.
5. Treat sections with normal swine serum diluted 1:20 with tris buffer — 15 minutes (to reduce non-specific background staining).
6. Drain off excess serum and, without washing, replace with the *primary antiserum*, e.g. rabbit anti-human Kappa light chain, optimally diluted in 1:20 normal swine serum.
7. Repeat stage 4.
8. Treat sections with *peroxidase-conjugated antiserum* e.g. peroxidase-conjugated swine anti-rabbit immunoglobulin, at working dilution, usually about 1:20.
9. Repeat stage 4.
10. Treat sections with freshly prepared diaminobenzidine tetrahydrochloride — 5–10 minutes.

    Solution

DAB reagent	12 mg
Tris buffer	20 ml
30% H_2O_2	0.05 ml

11. Wash well in running tap water.
12. Counterstain lightly in Mayer's haematoxylin — 30 seconds.
13. Blue in running tap water.
14. Dehydrate, clear and mount in DPX.

Results

Sites of specific antibody	dark brown
Nuclei	blue

Although more sensitive than the direct method, the indirect method has largely been superseded by the PAP method.

The peroxidase anti-peroxidase (PAP) method

The PAP method depends on the addition of an

excess of an *unconjugated second antibody* to link the primary antibody, directed against the tissue antigen, to the animal immunoglobulin of the PAP complex. One Fab 'arm' of the second antibody links to the Fc component of the first antibody, while the other Fab 'arm' is free to attach to the Fc portion of the PAP complex, thus forming a link between the primary antiserum and the PAP reagent.

The PAP complex–soluble peroxidase antiperoxidase complex, should be prepared in the same species as the primary antiserum, e.g. *rabbit* anti-human primary antiserum, — *rabbit* PAP.

Method

Steps 1–4 as in the previous method.

5. Remove excess fluid but do not allow the sections to dry, and replace with normal swine serum diluted 1:20 with tris buffer saline — 15 minutes (to reduce non-specific background staining). Drain off excess serum.
6. Treat sections with the *primary antiserum*, (e.g. rabbit anti-human muramidase) optimally diluted in 1:20 normal swine serum — 30 minutes.
7. Repeat stage 4.
8. Treat sections with *swine anti-rabbit immunoglobulins* diluted with tris buffer (usually 1:20) — 30 minutes.
9. Repeat stage 4.
10. *PAP* (*rabbit*) *complex* at optimal dilution, e.g. 1:100 in tris buffer saline — 30 minutes.
11. Repeat stage 4.
12. Treat with freshly prepared diaminobenzidine hydrochloride — 5–10 minutes.

    Solution

DAB reagent	12 mg
Tris buffer	20 ml
30% H_2O_2	0.05 ml

13. Wash well in running tap water — 5 minutes.
14. Counterstain lightly in Mayer's haematoxylin — 30 seconds.
15. Blue in running tap water — 10 minutes.
16. Dehydrate, clear and mount in DPX.

Results:

Sites of specific antibody	dark brown
Nuclei	blue

Control sections should always be carried through in parallel with the test sections. These should consist of:

(a) A known positive and a known negative section.
(b) An absorption control, i.e. an antigen-absorbed immune serum in place of the primary antiserum.
(c) A normal serum control of the same animal species in which the primary antiserum was raised.
(d) A substitution control. The primary specific antibody stage is omitted, the section remaining in tris buffer saline during Step 6.

Notes

1. Trypsinisation of formalin fixed tissue has been advocated by some workers to 'unmask' antigens in tissue sections (Curran & Gregory, 1977). This procedure is carried out after endogenous peroxidase activity has been blocked and the sections washed in tris buffer saline, i.e. after stage 4. Sections are incubated in 0.1% trypsin in 0.1% calcium chloride (adjusted to pH 7.8 with N/10 NaOH) for up to 2 hours. The sections should be pre-heated to 37°C in tris buffer saline before placing in trypsin. Several sections should be taken through to find the correct time for trypsinisation, as this may vary for each batch of sections. In our experience, trypsinisation is unnecessary when the tissue has been fixed in formal sublimate solution and is rarely required after adequate fixation in ordinary formol saline.

2. Specific background staining may occur in cases of myeloma, due to the increase of immunoglobulin in the serum (Taylor, 1978). This will result in an overall dark brown colouration in which both the myeloma cells and the background stain intensely. A similar type of background staining is caused by the diffusion of antigen from the cells prior to fixation. Prompt fixation of tissue will help to overcome the latter problem.

3. Unwanted non-specific antibodies may be present in the primary antisera; they are usually of a low titre and their effects can be minimised by using a high titre antiserum and diluting

until only the specific antibody is detected. Further reduction of the background staining can be achieved by treating the sections with a non-reacting serum, both prior to and combined with the primary anti-serum. This will occupy many of the non-specific binding sites.

4. A useful modification of the PAP technique, which helps to reduce background staining, is to apply the primary antiserum to the sections at 4°C for 18–24 hours. Very high dilutions of the antiserum are then effective, e.g. 1:500–1:5000.

Although background staining can be reduced by these various methods, it is impossible to eliminate it completely. With the increasing availability of monospecific antibodies some at least of these problems may be overcome. Other modifications, e.g. the avidin–biotin method, have further increased the sensitivity of the immunoperoxidase technique (see Ch. 4).

PARAFFIN SECTIONS

Different laboratories have their own preferred methods of preparing and staining sections. The methods advocated are those that have been found satisfactory in practice.

Fixation

Formol sublimate is an ideal fixative for lymph nodes since it preserves the cells well, with minimal shrinkage, and allows good subsequent staining. It is particularly useful when immunoperoxidase methods are to be employed and gives greatly superior results to formol saline fixation for this purpose. Fixation is usually complete in 6–8 hours with a slice of lymph node of 3 mm thickness. The chief drawback of formol sublimate as a fixative is the intensely poisonous nature of the solution and strict safety precautions should be observed in its handling and use.

Formol saline or *buffered formalin* are adequate for most general purposes, although fixation time is longer (12 hours for a slice of lymph node 3 mm thick). It is preferable to use freshly prepared fixatives and to keep the fixation time to a minimum, especially if immunoperoxidase studies are likely to be required.

Dehydration and embedding

After adequate fixation, tissue blocks are transferred to an automatic tissue processor timed to the following type of schedule:

70% alcohol	2 hours
90% alcohol	2 hours
absolute alcohol	4 changes of 1 hour each
toluene	2 changes of 2 hours each
paraffin wax	2 changes of 2 hours each

Vacuum embedding is carried out in fresh paraffin wax 1–2 hours. Lymph nodes are embedded in filtered paraffin wax (melting point 56°C).

Section cutting

Lymph node sections are routinely cut at 4 μm using a sharp knife kept specifically for this purpose. The disposable blade type of knife is ideal. Six sections are taken from each block, they are floated out using warm water only, as cracking and lifting of the section will occur if the water is too hot. Drying of the sections should take place at a low temperature — 37°C for the first half hour, 50°C for the remaining drying time.

Methods for paraffin sections

The following five methods, together with the chloroacetate esterase method (p. 35) have been found to be of value in the routine staining of lymph nodes.

1. Haematoxylin and eosin

Standard routine procedure. Differentiation of the haematoxylin should be adequate to show the nuclear chromatin structure, and the cytoplasm of histiocytes should be pale pink with the eosin counterstain. Heavy uneven staining is usually attributable to sections having been cut too thick.

2. Gordon and Sweets method for reticulin fibres (Gordon & Sweets, 1936)

Silver solution

To 5 ml of 10% analar silver nitrate, add fresh ammonia drop by drop until the precipitate first formed is just dissolved. Add 5 ml of 3% sodium hydroxide and re-dissolve the precipitate with a few more drops of ammonia. Make up to a volume of 50 ml with distilled water.

Method

1. Dewax sections in xylene, hydrate in alcohol and take to distilled water.
2. Oxidise in:
   0.5% potassium permanganate 47.5 ml
   3% sulphuric acid 2.5 ml— 5 minutes
3. Wash briefly in distilled water.
4. Bleach in 1% oxalic acid.
5. Wash well in distilled water.
6. Sensitise in 2.5% iron alum — 15 minutes.
7. Wash thoroughly in distilled water.
8. Silver solution — until sections become transparent — approximately 10 seconds.
9. Wash briefly in tap water.
10. Reduce in 10% formalin in tap water — 5 minutes.
11. Rinse in distilled water.
12. Tone in 0.2% gold chloride — 5 minutes.
13. Rinse in distilled water.
14. Fix in 5% sodium thiosulphate — 5 minutes.
15. Wash well in tap water.
16. Lightly counterstain nuclei in 1% neutral red — 30 seconds.
17. Rinse in tap water, dehydrate, clear and mount in DPX.

Results

Reticulin fibres	black
Nuclei	red

Silver impregnation methods are excellent for displaying the architecture of lymph nodes and revealing disturbances of pattern and vasculature.

3. *Giemsa* (Modification by Lennert, 1952, 1961)

Solutions

A. Sörensen's buffer pH 6.8
B. Giemsa solution (Merck ART 9204, marketed in Great Britain by BDH Ltd)

Method

1. Dewax sections in xylene, hydrate in alcohol, and rinse in pH 6.8 buffer.
2. Stain for 1 hour in diluted Giemsa solution.
   Stock Giemsa 20 ml
   pH 6.8 buffer 100 ml
3. Rinse sections in pH 6.8 buffer.
4. Differentiate in distilled water to which 4–5 drops of concentrated glacial acetic acid/50 ml have been added — 10–15 seconds.
5. Continue differentiation in 95% isopropyl alcohol (control microscopically until the correct differentiation is reached).
6. Stop differentation and dehydrate in 3 changes of absolute isopropyl alcohol — 1 minute each.
7. Clear in xylene, mount in DPX.

Results

Mast cell granules	violet
Nuclei	blue
Cytoplasm	varying shades of grey-blue, blue, mauve-blue and pink
Eosinophils	orange-red
RBC's	red-pink

Giemsa is an excellent cytological stain and the results are more directly comparable with those obtained with Romanowsky staining of blood or marrow films or lymph node imprints.

4. *Methyl green-pyronin Y, alcian blue method* (Bowers & Chadwin, 1966)

Solutions

A. Alcian blue 1 g
   70% alcohol 90 ml
   Conc. HCl 10 ml
B. Methyl green-pyronin Y solution:
   2.6 g of pyronin Y and 1.4 g methyl green (washed in chloroform) are stirred into 40 ml glycerol. To this 10 ml absolute alcohol and 400 ml 0.5% phenol are added. Mix well. It is advisable to allow this solution to ripen for 1 week before use. Specificity is lost after approximately 8 weeks.

Method

1. Dewax sections and take to 70% alcohol.
2. Immerse sections in 1% acid alcohol (1% HCl in 70% alcohol) — 2 minutes.
3. Stain in alcian blue solution (A) — 10 minutes.
4. Wash off stain in 1% acid alcohol — 3 changes — 1 minute each.
5. Wash in running tap water for at least 10 minutes.
6. Rinse in distilled water and stain in methyl green-pyronin Y solution — 10 minutes.
7. Differentiate in absolute alcohol until no more colour is removed (use a drop-bottle), clear in xylene and mount in DPX.

Results

Cytoplasm and granules of mast cells	bright azure
Other sulphated mucopolysaccharides, e.g. connective tissue mucins	blue-green
RNA in cytoplasm (e.g. of plasma cells)	magenta
Nuclei	purplish green
Nucleoli	magenta

Notes

1. The methyl green-pyronin Y method is excellent for demonstrating B-immunoblasts and plasma cells, the intensity of the pyronin staining increasing as the cell matures. The cytoplasm of T-immunoblasts is less strongly pyroninophilic. The advantages of combining the methyl green-pyronin Y method with alcian blue are in the overall intensification of the staining and the simultaneous demonstration of plasma cells and mast cells in contrasting colours. With the ordinary methyl green-pyronin Y (Unna Pappenheim) stain, mast cell granules appear an orange vermilion colour but this is less distinctive than the blue-green colour after alcian blue staining.
2. Occasionally difficulty can be encountered with the method after fixation in formol saline of acid pH. Results after acid decalcification are likewise generally unsatisfactory.

5. *Periodic acid Schiff method (PAS)*

The standard PAS method is used both with and without prior diastase digestion. Glycogen (present in lymphoblasts and certain metastatic tumours, e.g. hypernephroma and seminoma), is removed by diastase digestion, but immunoglobulin and Russell bodies are generally PAS positive and resistant to diastase digestion. PAS is also useful in displaying the lymph node architecture, collagen and reticulin being weakly PAS positive.

Other methods may be required in addition to the above recommended methods for the demonstration of specific features, e.g. Van Gieson's stain for collagen, congo red for amyloid and Perl's Prussian blue for haemosiderin. These and the standard methods for micro-organisms will be found in any textbook of histological techniques.

Trichrome methods are sometimes useful, not only for the demonstration of collagen and fibrin, but also when cytoplasmic Ig has been demonstrated by PAS staining. As Lennert (1978) has pointed out, the heavy chain class of cytoplasmic Ig may often be determined by means of Ladewig's modification of Mallory's aniline blue method (Ladewig, 1938) or Goldner's modification of Masson's trichrome method (Goldner, 1938). With the Ladewig and Goldner methods, IgM stains grey-blue or green respectively, while IgG and IgA usually stain orange-red to bright crimson with both methods (Lennert, 1978).

Marshall's 'metalophil' method (Marshall, 1948), which is a modification of the Weil-Davenport method, can be used to show up the dendritic processes of dendritic reticulum cells, but like many silver methods it is a capricious technique. Methods like this and the trichrome stains mentioned above are today being largely superseded by specific immunostaining techniques.

RESIN EMBEDDING

The resins employed for this purpose, being much harder than paraffin wax, give greater support to the embedded tissue and therefore much thinner sections can be cut than are possible after paraffin embedding. Resin embedding was first developed for cutting ultra-thin sections for electron microscopy (EM) on an ultramicrotome. More recently it has come to be widely used for embedding larger sized blocks (up to 1 cm^2) from which 'semi-thin' sections (0.5–2μm) may be cut on a purpose built microtome using a glass knife. Blocks of the fresh lymph node are taken at the time of receipt of the specimen and fixed in formol saline.

Tissue blocks for EM should not be more than 2 mm in maximum diameter; they are fixed in 4% glutaraldehyde, and later post-fixed in osmium tetroxide prior to embedding in araldite or one of the several commercially available resins.

It is not proposed to discuss here the ultrastructure of lymphoid cells. Most lymphoid cells have relatively few organelles (see Ch. 1) and whilst electron microscopy has been of great assistance in revealing, for example, the intricate ramifications and distribution of the dendritic reticulum cells of the follicles, in diagnostic practice, there is not much additional information to be gained from electron microscopy which is not disclosed on light microscopic examination of semi-thin sections. These sections have the added advantage of covering a larger field and thus of overcoming one of the pitfalls in EM interpretation, that of inadequate sampling.

Details of nuclear and cytoplasmic morphology are much more clearly seen with semi-thin sections than with conventional paraffin sections. For example the nuclear convolutions of T-lymphoblastic lymphoma or Sézary cells are readily visualised, as are the fat vacuoles in Burkitt's lymphoma. Staining is, of course, much fainter than it is in paraffin sections and some people find they miss the '3-D' effect imparted by the latter, which can be useful on low power examination of the section. Immunostaining can be carried out satisfactorily after removal of the resin.

REFERENCES

Barka T, Anderson P J 1962 Histochemical methods for acid phosphatase using hexazonium as coupler. Journal of Histochemistry and Cytochemistry 10: 741–753

Bowers D, Chadwin C G 1966 Simultaneous demonstration of mast cells and plasma cells. Journal of Clinical Pathology 19:298

Catovsky D, Pettit J E, Galton D A G, Spiers A S D, Harrison C V 1974 Leukaemic reticuloendotheliosis (hairy cell leukaemia): A distinct clinico-pathological entity. British Journal of Haematology 26: 9–27

Curran R C, Gregory J 1977 The unmasking of antigens in tissue sections by trypsin. Experientia 33: 1400–1401

Davis B J, Ornstein L 1959 High resolution enzyme localisation with a new diazo reagent hexazonium pararosaniline. Journal of Histochemistry and Cytochemistry 7: 297–301

Drury R A B, Wallington E A 1980 Carleton's histological technique, 5th edn. Oxford Medical Publications, Oxford University Press

Feller A C, Parwaresch M R 1981 Specificity and polymorphism of diaminopeptidase IV in normal and neoplastic T μ lymphocytes. Journal of Cancer Research and Clinical Oncology 101: 59–63

Goldner J 1938 A modification of Masson's trichrome technique for routine laboratory purposes. American Journal of Pathology 14: 237–243

Gordon H, Sweets H H 1936 A simple method for the silver impregnation of reticulin. American Journal of Pathology 12:545

Graham R C, Karnovsky M J 1966 The early stages of absorption of injected horseradish peroxidase in the proximal tubules of mouse kidney. Ultrastructural chemistry by a new technique. Journal of Histochemistry and Cytochemistry 14: 291–302

Heyderman E 1979 Immunoperoxidase technique in histopathology: applications, methods, and controls. Journal of Clinical Pathology 32: 971–978

Janckila A J, Li C–Y, Lam K–W, Yam L T 1978 The cytochemistry of tartrate resistant acid phosphate. American Journal of Clinical Pathology, 70: 45–55

Kulenkampff J, Janossy G, Greaves M 1977 Acid esterase in human lymphoid cells and leukaemic blasts: a marker for T lymphocytes. British Journal of Haematology 36: 231–240

Ladewig P 1938 Über eine einfache und vielseitige Bindegewebsfärbung (Modifikation der Mallory-Heidenhainschen Methode) Zeitschrift für wissenschaftlicher Mikroscopie 55: 215–217

Leder L D 1964 The selective enzocytochemical demonstration of neutrophil myeloid cells and tissue mast cells in paraffin sections. Klinische Wochenschrift 42: 11:553

Lennert K in collaboration with Mohri N, Stein H, Kaiserling E, Müller-Hermelink H K 1978 Malignant lymphomas. Springer-Verlag, Berlin

Lillie R D, Ashburn L L 1943 Supersaturated solutions of fat stains in dilute isopropanol for demonstration of acute fatty degeneration not shown by Herscheimer technic. Archives of Pathology 36: 432–435

Marshall A H E 1948 A method for the demonstration of reticuloendothelial cells in paraffin sections. Journal of Pathology and Bacteriology 60: 515–517

Mason D Y, Sammons R 1978 Alkaline phosphatase and peroxidase for double immunoenzymatic labelling of cellular constituents. Journal of Clinical Pathology 31: 454–460

Müller J et al 1975 Non-specific acid esterase activity: a criteria for the differentiation of T and B lymphocytes in

mouse lymph nodes. European Journal of Immunology 5:270
Nachlas M M, Seligman A M 1949 The histochemical demonstration of esterase. Journal of the National Cancer Institute 9: 415–425
Pearse A G E 1972 Histochemistry: theoretical and applied, 3rd edn. Churchill Livingstone, Edinburgh
Pinkus G S Hargreaves H K, McLeod J A, Nadler L M, Rosenthal D S, Said J W 1979 α-naphthyl acetate esterase activity. A cytochemical marker for T lymphocytes. American Journal of Pathology 97: 17–42
Streefkerk J G 1972 Inhibition of erythrocyte pseudoperoxidase activity by treatment with hydrogen peroxide following methanol. Journal of Histochemistry and Cytochemistry 20: 829–831
Taylor C R 1978 Immunoperoxidase techniques: theoretical and practical aspects. Archives of Pathology 102: 113–121
Taylor C R 1978 Immunocytochemical methods in the study of lymphoma and related conditions. Journal of Histochemistry and Cytochemistry 26: 496–512

4

J. A. Habeshaw

Specialised laboratory methods

INTRODUCTION

In addition to the standard techniques of investigating lymph node biopsies outlined in the last chapter there are other, more sophisticated investigations which require special facilities for their prosecution. Most of the procedures are only suitable for research laboratories, since few routine laboratories have either the time or the expertise to correlate and interpret the results. However, since much of our current knowledge about lymphoid cells and the neoplasms derived from them has been gained from the use of such techniques, it may be useful to give an outline of them here. Technical details would clearly be out of place, and it is proposed rather to indicate the scope of the methods cited, the information that can be gleaned from them, and how this relates to the morphological appearances seen in routine lymph node sections.

The investigations to be discussed are: 1) phenotyping of lymphoid and other cells found in lymphoreticular tissues, using specific antibodies to individual cell markers; 2) cytogenetic studies to detect chromosome aberrations, and the significance of the principal chromosomal defects in non-Hodgkin lymphoma.

PHENOTYPING

There is enormous cellular diversity within the immune system, first within the functionally different T and B lymphocyte sub-populations, secondly within the different classes of antigen receptor expressed by these cells, thirdly because of the variable functional states of lymphocytes during phases of reaction or inaction, and finally because of the different genetic background of each individual patient studied. Nonetheless, it is possible to describe the types of lymphocyte encountered in lymph nodes, by phenotyping.

The meaning of 'phenotype' as applied to phenotypic studies of lymphoma

The differentiated features of a cell are determined by activation of a 'programme' coded in the nuclear DNA. Initially the zygote can develop only by restricting, selectively, the programme it has inherited, at each cell division producing cells which are of specialised function — hence differentiated. Differentiated functions of cells include the production of specific enzyme proteins which control specialised metabolism and proteins which have no known enzymic function but which maintain the homeostatic balance between the differentiated cell and the organism as a whole. Many of these proteins, particularly glycoproteins, are expressed on the cell surface, and they can be subdivided on a broad basis into three main classes:

a) Marker proteins specific for a tissue or differentiated cell class (class specific marker). Examples are glycophorin, found in red cells and their precursors, and immunoglobulin, found only in B lymphocytes.
b) Receptor proteins which act as receptors for ligands important for differentiated cell function (e.g. oestrogen receptors on mammary epithelium). These are not specific for any one class of cell, but tend to be common to cells having common functions. In the lympho-myeloid cell system, receptors for the Fc portion of IgG,

and receptors for complement components are examples of receptors linking cells of connected function but different class.

c) Marker proteins which are species specific and form the 'self non-self' recognition system, e.g. the HLA allo-antigens.

Cells can be classified according to the expressed marker proteins on the cell membrane — this identifies cells on the basis of their *phenotype* (i.e. as expressing some part of the *genotype* — the total potential biological programme). Phenotypic features of cells are a measure of their differentiation (the differentiation compartment to which the cells belong) and their maturation (within that differentiation compartment, whether the cells are early (immature) or late (mature)). Change in a phenotypic feature not accompanied by a change in the differentiated state of the cell (modulation) indicates a response to a change in environment — a homeostatic adjustment of the cell.

The phenotypic markers used

The production of a phenotypic profile of lymph node tissue, in either cell suspension or in frozen section, uses, essentially, the same reagents. Of late, most of these reagents are monoclonal antibodies which have technical advantages over the previously available heteroantisera. With these reagents have been developed techniques employing second antibodies labelled with fluorochromes, enzymes, or biochemical ligands such as avidin/biotin or arsenilate. A discussion of the advantages of each system is beyond the scope of this chapter; it is sufficient to say that, properly employed, any of the available techniques will produce valid results.

The phenotypic markers in current use are (1) *Rosetting*, with coated or uncoated red cells. These techniques are applied in suspension and detect receptors for the immunological intermediates Fcγ, Fcμ, C3b, C3d expressed on more than one cell class, but which correctly applied can be interpreted as class specific markers; (2) *Heteroantisera*: use is mainly for the detection of surface immunoglobulin heavy and light chain classes and subclasses; (3) *Monoclonal antibodies* which are cell subset specific, or are important markers of other cell functions. The specificities of these markers are summarised below, and in Tables 4.1. and 4.2.

Rosettes

1. E rosettes. Sheep erythrocytes used fresh, neuraminidase treated, or treated with AET (2-aminoethylisothiouronium bromide hydrobromide), bind spontaneously to a major population of human T lymphocytes expressing the sheep erythrocyte receptor (SER) (Kaplan &Clark, 1974). Different conditions of incubation (at 4°C or 37°C) illustrate heterogeneity of SER, with weak and strong binding T-cell subsets (Bentwich et al, 1973; Brain et al, 1970; Jondal, 1976). Use of sheep erythrocyte binding on frozen sections has also been described (Jaffe et al, 1975). Equivalent results are produced using the monoclonal OKT11 which reacts with the 'receptor' for sheep red cells (Verbi et al, 1982).

2. Mouse RBC rosettes. Mouse red cells, prepared by mild papain treatment, will form spontaneous rosettes with a few per cent of neuraminidase treated normal lymphocytes in tonsil, node and cord blood. MRBC rosetting cells are early (immature) cells of B lineage and, although a minor subset of normal B-cells, are prominent components of lymphocytic lymphoma and chronic lymphocytic leukaemia (Gupta & Grieco, 1975).

3. Rosetting with Ig coated red cells. Ox red blood cells coated with IgG or IgM antibodies react with subsets of mononuclear cells. These cells possess receptors for the Fc piece of the relevant immunoglobulin, designated Fcγ, Fcμ receptors. Receptors for Fcα, Fcδ and Fcε have also been described. T cells can express receptors for Fcγ, Fcμ, Fcα, Fcδ and Fcε: in each case only a subset of T-cells can expresses the receptor (Gupta & Good, 1981). Receptors for Fcμ can be inhibited by pentameric serum IgM, thus serum should not be present when evaluating these receptors. Fcγ receptors bind preferentially to 'complexed' or aggregated IgG. Mononuclear phagocytes, and polymorphs express Fcγ receptors rather strongly (Natvig & Froland, 1976). Natural killer cells are also said to express Fcγ receptors. B-cells express Fcγ receptors weakly, and a relatively small proportion of normal B-cells is Fcγ receptor

Table 4.1 Distribution of B-cell associated phenotypic markers in normal lymphoid and accessory cell populations

Antigen/Marker Reference	Molecular Characteristics	Pre B	Follicular B	Mantle zone B	'CLL' like
BI Pan B cell (Stashenko et al 1980)	70K MW Dimeric glycoprotein antigen				
B2 Peripheral B cell (Nadler et al 1981)	140 K (reduced 120 K) glycoprotein antigen				
Bal "early" B cell (Abramson et al 1981)	30 K glycoprotein				
Ba2 (Kersey et al 1981)	24 K non integral glycoprotein				
RFA$_2$ (Caligaris Cappio et al 1982)	Not known				
OKT 10 (Von Camp et al) 1982)	40 – 45 K glycoprotein				
Fmc7 (Brooks et al 1980)	Non precipitable ? glycolipid				
P1153/3 (Greaves et al 1980)	Antigen Co Caps with SIg				
F8 : 11 : 13 (Dalchau & Fabre 1981)	215 K glycoprotein 190 K glycoprotein				
33.1 (Marti & Kindt 1982)	HLA "DR" related				
Surface IgM					
Surface IgM + D					
Surface IgG/IgA					
Cytoplasmic μ					
Cytoplasmic IgM					
Cytoplasmic IgG/IgA					

Pre-B — Pre B cell
Thymic LB — Thymic cortical lymphoblast
T_H — Peripheral T 'helper' subset
T_S — Peripheral T 'suppressor' subset
Neutral T — T-cell expressing Pan-T lineage markers but not subset specific markers
NK — Natural killer cell (includes a proportion of Leu 7 positive T cells)

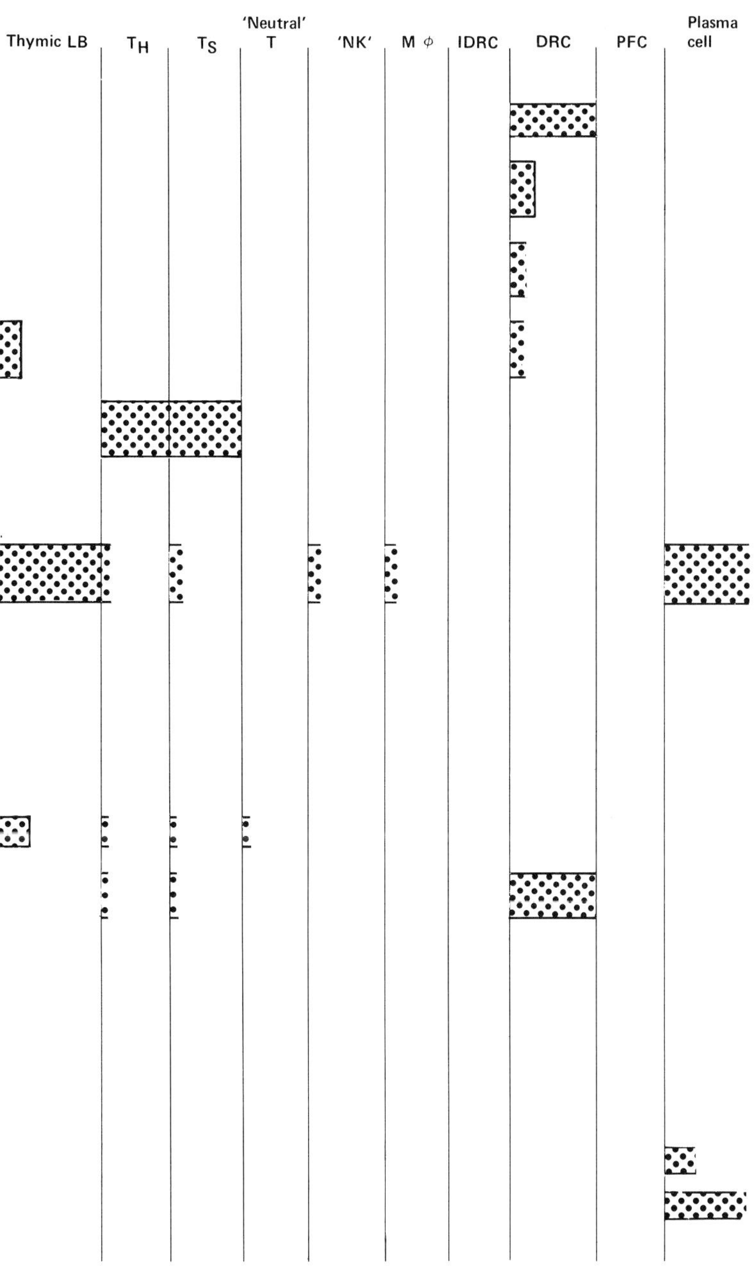

IDRC	Interdigitating reticulum cell of the paracortex
DRC	Dendritic reticulum cell of the follicle
PFC	Perifollicular cell
M	Macrophage

Closed boxes show the proportion of cells expressing the determinant. Open ended boxes show that some cells of the class described express the determinant, but the exact proportion is not known. Incompletely filled, closed boxes represent expression on a subset but not all cells of the class described.

Table 4.2 Distribution of T-cell and accessory cell associated phenotypic markers in normal lymphoid and accessory cell populations

Antigen/Marker Reference	Molecular Characteristics	Pre B	Follicular B	Mantle zone B	'CLL' like B c
C–ALL A (Ritz et al 1980)	95–100 K MW glycoprotein				
HLA–DR/DA$_2$, CA$_2$ (Brodsky et al 1979) (Charron & McDevitt 1979)	p28 p33 K MW glycoprotein				
Cortical thymic/OKT6/ NA 134 (Reihnertz et al 1980a)	49 K MW glycoprotein				
PAN T-cell/OKT1/Leu I (Wang et al 1980)	69–71 K MW glycoprotein				
PAN T-cell/OKT3 (Kung et al 1979)	19 K MW glycoprotein				
E Receptor/OKT11 (Verbi et al 1982)	E Rosette receptor				
T Helper/OKT4 Leu 3a (Reinhertz et al 1979)	55–62 K MW glycoprotein				
T cytotoxic/supressor OKT8/Leu 2a (Reinhertz et al 1980b)	32–43 K MW glycoprotein				

Antigen/Marker Reference	Molecular Characteristics	Pre B	Follicular B	Mantle zone B	'CLL' like B c
OKMI (Berard et al 1980)					
MO2 (Todd et al 1981)					
KI (Schwab et al 1982)	? 110 K MW glycoprotein				
HLeI (2DI) (Beverly et al 1980)	Common leukocyte antigen				
HLA/ABC (W6/32) (Parnham et al 1979)	"Core" determinant HLA				
OKT9 (Sutherland et al 1981)	Transferrin receptor				
PNA (Rose et al 1981)	Asialo glycoprotein				

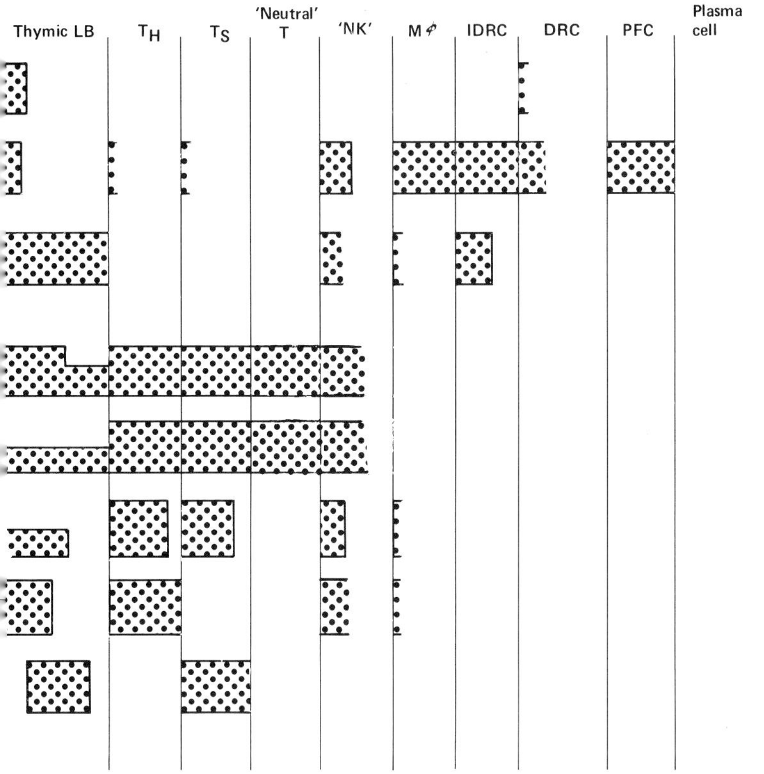

Thymic LB | T_H | T_S | 'Neutral' T | 'NK' | Mϕ | IDRC | DRC | PFC | Plasma cell

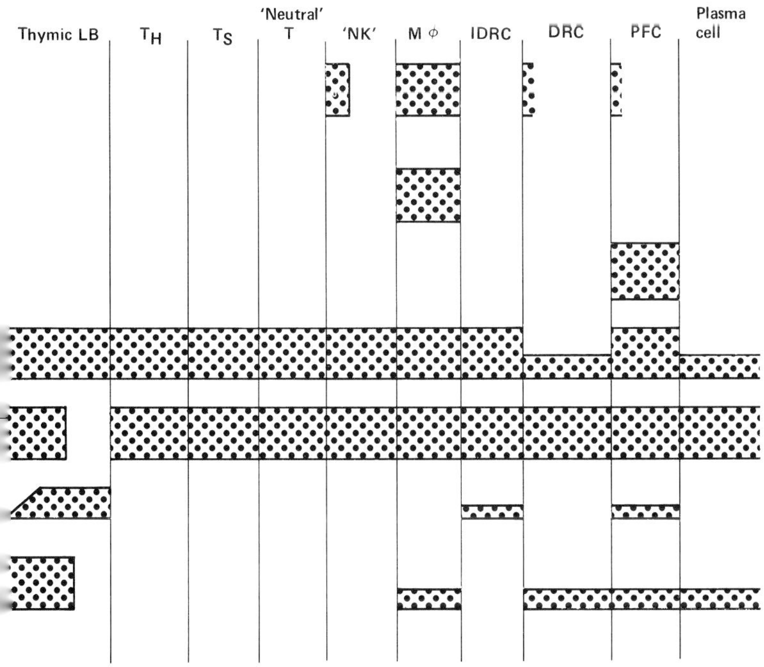

Thymic LB | T_H | T_S | 'Neutral' T | 'NK' | Mϕ | IDRC | DRC | PFC | Plasma cell

positive. Other cell types with Fc receptor expression include basophils, and eosinophils (which have high affinity receptors for IgE). Optimal conditions for Fc rosetting vary widely, especially on T-cells. In tissue frozen sections IgG sensitised ox red cells bind strongly to the interfollicular areas, sinus margins and mantle zones, and only weakly to germinal centres.

Rosetting to detect complement receptors

To the purist, complement receptors are detected using only systems which provide red cells coated with biochemically characterised individual complement components C3b, $C3b_i$, C3d. Those most commonly evaluated in phenotyping are the 'C3b' receptor and the 'C3d' receptor (Bianco & Nussenzweig, 1977).

The 'C3b' sensitised red cell binds strongly to neutrophils, mononuclear phagocytes, and some B lymphocytes. The 'C3d' sensitised red cell binds weakly to neutrophils and mononuclear phagocytes but strongly to B-cells (particularly of germinal centres) and to fetal (and some immature) thymocytes. The different methods of preparing these reagents (Lachmann et al, 1973) and the detailed analysis of their use are as described by McConnell & Lachmann (1976).

Functional tests for phagocytes

Functional tests for phagocytes employ latex beads (opsonised with serum) starch particles, or vital dyes. The use of the vital dye neutral red is an excellent way of determining pinocytotically active macrophages, which show rapid coarse granular uptake of the dye, myeloid cells which show finer 'stippled' uptake, and transformed lymphocytes, which show characteristic single dot uptake of dye. More recently, monoclonal antibodies OKM1 and MO2, which are myeloid and monocyte specific, have been introduced.

Antibodies and their use in phenotyping

The recently introduced monoclonal antibodies are significantly different reagents from classical heteroantisera. Monoclonal antibodies react with a single antigenic determinant (epitope) only, whereas heteroantisera bind to many different epitopes on a single antigen. For example, an antiserum against IgM raised in rabbits contains antibodies which bind to all the epitopes expressed by the immunising IgM, including the constant region epitopes (μ heavy chain specific), light chain epitopes, allotypic determinants, and variable region epitopes. The antiserum can be made specific for, say, μ chain by absorbing out antibodies which might cross react — e.g. the light chain reactive component can be removed by absorbing on insoluble light chains prepared from Bence Jones protein. Monoclonal anti-μ chain antibody, on the other hand, will react with only one epitope of IgM, since it is produced by fusing a single antibody forming cell with a HAT (hypoxanthine aminopterin thymidine) sensitive plasmacytoma cell from a mouse ('hybridoma'). A single epitope being recognised, it follows that *any* molecule bearing that epitope will react with the hybrid product. The skill in preparing monoclonal reagents lies in detecting the single clone which produces an antibody reacting with the required epitope. Thus a monoclonal antibody reactive with IgM (μ chain specific) will recognise only a C region epitope on IgM (it has to react with all μ heavy chains, but not with any part of the κ, λ, γ, α, δ, ε chains). Once selected, the required hybrid clone will produce any amount of monoclonal antibody of unalterable specificity.

Probably no two monoclonal antibodies are exactly alike, although they may react with the same antigen. For example, antibodies which are thought of as 'B-cell specific' may react with a similar epitope shared between, say, B-cells and the proximal convoluted tubule in kidney. Whilst working with monoclonals the user must be aware of these possible 'cross reactions'. Monoclonal antibodies represent not merely a new technological advance, but their use involves new ways of thinking about cell surfaces, cell lineages, and the functional significance of the surface markers.

Heteroantisera

Heteroantisera raised in rabbits, sheep, swine or goats have advantages over single monoclonal reagents for the detection of surface and cytoplasmic immunoglobulin. Heteroantisera made against T cells are the only true 'pan-T-cell' reagents, but have the drawback that they are difficult to prepare and are of low titre. Heteroantisera are used to detect the enzyme TdT (terminal deoxynucleotidyl transferase) since no monoclonal anti-TdT has so far been made.

In staining for surface membrane Ig, cells may require washing in acetate buffer, trypsinisation, or 'capping off' to delete non-specific membrane bound Ig. To avoid Fc receptor binding, heteroantisera from rabbits should always be used as $F(ab)_2$ preparations of IgG. For preference, all heteroantisera should be prepared by (1) affinity chromatography against the target antigen; (2) cross absorption against cross reactive antigen (e.g. anti-δ chain should be cross-absorbed against pooled human IgGκ and IgGλ); (3) used as $F(ab)_2$ fragments to avoid binding to Fc receptors. When using heteroantisera against heavy and light chains of immunoglobulin in tissue sections, these preparative steps are essential for the production of consistent results. A guide to the relevant techniques is given by Forni (1979). The binding of anti-heavy chain and anti-light chain antisera is usually assessed by direct staining (FITC or TRITC labelled product) in suspension, and by the PAP or sandwich technique in tissue sections (direct sandwich, e.g. rabbit $F(ab)_2$-anti-μ detected with goat anti-rabbit $F(ab)_2$-HRP labelled; PAP technique: rabbit $F(ab)_2$-anti-μ + swine anti-rabbit-IgG + rabbit anti-horseradish-peroxidase-HRP complex (PAP)).

Monoclonal antibodies are rarely available as directly labelled reagents. Most are IgG antibodies from mice, but a few are IgM in class. A guide to those monoclonal antibodies in current use together with their specificities is given in Table 4.1. The systems for detecting monoclonal antibody binding in cell suspension studies or in tissue sections are briefly as follows.

1. *Sandwich technique* using fluorescein or rhodamine labelled goat anti-mouse Ig. The goat anti-mouse Ig must be prepared by affinity chromatography on mouse (or rat) Ig CNBr Sepharose, and must be cross-absorbed against pooled human IgG and IgM (otherwise significant cross reactivity with human Ig is generally observed). If double staining techniques are to be used, the goat anti-mouse Ig may also need to be absorbed against the other antibody (e.g. with rabbit immunoglobulin).

2. The use of biotinylated monoclonal antibody with fluorochrome or enzyme labelled avidin (the *avidin/biotin system*). Avidin is an egg white protein with high affinity for the vitamin biotin. Biotin is readily coupled to antibody, the binding of which can then be detected using labelled avidin. Since neither avidin nor biotin has spontaneous binding specificity for cells, or immunoglobulins, the problems of using a second, potentially cross-reactive, antibody are avoided, allowing double staining to be more easily carried out. Several variants of the avidin/biotin system have been developed, including one (ABC system) using biotinylated goat-anti-mouse-Ig which can be used on frozen sections (Hsu et al, 1981). Use of a biotinylated primary monoclonal antibody is somewhat restrictive: if a goat anti-mouse reagent itself is coupled to biotin, and the tracer enzyme (horseradish peroxidase or alkaline phosphatase) likewise is biotinylated, the linking avidin then produces specific coupling between antibody binding sites and the enzyme.

3. The use of *arsenilated primary antibody* and rabbit anti-ARS antibody. ARS (arsenilate) is a haptene easily coupled to a wide range of proteins. Antibodies reactive with ARS are specific and easy to produce. The anti-ARS antibody is devoid of reactivity to mouse Ig, and the system can therefore be used to study double marking, when one monoclonal only carries the ARS haptene (Wofsy et al, 1978).

These systems have come into use for four reasons:

1. In order to economise on expensive monoclonal antibodies of varying and sometimes low affinity, some degree of amplification is needed to detect monoclonal binding.

2. Although it is relatively easy to study double staining with a direct labelled heteroantiserum together with a monoclonal antibody, obviously two monoclonal antibodies cannot be studied together using a single species second antibody. This is avoided in the ABC and arsenilate systems since the specificity of one of the reagents is not anti-mouse Ig (i.e. avidin in the ABC system, anti-ARS in the ARS system).

3. In tissue section staining where two different enzyme systems are used (e.g. horseradish peroxidase and alkaline phosphatase), the amplification for one enzyme (usually alkaline phosphatase) needs to be higher than for the other. To produce a balanced result, higher amplification using the ABC system can be obtained for the alkaline phosphatase than for the HRP using the direct sandwich technique.

4. The length of the procedure is curtailed when two indifferent systems can be used (as when anti-ARS antibody and avidin can be added in one step).

Frozen section technique

When using monoclonal antibodies on frozen sections of lymphoid tissue, the use of thin sections (4–6μ) is essential if the binding of individual cells is to be assessed. Sections are air dried and post fixed in acetone, and can be stored at −40°C for up to 3 months. After this time deterioration in some antigens is seen.

The availability of monoclonal antibodies specific for B and T cell subsets, together with increased technical flexibility conferred by the use of enzyme or biotin coupled second antibodies has had a profound impact upon the demonstration of organisation in lymphoid tissues in the normal or reactive node and in malignant lymphomas.

In cases where suspension phenotyping and frozen section histology are performed on the same material, there is a high degree of correlation between the findings. The advantage of the frozen section is that it demonstrates the anatomical distribution of subsets defined by surface phenotyping. It is inferior to surface phenotyping in demonstrating SIg in some cases, since a contribution to background staining from circulating Ig, and Ig present in tissues, cannot be avoided. Surface phenotyping has the advantage that manipulations (such as removal and regeneration of surface Ig, cell subset preparations, and tissue culture techniques) can be applied. The ideal condition is to perform suspension phenotyping *and* immunohistology on the same tissue in all cases.

The phenotype of normal lymphoid tissues

Values obtained with the different rosetting techniques vary from laboratory to laboratory, which is one of the features making the interpretation of phenotyping data difficult. Using standardised techniques, the results from any single laboratory should be reproducible. The data shown in Table 4.3 (normal blood mononuclear cells), Table 4.4 ('normal' or 'reactive' lymph nodes) and Table 4.5 (spleen) are derived from this laboratory. The type of cell expressing each 'receptor' is given alongside the data for blood (Table 4.3). In our laboratory, the routine mononuclear cell recovery following density gradient separation of blood, or spleen cell suspension, is of the order of 60% of the total starting number of mononuclear cells. This implies that a variable proportion of mononuclear cells of unknown phenotype is lost during separation procedures. Experiments with tonsil cell suspensions have shown that plasma cells are preferentially lost when the cell suspension is spun on a ficoll/triosil density gradient. When phenotyping lymph nodes, the use of preliminary gradient separations is to be avoided.

The values given for normal tissues vary widely. For example, the B cell population in man shows

Table 4.3 Phenotype of normal blood: percentage distribution of cells by phenotypic criteria

Cell type	Mean % ± S.D.	Range
T cells		
E rosettes	57±4.3	(33–82)
αLeu 1/OKT1	51±4.0	(36–61)
OKT3/UCHT1	62±4.0	(41–77)
OKT4/αLeu3a	43±2.0	(28–58)
OKT8/αLeu2a	21±2.0	(9–33)
Ratio T_H/T_S	2.0	
B cells		
SIg+ cells	11±2.1	(6–33)
HLA DR+	17±1.0	(13–22)
Other markers		
C3d	11±1.2	(4–23)
C3b	17±5.0	(1–43)
Fcγ	28	(8–40)
Fcμ	14–	(<1–29)
Functional phagocytes	14–	(5–27)
Cytoplasmic Ig+ cells		
IgM	3.2±1.4	
IgG	0.6±0.4	
IgA	0.8±0.6	

Table 4.4 Phenotype of three sets of 'normal' lymph node cell suspensions: percentage distribution of cells by phenotypic criteria

	% Mean value of 10 samples	±S.D.	Range	% Mean value of 12 samples	Range	% Mean value of 17 samples	Range
E rosettes	42	±2	(36–55)	42	(18–56)	40	(9–57)
αLeula/OKT1	59	±6	(41–69)	—	—	—	—
OKT3/UCHT1	58	±5	(38–71)	—	—	—	—
OKT4/αLeu3a	31	±7	(12–54)	—	—	—	—
OKT8/αLeu2a	18	±3	(9–30)	—	—	—	—
Ratio T_H/T_S	2.1		(0.9–4.2)				
SIg+ cells	35	±5	(18–76)	33	(15–57)	31	(17–53)
HLA-DR positive	31	±5	(18–51)	—	—	—	—
C3d rosetting	32	±5	(6–60)	24	(2–40)	27	(4–52)
C3b rosetting	11	±3	(1–20)	—	—	—	—
Fcγ rosettes	15	±6	(2–28)	15	(5–40)	15	(8–38)
Functional phagocytes (N Red test)	8	±6	(1–18)	10	(3–27)	8	(2–27)
Fcμ	—	—	—	2	(<1–6)	—	—
Peanut agglutinin	18	±3	(5–36)	—	—	—	—
Cytoplasmic Ig+ plasma cells	—	—	(2–11)	—	—	—	—
'Null' cells	—	—	(5–35)	—	—	—	—

Table 4.5 Phenotype of 'normal' spleen cell suspension: percentage distribution of cells by phenotypic criteria

	Mean value %	Range	No. of determinations
E rosettes	51	(25–63)	(9 samples)
OKT1/αLeula	31	(26–37)	(4 samples)
OKT3/UCHT1	46	(43–49)	(4 samples)
OKT4/αLeu3a	28	(24–35)	(5 samples)
OKT8/αLeu2a	21	(18–27)	(5 samples)
Ratio T_H/T_S	1.1		
SIg+ cells	30	(11–43)	(9 samples)
HLA DR positive	30	(26–36)	(5 samples)
C3b rosetting	31	(17–46)	(9 samples)
C3d rosetting	14	(7–26)	(4 samples)
Fcγ rosetting	26	(18–37)	(9 samples)
Fcμ rosetting	7	(<1–17)	(5 samples)
Phagocytes (NR test)	11	(9–26)	(9 samples)

an average κ to λ ratio of 2.4 : 1. In any given sample, the exact ratio varies over a range from 5 : 1 to 1 : 2.5. This is of significance when attempting to establish objective criteria for light chain restriction (monoclonality) in pathological samples. Those in which the κ to λ ratio is $>10 : 1$, or in which the λ to κ ratio is $>5 : 1$ are found to show histological evidence of malignant lymphoma in virtually all cases.

The phenotype of lymphoid cell subsets in malignant lymphoma of non-Hodgkin's type (NHL)

A guide to the phenotypes of normally present classes of B, T and other types of lymphoid cell is given in Table 4.6. The corresponding NHL classes in which these phenotypes are found are also shown. These tables are a summary of the data and do not indicate the accompanying cell populations (such as the T-cells in B-cell lymphomas, or B-cells which may accompany T-cell lymphomas) (Habeshaw et al, 1979, 1983). In Table 4.7, the phenotype of the accompanying cell populations which occur with the neoplastic population are shown.

It must be stressed that a given population of cells from a lymphoma may be homogeneous in respect of a lineage marker (e.g. B cell, or T cell), but within that group of cells occur subpopulations which can vary in respect of subclass specific markers. Thus 80% of lymph node cells may be IgM κ surface Ig positive, but only 20% express Fc or C3d receptors, 50% may react with Ba1 and 10% express cytoplasmic Ig. Similarly in frozen section immunoperoxidase reactions, the distribution of a marker like anti-HLA DR can show some areas strongly positive, while other areas of apparently identical cells are weakly positive or negative. So lymphomas composed principally of a single subset of B- or T-cells show phenotypic variants of the predominant clone occurring within the lymphoma.

It is particularly apparent that certain classes of lymphoma (especially those of the follicular group, and the immunoblastic lymphomas) are infre-

Table 4.6 Phenotypes of normal lymphoid cells at different stages of differentiation and the histological class of malignancy associated with them

Cell class	Phenotype	Type of malignancy
T cells		
'Pre T cell' (Bone marrow derived prethymic T cell).	HLA DR+ (Ia+) TdT+ OKT10+ Leu1+ OKT9+ (Markers in this group may not be present on all cells)	C-ALLA negative ALL. Rarely lymphoblastic lymphoma, with mediastinal mass.
Thymic cortical T lymphocytes (these can be classed as early (TdT+, OKT10+, Leu1+, PNA+, HLA ABC−) Intermediate (TdT+, Leu1+, OKT6+, PNA±), or Late (TdT+ OKT6+, OKT11+, E rosette+, OKT3, T4, T8+ variable))	TdT+ OKT6+ Leu1+ E rosette + OKT11+ Usually OKT10+ OKT9 >5% PNA± HLA ABC± HLA DR− Acid phosphatase+ OKT3± OKT4 (−) or (+) or (+) or (−) OKT8 (−) or (−) or (+) or (+)	T lymphoblastic lymphoma/leukaemia. (Note: these tumours contain mixtures of cells of thymic cortical phenotypes. Thus OKT6 may mark only a minority of cells which are Leu1+ or OKT11+. In 'later' tumours fewer PNA+ cells occur, and there may be expression of OKT3, T4 and/or T8. In some lymphomas a population of C-ALLA+ cells occurs).
Peripheral T cells:		
T_H Subset: Normally present in blood, nodes and spleen in T areas. A subpopulation is associated with germinal centres. Predominant interfollicular (paracortical) population.	Leu1+, OKT3+, OKT4+ Usually E+, OKT11+ TdT− HLA DR+ if 'transformed' OKT9+ in proportion to growth rate.	Most cases of cutaneous T cell lymphoma, T zone lymphoma, T lymphomas of Japanese or Caribbean type. Visceral T cell lymphomas. (HLA DR may be positive on T lymphomas of 'Immunoblastic' type.)
T_S Subset: Normally the minor population in blood and node. In spleen roughly equal proportions of T_H and T_S subset. Normally restricted to interfollicular and paracortical area (node).	Leu1+ OKT3+ E rosette+ OKT11+ OKT8+ TdT−	Various T cell leukaemias (T CLL, T PLL and occasional T cell lymphomas have been described. In AILD T suppressor cells are frequently the dominant T cell population.
'Neutral' T cell. Cells of T lineage which do not express T4 or T8 subset markers. Found as a normal population in spleen and blood and as a minor population in lymph nodes.	Leu1+ OKT3+ E Rosette+ OKT11+ OKT4− OKT8−	Some cases of adult T cell lymphoma, of T zone type. (Phenotypes Leu1+ OKT3+, E rosette− or Leu1+ E rosette+ OKT3−).
Double marked T cell. This population normally present only in thymic medulla. Small numbers of normal double marked cells may be present in nodes or spleen.	Leu1+ OKT3+ E rosette+ TdT− OKT4+ OKT8+	Cases of T-cell leukaemia of TdT negative type (T-PLL) described. Some cases of T immunoblastic lymphoma.

Table 4.6 (*contd*)

Cell class	Phenotype	Type of malignancy
B cells		
Pre-B cell. Normally present in bone marrow only.	TdT+ C-ALLA+ B1± Ba1± Cyμ chain+ HLA DR+ PI 153/3+ OKT10±	Pre-B ALL: variant of common ALL with cytoplasmic μ heavy chain. Lymphoblastic lymphomas with this phenotype are cytologically common ALL. (FAB-LI type)
'Early' B cell, showing some affinities with pre-B cells, but different morphology (FAB L-3)	Surface IgM+ B1+ C-ALLA± TdT− HLA DR+ PNA± No expression of Fcγ or C3d/C3b receptor	Most cases of childhood lymphoblastic lymphoma of B cell type. (B lymphoblastic lymphomas can be C-ALLA+ with surface Ig. Some show cytoplasmic Ig staining. Never TdT positive).
Germinal centre 'centrocyte' class is restricted to germinal centres: precursor is unknown.	Surface IgM+ (May express other single Hc classes) Ba2+ OKT10+ PNA+ (in g.c.) C-ALLA± B1+ C3d receptor±	In one form of centroblastic and centrocytic follicular lymphoma may be the predominant cell type: is then C-ALLA positive. Some centroblastic lymphomas with similar phenotype but usually PNA−, are C-ALLA negative. Cytoplasmic Ig is usually negative.
B cell of the mantle zone. Restricted in distribution to the lymphocyte corona around germinal centres, and inner B cell areas of the spleen.	Surface IgM+ and IgD+ B1+ Ba1+ B2+ RFA-2+ PNA C-ALLA− C3b, C3d± HLA DR++	Cells of similar phenotype occur in centrocytic lymphoma (where IgD expression may be lost). A cellular component of most cases of centroblastic and centrocytic follicular lymphoma. Cytoplasmic Ig always negative.
CLL B cell. This B cell subset is normally present in cord blood, fewer in adult blood or node. Present in spleen and possibly marrow.	Surface Ig weak Usually M+ or M+D (can be other Hc) Mouse RBC+ Fcγ+ Fcμ± OKT1/Leu1+ HLA DR+ Ba1± B1± (weak) PNA− C3d±	The cell of CLL/MLL. (Phenotypically distinct from the coronal B lymphocyte). Has a null cell component (HLA DR+ SIg−). Related to (but distinct from) myeloma, lymphoplasmacytoid lymphoma, and the 'hairy cell' (about half are FMC7 positive).
'Lymphoplasmacytoid' cell. Small non-cleaved cell with some features of plasmacytoid differentiation. Medullary cords and interfollicular areas of node.	Single Hc isotype M, or G, or A. Cytoplasmic Ig present. Strong surface Ig staining. B1+ B2± Ba1± HLA DR++/± PNA+ C3b/C3d± Fcγ± MRBC+ (some cases)	Lymphoplasmacytoid lymphoma. (These lesions contain variable numbers of SIg% and cytoplasmic Ig positive cells, in addition to true plasma cells) HLA DR expression is variable. Circulating cells frequently present. Related to CLL/MLL

Table 4.6 (*contd*)

Cell class	Phenotype	Type of malignancy
Immunoblast of B cell type. The term immunoblast embraces transformed B cells of most of the above categories (except centrocytes which do not appear to transform). The phenotype is variable. Most are identifiable as plasma cell precursors.	Plasma cell precursor variant. Strong, non-capping SIg, single Hc isotype plus cytoplasmic Ig. B1+/weak B2− Bal± HLA DR weak OKT9 usually >5% PNA±	Cell of B immunoblastic lymphoma. (The most common B phenotype associated with T cell predominance in a transformed progression of centroblastic and centrocytic lymphoma. Rarely, B cells in such cases can show presence of OKT3 with surface and/or cytoplasmic Ig.)
	Other types can be HLA DR−/SIg− CyIg+ (Plasmablasts) or	Plasmablastic variant of immunoblastic lymphoma.
	Leu1/OKT1/RFA1+ B1− RFA 2+ C3d+ PNA−	Phenotype of immunoblastic transformation of CLL (Richter's Syndrome).
Plasma cell	Surface Ig− Cytoplasmic Ig++ HLA DR− B1/B2/Bal− PNA+ OKT10+	Plasmacytoma. (Plasma cells of myeloma are of different phenotype and associated with a 'null' cell component. Most B markers −; PNA and OKT10 usually +).
Hairy cell of leukaemic reticuloendotheliosis	Single Hc isotype SIg+ Fcγ+, Fcμ+ C3b+, C3d+ MRBC± FMC 7+ B1+ PI 153/3+	Phenotype bears some relationship to CLL, the diseases are related and probably of B type. The relationship of HCL to other classes of lymphoma not known.

Table 4.7 Types of malignant lymphoma and the accompanying cell populations

Histological class	Primary (predominant or objectively abnormal component	Accompanying cell types
B cell lymphomas		
Centroblastic centrocytic follicular	B cell of follicular centre. Monoclonal SIg. Usually single H chain isotype. Usually IgM. Sometimes multiple H chain isotypes. Occasionally Leu-1+ SIg+ phenotype predominates.	T cells. Levels vary from 10–60%. Usually normal T_H:T_S ratio. Occasionlly T_S predominant. B cells of lymphocyte corona (if present) polyclonal, express M+D. Frequently 5–10% of total B cells.
Centroblastic lymphoma	B cell. Monoclonal SIg. Single H chain isotype. Usually IgM.	60% of cases show >50% T cells with normal T_H:T_S ratio. T cells may be HLA DR+ and transformed. Occasional cases have minor population of plasma cells.
Centrocytic lymphoma	B cell. Monoclonal SIg. Single H chain isotype. Usually IgM with λ light chain.	Low levels of T cells in all cases studied (<10%)

Table 4.7 (*contd*)

Histological class	Primary (predominant or objectively abnormal component	Accompanying cell types
Lymphocytic lymphoma	B cell. Weak SIg (IgM or IgM+D). Occasionally other multiple H chain isotypes. Monoclonal with strong $\varkappa$ predominance.	Significant 'null' populations of Leu1+ HLA DR+ phenotype. T cell levels very variable but usually low.
Immunoblastic lymphoma (B cell type)	B cell of one of three main subtypes: 1. Non capping. SIg+, single H chain isotype (M or G or A). Sometimes mixed H chain class. Cytoplasmic Ig present in <10% of cells.	T cells: about 50% cases are T predominant. Both T_H and T_S present. T_H often more predominant. Macrophages (histiocytic) component can be present occasionally up to 20%.
	2. Plasmacytoid form. Most cells SIg negative. Cytoplasmic Ig positive (sometimes only L chain or H chain present). Only 1 class of H chain. HLA DR: low or negative. PNA+.	T cells 20–40%. T_H and T_S both present. Sometimes 'neutral' T cell (T4, T8 negative). 'Null' population, not objectively plasma cell (CyIg−) can be a major component.
	3. Leu1+SIg+phenotype. HLA DR+. Surface Ig strong, non capping. Usually single, occasionally multiple H chain isotype. Cytoplasmic Ig not present. Clonality difficult to establish. PNA−	T cell levels generally low (10–15%). Null populations occur, expressing HLA DR (SIg− HLA DR+).
B lymphoblastic lymphoma	SIg+ single H chain usually M. Monoclonal. Some express CyIgM as well. Some cases PNA+. Fcγ, Fcμ, C3d not expressed.	C-ALLA+ Ia+ population may be present. Small numbers of C-Alla+ Cyμ+ cells also found. T cells insignificant.
Lymphoplasmacytoid lymphoma	Single H chain isotype. Monoclonal SIg+ populations. May be Fcγ+ C3d+. Strong SIg expression.	T cells low in all cases studied (10%). Both classes T_HT_S present. Plasma cell derivatives of the objectively neoplastic clone also present but very variable in number.
T cell lymphomas		
Cutaneous T cell lymphoma T zone lymphoma	Commonest phenotype is of OKT1, OKT3, OKT4 positive T cells (T_H subset) SER±.	Plasma cells of polyclonal type (CyIgK and CyIgL).
Epidermotrophic or visceral T cell lymphomas of high grade histology	Other phenotype seen less commonly is the 'neutral' T cell (OKT1+ OKT3+ OKT4− OKT8−). E rosette±.	SIg B cells polyclonal type.
Lymphoepithelioid lymphoma (Lennert's lymphoma)	In 2 cases seen the predominant phenotype was 1. neutral T cell type 2. T suppressor (OKT3+ OKT8+)	A small number of T_S cells usually persent as 'contaminants'. T_H:T_S ratios in T_H lymphomas should exceed 10. In 'neutral' T cell phenotypes, the T_H:T_S ratio is not relevant.
T lymphoblastic lymphoma	Cortical thymocyte phenotype TdT+ OKT6+ Leu1/OKT1+. May be PNA+ OKT10+ OKT11± OKT4+ and/or OKT8+. May be HLA− ABC negative. HLA DR always negative.	In a third of cases a C-ALLA+ population is present (J5+ HLA DR+). Occasionally C-ALLA+ and OKT6+ overlap is seen. The major population may be 'null' with a minor OKT6+ OKT1/Leu1+ population. PNA positivity appears reciprocally related to HLA ABC expression.

quently composed of a 'pure' neoplastic clone. High levels of accompanying T-cells are a constant feature of B-cell lymphomas showing follicular (nodular) organisation. All such tumours also contain dendritic reticulum cells, visible in appropriately stained frozen section preparations. The diffuse forms of B-cell lymphoma (with the exception of some centroblastic and some immunoblastic lymphomas) are less frequently associated with significant T-cell populations. Progression in follicular lymphoma from the follicular to the diffuse phase is accompanied by decreasing levels of T-cells within the tumour, and increasing dominance of the light chain class restricted B-cell clone. Transformation from a centrocyte predominant centroblastic-centrocytic lymphoma, into an immunoblastic or centroblastic lymphoma is accompanied by an initial increase (often to predominance) of T lymphocytes, later followed by expansion and blast transformation of the dominant B-cell clone. These examples show that even within a malignant condition, characterised by the presence of an objectively neoplastic, single clonal element, other functionally related cells are an integral part of the neoplastic process. During transformation, the B-cell clone itself can undergo phenotypic changes and this indicates (e.g. in immunoblastic transformation) a shift to the functional end cell (immunoblast-plasmablast). The 'maturation block' within lymphomas is not absolute: in most instances at least a proportion of the malignant clone has the capacity for further differentiation, as seen for example in ALL (Cossman et al, 1982).

B-cells can express multiple heavy chain isotypes on the cell surface, associated with a single light chain class. When a B-cell becomes committed to terminal differentiation, a single class of heavy chain (HC) only is expressed. In serial biopsies from NHL patients (usually with centroblastic-centrocytic follicular lymphoma) immunoglobulin heavy chain class switching is observed. Multiple HC isotype expressing cells become committed to single heavy chain isotype expression in a manner which can be predicted from the known sequence of heavy chain expression in ontogeny. Although the details of this complex process are beyond the scope of this chapter, there is (a) experimental evidence that T-cells influence the switch (Kawanishi et al, 1983) and (b) in serial biopsies, HC isotype switching is seen during phases of T-cell predominance which precede or accompany blast cell transformation.

Therefore, we must conclude that at least a proportion of non-Hodgkin's lymphomas represent a progressive proliferation of mutually dependent cells of different lineages, in which only one component (the B-cell) is classified (or classifiable) as objectively neoplastic. These conditions do not conform to the idealised concept of a neoplasm as a single clone of functionally abnormal cells which show progressive and uncoordinated growth (Habeshaw et al, 1979).

The immunohistology of normal lymph nodes and malignant lymphomas in frozen section

B-cells in normal nodes occupy areas of the cortex (primary follicles, or secondary follicles with germinal centres) and the medullary cords. Scattered amongst the T-cells of the paracortical area, and in the interfollicular areas are found a B-cell subpopulation, and the major areas of localisation of plasma cells. The germinal centre itself shows the presence of IgM positive B-cells in the pale staining segment subjacent to the lymphocyte corona. The basal or dark segment of the germinal centre shows weaker staining SIgM+ cells; isolated strongly staining SIg+ B-cells do occur in this location. Staining for IgG and IgA shows these two SIg bearing classes to be localised to the pale segment of the germinal centre. Cells of the lymphocyte corona react with IgM and IgD antisera, and IgD staining occurs on very few germinal centre cells. The interfollicular B-cells are IgM, IgG or IgA positive; in our experience IgA positive B-cells are frequently localised around small vessels.

The OKT4 T-cell subset is found predominantly in the paracortical area, and is also localised in a narrow band 1–2 cells deep between the germinal centre and the corona. Where the lymphocyte corona is absent, this T_H subset infiltrate is not seen. In some examples, quite extensive areas of the lymphocyte corona can be replaced by T_H subset lymphocytes. These areas fail to stain with anti-IgD antiserum giving a 'gaptoothed' appearance to the corona. In especially large germinal centres, islands or inclusions of small lymphocytes can occur. Immunohistochemistry shows these to be occupied largely by IgM+ IgD+ mantle B-lymphocytes, with associated T-cells, usually of T_H subset.

Plasma cells, recognised by cytoplasmic Ig staining, have a markedly eccentric distribution within the germinal centre, being limited to the pale staining area. The numbers are very variable.

The dendritic reticulum of normal nodes or tonsil is distributed throughout the germinal centre: it appears more frequently 'condensed' towards the pale zone. Antisera against Ig of all subclasses (except IgD and IgE) will react more or less strongly with this dendritic component, as will monoclonal antibodies specific for dendritic reticulum cells.

Peanut agglutinin (PNA) staining, particularly in weakly stained specimens, shows a very similar distribution to that of plasma cells (which are PNA positive) and to centrocytes. In more heavily stained specimens, the whole germinal centre, including the dendritic reticulum, appears to stain, although close examination shows individual positive and negative B-cells within the centre.

Tingible body macrophages, particularly in highly active germinal centres, sometimes show strong cytoplasmic staining with OKT4, but this is a variable feature.

Monoclonal anti-HLA DR reagents stain virtually all follicular cells, but the staining of the germinal centre proper is noticeably weaker than staining of the lymphocyte corona. The monoclonal antibody OKT9 shows staining largely restricted to the germinal centre. The monoclonal antibody J5 (C-ALLA) stains the normal germinal centre weakly, if at all. This staining appears as non-specific 'background' staining of the reticulum with rather weak specific membrane staining of a few individual cells. The differential staining of the follicle (germinal centre and corona) with monoclonal anti-B-cell antibodies reveals clear distributional differences between the germinal centre B-cells, and those of the lymphocyte corona (Table 4.8). These data show that the normal germinal centre, and its lymphocyte corona, are composed of phenotypically heterogeneous B-cells.

In the spleen, the B-cell area surrounds, and is often eccentric to, the periarteriolar lymphocytic sheath (PALS) which is the main T-cell area. B cells in spleen are mainly present in an outer marginal zone of the white pulp, subjacent to the marginal sinus, and represent a specific B-cell sub-population which also occurs in the outer mantle zone of the germinal centre and the interfollicular areas of lymph nodes. Internal to this zone occurs an indistinct accumulation of B-cells which express IgM and IgD. B-cells of both zones are B1+ and Ba1+, but clearly differ in their heavy chain isotype expression. When germinal centres are present, they appear to develop within the area occupied by IgM+D lymphocytes, and hence acquire a corona of IgM+ and IgD+ lymphocytes, as occurs with lymph node germinal centres. Dendritic reticulum cells occur in these centres (or pre-existing DRC proliferate in these sites). In the absence of germinal centres in spleen, the splenic B cell sub-populations are PNA negative.

The predominant B-cell population in a reactive lymph node therefore depends upon which subset of B-cells (e.g. germinal centre or corona), is present in greatest proportion. In suspension, the phenotype obtained from a lymphomatous lymph node will also depend upon the degree of similarity between the lymphoma B-cell population and

Table 4.8 B cell specific markers distinguishing germinal centre from mantle zone B cell subsets (data from Lesley Murray, by kind permission)

Monoclonal antibody	Germinal centre		Lymphocyte corona
	Centroblasts	Centrocytes	MZ cells
B1	+	++	+/−
HLA DR	+	+	++
RFA-2*	−	−*	++
OKT10	+	+	−
Ba1	−	+	++
Ba2	++	+	−
J5	+	±	−
B2	+	+	+/−(weak)
OKT9	±	+/−	−
PNA	+	+	−
F8, 11, 13	+/−	++	++
IgM	−	+	++
IgD	−	−	++/−
IgD		−	−
FMC 7			

RFA-2* reacts with T cells in addition to B cells. In GC, RFA-2+ cells are probably T cells.
+/− = positive or negative
± = weak staining
\+ = positive
++ = strong positive
− = negative

some normal B-cell subset, and the extent to which the malignant condition reflects the normal organisation and arrangement of the node. The suspension phenotype of the involved node in centroblastic-centrocytic follicular lymphoma is frequently indistinguishable from the profile of a reactive lymph node, and in Hodgkin's disease the presence of T-lymphocyte predominance is frequently the only clue to the nature of the underlying process, even when the histological appearances are unequivocal.

In the following pages individual cases of suspension/section phenotyping are shown. These have been selected as fairly typical examples of the class of disease portrayed, but there is no 'right' phenotypic profile for each histological class of lymphoma. In most of the presented cases, the histological diagnosis was also typical of the class of lymphoma.

CASE 1

P.J. Male aged 48. Inguinal lymphadenopathy with hepatosplenomegaly; no involvement of skin. Histology 'diffuse lymphoma of uniform, medium sized angular cells'. This was originally interpreted as a centrocytic lymphoma, but the suspension phenotype clearly indicated the erroneous nature of this diagnosis.

Phenotype

T cells		*B cells*	*Other markers*	
OKT3	93%	B subset markers all negative	Phagocytes	2%
OKT1/Leu 1	90%		HLA DR	4%
OKT4	94%			
OKT8	1%	SIg positive cells <1%	2 DI positive	all cells
E rosettes/OKT11	8%	C-ALLA negative		
OKT6 negative				
TdT negative				

The phenotypic features are quite clear cut. They indicate a mature T-helper subset phenotype, (Leu1+, OKT3+, OKT4+, OKT8−) which is E rosette negative. The absence of OKT6 positivity and terminal deoxynucleotidyl transferase reactivity excludes an intrathymic origin for the lymphoma cells. In lesions of this type it is surprising how few 'contaminating' other cell types there are, even in a node biopsy. This is in marked contrast to the complex mixed phenotypes of T-cell predominant follicular or immunoblastic lesions.

Final diagnosis: Peripheral T-cell lymphoma of medium-sized cells and T-helper subset. (The clinical course was that of an aggressive T-cell lymphoma.)

CASE 2

G.M. Male aged 71. Biopsy of node on chest wall. Hepatosplenomegaly. Histology: malignant lymphoma, centrocytic, small cell type. (Phenotype consistent.)

Phenotype

T cells		*B cells*		*Other markers*	
Leu1	13%	B1	35%	OKT9	>1%
OKT3	>1%	Ba1	58%	OKT10	9%
OKT4	>1%	Ba2	Nil	HLA DR	59%
OKT6	Nil	33.1	45%	OKM1	6%
OKT8	1%	FMC7	Nil	PNA	Nil
OKT11	1%	J5	Nil		
Leu 7	1%	SIgM	77%		
		K chain	66%		
		L chain	5%		
		SIgD	26%		

The node suspension is B cell predominant, with monoclonal SIgMκ, and SIgM+Dκ B-cell populations. A small population is Leu 1 positive, and overlapping with SIg expression. The expression of Ba1, without Ba2, characterises a B-cell of coronal rather than GC type. The lack of J5 expression suggests a 'late' or 'mature' peripheral B cell type. Not CLL-like (lacks FMC 7) although the weak expression of HLA DR, 33.1, and OKT1/Leu 1 is a feature shared by some CLL. Cytoplasmic Ig was not a feature, though a few plasma cells were present.

CASE 3

F.H. Male aged 3 years 6 months. Abdominal mass: mesenteric node biopsy, ileum involved with lymphoma. Histology: B lymphoblastic lymphoma of Burkitt type.

Phenotype

T cells		*B cells*		*Other markers*	
OKT3	6%	B1	64%	2DI	All cells
OKT4	3%	Ba1	94%	W6/32	All cells
OKT8	3%	Ba2	88%	OKT10	90%
OKT6	Nil	PI/153/3	44%	OKMI	2%
OKT11	6%	J5	7%	MO2	4%
		SIgM	94%	PNA	1%
		λ chain	93%		

The node profile is B-cell predominant, with few T cells, and none showing OKT6 expression. B cell component is monoclonal (for IgMλ) OKT10, Ba1, Ba2, B1 and PI/153/3 positive indicating an 'early' B-cell phenotype. Other features which can be positive in this type of lesion are J5 (C-ALLA) and PNA. Some cases are also CyIgM positive.

CASE 4

E.B. Female aged 56. Histology: centroblastic-centrocytic follicular lymphoma. (Repeat biopsy: stable histology and phenotype 6 years.)

Phenotype

T cells		*B cells*		*Other markers*	
OKT1/ Leu1	21%	SIgM	63%	HLA DR	56%
OKT3	21%	SIgD	20%	2DI	Positive
OKT4	15%	SIgA	3%	OKT9	1%
OKT8	6%	SIgϰ	62%	'C3d' rosettes	23%
E rosettes/ OKT11 KT11	9%	SIgλ	13%		
		PNA	51%	'C3b' rosettes	17%
OKT6	Nil	C-ALLA (J5)	35%		

This is a typical phenotype of the most common form of follicular lymphoma. The T-cell profile is of helper (15%) and suppressor (6%) T-cells of mature type. There are 2 B-cell components: 1) SIgM+ϰ+ follicular component expressing C-ALLA antigen, PNA and HLA DR positivity; 2) a polyclonal SIgM+D ϰ and λ component which represents the residual coronal lymphocytes. Frozen sections confirm the localisation of J5 positivity and PNA positivity to the follicular cells. B-cell subset monoclonals were not utilised in this case. B-cells expressed both C3b and C3d receptors. The only anomaly is the low level of OKT11/E rosette expression.

CASE 5

I.C. Female aged 50. In relapse. Previous biopsy with similar histology 2 years ago. Histology: high grade malignant lymphoma of polymorphic centroblastic type.

Phenotype

T cells		*B cells*		*Other markers*	
OKT I/ Leu I	49%	SIgM	9%	HLA DR	18%
OKT3	67%	SIgG	16%	OKT9	5%
OKT4	21%	SIgD	Negative	2DI	Positive
OKT8	41%	SIgϰ	16%	W6/32	Positive
E rosettes	40%	SIgλ	Negative		
		PNA	10%		

The phenotype is that of a clearly T8 predominant lesion, containing a monoclonal B-cell population marking as (SIgM+G+, SIgG+, HLA DR+ and PNA+). C-ALLA was not expressed. Only occasional plasma cells were present, all of Gϰ CyIg+ type. This phenotype of T-cell predominance with monoclonal B-cells is the most common presentation (in our experience) of centroblastic lymphoma.

CASE 6

J.M. Female aged 59. Retroperitoneal mass involving lymph nodes and pancreas. Histology: high grade malignant lymphoma of unusual type, most suggestive of immunoblastic lymphoma.

Phenotype

T cells		*B cells*		*Other markers*	
OKT1/ Leu1	85%	SIgM	45%	OKT9	6%
OKT3	64%	SIgG	2%	HLA DR	55%
OKT4	44%	SIgD	3%	MRBC rosettes	9%
OKT8	9%	SIgA	8%		
OKT6	<1%	SIgϰ	51%		
OKT11/ E rosettes	31%	SIgλ	1%		
		C-ALLA (J5)	28%		
		PNA	45%		

Phenotypes from immunoblastic lymphoma are difficult to interpret, being very variable. T-cell levels are often high (in this case 53% given by OKT4+OKT8, 64% by OKT3). There is a clear monoclonal B-cell population SIgMϰ positive, C-ALLA positive, HLA DR positive and PNA positive, similar to that seen in centroblastic-centrocytic follicular lymphoma. Leu 1 positivity must be present on some B-cells, and some B-cells are MRBC rosetting. The presence of some OKT3+ SIg+cells cannot be exluded either. The B-cell subset markers were not used in this case, but the phenotype does indicate a possible origin from pre-existing follicular lymphoma.

CASE 7

S.B. Male aged 16. Infraclavicular lymph node. Histology: T lymphoblastic lymphoma — convoluted cell type (acid phosphatase positive).

Phenotype

T cells		*B cells*		*Other markers*
OKT1/ Leu1	100%	All B cell markers negative		HLA ABC Positive
OKT3	Most cells weak positive			OKT9 10% HLA DR Negative
OKT 4	Positive	J5	Negative	
OKT8	2%	PNA	Negative	
OKT6	Positive			
E rosettes	2%			
TdT	Positive			

In this node, virtually all cells were positive for OKT1, OKT4, OKT6 and stained for TdT. No B-cells were detected by SIg staining or cytoplasmic Ig staining. The expression of OKT3 was noticeably weak, but most cells were rated positive. This is typical of only one of the many variants of phenotype in T-cell lymphoblastic lymphoma: most have in common the expression of Leu1, OKT6 and TdT positivity. Accompanying J5 positive HLA DR positive populations can occur, and HLA ABC can be negative on a substantial proportion of lymphoma cells.

These illustrative cases show that the 'mix' of cells in any single class of lymphoma is variable. Nonetheless, phenotypic studies of normal B-cells from blood, bone marrow, spleen and lymph node germinal centre and mantle zone show the existence of possibly five phenotypically distinct maturation phases or even sub-classes of B-cells. The different histological types of NHL can be composed of any single sub-class alone (as in, for example, Burkitt lymphoma), but more commonly several B-cell sub-classes of the malignant clone appear together in the lesion, with one being predominant (as in follicular lymphoma). Consequently the dominant B-cell phenotype in centroblastic-centrocytic follicular lymphoma can be of CALL+, SIgM+, PNA+ type (like Burkitt) or can be of MRBC+, weak SIgM+, Leu1+ type (like CLL) with the majority of cases showing a mixture of these B-cell phenotypes (as in the normal germinal follicle). In adults, the most common types of B-cell malignancy are centroblastic-centrocytic lymphoma, lymphocytic lymphoma (CLL) and malignancies of immunoglobulin secreting cells (lymphoplasmacytoid lymphoma/myeloma). These classes of lymphoma are virtually unknown in children, although B-cells of these types, well developed germinal centres, and mature plasma cells are normally present. Conversely, B lymphoblastic lymphoma, and the related common ALL, and pre-B ALL, are rare in adults, but are the most frequent B-cell lineage malignancies of children (Berard et al, 1981; Greaves, 1982). Since the same 'target' cell populations for neoplastic transformation exist in both children and adults the difference in presentation must be accounted for by differences in the way the adult immune system influences B-cell differentiation and function (i.e. the histological class of lymphoma is a function of the age of presentation). One obvious possibility is that the lymphomas of children might belong to a 'T independent' line of B-cell development, whilst those of adults are mainly of 'T dependent' lines of B-cell differentiation.

Although the data are inadequate, one logical view is that lymphomas are proliferations of a functional 'unit' composed of T-cells, B-cells and the relevant accessory cells, in which the controlling mechanisms have gone wrong. The resulting phenotype and histology indicate the class of defect in the patient. The monoclonality exhibited by the neoplastic B-cells is the result of the clonal selection process, and the lack of an effective immune response indicates that some error in the coordination of proliferation, cell elimination and functional differentiation has occurred. Whether this is due to some intrinsic B-cell defect, or is a consequence of 'immune system malfunction' is a topic for further investigation.

CHROMOSOMAL ABNORMALITIES AND THEIR SIGNIFICANCE IN LYMPHOMA

A detailed technical account of current cytogenetic methods, including banding nomenclature and chromosome staining, would be out of place here. This topic is adequately covered in several texts, notably in Priest (1977). As phenotyping has extended our descriptive power in relation to the types of cell encountered in NHL and in the normal node, so chromosomal analysis has enhanced our understanding between the frequently abnormal karyotypes of lymphoma cells, and their possible significance. This has been made possible by the techniques of phenotyping (applied to gene mapping in mouse/human hybrids) and more recently by the introduction of C DNA probes which allow detection of individual genes. The scope of such investigations will be broadly outlined here, in an effort to convey the real excitement and interest which accompanies the urge to explore the internal mechanisms of cell growth, differentiation, and function.

When standard cytogenetic techniques are applied to the study of lymphomas the results are disappointing for three reasons: (1) the growth fraction of low grade (the most common) lymphomas is low, yielding in primary culture only 1 in 1000 mitoses capable of being analysed; (2) the morphology and compact nature of lymphocyte chromosomes makes banding difficult, and (3) until recently it was not possible selectively to grow the B-cell (neoplastic) component in vitro, and mitogens employed (usually PHA) stimulate growth of T-rather than B-cells. Thus the range of NHL in which the karyotype could be studied was narrow, including Burkitt lymphoma, some high grade lymphomas, and T-cell lymphomas responsive to PHA. As a result, knowledge of specific (i.e. non random) chromosomal abnormalities in NHL was patchy. Recent technical advances have now established that (1) consistent karyotypic profiles can be obtained from 90% of involved lymph node biopsies, (2) node tissue must be studied as results from blood are inconsistent, (3) it is important to have adequate histological and phenotypic characterisation of the tissue studied and (4) appropriate techniques of culture should be used to enhance chromosome banding and stimulate mitosis in the neoplastic cell population.

Banding lymphocyte chromosomes effectively depends upon the technique of methotrexate synchronisation, which results in longer, less compact, chromosomal structure. Briefly, in this technique cells are first cultured, then synchronised by addition of methotrexate (17 hours) and incubated with thymidine (6 hours) before exposure to colcemid. B-cell growth may be enhanced by the use of T-cell conditioned medium (PHA-TCM, PHA-TCM-TPA), and it is now possible to use T-cell depleted cultures of B-cells for karyotyping.

Non-random chromosome changes in NHL occur in a consistent fashion in lymphomas of one phenotypic/histological class. These involve chromosome 14 in Burkitt lymphoma and some lesions of non-Burkitt type (Fokuhara & Rowley, 1978), where translocations occur between chromosomes 8 and 14 ($8q-/14q+$) (Manolov & Manolova, 1972). Similar abnormalities involving the long arm of chromosome 14 occur in ataxia telangiectasia, and sometimes in normal blood lymphocytes (McCaw et al, 1975). Less frequently, translocations between chromosomes 8 and 2 ($8q^+/2p^-$) and 8 and 22 ($8q^+/22p^-$) are observed. In lymphomas of follicular type, the most common abnormality is translocation between chromosome 18 and 14 (T 14: 18, q32.3: q21.3) (Yunis et al, 1982). In malignant lymphoma, lymphocytic (CLL) the principal abnormality is trisomy of chromosome 12 (Yunis et al, 1982; Gharton et al, 1980) with translocations between 11 and 14 (T11: 14, q13: q32) also occurring. Trisomy, or polyploidy of chromosome 12 also occurs in follicular lymphoma, and has been shown in Sternberg-Reed cell lines (Diehl et al, 1981).

The significance of non-random chromosomal abnormalities is difficult to assess. Before the advent of gene mapping by somatic cell hybridisation or other means, the connection between a certain break point on a chromosome, and some relevant cell functions, could not be made. It has now been established that abnormalities involving chromosomes 14, 2 and 22 are connected to the state of immunoglobulin synthesis in Burkitt lymphoma cell lines. Chromosome 14 carries the heavy chain genes, chromosome 2 the kappa chain genes, and chromosome 22 the lambda chain genes. The band 14q32 localises the heavy chain gene cluster (Kirsch et al, 1982). The translocations associated with B lymphoma cells, therefore, commonly (in Burkitt lymphoma, invariably) involve chromosomes, and break points associated with at least one of the chromosomes carrying immunoglobulin genes (Erikson et al, 1982).

It was suggested and confirmed that the karyotypic abnormalities in Burkitt cell lines ($8q_{-}/14q^{+}$, $8q^{+}/2p^{-}$,$8q^{+}/22p^{-}$) correlated with the expression of the appropriate $\varkappa$ ($2p^{-}$) or λ ($22p^{-}$) light chain surface Ig by the tumour cells (Lenoir et al, 1982). Evidence is accumulating that heavy chain genes involved in the 8: 14 translocation are functionally abnormal (McIntosh et al, 1983), suggesting that the translocation involves the heavy chain gene site.

Less is known in detail of chromosome 12, or the significance of abnormalities of this chromosome in NHL. At least one known B cell differentiation antigen and the gene for interferon (IFN) map to this chromosome (Naylor et al, 1983).

Karyotypic abnormalities, therefore, in human lymphoma certainly relate to the normal functional attributes of the cells involved. However, these karyotypic anomalies may have further significance. The hypothesis proposing primary (genetic) causation of cancer proposes that significant disturbances in the arrangement of genetic material within cells are the initiating cause of neoplastic transformation in cells. The strongest candidate for the initiation of transformation is the oncogene. The chromosomal locations for several oncogenes in man have been established; they are: C-myc (chromosome 8q24), C-sis (chromosome 22q), C-abl (chromosome 9q34), V-fes (V-fps) (chromosome 15). Klein (1982) has proposed that in Burkitt's lymphoma the oncogene (C-myc) on chromosome 8 becomes translated to the heavy chain gene region of chromosome 14, or the light chain regions of chromosomes 22 or 2, and thereby becomes 'activated' in a way that induces neoplastic transformation and growth. Many questions, of course, remain to be answered, not least the function of the oncogenes normally present in the DNA of all eukaryotic cells.

'Untying the string' of the lymph node is no more than the first stage in the unravelling of those messages in the long strands of DNA, which some believe will hold the key to understanding cancer. There is a more important message conveyed in the chapters of this book: new ways of looking at old problems invariably mean evolving new patterns of thought, in which the older conventional frontiers need to be redrawn. Thoughts about lymphoid malignancy are slowly moving away from the malignant cell concept to address the more significant question of what constitutes malignant behaviour of cells in their host, the cancer patient. The varying appearances of lymphoma in a lymph node section are something to be explained, not debated about. Morphology is far from trivial, but can appear so to the scientist who needs to believe that neoplastic transformation is the only concept required to explain cancer. The pathologist might regard the scientific approach as trivial, since he, not science, is the judge of what is or is not a cancer in the patient. Perhaps it is just that neither attitude will long survive untouched in the new world which these specialised techniques are now allowing us to explore.

REFERENCES

Abramson C S, Kersey J H, LeBien T W 1981 A monoclonal antibody (BA1) primarily reactive with cells of human B lymphocyte lineage. Journal of Immunology 126: 83–88

Bentwich Z, Douglas S D, Skutelsky E, Kunkel H 1973 Sheep red blood cells binding to human lymphocytes treated with neuraminidase: enhancement of T cell binding and identification of a subpopulation of B cells. Journal of Experimental Medicine 137: 1532–1537

Berard C W, Greene M H, Jaffe E, Magrath I, Zeigler J 1981 A multidisciplinary approach to non-Hodgkin's lymphomas (NIH Conference) Annals of Internal Medicine 94: 218–235

Berard J, Reinherz E L, Kung P C, Goldstein G, Schlossman S F 1980 A monoclonal antibody reactive with human peripheral blood monocytes. Journal of Immunology 124:1943

Beverly P, Lynch D, Delia D 1980 Isolation of human haematopoetic progenitor cells using monoclonal antibodies. Nature 287:332

Bianco C, Nussenzweig V 1977 Complement receptors. Contemporary Topics in Molecular immunology 6: 145–176

Brain P J, Gordon J, Willets 1970 Rosette formation by peripheral blood lymphocytes. Clinical and Experimental Immunology 6: 681–688

Brodsky F M, Parnham P, Barnstable C J, Crumpton M J, Bodmer W F 1979 Hybrid myeloma monoclonal antibodies against MHC products. Immunological Reviews 47: 3–61

Brooks D A, Beckman I, Bradley J, McNamara P J, Thomas M E, Zola H 1980 Human lymphocyte markers defined by antibodies derived from somatic cell hybrids I. Hybridoma secreting antibody against a marker for human B lymphocytes. Clinical and Experimental Immunology 39: 477–485

Caligaris-Cappio F, Gobbi M, Bofill M, Janossy G 1982 Infrequent normal B lymphocytes express features of B chronic lymphocytic leukaemia. Journal of Experimental Medicine 155: 623–629

Charron D J, McDevitt H O 1979 Analysis of HLA D region associated molecules with monoclonal antibody. Proceedings of the National Academy of Sciences of the United States of America 76: 6567–6571

Cossman J, Neckers L M, Arnold A, Korsmeyer S J 1982 Induction of differentiation in a case of common acute lymphoblastic leukaemia. New England Journal of Medicine 307: 1251–1254

Dalchau R, Fabre J W, 1981 Identification with a monoclonal antibody of a predominantly B lymphocyte specific determinant of the human leukocyte common antigen. Journal of Experimental Medicine 153: 753–765

Diehl V, Kirchner H H, Schaadt M, Fonatsch C, Stein H, Gerdes J, Boie C 1981 Hodgkin's Disease: establishment and characterisation of four in vitro cell lines. Journal of Cancer Research and Clinical Oncology 101: 111–124

Erikson J, Finan J, Nowell P C, Croce C M 1982 Translocation of immunoglbulin VH genes in Burkitt lymphoma. Proceedings of the National Academy of Sciences of the United States of America 79: 5611–5615

Forni L 1979 Reagents for immunofluorescence and their use for studying lymphoid cell products. In: Lefkovits I, Pernis B (eds) Immunological methods. Academic Press, New York, p 151–166

Fukuhara S, Rowley J D 1978 Chromosome 14 translocations in non Burkitt lymphomas. International Journal of Cancer 22: 14–21

Gharton G, Robert K-H, Friberg K, Zech L, Bird A G 1980 Non random chromosomal aberrations in chronic lymphocytic leukaemia revealed by polyclonal B cell mitogen stimulation. Blood 56: 640–647

Greaves M F 1982 Leukaemogenesis and differentiation: a commentary on recent progress and ideas. Cancer Surveys 1: 189–204

Greaves M F, Verbi W, Kemshead J, Kennett R 1980 A monoclonal antibody detecting an antigen shared by common acute lymphoblastic leukaemias and B lineage cells. Blood 56:1141

Gupta S, Good R A 1981 Subpopulations of human T lymphocytes: laboratory and clinical studies. Immunological Reviews 56: 89–114

Gupta S, Grieco M H 1975 Rosette formation with mouse erythrocytes. Probable marker for human B lymphocytes. International Archives of Allergy and Applied Immunology 49: 734–739

Habeshaw J A 1979 Hypothesis: non-Hodgkin lymphomas are abnormal immune responses. Cancer Immunology and Immunotherapy 7: 37–42

Habeshaw J A, Bailey D, Stansfeld A G, Greaves M F 1983 The cellular content of non-Hodgkin lymphomas: a comprehensive analysis using monoclonal antibodies and other surface marker techniques. British Journal of Cancer 47: 327–351

Habeshaw J A, Catley P F, Stansfeld A G, Brearley R L 1979 Surface phenotyping, histology, and the nature of non-Hodgkin lymphoma in 157 patients. British Journal of Cancer 40: 11–34

Hsu S-M, Raine L, Fanger H 1981 Use of avidin-biotin-peroxidase complex (ABC) in immunoperoxidase techniques: a comparison between ABC and unlabelled antibody (PAP) procedures. Journal of Histochemistry and Cytochemistry 29: 577–580

Jaffe E S, Shevach E M, Sussman E H, Frank M, Green I, Berard C W 1975 Membrane receptor sites for the identification of lymphoreticular cells in benign and malignant conditions. British Journal of Cancer 31 (Suppl. II): 107–120

Jondal M 1976 SRBC rosette formation as a human T lymphocyte marker. Scandinavian Journal of Immunology 5 (Suppl. 5): 69–76

Kaplan M E, Clark C 1974 An improved method for the detection of human T lymphocytes. Journal of Immunological Methods 5: 131–135

Kawanishi H, Saltzman L E, Strober W 1983 Mechanisms regulating IgA class-specific immunoglobulin production in murine gut-associated lymphoid tissues. Journal of Experimental Medicine 157:433

Kersey J H, LeBien T W, Abramson C S, Newman R, Sutherland R, Greaves M 1981 p24: a human haematopoetic progenitor and acute lymphoblastic leukaemia associated cell surface structure identified with monoclonal antibody. Journal of Experimental Medicine 153: 726 731

Kirsch I R, Morton C C, Nakhara K, Leder P 1982 Human immunoglobulin heavy chain genes map to a region of translocations in malignant B lymphocytes. Science 216: 301–303

Klein G 1982 The role of specific chromosomal translocations and trisomies in the origin of some murine and human tumours of lymphoid origin. Cancer Surveys I: 299–309

Kung P C, Goldstein G, Reinherz B L, Schlossman S F 1979 Monoclonal antibodies defining distinctive human T cell surface antigens. Science 206:347

Lachmann P J, Hobart M J, Aston W D 1973 Complement technology. In: Weir D M (ed) Handbook of Experimental Immunology, 2nd edn. Blackwell Scientific Publications, London

Lenoir G M, Preud'Homme J L, Bernhein A, Berger R 1982 Correlation between immunoglobulin light chain expression and variant translocation in Burkitt's lymphoma. Nature 298: 474–476

Manolov G, Manolova Y 1972 Marker band in one chromosome 14 from Burkitt lymphomas. Nature 237: 33–34

Marti G E, Kindt T J 1982 A monoclonal antibody with reactivity for lymphoid cells transformed or activated by EBV. Journal of Cellular Biochemistry (Abst.) Supp. 6:39

McCaw B K, Hecht F, Harnden D G, Teplitz R L 1975 Somatic rearrangement of chromosome 14 in human lymphocytes. Proceedings of the National Academy of Sciences of the United States of America 72: 2071–2075

McConnell I, Lachmann P J 1976 Complement and cell membranes. Transplantation reviews 32: 72–92

McIntosh R V, Cohen B B, Steel C M, Read H, Moxley M, Evans J H 1983 Evidence for the involvement of the immunoglobulin heavy chain gene locus in the 8:14 translocation of human B lymphomas. International Journal of Cancer 31: 275–279

Nadler L M, Stashenko P, Hardy R, Van Agthoven A, Terhorst C, Schlossman S F 1981 Characterisation of a human B cell-specific antigen (B-2) distinct from B1. Journal of Immunology 126: 1941–1947

Natvig J B, Froland S S 1976 Detection of a third lymphocyte-like cell type by rosette formation with erythrocytes sensitised by various anti Rh antibodies. Scandinavian Journal of Immunology 5 (Suppl. 5): 83–90

Naylor S L, Sakaguchi A Y, Shows T B, Law M L, Goeddel D U, Gray P W 1983 Human immune interferon gene is located on chromosome 12. Journal of Experimental Medicine 157: 1020–1027

Parnham P, Barnstable C J, Bodmer W F 1979 Properties of an anti-HLA ABC monoclonal antibody. Use of a monoclonal antibody W6/32 in structural studies of HLA ABC antigens. Journal of Immunology 123:342

Priest J H 1977 Medical cytogenetics and cell culture; 2nd edn. Lea & Febiger, Philadelphia

Reinherz E L, Kung P C, Goldstein G, Levy R H, Schlossman S F 1980 Discrete stages of human intrathymic differentiation: analysis of normal thymocyte and leukaemic lymphoblasts of T cell lineage. Proceedings of the National Academy of Sciences of the United States of America 77: 1588–1592

Reinherz E L, Kung P C, Goldstein G, Schlossman S F 1979 Further characterisation of the human inducer T cell subset defined by monoclonal antibody. Journal of Immunology 123: 2894–2896

Reinherz E L, Kung P C, Goldstein G, Schlossman S F 1980 A monoclonal antibody reactive with the human cytotoxic/suppressor T cell subset previously defined by a heteroantisera termed TH2. Journal of Immunology 124:1301

Ritz J, Pesando J M, Notis-McConarty J, Lazarus H, Schlossman S F 1980 A monoclonal antibody to human acute lymphoblastic leukaemia antigen. Nature 283: 583–585

Rose M L, Habeshaw J A, Kennedy R, Sloane J, Wiltshaw E, Davies A J S 1981 Binding of peanut lectin to germinal centre cells. A marker for B cell subsets of follicular lymphoma. British Journal of Cancer 44: 68–74

Schwab U, Stein H, Gerdes J, Lemke H, Kirchner H, Schaadt M, Diehl V 1982 Production of a monoclonal antibody specific for Hodgkin and Sternberg-Reed cells of Hodgkin's Disease and a subset of normal lymphoid cells. Nature 299: 65–67

Stashenko P, Nadler L M, Hardy R, Schlossman S F 1980 Characterisation of a human B lymphocyte-specific antigen. Journal of Immunology 125: 1678–1685

Sutherland R, Delia D, Schneider C, Newhan R, Kemshead J T, Greaves M F 1981 Ubiquitous cell surface glycoprotein on tumour cells is proliferation associated receptor for transferrin. Proceedings of the National Academy of Sciences of the United States of America 78: 4515–4519

Todd R F, Nadler L M, Schlossman S F 1981 Antigens on human monocytes detected by monoclonal antibodies. Journal of Immunology 126:1435

Trucco M M, Garotta G, Stoker J W, Ceppelini R 1979 Murine monoclonal antibodies against HLA structures. Immunological Reviews 47: 219–252

Van Camp B, Thielemans C, Dehou M F, Demey J, Dewaele M 1982 Two monoclonal antibodies OKIal and OKT10 for the study of the final B cell maturation. Journal of Clinical Immunology 2: 67–74 (suppl)

Verbi W, Greaves M F, Schneider C, Koubek K, Janossy G, Stein H, Kung P, Goldstein G 1982 Monoclonal antibodies OKT11 and OKT11a have pan T cell reactivity and block sheep erythrocyte receptors. European Journal of Immunology 12: 81–84

Wang C Y, Good R A, Ammirati P, Dymbort G, Evans R L 1980 Identification of a P69–71 complex expressed on human T cells sharing determinants with B-type chronic lymphatic leukaemia. Journal of Experimental Medicine 151:1539

Wofsy L, Henry C, Cammisuli S 1978 Hapten-sandwich labelling of cell surface antigens. Contemporary Topics in Molecular Immunology 7: 215–237

Yunis J J, Oken M M, Kaplan M E, Ensrud K M, Howe R R, Theologides A 1982 Distinctive chromosomal abnormalities in histologic subtypes of non-Hodgkin lymphoma. New England Journal of Medicine 307: 1231–1236

5

A.G. Stansfeld

An introduction to biopsy interpretation

In this chapter we shall consider the various features which should be looked for in a lymph node biopsy. The macroscopic appearances of the node will be examined first and then the microscopic appearances. For the novice this will serve as an introduction to the various pathological conditions to be described in subsequent chapters, but more experienced readers will be able to skip much of the contents. The chapter concludes with a summary of some of the more commonly encountered difficulties in lymph node biopsy interpretation.

MACROSCOPIC FEATURES

Although the amount of information that can be gleaned from macroscopic examination of an excised lymph node is limited, this aspect of the examination should never be neglected. Note should be taken of the size, shape, consistency and surroundings of the node (where relevant) and of the appearance of the cut surface. If more than one node has been excised, the appearances of each should be noted and compared.

Size

This is of little value in deciding whether a lymph node is reactive or neoplastic. A very large node, 4 or 5 cm in length, may sometimes prove to be reactive, just as a tiny node may contain neoplasm. The overall diameter of the node may be misleading, since a node which may be obviously enlarged on palpation, may prove on section to consist largely of adipose tissue surrounded by only a narrow rim of lymphoid tissue. This phenomenon is most often seen in axillary nodes and this is one reason why clinical staging of mammary carcinoma is unreliable.

Shape

Of greater value is the shape of the node, for a globular node is more likely to contain neoplasm than one which is flattened or retains its usual reniform shape.

Consistency

A soft or friable consistency may sometimes be found in reactive nodes, especially those which have enlarged rapidly or which contain many polymorphonuclear leucocytes. Friability is, however, more characteristic of neoplastic nodes, whether lymphomatous or metastatic. An increased consistency is found particularly in tuberculosis, Hodgkin's disease and metastatic carcinoma and is due to the fibrosis which commonly accompanies these lesions.

Surroundings

Often the lymph node is excised cleanly and surrounding tissue is not included in the specimen. If surrounding adipose tissue is included, this may be because the node was adherent to neighbouring structures as a result of inflammation or neoplastic infiltration. Several nodes may be 'matted together' for the same reasons.

Cut surface

The most helpful feature of the macroscopic examination is the appearance of the cut surface of the node or nodes. Normal and simple reactive nodes are generally pink in colour when fresh, and grey or pinkish-grey after formalin fixation, depending on the length of time the tissue has been in fixative. Normal mesenteric nodes are often yellow due to the lipid contained in chyle. It is seldom that a follicular pattern can be made out on the cut surface of normal or reactive nodes unless a hand lens is used.

In pathological states the cut surface may be uniform or variegated. A uniform pale pink or whitish appearance is particularly characteristic of lymphomas and the cut surface of the incised node often bulges when fresh (Fig. 5.1). In sarcoidosis, the fresh node has a pale tawny or buffish colour. A distinct follicular pattern may sometimes be seen on the cut surface in follicular lymphoma or in Hodgkin's disease but in nodular sclerosing Hodgkin's disease, the pattern is generally nodular rather than follicular, that is, the 'nodules' are, on average, larger and less uniform. A variegated pattern, sometimes with distinct nodules, may also be seen with metastatic tumours. Metastatic melanoma is often readily identified by the black, or mottled, grey-black colour, but brown or yellow mottling may denote haemosiderin pigmentation in an infarcted lymph node. Nodes which are totally infarcted generally show a dull, lustreless, reddish-brown or yellowish-brown cut surface. A little later, the necrotic centre becomes demarcated by a thick 'capsule' of grey translucent fibrous tissue. Partial necrosis, seen as opaque yellowish-white patches on the cut surface, is particularly characteristic of metastatic carcinoma, and less so of Hodgkin's disease. The caseous necrosis of tuberculosis is white rather than yellow and is generally quite distinctive, the necrotic foci being surrounded by a grey or pink, slightly translucent zone of granulation tissue. Calcification in lymph nodes is generally indicative of healed tuberculosis, or of histoplasmosis in countries where that disease is rife.

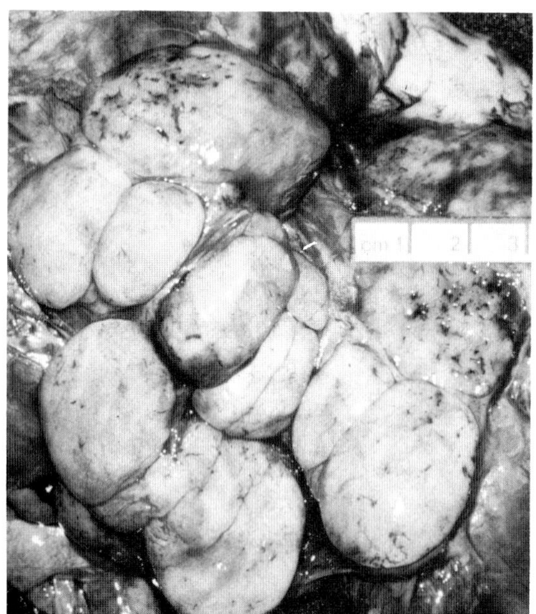

Fig. 5.1 Incised mesenteric lymph nodes in malignant lymphoma of lymphocytic type (B-CLL). Note bulging of cut surfaces.

Although necrosis with suppuration may occur in mesenteric nodes with *Yersinia* infections, in inguinal nodes in lymphogranuloma venereum and in superficial nodes in cat scratch disease, abscess formation may not be apparent to the naked eye, since the abscesses are often very small. They may appear rather as punctate foci of necrosis on the cut surface of the node.

Haemorrhage on the cut surface of the node is sometimes seen in acute infections, e.g. infectious mononucleosis, but is particularly characteristic of some types of leukaemia and high grade malignant lymphoma, especially in the presence of thrombocytopenia.

MICROSCOPIC EXAMINATION

In the interpretation of a lymph node biopsy section, two aspects demand attention:

1. the pattern of the node, and
2. the cellular constituents.

The pattern

This will naturally be examined first, since observation of the pattern is really an extension of the macroscopic examination. Many features can be readily seen with a hand lens and disturbances of the normal pattern can best be appreciated at a low magnification — either with a hand lens or with the scanning objective of the microscope.

In studying the architecture of a lymph node at a low magnification, the trained eye takes note of many features at once, as an artist may take in the varied features of a landscape without consciously analysing its constituent parts. It is, however, only a subconscious awareness of these parts that allows such a synthesis to be made. So here we must look at the architectural features one by one.

Capsule and trabeculae

A normal lymph node has only a thin collagenous capsule from which a few slender trabeculae pass towards the hilum. The trabeculae carry the main blood vessels of the node as they radiate out from the hilum. Occasionally, as an anatomical variant, the node may appear to be subdivided into lobules by more clearly defined fibrous septa, but this picture is readily distinguishable from pathological fibrosis of the capsule and trabeculae (Fig. 5.2). Marked fibrous thickening of the capsule is always pathological and is commonly observed in chronic inflammatory conditions and in Hodgkin's disease. In nodular sclerosing Hodgkin's disease there are often fibrous septa in continuity with the thickened capsule, producing a readily visible lobulated or nodular appearance (see Fig. 9.14, p. 208).

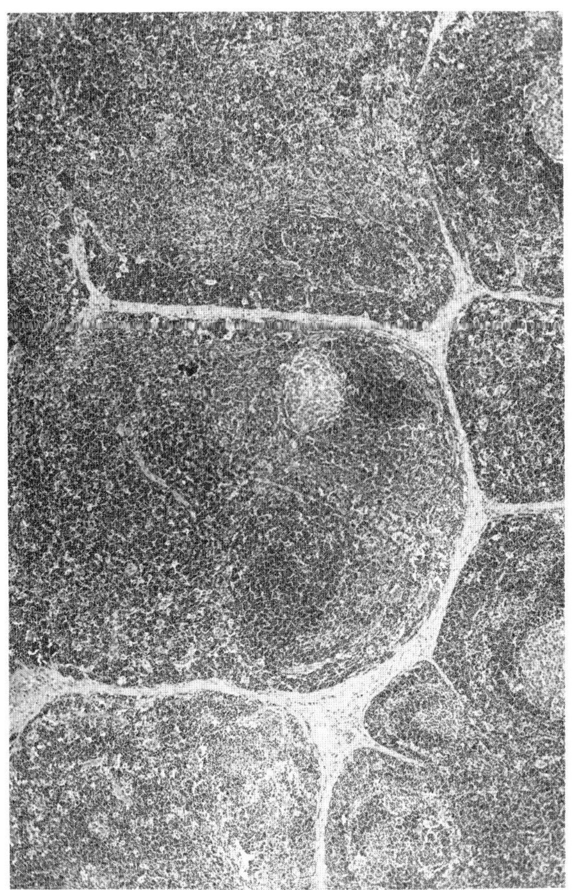

Fig. 5.2 Fibrous septation of lymph node as an anatomical variant (H E × 60)

Widening and cellular infiltration of the node capsule and trabeculae is a commonly observed phenomenon. In these circumstances it is important to look carefully at the infiltrating cells. If they consist of a mixed population, and especially if they are predominantly small lymphocytes and plasma cells, then it is likely that the process is inflammatory. If, on the other hand, the infiltrating cells are monomorphic and a similar infiltrate is seen in the node pulp, then a leukaemic or lymphomatous process must be considered likely, especially when there is blurring or actual destruction of the capsule. Extra-nodal infiltration, that is, spread of lymphoid cells through the capsule and into the surrounding adipose tissue, may arouse a suspicion of malignant lymphoma, but the same phenomenon may also be seen in lymphadenitis and is one of the characteristic features of angioimmunoblastic lymphadenopathy (AIL) (Ch. 8, p. 176). Once again, detailed examination of the infiltrating cells will generally make the distinction clear.

Lymph follicles

The lymph follicles are often the most obvious feature on low power examination of a normal node and their disappearance contributes more to the effacement of pattern than the loss of any other architectural feature. Sometimes, however, follicles are absent, or at least inapparent, in an unstimulated node. The follicles tend to be concentrated at the periphery of the cortex and they may lie so superficially that they give a knobbled aspect to the surface of the node (Fig. 5.3). The appearance of the follicles varies according to their state of activity which in turn depends upon antigenic stimulation. Primary follicles, which ap-

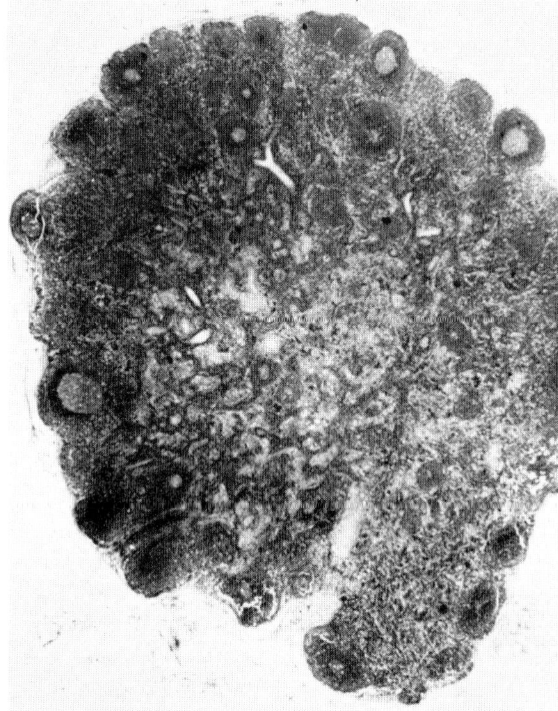

Fig. 5.3 A 'normal' lymph node showing cortex with secondary follicles and medulla with anastomosing sinuses (H E × 8)

pear as rounded aggregates of small lymphocytes, represent follicles in their unstimulated state. After antigenic exposure, the primary follicles develop germinal centres to become secondary follicles (see Ch. 1). The size, shape and appearance of these germinal follicles varies greatly (see Ch. 6). Their cellular ingredients are considered below, but it may be noted at this stage that the germinal centre stains more lightly than the surrounding mantle of small lymphocytes since the germinal centre cells (centroblasts and centrocytes) are larger and have more cytoplasm than lymphocytes. In a silver impregnation preparation, the follicles are traversed by only scanty reticulin fibres in contrast with the surrounding pulp. As the germinal centres expand, due to cell accumulation and proliferation within them, there may occur a condensation of reticulin fibres around each follicle, enclosing the peripheral lymphocyte mantle as well as the germinal centre. One or two small blood vessels may sometimes be seen in the middle of the follicle.

Paracortex (deep cortex: thymus-dependent cortex)

In human lymph nodes, the follicles (B-lymphocyte zone) are generally a much more obvious architectural feature than the paracortical areas (T-lymphocyte zone). This is no doubt mainly due to the generally clear definition of the cortical follicles with their contrasting germinal centres, whilst the paracortex is often diffuse and poorly defined. In nodes from certain sites, however, especially mesenteric nodes, the T cell areas may be much more prominent and well defined, forming nodular masses which project into the medulla from the deep aspect of the cortex (Fig. 5.4). Expansion of the paracortex is commonly seen in early Hodgkin's disease. Enlargement of this zone is also characteristic of certain viral infections, but here the picture is complicated by other changes in the node (see Ch. 6).

The chief distinguishing feature of the paracortex is the presence of post-capillary venules which

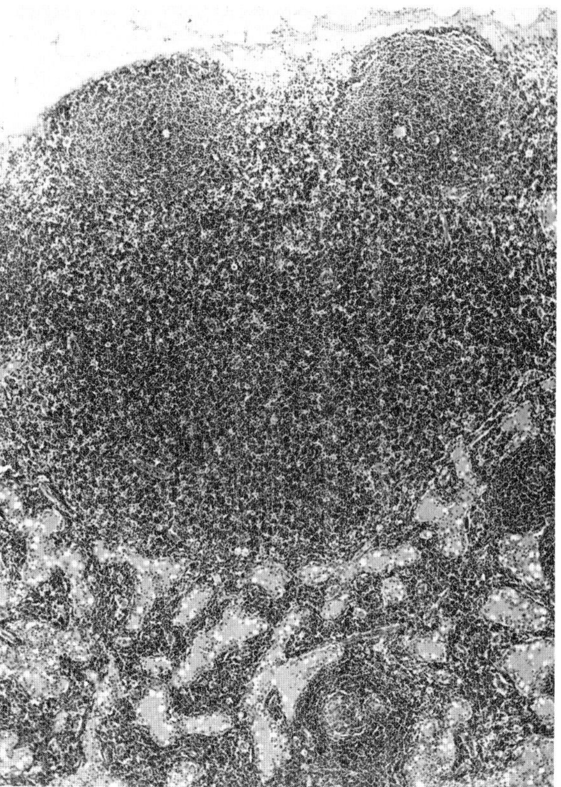

Fig. 5.4 Mesenteric lymph node showing paracortical nodule ('deep cortex') projecting into medulla (H E × 63)

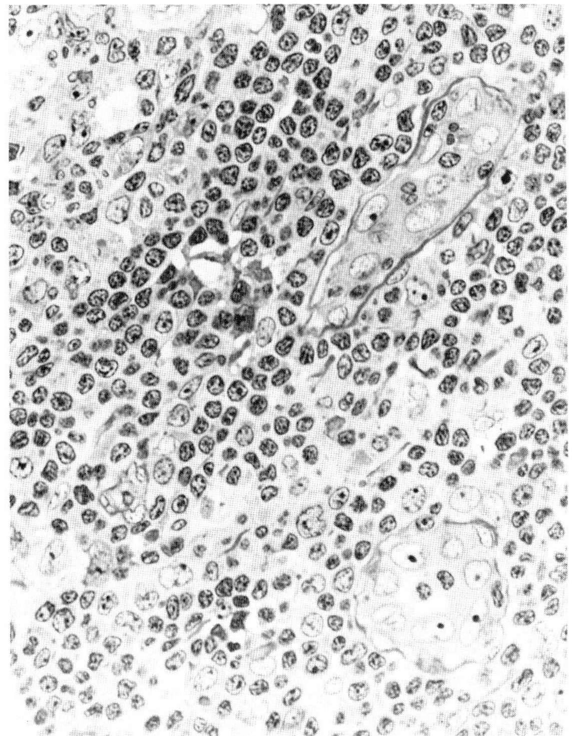

Fig. 5.5 Semi-thin section (resin embedded) of a reactive lymph node showing two post-capillary venules in the T-zone — one is cut transversely, the other longitudinally. Note lymphocytes traversing the walls. The edge of a secondary follicle (B-zone) is seen (top left). (H E × 600)

are lined by plump endothelial cells and which often show lymphocytes in their walls (Fig. 5.5). In the resting state, these vessels are inconspicuous, but they become much more obvious in the conditions enumerated above and their disposition can be better appreciated with PAS staining or in a silver impregnation preparation.

Lymph sinuses

The clarity with which the lymph sinuses can be seen is very variable, even in normal lymph nodes, nevertheless these irregular channels constitute an important architectural landmark. The plane of section as well as the site of origin of the lymph node will influence the number of sinuses that are visible, and since they are very thin-walled, collapsible structures, their visibility will often depend on the lymph flow through the node at the time of its removal. The deep cortical or intermediate sinuses are commonly collapsed and inconspicuous even when the marginal and medullary sinuses are clearly visible and even dilated.

Again much will depend upon whether the lymph sinuses are relatively empty, except for clear lymph, or whether they are choked with cells. In the latter event, they may be invisible on hand lens inspection and easily missed, even under the microscope. This is particularly so when the cells are predominantly small lymphocytes — a frequent finding in the lymph nodes of children. When the sinuses become filled with histiocytes, as in the various forms of sinus histiocytosis (see Ch. 14), these cytoplasm-rich cells contrast with the prevailing colour of the stained section and the sinuses are clearly visible on scanning the node. Likewise, the sinuses may be rendered conspicuous by injected lymphangiographic oil contrast medium (see Fig. 14.8, p. 349), phagocytosed material or secondary neoplastic infiltration. On rare occasions, dilated, empty-appearing, lymph sinuses may occupy the greater part of the tissue section — a picture which suggests lymphatic obstruction (lymphangiectasis). The lymph sinuses are often obliterated in a node occupied by malignant lymphoma, but not invariably so, indeed they may rarely be dilated due to lymphatic obstruction by the neoplasm (see Figs 10.49 & 10.51, pp. 261 & 262).

Blood vessels

It is seldom that the larger blood vessels of a lymph node stand out as a conspicuous architectural feature. The trabecular arteries may be thrown into relief by adventitial inflammatory oedema, e.g. in cat scratch disease, or by concentric periarterial fibrosis in nodular sclerosing Hodgkin's disease and occasionally these vessels stand out because of an arteritic reaction.

Infarction or patchy ischaemic necrosis of a lymph node should encourage a search for vasculitic or thrombotic lesions of blood vessels, as may be found in certain drug reactions or systemic lupus erythematosus (SLE). Increased prominence of post-capillary venules is generally associated with increased activity of T lymphocytes or, less commonly, T-cell neoplasia.

Regional and age differences in lymph nodes

It should be pointed out that the architectural and cellular details normally vary in some degree in lymph nodes from different sites and it is therefore helpful to know the origin of the biopsy. Thus, for example, the follicles, paracortical areas and medullary sinuses are commonly much more clearly delineated in mesenteric nodes than they are in cervical nodes. As mentioned earlier, axillary nodes commonly undergo fatty involution at the centre with advancing age (Fig. 5.6), whilst inguinal nodes in adults are often scarred and sometimes show focal calcification in areas of hyaline fibrosis (Fig. 5.7). Again, whereas axillary and

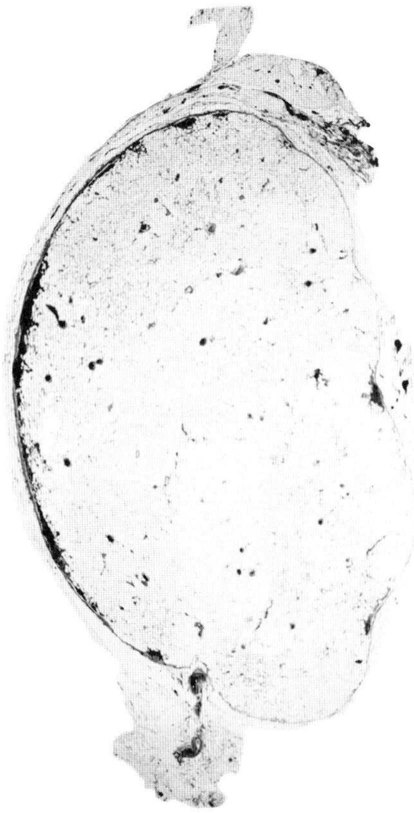

Fig. 5.6 Axillary lymph node showing advanced fatty involution with only a narrow rim of lymphoid tissue remaining. Biopsy was performed because of the large size of the node. (H E × 3)

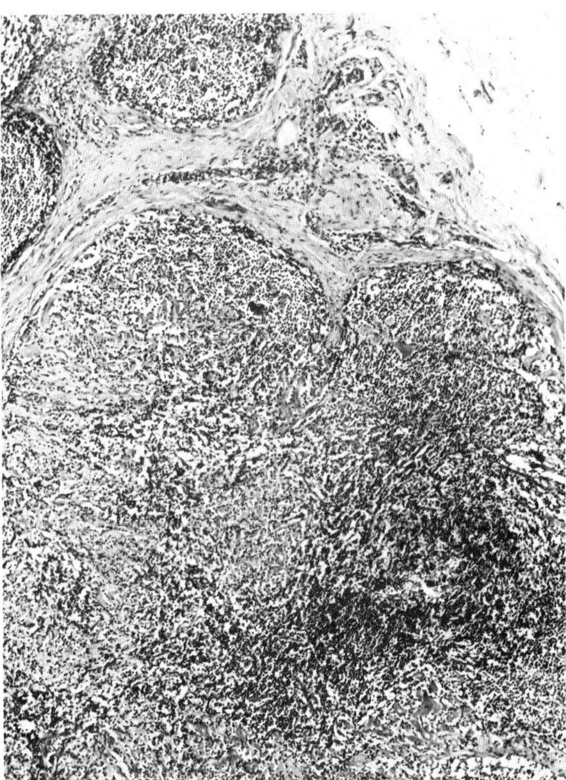

Fig. 5.7 Heavily scarred inguinal lymph node (H E × 120)

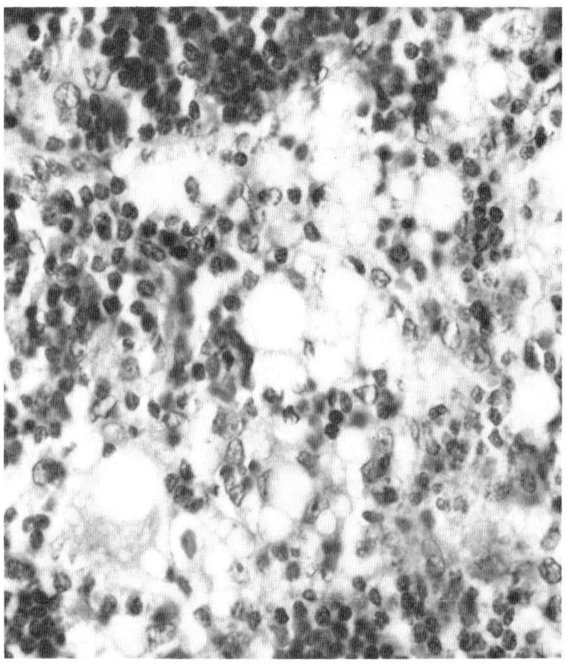

Fig. 5.8 Cystic lymph node removed at cholecystectomy, showing foamy macrophages in the node pulp (H E × 470)

other superficial nodes frequently exhibit reactive sinus histiocytosis, the mediastinal nodes more commonly show pulp histiocytosis with the accumulation of dust or carbon filled macrophages. Clusters of foamy, lipid-filled macrophages are often a feature of coeliac nodes and of the cystic lymph node at the neck of the gall bladder (Fig. 5.8). Nodes from the parotid region frequently contain normal salivary gland elements and a variety of benign epithelial inclusions are encountered from time to time in lymph nodes from other regions (see Ch. 15). It is important not to mistake heterotopic epithelial structures in lymph nodes for metastatic carcinoma. Nests of cells which have been variously interpreted as naevus cells and glomus cells are sometimes found in the capsule of axillary nodes and these again may be misinterpreted as malignant cells (see Ch. 15).

The age of the subject must also be taken into consideration when a lymph node biopsy is being examined, for the normal appearances of lymph nodes in children differ from those in adults, chiefly in the greater number of lymphocytes to be seen in the pulp and sinuses during childhood. The lymph follicles too are generally more conspicuous in lymph nodes from young people. Due allowance for these differences must be made in deciding whether or not a given lymph node is pathological.

Artefacts affecting the pattern

Finally, a word of warning is necessary concerning artefacts in the section which can distort or destroy the normal pattern. The importance of good quality, thin, unlined sections has already been stressed. Even good sections cannot, however, compensate for rough handling of the tissue prior to fixation, poor fixation, or faults in embedding.

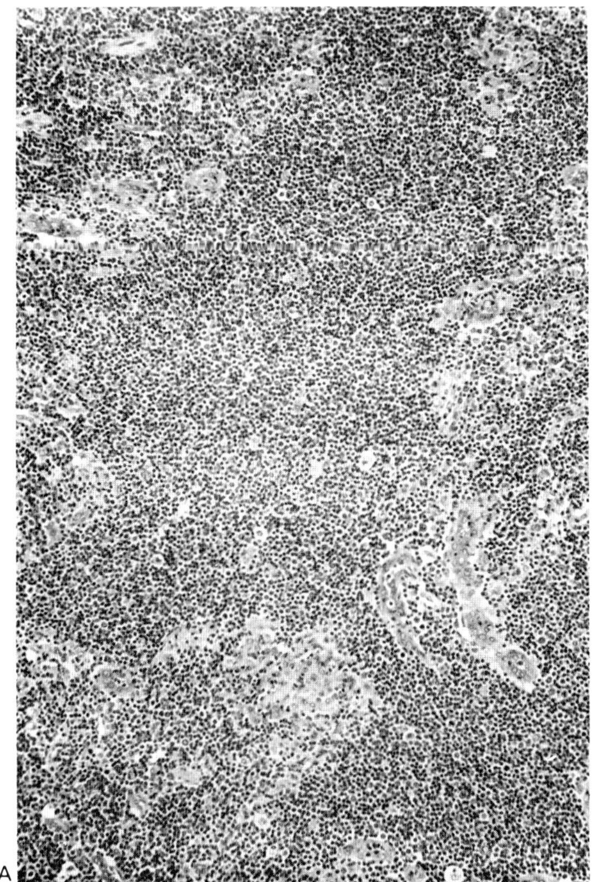

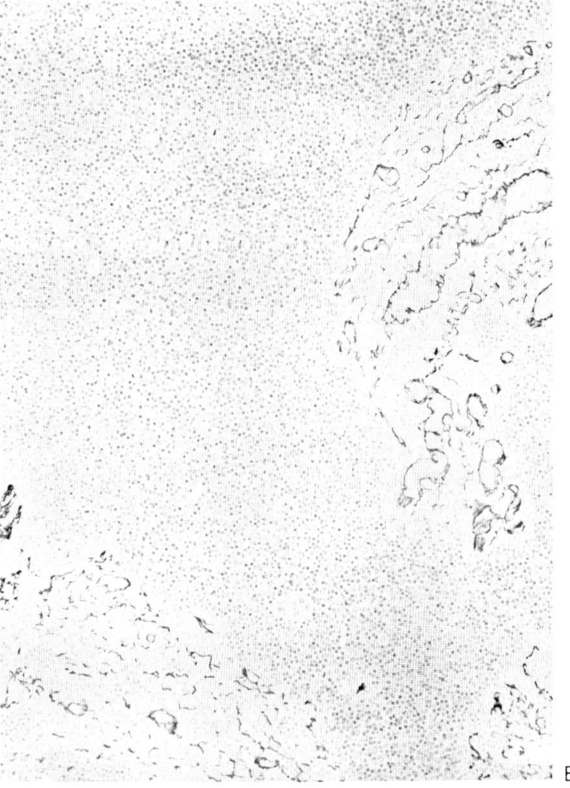

Fig. 5.9 Artefact caused by internal splitting of lymph node during removal, the capsule remaining intact (see text). (a) H E, (b) Reticulin stain — both × 120.

Two artefacts deserve mention here. One is the internal disruption of a lymph node due to rough handling of the node before it is put into fixative. This may occur even when the capsule remains intact and may result in an appearance which can be very confusing, for lymphocytes may pour into splits in the tissue and, after fixation and sectioning, the loss of continuity may not be apparent in routinely stained sections (Fig. 5.9a). A false impression may be gained of a diffuse, patternless lymphocytic infiltration in parts of the node. Silver impregnation will quickly dispel this illusion, for it will reveal the tears and loss of continuity in the reticulin framework (Fig. 5.9b). The second artefact is attributable to the fact that the lymphoid cells of the germinal centres tend to adhere to one another much more strongly than the lymphoid cells around them. Consequently, trauma, or poor fixation, or both, sometimes results in the detachment of clumps of germinal centre cells from their surroundings and, seen out of context, they may be difficult to recognise for what they are and may even be mistaken for carcinoma cells (Fig. 5.10).

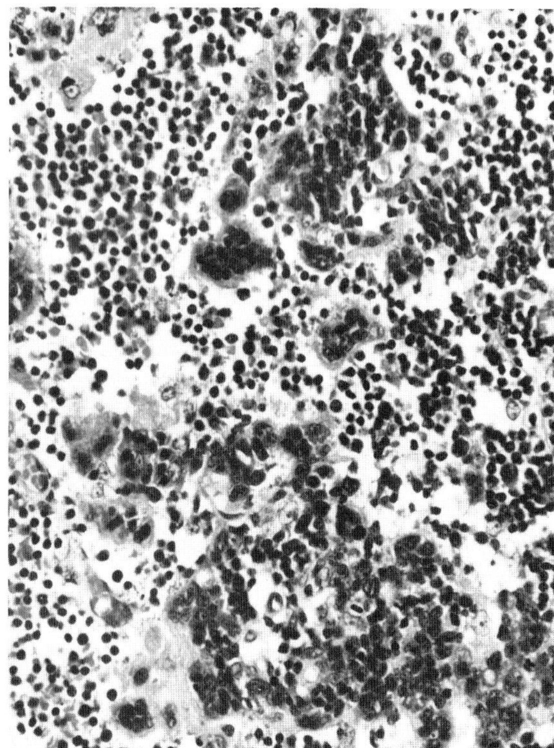

Fig. 5.10 Lymph node biopsy showing cohesive clusters of germinal centre cells separated from their normal surroundings by trauma during removal (H E × 300)

The cellular constituents

After assessment of the pattern of the lymph node section with a hand lens or scanning objective of the microscope, attention should be turned to the details of the cell picture. The pattern is, of course, largely determined by the character and organisation of the constituent cells and some idea of the cell picture can often be gained from naked eye inspection of the section. With haematoxylin and eosin (HE) staining, a lymph node filled with small lymphocytes, as in chronic lymphocytic leukaemia, will appear a uniform dark blue colour. By contrast, a node containing many histiocytes (e.g. sarcoidosis) stains a lighter, predominantly pink, colour. The different types of cell normally encountered in lymph nodes have already been mentioned in Chapter 1. Here we shall consider in more detail the morphological appearances and distribution of the individual cell types, particularly as they may be seen in a HE stained section of a fixed lymph node. The cells to be considered are: lymphocytes and their 'blast cell' derivatives (immunoblasts), the lymphoid cells of the germinal centres (centroblasts and centrocytes), plasma cells, histiocytes and other types of reticulum cell, vascular endothelial cells, mast cells and granulocytes, especially eosinophils.

Morphology of the cells on light microscopy:

Lymphoid cells

Small lymphocytes ordinarily make up the bulk of the cells in a lymph node, filling the interstices of the reticulin framework and thus tending to obscure in a section the more dispersed reticulum cells. As has been said earlier, normal T and B lymphocytes cannot be distinguished from one another by light microscopy, still less can the different sub-populations of T lymphocytes, such as helper and suppressor cells, be separated in routine stained sections. However, monoclonal antibody studies have now confirmed what had long been suspected, namely, that a majority of the small lymphocytes forming the mantle zone around the germinal centres are B-cells, whilst a considerable proportion of the lymphocytes in the paracortex are T-cells.

Cells of the germinal centre

Only the B lymphoid cells of the germinal centres are sufficiently different to be clearly distinguished from lymphocytes by straight morphological criteria. These cells are of two main kinds, namely, centroblasts and centrocytes, and together they make up the bulk of the germinal centres. The weight of experimental evidence supports the assumption that, in the development of a germinal centre, the centroblasts appear first and centrocytes develop from them at a later time (Nieuwenhuis & Keuning, 1974). Indeed, in the early stage of germinal centre formation, the cells are exclusively centroblasts and these appear to be the actively dividing cells of the reactive follicle. This sequence of events has, however, been contested by some authors (Lukes & Collins, 1975), who believe that centrocytes are the precursors of centroblasts. There can be no doubt that these two cell types are different phases in the life cycle of the B-lymphocyte and the fact that one transforms into the other is attested by the consistent finding of cells of intermediate character within the fully established germinal centre. Both types of cell vary a good deal in size. In lymph nodes, as in tonsils, it is often possible to make out a definite zonal arrangement of the germinal centre cells, with concentration of centroblasts (dark zone) at the lower pole, furthest away from the marginal sinus. A crescentic cap of more thinly disposed centrocytes (pale zone) occupies the upper pole of the germinal centre and this in turn is enveloped by the lymphocyte corona (Fig. 5.11). Plasma cells are not often recognised in germinal centres, though they are frequently present there, especially in briskly reacting lymph nodes.

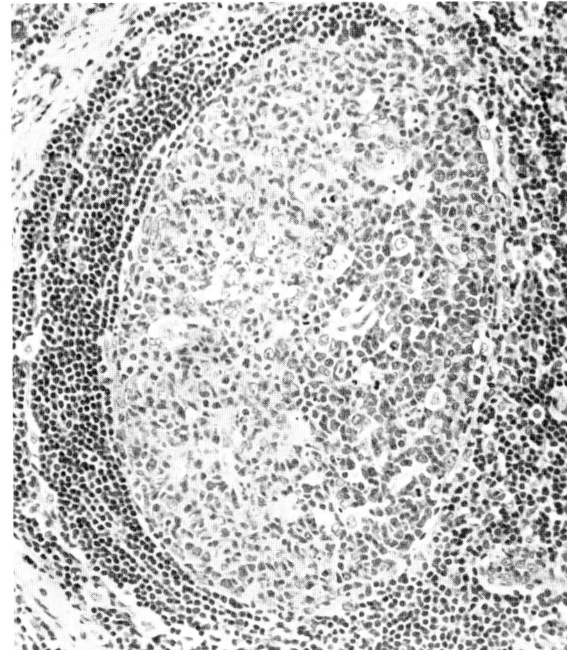

Fig. 5.11 A reactive lymph follicle showing zonation of germinal centre. The 'dark' zone (right) is composed predominantly of centroblasts, the 'pale' zone (left) predominantly of centrocytes. The lymphocyte corona covers the latter. (H E × 240)

Lymphocytes

The appearance of small lymphocytes, whether viewed in smears and imprint preparations or in lymph node sections, is too well known for much description to be required. They are typically small cells, 7–9 μm in diameter, round or ovoid in shape, with a round nucleus occupying most of the cell, enclosed by a very narrow rim of cytoplasm. The nucleus shows a coarsely clumped chromatin pattern so that it stains darkly and a nucleolus is seldom visible. The cytoplasm, barely visible in tissue sections, is a clear, light blue in smears or imprints stained by the Romanowsky methods. Larger lymphocytes, with similar nuclear characteristics, but with a greater amount of cytoplasm are less frequently encountered in the peripheral blood, but cells of this type often form a minority population in normal lymph node sections or imprints. Some of these large lymphocytes display an obvious central nucleolus. On exposure to certain plant lectins in vitro, or to specific antigenic stimulation in vitro or in vivo, a proportion of the small lymphocytes will transform into large, blast-type cells, which may then undergo mitotic division (Ch. 1). Blast cells of this type (immunoblasts) are commonly recognised in sections of reactive lymph nodes. They may be either of B lymphocyte or T lymphocyte origin and both types of immunoblast have broadly similar characteristics (Fig. 5.12). In both, the nucleus is large and 'vesicular'* with a prominent, often central, nucleolus. The cytoplasm, scanty at first, but increasing in amount later, is basophilic when stained by Giemsa. However, whilst the cytoplasm of the T immunoblast is rich in polyribosomes, that of the B immunoblast contains also increasing amounts of rough endoplasmic reticulum, which tends to

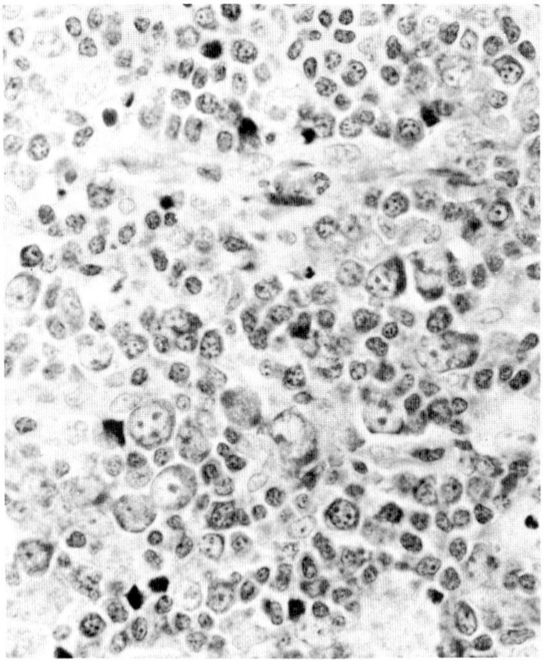

Fig. 5.12 Reactive lymph node showing large immunoblasts with basophilic cytoplasm (Giemsa × 470)

intersify the basophilia of the cytoplasm in reactive immunoblasts of B-type. The resemblance of such cells to plasma cells increases as the cells mature. It is worth noting that intense cytoplasmic basophilia or pyroninophilia is much more characteristic of reactive immunoblasts than of their neoplastic counterparts.

* The vesicular (= bladder-like) appearance is undoubtedly a fixation artefact, since it is not seen in imprints or in well fixed tissue, but fixation is rarely so good in lymph node sections that the artefact is wholly absent. (See section on artefacts on p. 82)

Centrocytes

('Cleaved follicle-centre cells' of Lukes)

These cells are somewhat larger than small lymphocytes and vary quite markedly in size, ranging between 8 and 15 μm in diameter. In sections and in imprints, centrocytes stain more lightly than lymphocytes for two reasons. First, the larger nucleus has a more open, i.e. less dense, chromatin structure and secondly, the cell generally has a greater amount of cytoplasm than the lymphocyte. The nucleus is chiefly remarkable for its irregular contour. More often ovoid or elongate than round in shape, the nuclear outline often shows notches or indentations which are more readily visible in thin sections than in smears or imprints as a rule (Fig. 5.13). When viewed *en face* these clefts appear as darker streaks which are quite characteristic of the centrocyte nucleus. Since the nuclear chromatin is more dispersed, a small nucleolus is often visible. On electron microscopy, 'nuclear pockets', i.e. invaginations of cytoplasm, are often seen.

The nucleus varies in size with the size of the cell, but proportionately the amount of cytoplasm varies even more. That is, the large centrocyte has considerably more cytoplasm in proportion to its size than the small centrocyte. The cytoplasm, in contrast to that of the centroblast, is very weakly basophilic and stains a light grey-blue with Giemsa.

In normal lymph nodes, centrocytes seem to be confined to the germinal centres of the follicles, although sometimes in reactive states (see Ch. 6) similar cells may be seen outside follicles.

Centroblasts

('Non-cleaved follicle-centre cells' of Lukes)

Like centrocytes, centroblasts show much variation in size (range 9 to 18 μm). They are, however, typical 'blast' cells with proportionately much larger 'vesicular' nuclei (see footnote on this page) and only a narrow rim of basophilic cytoplasm (Fig. 5.13). The nucleus is round or ovoid in shape and regular in outline with widely dis-

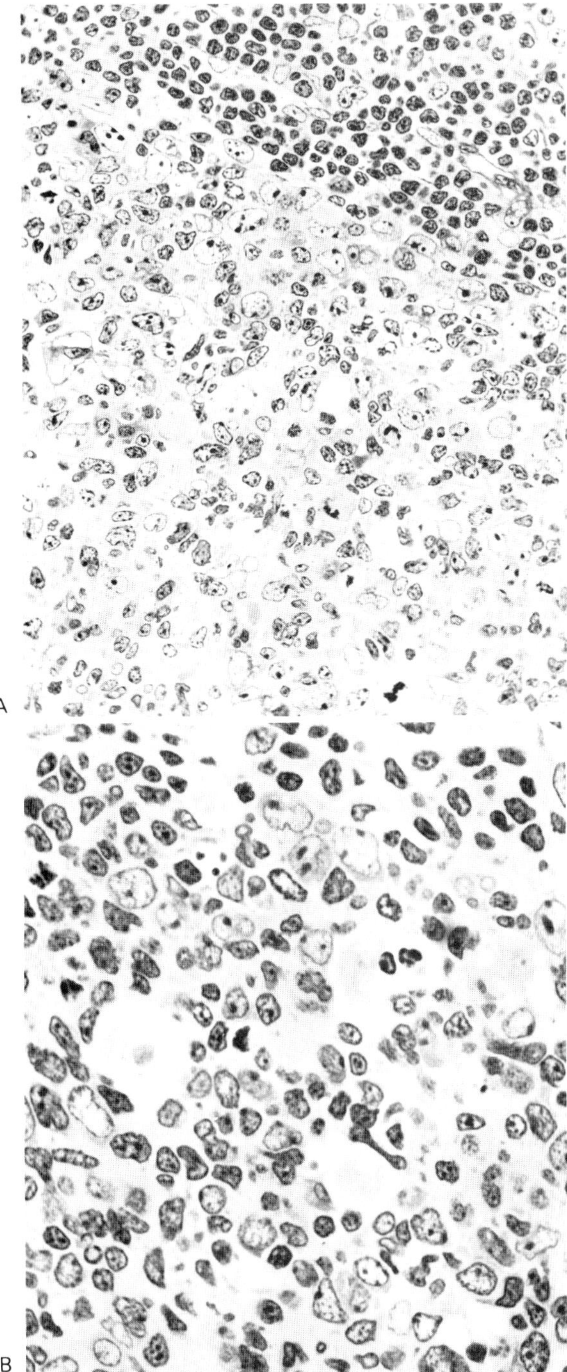

Fig. 5.13 (a) Reactive lymph follicle showing part of germinal centre and lymphocyte corona. Centroblasts predominate near the rim of the germinal centre, centrocytes beneath this with some 'tingible-body' macrophages. Some cells of intermediate character are seen. (Resin embedding H E × 470) (b) Higher power view of reactive germinal centre showing centroblasts and centrocytes. The large pale cells are macrophages. (Resin embedding H E × 600)

persed chromatin, more condensed round the nuclear membrane where two or three or more conspicuous nucleoli may often be seen. Mitoses can frequently be seen in cells of this type. In reactive germinal centres, centroblasts often outnumber centrocytes, but there is considerable variation in the proportions of the two cell types present and, as already mentioned, intermediate cell types are commonly found.

Plasma cells

Plasma cells in small numbers may be considered a normal feature of lymph nodes in post-natal life. They may be found almost anywhere within the node but are most frequent in the pulp cords which lie between the medullary sinuses. It is in this situation that plasma cells first appear in the experimentally antigen-stimulated node. With continued stimulation by an antibody-provoking antigen, plasma cells progressively increase in number, spreading to the cortex and even to the germinal centres, until they sometimes become the dominant cell in the node.

The normal plasma cell is one of the most easily recognised cells in the body. Its round, eccentric nucleus with typical 'clock-face' nuclear chromatin pattern, deeply staining, amphophilic cytoplasm and characteristic perinuclear '*hof*' enable this cell to be recognised wherever it is found. Even binucleate or multinucleate plasma cells are readily identifiable and call for no further description.

Plasmacytoid T cells

(T-associated plasma cells)

In 1973 Müller-Hermelink, Kaiserling and Lennert published a light and electron microscope study of these distinctive cells which had been described by Lennert more than 12 years earlier as 'lymphoblasts' occurring in 'nests' (Lennert & Remmele, 1958; Lennert, 1961). Although these cells show a certain resemblance to plasma cells, having round, sometimes excentric, nuclei and well developed rough endoplasmic reticulum in the cytoplasm, they are in fact only found in the T cell areas of the node, often in close juxtaposi-

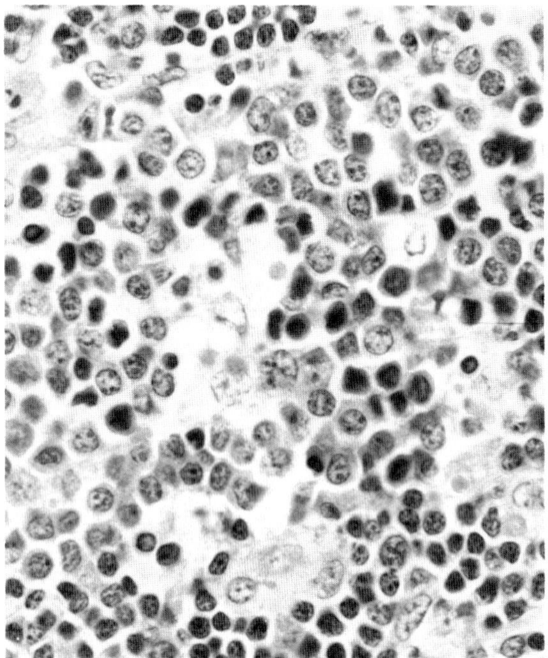

Fig. 5.14 Reactive lymph node in secondary syphilis showing many plasmacytoid T cells (T-associated plasma cells) in T zone. Note cells with pyknotic nuclei. (H E × 590)

tion to the post-capillary venules. From their distribution in the node, their common association with T-zone reactions and their phenotypic expression (Feller et al, 1983), these 'T-associated plasma cells' appear to be a special form of secreting T-cell, perhaps secreting lymphokines as Feller and co-workers (1983) suggest. Plasmacytoid T cells differ from typical plasma cells in having leptochromatic nuclei with a small, central nucleolus and less strongly staining cytoplasm which is grey-blue rather than violet with Giemsa staining (Fig. 5.14).

Reticulum cells

Histiocytes (i.e. mononuclear phagocytes) and other types of reticulum cell are here considered together, partly because they look alike on light microscopy and partly because there is not universal agreement at the present time on the exact relationships of the cell types to one another, or indeed on the number of separate types of reticulum cell that exist. Four distinct types of reticulum (reticular) cell may be distinguished by electron microscopy and enzyme histochemistry (see Lennert et al, 1978) (Table 5.1). These are histiocytes (macrophages), dendritic reticulum cells, interdigitating reticulum cells, and fibre-forming reticulum cells (fibroblasts). Little is known of the precise function of the non-phagocytic reticulum cells, although it is widely believed that the specialised dendritic reticulum cells of the follicles are probably concerned in the presentation of processed antigen to the B lymphoid cells. The distinctive interdigitating reticulum cells of the T-zones may have a similar role in the 'instruction' of T lymphocytes (Sunshine et al, 1980).

Histiocytes

The somewhat negative morphological attributes of resting histiocytes, when stained by conventional methods and examined under the light mi-

Fig. 5.15 Frozen section of a 'normal' lymph node stained for non-specific esterase to show the very large number of histiocytic reticulum cells (appearing black) normally present. The large cells in a secondary follicle (right) are tingible body macrophages. Part of a lymph sinus is shown on the left. (× 120)

Table 5.1 Localisation and enzyme pattern of reticulum cells in normal lymphatic tissue (Reproduced by kind permission from Lennert K, Kaiserling E and Müller-Hermelink H K, 1978, Malignant Lymphomas: models of differentiation and cooperation of lymphoreticular cells. Cold Spring Harbor Laboratory)

Reticulum cell	Localisation	Surface membrane-bound enzymes			Intracytoplasmic enzymes	
		Alkaline phosphatase	5'-nucleotidase	ATPase	Acid phosphatase	Non-specific esterase
Dendritic	B-cell regions	–	+	–	–	+
Interdigitating	T-cell regions	–	–	+	focally (+)	(+)
Histiocytic	All areas	–	–	(–)	++	++
Fibroblastic	Predominantly at borders of T-cell regions	+	–	–	(+)	(+)

– = negative; (–) = usually negative; (+) = weakly positive; + = moderately positive; ++ = strongly positive

croscope, means that they are generally inconspicuous and often overlooked. To appreciate the numbers of such cells in a normal lymph node, it is necessary to employ an enzyme histochemical method (e.g. non-specific esterase) on a fresh frozen section (Fig. 5.15). The histiocyte in its resting state has an elongate, ovoid or indented nucleus, with finely dispersed nuclear chromatin and generally a small, central nucleolus. The cytoplasm is relatively abundant, pale and weakly eosinophilic, but the cell boundaries are often indistinct. When actively engaged in phagocytosis, the cells tend to be much larger and rounded in shape (macrophages), having a round or oval nucleus and a large quantity of pale staining cytoplasm which may contain obvious vacuoles or ingested material. A typical example is the 'tingible body' macrophage of the germinal centres, containing ingested nuclear debris (Fig. 5.16). Brown, granular pigment in macrophages may be either haemosiderin, derived from ingested red cells, or melanin, which is commonly found in the superficial nodes of dark-skinned races.

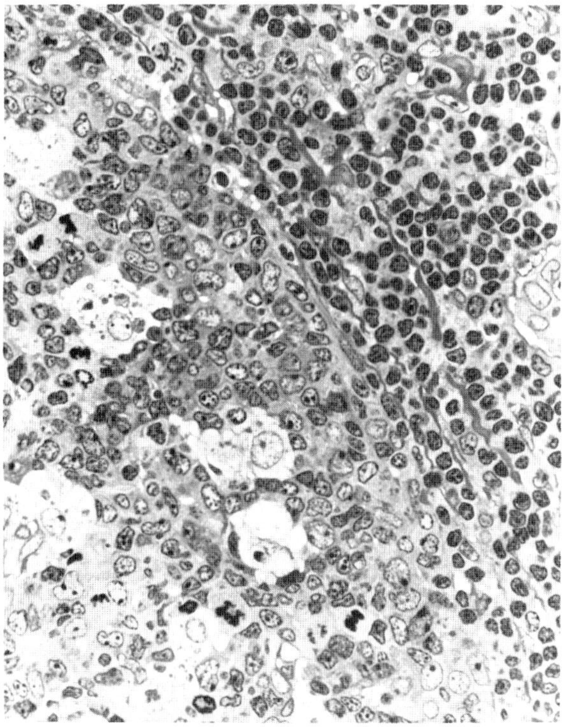

Fig. 5.16 Large 'tingible-body' macrophages in the germinal centre of a briskly reactive follicle. Note mitotic activity. (H E × 600)

Although histiocytes are widely dispersed throughout the normal node, they are found in highest concentration along the course of the lymph sinuses (littoral cells) where they are well placed to phagocytose particulate material carried in the lymph stream.

Dendritic reticulum cells

These inconspicuous cells are confined to the follicles and may be found both in the germinal centres and in the mantle zones. On light microscopy of conventionally stained sections, they are easily overlooked for the cytoplasm is not visible and the cell appears as a small 'naked' nucleus. It is only on electron microscopy that the complex dendritic ramifications of the cytoplasm can be seen. When one is familiar with the distinctive features of the nuclei, these dendritic reticulum cells can often be picked out in the follicles, even in routine stained lymph node sections. The nucleus is small, sometimes round, but often triangular, with a thick, well defined, nuclear membrane, a clear nuclear sap and a prominent round, central nucleolus, like the bull's-eye in a target (see Fig. 10.63, p. 268). The cytoplasm is weakly positive for non-specific esterase (see Table 5.1). Dendritic reticulum cells are well shown up by Marshall's metalophil method (Marshall, 1948).

Interdigitating reticulum cells

The interdigitating reticulum cell is as specific for the T-zones of the node as the dendritic reticulum cell is for the B-zones and, as stated above, it seems likely that both types of cell exercise similar functions in respect of either T or B lymphocytes. Within the T-zones, the interdigitating reticulum cells are much more obvious than are the dendritic reticulum cells within the follicles, but they are readily mistaken for histiocytes when viewed in conventionally stained sections by the light microscope. In a 'normal', non-reactive, lymph node, interdigitating reticulum cells are relatively few in number, but in situations evoking a T lymphocyte response, these reticulum cells may appear in greatly increased numbers, first as isolated cells, then in small clusters and finally in confluent masses, such as may classically be seen in dermatopathic lymphadenitis (p. 354).

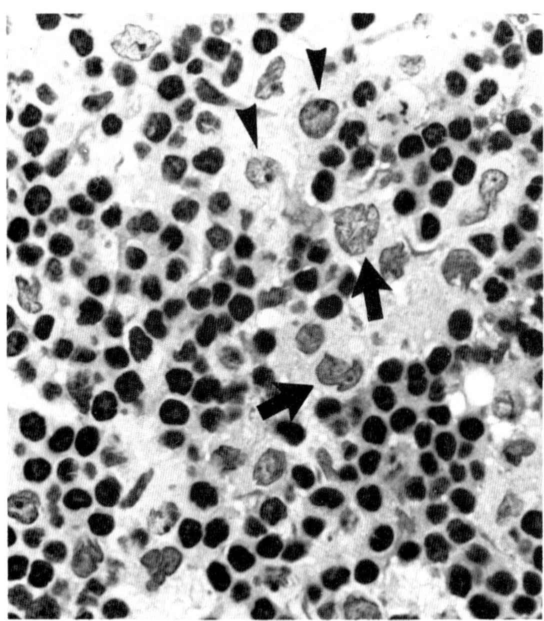

Fig. 5.17 Interdigitating reticulum cells in T zone of lymph node (arrows). Note irregular, folded nuclei and inconspicuous nucleoli, in contrast with histiocytic reticulum cells (arrowheads). (Resin embedding Haematoxylin and Phloxine × 600)

The interdigitating reticulum cell has an irregular, elongate and often 'twisted-looking' nucleus, sometimes showing 'folds' in the nuclear membrane (Fig. 5.17). The nuclear chromatin is finely dispersed and one or more small nucleoli may or may not be visible. The cytoplasm is abundant and moderately eosinophilic. On electron microscopy, complex interdigitations of the cell membranes can be seen between one cell and another. Despite the resemblance of these cells at first sight to histiocytes, they are non-phagocytic and show different enzyme histochemical reactions to histiocytes (see Table 5.1).

Fibre-forming reticulum cells

(Fibroblasts)

There is now much evidence to suggest that different sub-populations of 'fibroblasts' exist in the body and it seems fairly certain that the fibre-forming cells of the lymphoreticular tissues are not the same as the fibroblasts of ordinary connective tissue, at least in normal circumstances. The most obvious difference is of course, that , in normal conditions, the fibre-forming reticulum cell forms reticulin fibre only and not fully mature collagen. Lymph node 'fibroblasts' are widely distributed in the node and, in common with other fibroblasts, they are often found in close relation to small blood vessels. Morphologically, they have much in common with fibroblasts elsewhere, but their cytoplasmic processes tend to be shorter and the cell is often stellate in form rather than spindle-shaped. The nuclear and cytoplasmic staining characteristics are the same as those of fibroblasts in general.

Vascular endothelium

It may seem unnecessary to discuss vascular endothelium as a specific cellular ingredient of the lymph node, but in fact the endothelium lining the post-capillary venules (PCV) is peculiar to these particular vessels and, in tissue sections, these plump endothelial cells are often mistaken for other types of cell. In contrast to the flattened endothelial cells lining blood vessels in general, the endothelium which lines the PCV is remarkably prominent (Fig. 5.18). Lennert prefers the term 'epithelioid venule' to post-capillary venule, to emphasise this difference in the lining cells, and the whole aspect of these cells suggests a higher degree of metabolic activity than one commonly associates with vascular endothelium. Lymphocytes are commonly seen within the walls of PCV and, as Gowans & Knight showed in 1964, there is a constant traffic of lymphocytes recirculating by this route (see Ch. 1). The degree of prominence of this type of endothelium varies with the activity of the lymph node at any particular time. In a quiescent node, the cells are relatively flattened, although still more conspicuous than vascular endothelium in ordinary venules. In an immunologically stimulated node, however, the venular endothelial cells are swollen and rounded and sometimes remarkably 'epithelial' in appearance. Their nuclei are large and round with a well defined nuclear membrane, rather delicate nuclear chromatin and a prominent central nucleolus. The cytoplasm is often relatively scanty and, being weakly eosinophilic, does not attract attention. The post-capillary venules are of course a specific feature of the T-zones, but in a briskly reactive node they are commonly surrounded by a variety of other cells besides lymphocytes and in this setting the swollen endothelial cells may be readily mistaken for carcinoma cells or 'blast' cells by the unwary. Commonly, in a small venule, the lumen is not visible and a close-packed clump of endothelial cells may assume the appearance of a giant-cell (Fig. 5.18). A reticulin preparation will of course instantly dispel such an illusion, but it is necessary constantly to be on one's guard against making such mistakes.

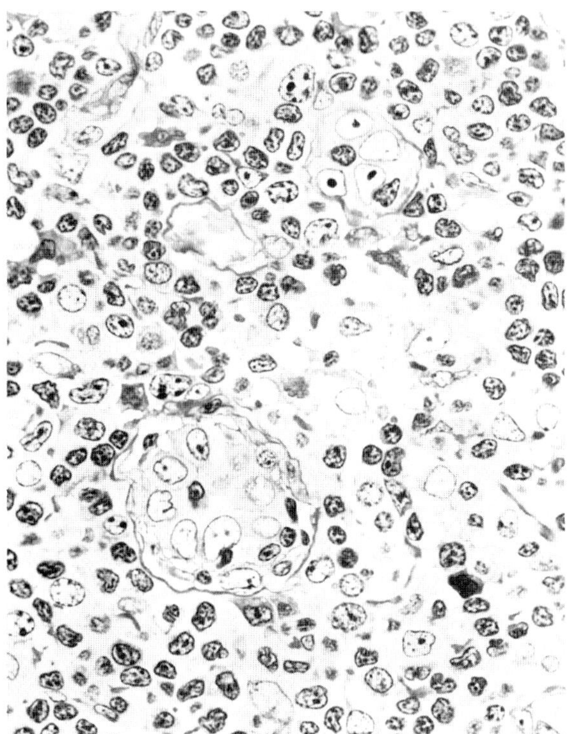

Fig. 5.18 Post-capillary (high endothelial) venules. Note very prominent endothelium and lymphocytes in walls. No lumen is visible in the upper vessel which might be taken for a multinucleate giant-cell if the basement membrane was not visible. (Resin embedding H E × 750)

Mast cells

Mast cells are generally found in small numbers in any lymph node and tend to increase in chronic reactive and inflammatory states. They are often present in relation to small blood vessels in the hilar region, as well as scattered throughout the pulp. In HE-stained sections they often look like large eosinophils, owing to the brightly staining granules in the cytoplasm, but the nucleus is ovoid and not bilobed.

Granulocytes

Neutrophil polymorphs are very commonly observed in small numbers even in 'normal' lymph nodes. A significant increase of polymorphs in the marginal sinus or node pulp generally points to an inflammatory process. These cells are readily identifiable under the high power and do not call for any description. Eosinophil polymorphs are even more easily recognised, even with the low power of the microscope. They are very frequently seen in small numbers in lymph nodes and in certain pathological conditions, their numbers may increase enormously (see Ch. 6, p. 88).

Artefacts at the cellular level

Grosser artefacts, affecting the node pattern, have been discussed already (p. 73). It is important, however, to be aware of artefacts at the cellular level resulting largely from differences in fixation. As Baker pointed out many years ago (1950), in the whole business of fixing, dehydrating, embedding, cutting and staining a tissue, one is introducing a series of artefacts, so that that the cell viewed down the microscope is a very different object from the living cell. This does not, of course, matter, since one is not comparing dead with living cells. What does matter is that the pathologist should become acquainted with the range of microscopical appearances which a single tissue may present, when fixed with different fixatives, for different periods of time, after differing intervals following removal from the body. With certain types of cell (e.g. squamous epithelium), the differences are slight, even with marked variations in the treatment of the tissue. With lymphoid cells, however, the differences may be very great, with but minor variations in procedure. Cell size and morphology are both profoundly modified by the fixation technique and, generally speaking, the nucleus is more subject to alteration than the cytoplasm.

Even in an *apparently* well-fixed lymph node (Fig. 5.19) the cells at the periphery (reached first by the fixative) may look very different from the cells at the centre (reached later, by a slowly penetrating fixative solution such as formalin). When such striking differences may be seen in a single section, showing the *same* population of cells, treated with the *same* fixative solution and the only variable has been a minor delay in fixation of the more centrally placed cells, it emphasises the need for caution in drawing conclusions when biopsy sections from different laboratories are compared. Further delay in fixation will produce shrinkage of the cells, sometimes very gross, and consequently

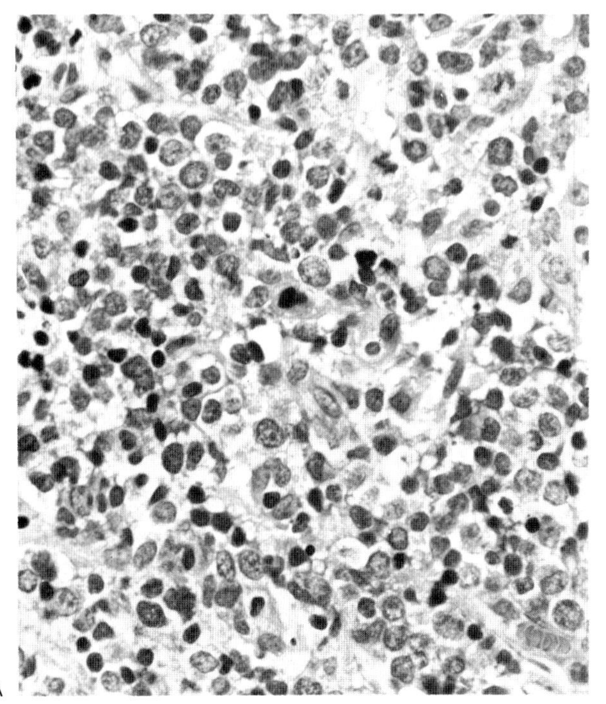

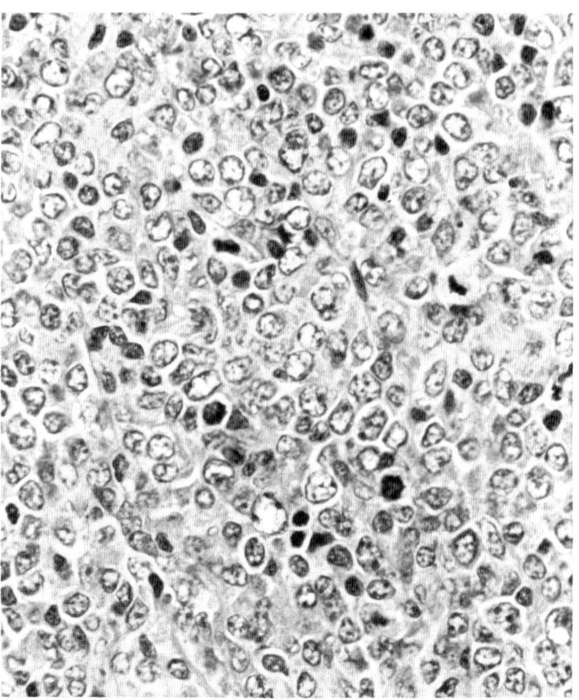

Fig. 5.19 High grade malignant lymphoma (centroblastic) (a) well fixed edge of tumour (b) less well fixed interior (same section). (H E × 480)

gaps appear between the individual cells in the tissue. All too familiar is the picture which results from a large node being put straight into fixative without being sliced. Only a narrow band of tissue around the periphery is at all adequately fixed, the cells in the centre may be unrecognisable. It is useful to compare the appearances seen in sections, when one-half of a lymph node biopsy has been fixed in formol saline and the other half in formol sublimate. The cells in the two sections look quite different and the latter produces less shrinkage.

Common problems in interpretation

Probably the most commonly encountered problem in lymph node biopsy interpretation is that of deciding between a reactive proliferation of lymphoid cells and a neoplasm — generally, of course, a malignant lymphoma. This may, at times, be extremely difficult, having regard to the extreme lability of lymphoid cells and their natural capacity to move around and hence to infiltrate tissues. Nevertheless, the decision is crucial, for upon it may depend whether the patient is dismissed with a smile and a pat on the back or whether unpleasant and potentially dangerous forms of treatment are administered in an attempt to rid the patient of the disease. There are those who argue that it is better to report the lesion as malignant, where doubt exists, but this approach means subjecting patients to a form of treatment which could lead to serious morbidity or even death, when perhaps the condition itself is quite benign. Reactive lymphoid proliferations may be mistaken for malignant ones, either because of a real or fancied resemblance of the lesion to some known form of malignant lymphoma or, less pardonably, because of the presence of 'atypical' (often 'blast') cells and frequent mitoses. Lukes (1968) was right in insisting that a histological diagnosis of malignant lymphoma should only be based on positive criteria which allow the pathologist to identify at least the broad category of lymphoma to which the tumour is thought to belong.

It would be impossible to lay down a complete set of rules on how to distinguish benign and malignant lymphoid proliferations and only a few guidelines can be given. The common problems which give rise to diagnostic difficulty may be subdivided, according to the prevailing pattern in the biopsy section, into: (1) follicular proliferations, (2) diffuse proliferations (i.e. nodes showing effacement of normal pattern) and (3) sinus proliferations. Each of these will be briefly considered here but more detailed descriptions of underlying disorders will be found in later chapters. Dorfman & Warnke (1974) have written a useful review of the types of lymphadenopathy which may be mistaken for malignant lymphomas.

Follicular proliferations

When the biopsy section shows an accentuated follicular pattern, the differential diagnosis is generally between follicular hyperplasia (p. 89) and follicular lymphoma of centroblastic-centrocytic type (p. 260). The differential features are discussed on page 263–4 (see also Table 10.2). Sometimes Hodgkin's disease of the nodular, lymphocytic predominant type poses a problem (p. 204) and angiofollicular hyperplasia (giant lymph node hyperplasia, Castleman's disease) may present difficulties to those unfamiliar with this uncommon lesion (p. 184).

Diffuse proliferations

Here, perhaps, the greatest difficulties are experienced in recognising reactive proliferations and in distinguishing them from diffuse malignant lymphomas, for disappearance of the normal architectural landmarks, especially the follicles, may be accompanied by very active proliferation of lymphoid cells, i.e. widespread blast-cell transformation and frequent mitoses. The confused and apparently disorderly cell picture may be compounded by an influx of reactive macrophages or epithelioid cells and sometimes by necrosis and the presence of neutrophil or eosinophil polymorphs in large numbers.

Reactive proliferations of this kind are most often met with in certain viral infections, especially infectious mononucleosis (p. 128) and in drug hypersensitivity states (p. 135). Most other infections are less of a problem in this regard, but necrotising lesions, such as are seen in 'histiocytic necrotising lymphadenitis without granulocytic infiltration' (p. 87) and systemic lupus erythematosus (p. 165) may sometimes be mistaken for malignant disorders. Extreme examples of reactive plasmacytosis in lymph nodes (p. 93) may be wrongly reported as plasma cell neoplasms — the reverse situation is less likely. Some cases of reactive plasmacytosis with many immature cells are due to infectious mononucleosis, but not infrequently the cause is undiscovered.

Finally, immunoblastic (angioimmunoblastic) lymphadenopathy (p. 175) needs to be distinguished from Hodgkin's disease and some other lymphomas. Here the distinction may be very difficult and indeed, sometimes impossible, for this bizarre disorder is widely believed to be pre-lymphomatous, so that transitional stages into malignant lymphoma are to be anticipated in a proportion of cases.

Sinus proliferations

Reactive sinus histiocytosis is a commonly observed change, but it is unlikely to be mistaken for malignant histiocytosis. The only lesion which may present difficulty in this regard is 'sinus histiocytosis with massive lymphadenopathy' (p. 350). Although the large cells encountered in this condition may appear alarming to those unfamiliar with the picture, the features are so distinctive and consistent that it is generally a case of 'once seen, never forgotten'.

Neoplastic disorders

If it is clear from the biopsy sections that one is dealing with a neoplasm, there remain the further questions of deciding between a primary lymphoreticular neoplasm or a metastatic tumour and of arriving at a specific diagnosis. The malignant lymphomas are discussed in Chapters 9, 10, 11 and 12, leukaemias in Chapter 13, malignant histiocytic neoplasms in Chapter 14 and metastatic neoplasms in Chapter 15.

REFERENCES

Baker J R 1950 Cytological Technique 3rd edn. Methuen, London, Ch 1, p 1–21

Dorfman R J, Warnke R 1974 Lymphadenopathy simulating the malignant lymphomas. Human Pathology 5: 519–550

Feller A C, Lennert K, Stein H, Bruhn H-D, Wuthe H-H 1983 Immunohistology and aetiology of histiocytic necrotizing lymphadenitis. Report of three instructive cases. Histopathology 7: 825–839

Gowans J L, Knight E J 1964 The route of re-circulation of lymphocytes in the rat. Proceedings of the Royal Society of London. Series B 159: 257–282

Lennert K 1961 Diagnostik in Schnitt und Ausstrich. Bandteil A: Cytologie und lymphadenitis. In: Lubarsch O, Henke F, Rössle R, Uehlinger D (eds), Handbuch d spez path Anat u Histol, Vol 1/3A. Springer, Berlin, p 168

Lennert K, Remmele W 1958 Karyometrische untersuchungen an lymphknotenzellen des menschen. 1 Mitteilung: germinoblasten, lymphoblasten und lymphozyten. Acta haematologica (Basel) 19: 99–113

Lennert K, Kaiserling E, Müller-Hermelink H K 1978 Malignant lymphomas: models of differentiation and cooperation of lymphoreticular cells. In: Clarkson B, Marks P A, Till J E (eds) Differentiation of normal and neoplastic hematopoietic cells, Book B. Cold Spring Harbor Conferences on Cell Proliferation, Cold Spring Harbor, Vol 5, p 897–913

Lukes R J 1968 The pathologic picture of the malignant lymphomas. In: Zarafonetis C J D (ed) Proceedings of the international conference on leukaemia-lymphoma. Lea and Febiger, Philadelphia, p 333–354

Lukes R J, Collins R D 1975 New approaches to the classification of the lymphomata. British Journal of Cancer Suppl 2: 1–28

Marshall A H E 1948 A method for the demonstration of reticulo-endothelial cells in paraffin sections. Journal of Pathology and Bacteriology 60: 515–517

Müller-Hermelink H K, Kaiserling E, Lennert K 1973 Pseudofollikulläre nester von plasmazellen (eines besonderen typs?) in der paracorticalen pulpa menschlicher lymphknoten. Virchow's Archiv B (Zellpath) 14: 47–56

Nieuwenhuis P, Keuning F J 1974 Germinal centres and the origin of the B-cell system; II Germinal centres in the rabbit spleen and popliteal lymph nodes. Immunology 26: 509–519

Sunshine G H, Katz D R, Feldmann M 1980 Dendritic cells induce T cell proliferation to synthetic antigens under Ir gene control. Journal of Experimental Medicine 152: 1817–1822

6

A.G. Stansfeld

Inflammatory and reactive disorders

INTRODUCTION

Substances of a wide variety may be carried to the lymph nodes in the lymph stream and the reactions evoked show a corresponding variation. Some substances are inert and if particulate or colloid in nature (e.g. carbon), they are merely taken up by phagocytes and are then stored in the node, perhaps slowly accumulating over a long period of time without producing any other effect (see Ch. 14). A great many transported substances are antigenic and evoke an immune response which may involve predominantly either the B-lymphocyte or the T-lymphocyte system, according to the nature of the antigenic stimulus. Many foreign antigens, as well as some more simple molecules which are not antigenic, excite an inflammatory reaction when they are introduced into the tissues or pass in the lymph stream to a lymph node. In an experimental situation it is possible to isolate effects attributable to inflammation alone, when a noxious stimulus is introduced, but in naturally occurring disease most of the agents which cause inflammation also carry antigenic determinants, so that the resulting histological picture in the lymph node is compounded of both inflammatory reaction and immune response and it is not easy to distinguish clearly the effects of each. For this reason, the effects of inflammation and the immune response are here considered together, sometimes one feature predominating, sometimes another. The repertoire of reactions is limited, so that a similar picture may result from a variety of infections. Nevertheless, many infectious agents produce a characteristic, rarely even a pathognomonic, histological picture. The milder reactions are generally 'non-specific', i.e. a similar picture may be produced by a variety of different agents.

In this chapter we shall consider first the main *types of reaction* which may be encountered in lymph nodes and then discuss in turn the more important specific causes of lymphadenitis*. Those reactions in which inflammation is the predominant feature will be discussed before those characterised mainly by an immune response. Broadly speaking, the primarily inflammatory lesions are more often caused by bacterial or fungal infections, whilst the predominantly immunological reactions are often associated with viral infections and drug reactions.

PREDOMINANTLY INFLAMMATORY REACTIONS

Acute lymphadenitis

Whilst acute inflammation of lymph nodes in certain sites is a common occurrence, the diagnosis is often apparent on clinical grounds, and such nodes are seldom removed for biopsy. Nevertheless, acute lymphadenitis of varying grades of severity is frequently encountered in biopsy material, especially in nodes draining ulcerated and infected lesions, e.g. malignant neoplasms of stomach or gut.

The most frequently observed change, even in mild inflammatory reactions, is so-called 'sinus catarrh' (Fig. 6.1). In this, the lymph sinuses of the node are dilated owing to the increased flow of

* The terms 'lymphadenitis' and 'lymphadenopathy' are often used interchangeably, but, strictly, the former should be reserved for lesions of an inflammatory nature, whilst the latter may be used of any lymph node enlargement.

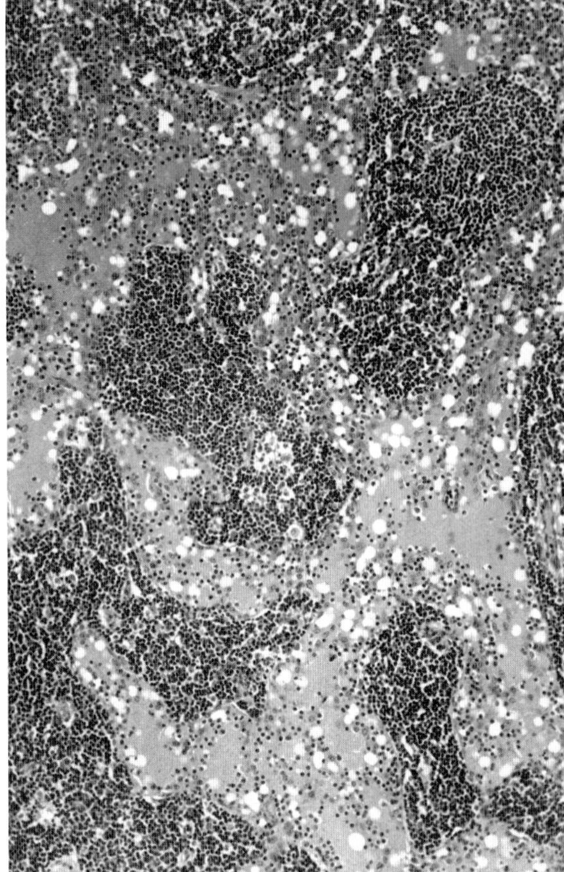

Fig. 6.1 Abdominal lymph node draining an ulcerated carcinoma of the colon, showing sinus catarrh. The dilated lymph sinuses contain proteinaceous fluid coagulated by the fixative, together with fat droplets and free cells, mainly lymphocytes. (H E × 120)

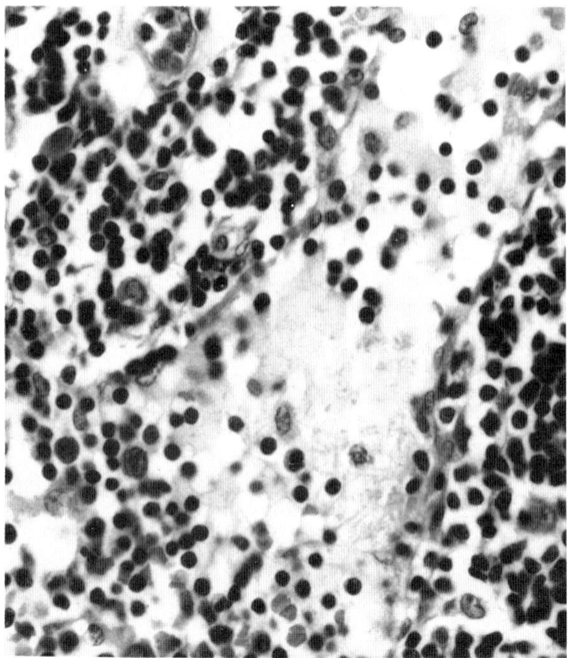

Fig. 6.2 Acute lymphadenitis. Dilated lymph sinus showing delicate threads of fibrin extending from the sinus wall. (H E × 470)

lymph through the node and the dilatation may be such as to cause marked enlargement of the node. The dilated sinuses may appear empty in a histological preparation, but they often contain, at least in part, a homogeneous, weakly eosinophilic coagulum of proteinaceous fluid and sometimes, in more severe reactions, a recognisably fibrinous exudate (Fig. 6.2). The cell content of the expanded sinuses varies from a few macrophages derived from the littoral cells (sinus-lining histiocytes) to large numbers of neutrophil polymorphs and many macrophages.

Whilst the sinuses commonly show the most conspicuous alteration in acute lymphadenitis, there are also changes to be seen in the dense pulp of the node. Dilatation of blood vessels may be a very prominent feature, revealing a far larger number of small vessels in the node than is ordinarily apparent. Polymorph emigration and infiltration of the node pulp may also be seen and, less frequently, actual suppuration. The capsule and trabeculae may be widened by oedema or inflammatory cell infiltration.

Suppurative lymphadenitis

Acute suppurative lymphadenitis is most often due to staphylococcal infections and is therefore most commonly seen in superficial nodes, especially axillary and inguinal groups. It has become much less frequent since the introduction of antibiotic therapy. In advanced cases the whole node may be destroyed by suppurative inflammation and the resulting abscess may show on biopsy no evidence of having originated in a lymph node.

Generally less acute and more localised suppurative lymphadenitis is a feature of many other infections, including yersiniosis (p. 98), listeriosis

(p. 107), some fungal infections (pp. 111–116), lymphogranuloma venereum (p. 123) and cat scratch disease (p. 124). Although the lesions caused by these organisms are often morphologically similar, the quite different sites of involvement, e.g. mesenteric nodes in yersiniosis, superficial nodes in cat scratch disease, help to distinguish them. Other organisms have from time to time been implicated in causing suppurative lymphadenitis.

It should also be remembered that massive polymorph infiltration is sometimes seen in association with neoplastic infiltration. Thus, nodular sclerosing Hodgkin's disease (Ch. 9), and less often, metastatic carcinoma or melanoma (Ch. 15), may occasionally be mistaken for suppurative lymphadenitis.

Acute necrotising lymphadenitis

This is the principal lesion in bubonic plague in which the buboes may subsequently break down and suppurate. Primarily necrotising lesions may also be seen in tularaemia (p. 97), anthrax (p. 97), typhoid (p. 100) tuberculosis (p. 101), melioidosis (p. 108), primary syphilis (p. 108), lymphogranuloma venereum (p. 123) and cat scratch disease (p. 124). It is important to distinguish these infective disorders not merely from one another but from lymph node infarction (p. 144) (sometimes associated with drug hypersensitivity, p. 135), SLE (p. 165) or Wegener's granulomatosis (p. 148), and particularly from necrotic neoplasms.

A previously unrecognised form of necrotising lymphadenitis, which may have been confused with SLE, has recently been described under the title of *histiocytic necrotising lymphadenitis without granulocytic infiltration* (Kikuchi, 1972; Pileri et al, 1982; Eimoto et al, 1983). This evidently distinct condition seems to be not uncommon and is certainly found in Britain and Continental Europe as well as the Far East. It may well turn out to be of world-wide occurrence. According to the reports cited above (and our own observations) the disease affects chiefly young women and is generally confined to a single node, or a small group of nodes, usually in the cervical region. The lymph node enlargement is of moderate degree, and may be accompanied by malaise and slight fever, but the disease is generally mild and self-limiting.

Histologically the nodes show conspicuous and sometimes extensive focal areas of necrosis which are not sharply demarcated from the surrounding sheets of pale 'histiocytic' cells (Figs 6.3, 6.4). Within the necrotic areas there is much nuclear debris, but polymorphs are conspicuously absent, in contrast with the findings in systemic lupus erythematosus and in bacterial infections (Pileri et al, 1982). The cellular infiltrate, within which the necrosis appears to have developed, includes a proportion of transformed lymphoid cells as well as histiocytes: plasma cells are usually scanty but Feller et al (1983) have demonstrated a high content of plasmacytoid T cells (see p. 77). Other parts of the node may appear relatively normal and follicular hyperplasia is not a feature (Eimoto et al, 1983). The lesions are almost certainly due to an

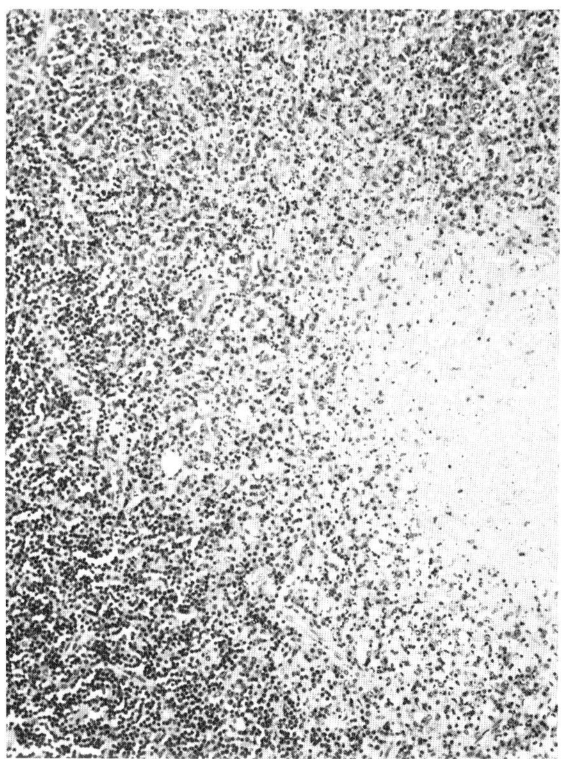

Fig. 6.3 Cervical lymph node biopsy from a young woman showing characteristic changes of histiocytic necrotizing lymphadenitis without granulocytic infiltration. A focus of necrosis (right) is surrounded by histiocytic cells. (H E × 120)

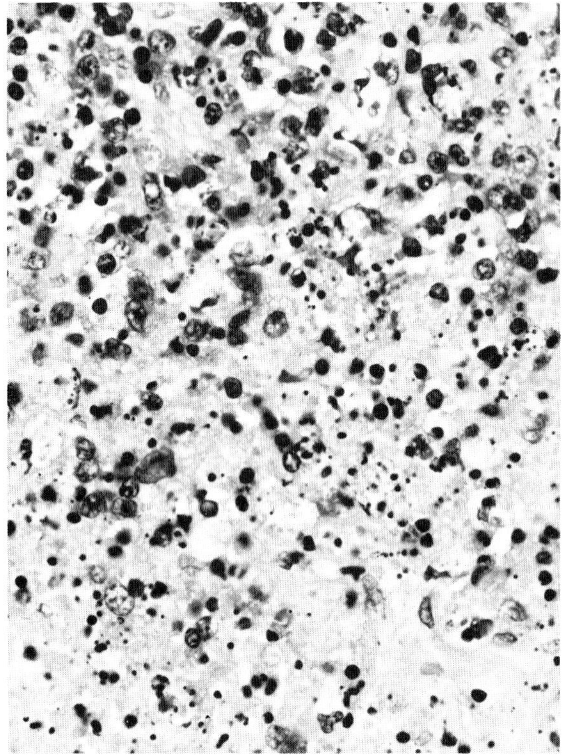

Fig. 6.4 Higher power view of the same lymph node as in Fig. 6.3 showing detail of cellular reaction at the edge of the necrotic area. There is much nuclear debris but polymorphs are absent. (H E × 470)

infection, but until the cause is discovered it is probably best to retain the descriptive but rather cumbrous title given above. Feller et al (1983) found evidence of Yersinial infection in three patients with this disease, but further studies are required to confirm this association.

Chronic lymphadenitis

Chronic inflammation is a much less precise concept than acute inflammation and in this context it is impossible to make a sharp distinction between chronic inflammation and reactive histiocytosis. For the purpose of this book, an arbitrary decision has been taken to include in this chapter most of those conditions known to be or thought to be of infective origin, however prominent the histiocytic component of the reaction, and to include in Chapter 14 mostly those forms of reactive histiocytosis, including granulomatous disorders, in which infection either does not play a part or remains unproven.

In the more chronic types of lymphadenitis, as would be expected, the inflammatory reaction is frequently combined with an immune response to the provoking agent or to products of tissue destruction. Thus one may see hyperplasia of lymph follicles, increased prominence of post-capillary venules, an increase of lymphocytes and the presence of immunoblasts and plasma cells, in addition to scarring which has resulted from tissue destruction and granulation tissue formation. A macrophage response may be interpreted as either a direct reaction to injury or as a part of the immune response.

The pattern of changes is very variable, depending to a great extent on the severity of the inflammatory reaction which, in turn, is determined by the aetiological agent. In the milder, 'non-specific' reactions there may be macrophages scattered throughout the pulp of the node, often combined with reactive sinus histiocytosis and an increase of plasma cells in the pulp or medullary cords. Sometimes there is focal or more generalised capsular thickening and scarring, again often accompanied by plasma cell infiltration. When healing occurs, there may be widespread scarring and replacement of much of the lymphoid tissue by hyaline collagen which may show focal calcification. This is a common finding in inguinal nodes in adults. There may be, on the other hand, evidence of continuing infection with chronic abscess formation or massive accumulation of macrophages with foamy cytoplasm, which often indicate previous suppuration or necrosis. An increase of mast cells is frequently seen in chronic lymphadenitis, sometimes associated with a notable increase of eosinophil leucocytes.

Tissue eosinophilia

Whilst small numbers of eosinophils are very commonly seen in lymph nodes in a variety of circumstances, a massive eosinophilia is uncommon. It may be seen in helminth infestations such as filariasis or with other metazoan parasites such as 'larva migrans' (p. 122). Heavy eosinophilia is sometimes a feature of drug reactions or other types of allergy (e.g. in mesenteric nodes in food

Table 6.1 Some conditions in which granulomas are found in lymph nodes

Infections	Lymphoproliferative disorders and other neoplasms	Other
Tuberculosis and other mycobacterial diseases	Drug reactions	Some immunodeficiency disorders
Tularaemia	Angioimmunoblastic lympadenopathy	Sarcoidosis
Brucellosis	Hodgkin's disease	Crohn's disease (abdominal nodes)
Syphilis — primary and secondary	T-cell lymphomas, especially lymphoepithelioid lymphoma	Primary biliary cirrhosis (abdominal nodes)
Histoplasmosis and other fungal diseases	B-cell lymphomas, especially lymphoplasmacytoid and immunoblastic lymphoma	Berylliosis and other minerals, e.g. zirconium
Kala-azar	Metastatic carcinoma, especially mammary and nasopharyngeal	Polyvinylpyrrolidone
Toxoplasmosis		
	Metastatic seminoma	Materials used in prostheses — silicone etc
Cat scratch disease		
Infectious mononucleosis		

allergies) and may be associated with vasculitis in the node (p. 147). In eosinophilic granuloma, whether of lymph nodes or bones, eosinophils are associated with sheets of distinctive, pale-staining 'histiocytes'. In this condition eosinophils may be very numerous, sometimes forming solid aggregates — so-called eosinophil abscesses (p. 366). In mastocytosis eosinophils are also found, although usually in smaller numbers. Finally, it should not be forgotten that heavy eosinophilia may mask the presence of an underlying neoplasm, whether Hodgkin's disease, other lymphoma or secondary carcinoma. An eosinophilic variant of chronic myeloid leukaemia also needs to be considered in the differential diagnosis of such cases.

Granulomatous lesions

The term granuloma implies a focal aggregation of histiocytes, which have undergone or are undergoing transformation into epithelioid cells, but it is not always easy to draw a hard and fast line between granuloma formation and simple reactive histiocytosis (see p. 345). The number and variety of granulomatous reactions in lymph nodes is very great and the list given in Table 6.1 is by no means exhaustive. In addition, small granulomas are sometimes found in association with non-specific reactive hyperplasia (p. 90), and in instances of unexplained lymphadenopathy. In some of the infective lesions, notably tuberculosis, histoplasmosis, cat scratch disease, tularaemia and kala-azar, granuloma formation is associated with pronounced necrosis and less conspicuous necrosis is often seen in sarcoidosis (p. 355). In some instances, granulomatous lesions undergo healing with subsequent fibrosis but granulomas are often remarkably persistent. Calcification is often a sequel of tuberculous caseation or the necrosis associated with histoplasmosis.

PREDOMINANTLY IMMUNE REACTIONS

The early changes in a lymph node which is draining a focus of infection or ulceration, are often characterised by predominantly exudative phenomena — hyperaemia and sinus catarrh. Over the course of a few days, however, features indicative of an immune response appear. These differ in detail depending upon the nature of the exciting antigen(s) and whether it is a primary or secondary response (see Ch. 1, p. 12). The observed phenomena in the lymph node may indicate a predominantly B-lymphocyte response or a predominantly T-lymphocyte response, depending again on the nature of the provoking antigen. Since, however, most reactions involve more than one type of antigen and the T and B cell systems act in concert, the observed immune reaction often has the features of a mixed type of response.

Predominantly B-lymphocyte response

Reactive follicular hyperplasia

This is characterised by the presence of enlarged lymph follicles with prominent germinal centres and by the appearance of plasma cells, initially in the medullary cords of the lymph node and, later, throughout the interfollicular pulp of the node. This picture is very commonly observed in lymph node biopsies and, in the absence of other, more specific histological features which may indicate the cause of the reaction, the term *non-specific reactive hyperplasia* is often applied. The picture is commonly seen, for example, in cervical nodes in relation to infected tonsils or in the nodes draining ulcerated lesions of the stomach or gut. In the latter, there is often associated 'sinus catarrh'. As might be expected, the same picture of a lymph node engaged in antibody production is characteristic of the lymphadenopathy commonly associated with rheumatoid arthritis (Fig. 6.5). It is not uncommon, however, for the cause to remain undiscovered in cases where solitary or even multiple lymph nodes show reactive follicular hyperplasia.

In the early stages of the process, the hyperplastic follicles may be restricted to the cortex of the node and at times reactive germinal centres may be confined to a very few, or even a single, follicle, whilst the remaining follicles appear dormant (Fig. 6.6). Later the follicular hyperplasia often extends and encroaches on the medullary region until, in extreme cases, the node appears to be filled with enlarged reactive follicles, obliterating or greatly reducing the number of visible lymph sinuses (Fig. 6.5). At this stage, the picture has to be distinguished from that of follicular lymphoma which it may sometimes closely resemble (see p. 263). The proportion of the node which is occupied by reactive follicles varies much from case to case and is independent of the size of the node. Sometimes follicles are closely packed and

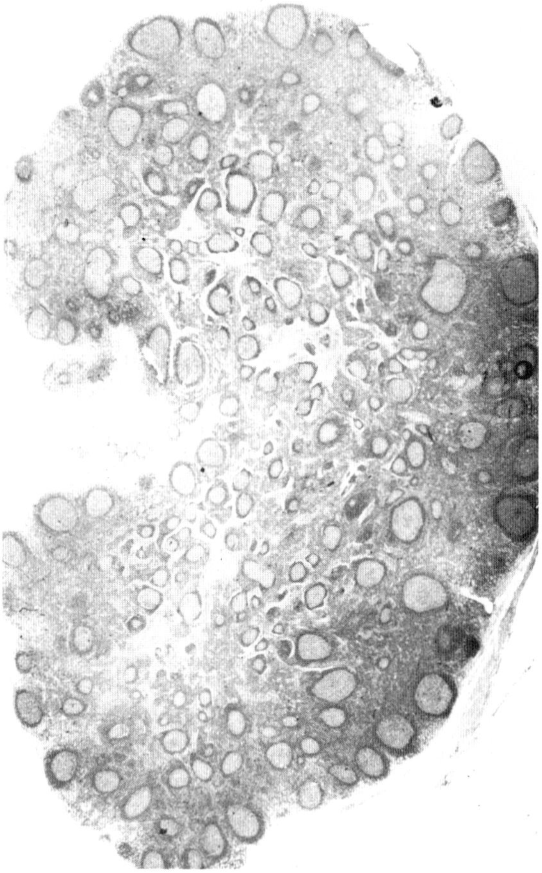

Fig. 6.5 Axillary lymph node in chronic rheumatoid arthritis showing follicular hyperplasia. The pale germinal centres are sharply outlined by the surrounding lymphocyte mantles. The interfollicular pulp of this node contained many plasma cells. (H E × 6)

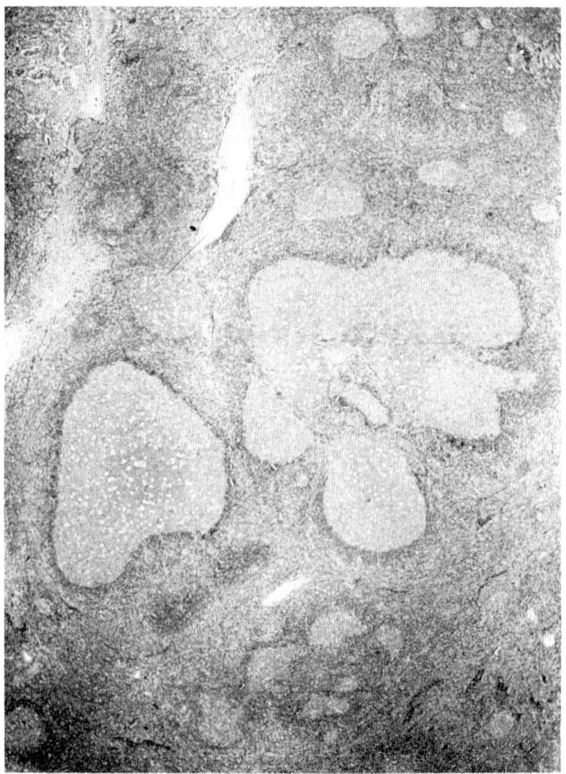

Fig. 6.6 Reactive lymph node in which hyperplasia is confined to two or three giant-sized follicles of irregular shape, whilst other follicles remain dormant. Note 'starry sky' appearance of germinal centres. (H E × 18)

even appear confluent, at other times, in a more 'mixed' immune response, prominent follicles with large germinal centres are separated from one another by broad tracts of interfollicular pulp containing often a mixture of cells, including plasma cells, as well as conspicuous post-capillary venules.

Follicular hyperplasia of striking degree is particularly characteristic of reactions in children or young adults and is much less often seen in the elderly. When antigenic stimulation provokes a follicular reaction in a previously atrophic node, germinal follicles may extend into the adipose centre of the node but only rarely do reactive follicles spread through the node capsule and, unlike the follicles of follicular lymphoma, they never infiltrate the surrounding adipose tissue to a significant degree.

It should be noted that reactive germinal follicles may grow to a very large size in cases where there is prolonged immune stimulation. Such giant follicles are often irregular in shape, resembling the pieces of a jigsaw puzzle (Fig. 6.7). In these circumstances, the germinal centres may contain a high proportion of centroblasts and may show many mitotic figures, but there are generally two features present which help to confirm the benign, reactive nature of the process. These are: (1) persistence, at least in part, of the small lymphocyte mantle zone around or at one pole of the germinal centre and (2) the presence of a 'starry sky' pattern within the germinal centre, due to scattered, large, 'tingible body' macrophages (Fig. 6.7). Sometimes, especially in superficially situated follicles, a zonal arrangement may be seen in the germinal centre (see p. 75). (For other features which help to distinguish reactive from neoplastic follicles, the reader is referred to Ch. 10, p. 264).

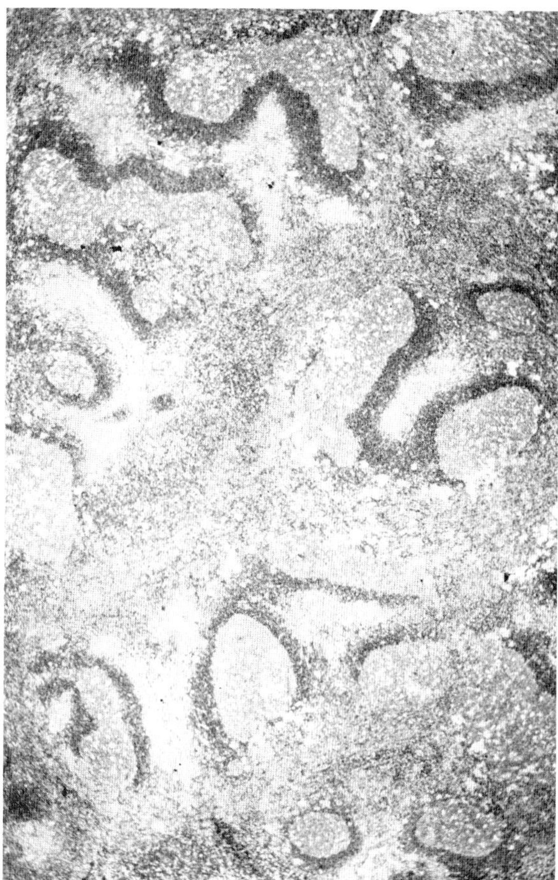

Fig. 6.7 Cervical lymph node from a youth of 19 showing follicular hyperplasia due to toxoplasmosis. This had been erroneously diagnosed as follicular lymphoma. Note irregular shape of follicles, 'starry sky' appearance of germinal centres and prominent lymphocyte mantles. (H E × 18)

So long as the germinal follicles of a reactive node remain intact, a diagnosis of simple reactive hyperplasia is generally not difficult. At times, however, one of two events may occur, which complicate the histological picture and make diagnosis more difficult. The first of these, most often seen in reactive nodes from children, is a progressive expansion of the germinal centres until the mantle zone (lymphocyte corona) disappears, so that the margin of the follicle is no longer defined. In these circumstances the follicles may become so large that they appear to coalesce, sometimes forming tumour-like masses, and the impression is gained that the normal architecture is effaced (Figs 6.8, 6.9, 6.10). Careful examination, however, will show that the expanded germinal centres can still be recognised by their starry sky pattern, whilst the intervening T zones are identifiable by their prominent venules (Fig. 6.11).

The second type of alteration, which may affect a proportion of the follicles in long continued reactive follicular hyperplasia, has been described by Lennert & Müller-Hermelink (1975) as 'progressive transformation' of germinal centres. The enlarged germinal centre appears to break up into fragments and lymphocytes in increasing numbers become interposed between the fragmented clumps of ger-

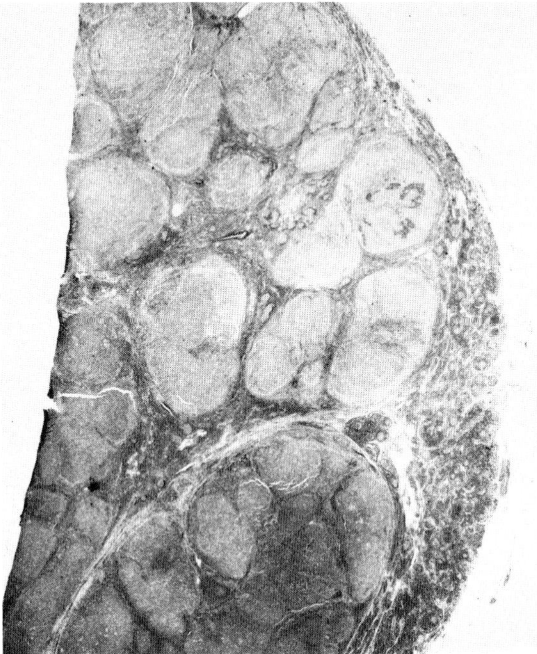

Fig. 6.8 Cervical lymph node from a boy aged 12, showing conglomerate tumour-like masses of reactive germinal follicles compressing a peripheral rim (right) of non-reactive lymphoid tissue. This was wrongly interpreted as a malignant lymphoma of follicular type. (H E × 6)

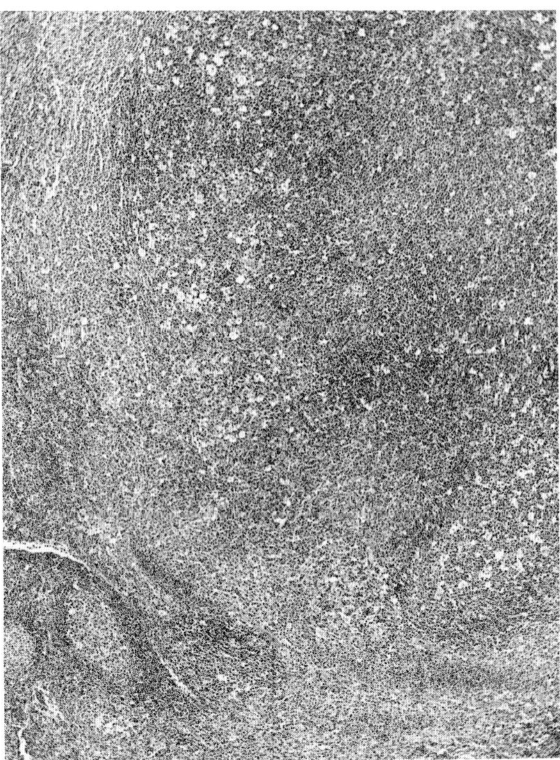

Fig. 6.9 Cervical lymph node from a boy of 6 in which coalescent reactive follicles have formed a tumour-like nodule (upper right), the lymphocyte mantles having disappeared. Note 'starry sky' pattern. (H E × 47)

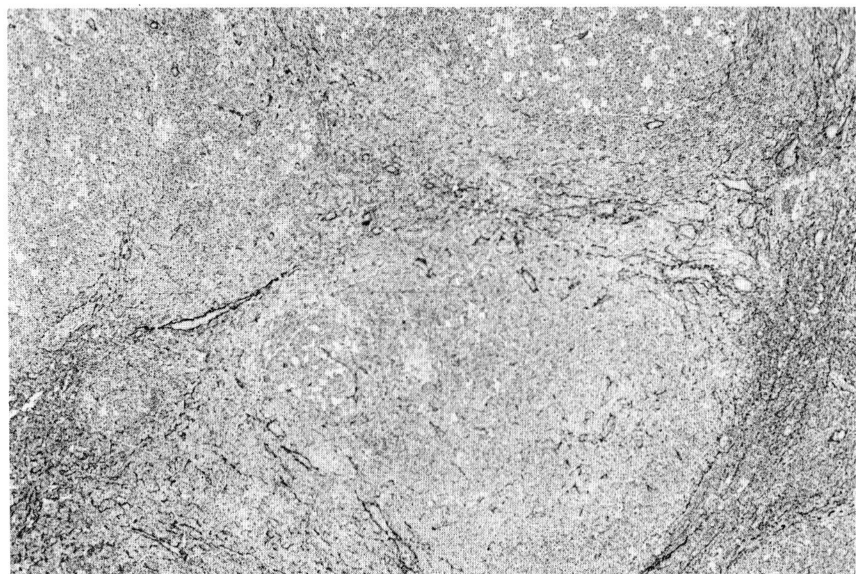

Fig. 6.10 Another field from the same node as Fig. 6.9. Silver impregnation delineates the follicles more clearly. (Gordon and Sweets reticulin × 47)

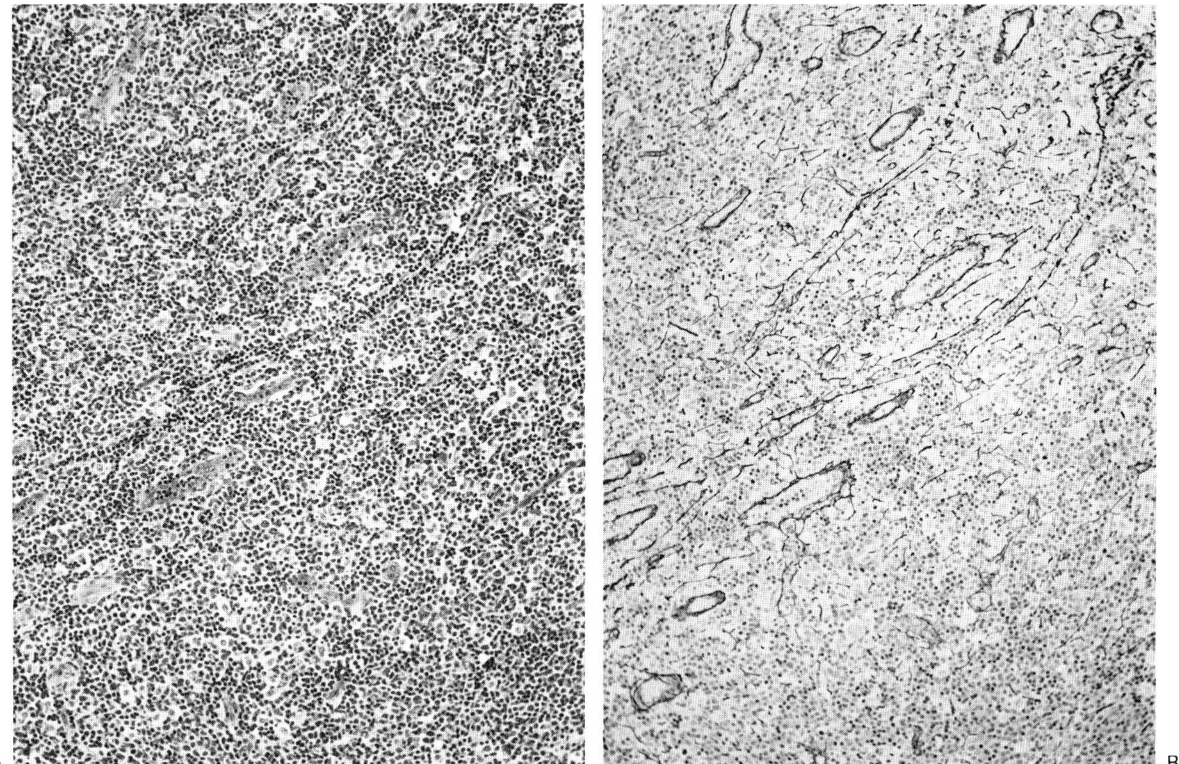

Fig. 6.11 (a) and (b) Axillary lymph node from a boy of 7 showing extreme follicular hyperplasia. The lymphocyte corona has disappeared so that the margin of the follicle (bottom right) is no longer discernible in (a). Silver impregnation shows the venules and reveals the follicular pattern more clearly. ((a) H E (b) Gordon and Sweets reticulin. Both × 120)

minal centre cells, until these are reduced to isolated centrocytes or centroblasts and the germinal centre is no longer recognisable (Fig. 6.12). At this stage the affected follicle has the appearance of a very large primary follicle and only on high power examination can scattered germinal centre cells be identified. Around the disintegrated germinal centre, a halo of small epithelioid cell clusters may develop, perhaps provoked by the release of entrapped antigen–antibody complexes (Fig. 6.13).

This event can be seen in lymph nodes from adults or children and whilst its precise significance is uncertain, it may on occasions presage the development of Hodgkin's disease (Poppema et al, 1979) (see p. 265).

Plasmacytosis

Although a plasma cell reaction is often accompanied by obvious follicular hyperplasia, this is not always the case and the two phenomena do not necessarily parallel one another in intensity. Indeed one may sometimes see a diffuse and massive plasma cell infiltration of the node pulp in the presence of quite small germinal centres, or even in the total absence of lymph follicles (Fig. 6.14). The picture then needs to be distinguished from that of a plasmacytoma or lymphoplasmacytoid lymphoma (see p. 249).

In some of the more acute examples of reactive plasmacytosis, the cellular infiltrate includes plasma cells of *all degrees of maturity*, even including plasmablasts and immunoblasts, there is, however, no cellular atypia (see Fig. 6.15). In more chronic cases, the plasma cells are all of mature type, although binucleate and sometimes multinucleate forms may be found. Russell bodies may also be a feature. There may be pronounced thick-

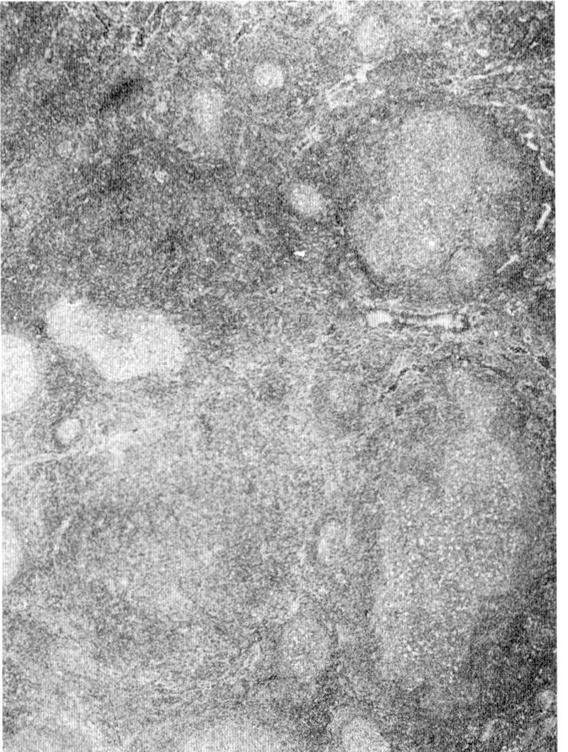

Fig. 6.12 Axillary lymph node from a boy of 9 showing progressive transformation of germinal centres. A hyperplastic germinal centre is seen at lower right. Other enlarged follicles have undergone transformation into less distinct nodules (top right and lower left). (H E × 18)

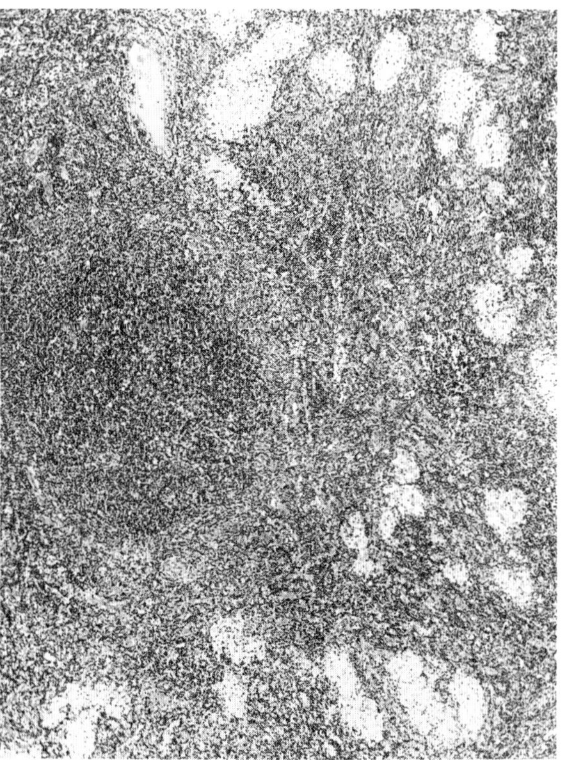

Fig. 6.13 A progressively transformed germinal centre (left) surrounded by small clusters of epithelioid cells. No trace of the original germinal centre can be seen. (H E × 47)

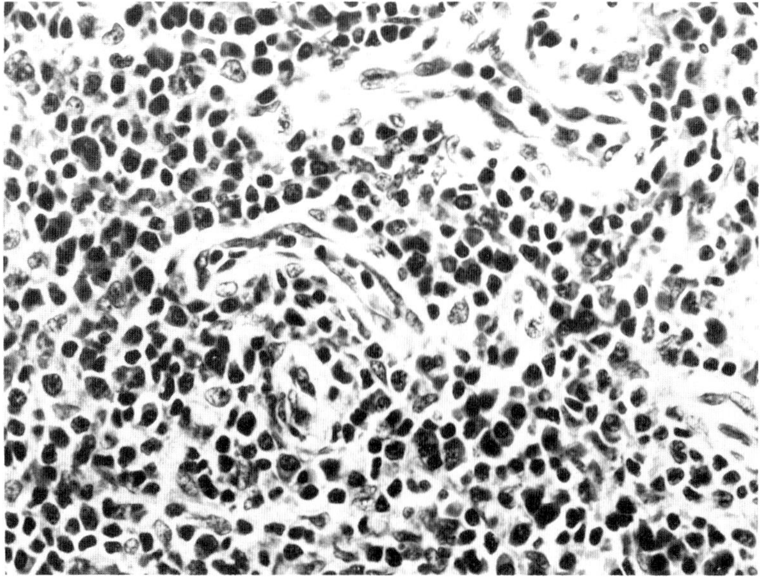

Fig. 6.14 Inguinal lymph node from a woman of 66 showing striking reactive plasmacytosis. Follicles were absent and the entire node pulp was filled with plasma cells of varying maturity. The thick-walled, hyalinised venules distinguish this picture from that of angioimmunoblastic lymphadenopathy. (H E × 470)

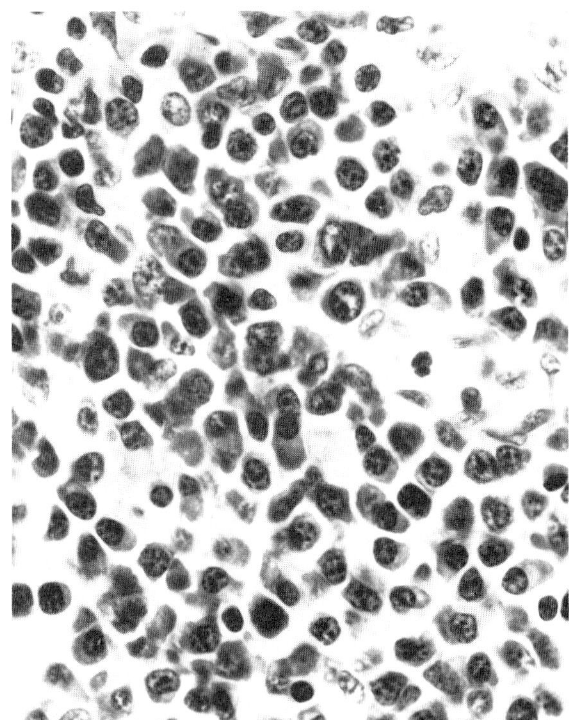

Fig. 6.15 Lymph node showing reactive plasmacytosis. Two plasmablasts (above centre) are seen, together with plasma cells of varying degrees of maturity. Contrast with Fig. 10.32 (p. 250) which shows the much greater uniformity of the cells in a plasmacytoma. (H E × 750)

ening of the walls of the venules which are often a prominent feature in such cases (Fig. 6.14). Striking reactive plasmacytosis is sometimes an accompaniment of Hodgkin's disease and is also seen in some cases of immunoblastic lymphadenopathy (p. 176). In all these instances the plasma cells are polyclonal, both types of light chain being represented when immunostaining is carried out.

Predominantly T-lymphocyte response

This type of reaction is perhaps most characteristically seen in certain viral infections but more chronic T-zone hyperplasia without obvious cause is sometimes encountered (Fig. 6.16). In the most acute type of reaction, e.g. infectious mononucleosis (see p. 129), the follicles may be suppressed and may disappear altogether whilst the paracortex is expanded and contains prominent post-capillary venules as well as many transformed lymphocytes (T-immunoblasts). The effect is often to convey an impression of effacement of normal architectural features and this, combined with the presence of blast cells and mitotic activity, may lead to an erroneous diagnosis of malignant lymphoma.

In less severe T-cell reactions, e.g. Herpes zoster, the presence of isolated T-immunoblasts, randomly distributed amongst small lymphocytes in the expanded paracortical areas, gives a distinctive 'spotty' appearance to the node at low magnification (see p. 134). A somewhat similar effect can also be brought about by the presence of increased numbers of interdigitating reticulum cells in the T-zones, as may be found in the early stages of dermatopathic lymphadenitis. Clusters of plasmacytoid T cells (see p. 78) may also impart a characteristic appearance to the node. In all these situations the T-zonal character of the response

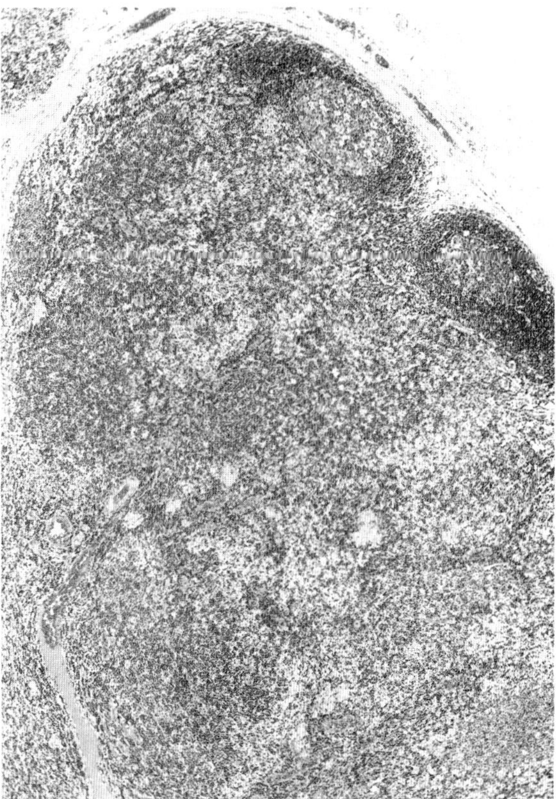

Fig. 6.16 Lymph node from a man of 38 showing small, inactive cortical follicles and marked hyperplasia of the paracortex (H E × 47)

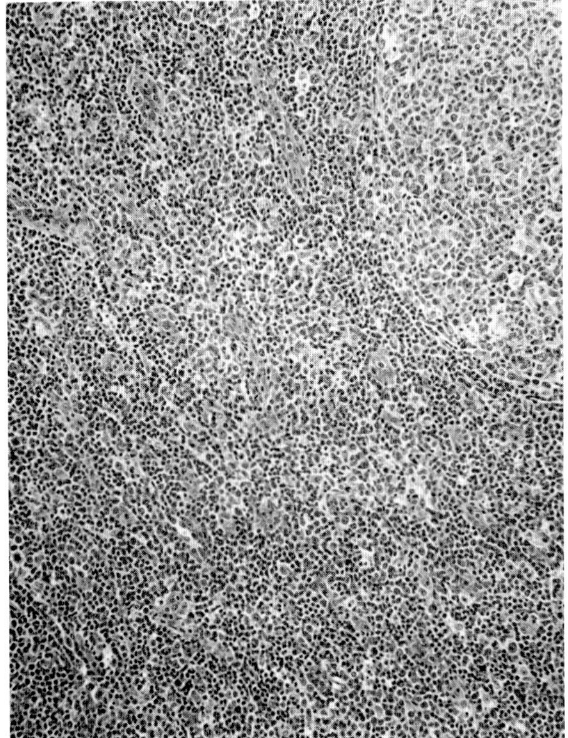

Fig. 6.17 Adult lymph node showing active hyperplasia in both B and T cell areas. Part of a reactive follicle is seen (upper right) with expanded paracortex below and to the left. (H E × 120)

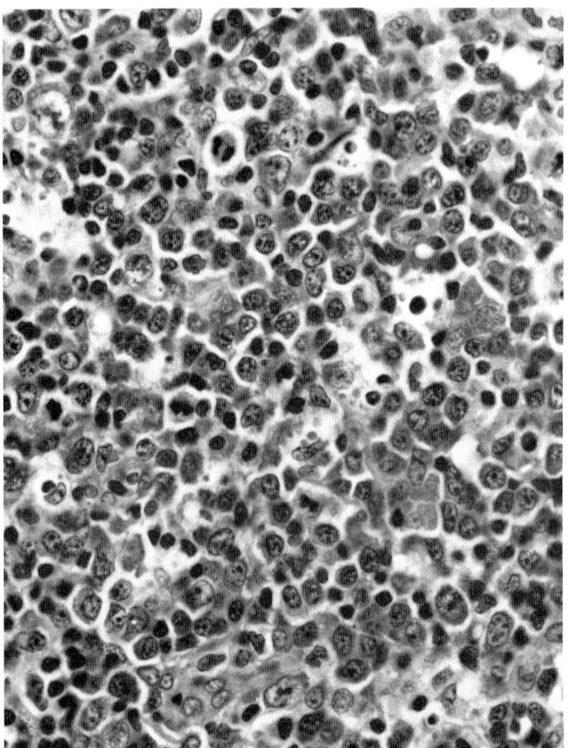

Fig. 6.18 High power views of same node as Fig. 6.17 showing detail of paracortical infiltrate. The mixed character of the infiltrate is apparent with 'blast' cells mingling with lymphocytes and plasma cells of varying maturity. Note mitoses. (H E × 470)

can be recognised not only by the absence or relative suppression of follicles, but also by the increased prominence of post-capillary venules.

In many instances of lymphadenitis the reaction seen in the lymph node bears the stamp of a mixed B and T cell response, that is, follicular hyperplasia of varying degree is associated with broad interfollicular zones containing prominent venules and a mixed cellular infiltrate which includes plasma cells as well as T lymphocytes and interdigitating reticulum cells (Figs 6.17, 6.18).

SPECIFIC TYPES OF LYMPHADENITIS

In this section an attempt will be made to describe some of the more important specific varieties of lymphadenitis of known aetiology. The number of known agents which may cause lymphadenitis is very great and a comprehensive account of all documented causes is beyond the scope of this book. For a fuller account the reader is referred to the Chapter on this subject in *Systemic Pathology* Volume 2 (Symmers, 1978).

It is difficult to tabulate the different varieties of lymphadenitis according to the type of histological reaction, e.g. granulomatous or non-granulomatous, for the same agent may at different times excite different reactions. We shall therefore classify the types of lymphadenitis in terms of the aetiological agent or agents concerned, in so far as these are known, starting with the infective causes. Stress will be laid on those conditions which commonly cause lymphadenopathy and, in particular, those in which lymph node biopsy is frequently performed for diagnostic purposes.

BACTERIAL INFECTIONS

Pyogenic cocci — anthrax — diphtheria

An acute lymphadenitis is a regular feature of these types of infection. The nodes involved are of course those which drain the primary source of infection, whether it be the skin, the throat or elsewhere. The nodes often enlarge rapidly, are painful and tender, and there is pronounced periadenitis and oedema of surrounding tissues. It is rare for lymph node biopsy to be performed in these diseases and in anthrax the procedure itself may be dangerous, for the organisms are often present in large numbers in the lymph node. The histological picture in each of these conditions is that of a severe acute lymphadenitis often with necrosis and haemorrhage and, except for the presence of the causative organism in the first two conditions, the picture is non-specific. *B.anthracis* may be identified in a Gram stain on a fresh imprint of the node draining a malignant pustule. Pyogenic coccal infection, especially that due to *Staphylococcus aureus*, if not treated promptly, may progress to suppuration and form an abscess, with total destruction of the original node.

Bubonic plague

The 'buboes' which characterise this condition are of course lymph nodal swellings. Since the infection is generally transmitted by the bites of rat fleas, the lymphadenitis affects primarily superficial groups of lymph nodes, usually in the inguinal region, less often the axilla. The nodal enlargement is often dramatic and is accompanied by fever and rapid prostration. Histologically the nodes show massive, confluent necrosis, often haemorrhagic, with variable polymorph infiltration, but without evidence of reaction on the part of the few residual lymphoid cells. *P.pestis* is a Gram negative organism but may be demonstrated by thionin or other appropriate stains, since it is generally present in large numbers. Death is accelerated by disseminated intravascular coagulation and venous thrombi may be readily detected in the tissues at post-mortem.

Tularaemia

As with plague, tularaemia is nowadays predominantly a disease of the tropics and sub-tropics and although it has been reported in Europe, it is much more frequently encountered in the Southern USA where it is prevalent among ground squirrels and other rodents. This disease in man has much in common with plague: it is transmitted chiefly by ticks and other biting insects and it is caused by a related organism — *Francisella* (formerly *Pasteurella*) *tularensis*. A similar pattern of nodal involvement is seen and again the histological features in the more acute cases are those of an acute lymphadenitis with widespread necrosis. Tularaemia is, however, generally less serious than plague and although rapidly fatal cases do occur, it is often a milder, more chronic disease, as exemplified by a European case (Wood et al, 1976). In the more chronic forms of the disease the lymph node reaction is granulomatous and may be frankly tuberculoid with central necrosis of caseous appearance and surrounding epithelioid cell reaction,

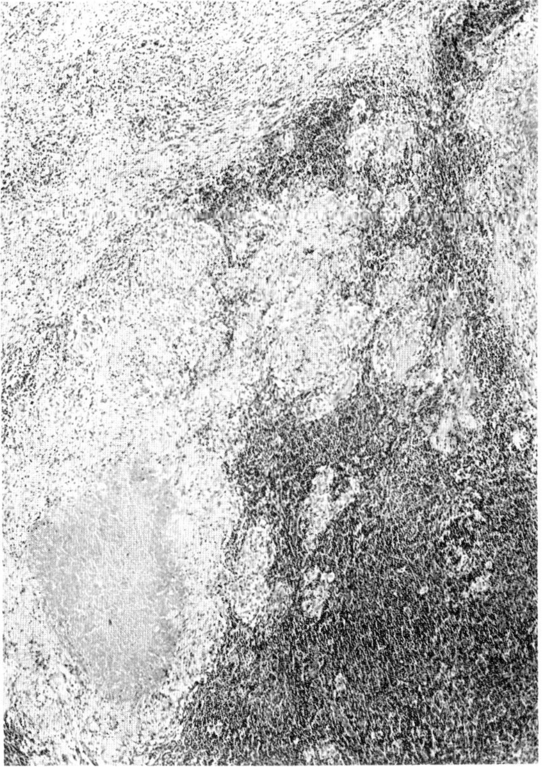

Fig. 6.19 Margin of lymph node in tularaemia showing focal granulomatous inflammation with caseous necrosis and gross capsular thickening (case of Wood et al, 1976). (H E × 47)

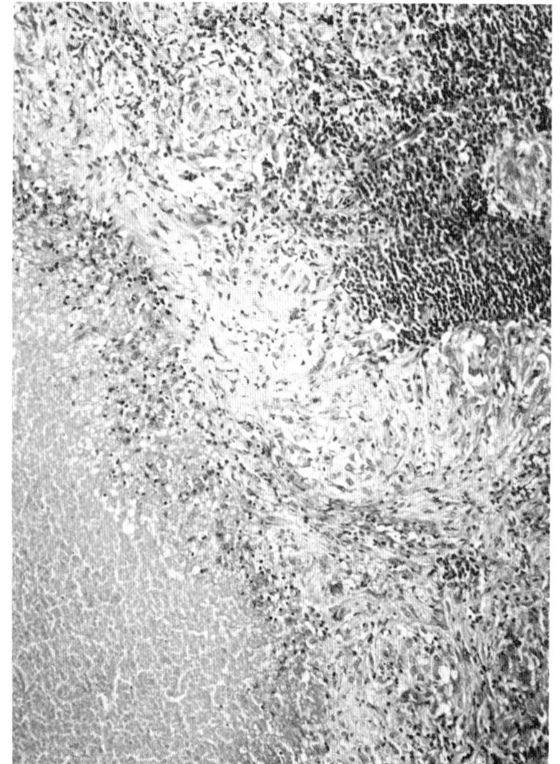

Fig. 6.20 Higher power view of same node as Figure 6.19. Note the general similarity to tuberculosis (HE × 120)

sometimes including multinucleate giant-cells of Langhans type (Figs. 6.19, 6.20).

Yersinia lymphadenitis

(Pseudotuberculosis)

Two closely related organisms, *Yersinia* (formerly *Pasteurella*) *pseudotuberculosis* and *Y. enterocolitica*, cause focal inflammatory lesions in the gut with a secondary mesenteric lymphadenitis which often dominates the clinical picture. The name pseudotuberculosis probably stems as much from the clinical similarity to tuberculosis of the mesenteric nodes, as from the similarity of the pathological features. The name dates from the time when tuberculosis was rife in Britain and 'tabes mesenterica' was frequently seen. Infection is probably due in most instances to ingestion of uncooked food contaminated by the organism which is often endemic in rodent populations and may also be carried by wood pigeons. Widespread in distribution, the disease is not uncommon in Britain and is probably more frequent than is generally realised. The primary lesion most often affects the Peyer's patches of the lower ileum or the lymphoid tissue of the appendix, but in many instances the primary lesion is insignificant and is overshadowed by the associated mesenteric lymphadenitis. There may be simulation of acute appendicitis with right iliac fossa pain and tenderness accompanied by fever. At laparotomy, the ileocolic nodes are swollen and hyperaemic with or without an overlying peritoneal reaction, but the appendix and intestine may appear outwardly normal. In these circumstances, lymph node biopsy may be performed to establish the diagnosis, which can be confirmed by culture of the organism or, more often, by serological tests for appropriate antibodies, which will identify the species of *Yersinia* involved. The distinction between infections caused by these two organisms cannot be made on histological grounds for the histological features are similar in both, but it now seems that infections in man are more commonly due to *Y. enterocolitica*. The microscopic features are sufficiently distinctive, when the picture is fully developed, to establish the diagnosis with reasonable certainty, taking into account the clinical features and the site of the involved nodes. Without this knowledge, there could be confusion with a variety of infections, but especially with cat scratch disease or lymphogranuloma venereum, in both of which the histological picture is somewhat similar.

Sharply defined 'geographical' foci of necrosis or actual microabscesses (Fig. 6.21) stand out against a background of non-specific inflammation and reactive follicular hyperplasia in the node. At an early stage the abscesses are poorly defined (Fig. 6.22) but later they become clearly demarcated and are thrown into relief by a surrounding border of macrophages (Fig. 6.23), sometimes with a palisaded arrangement and sometimes showing an occasional multinucleate giant cell (Fig. 6.24). The resemblance to tuberculosis is, however, not very close as a rule. The necrotic foci show complete cell breakdown and are often filled with degenerating polymorphs and nuclear debris. These foci may be small and sparse or may occupy

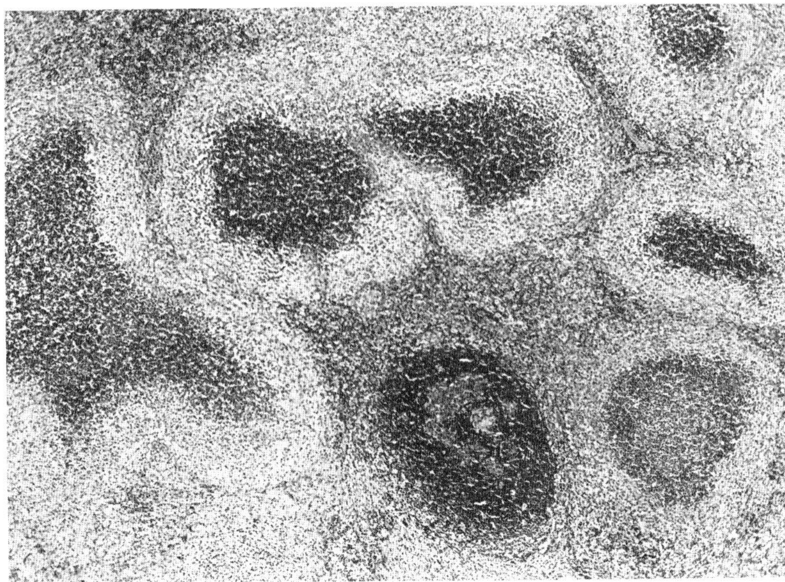

Fig. 6.21 Mesenteric lymph node in Yersinial lymphadenitis showing multiple micro-abscesses and a single residual lymph follicle (below) (H E × 47)

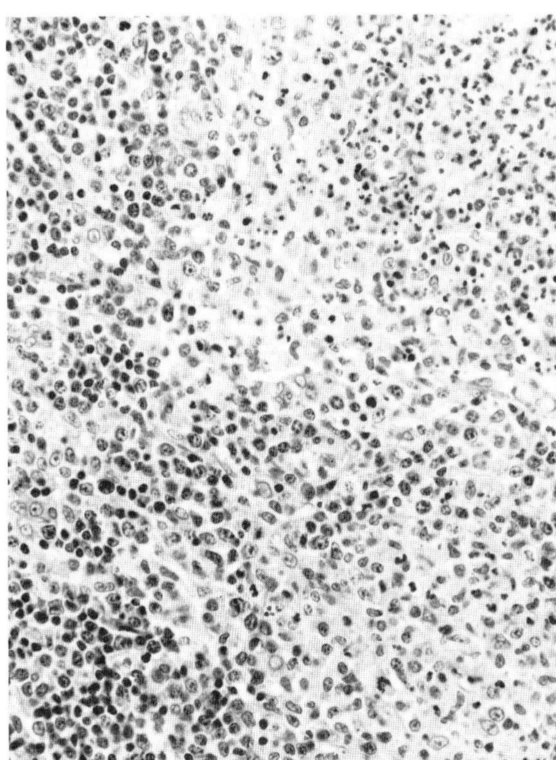

Fig. 6.22 Mesenteric lymph node showing early lesion of Yersinial lymphadenitis. The margin of a poorly defined microabscess is seen (top right). (H E × 300)

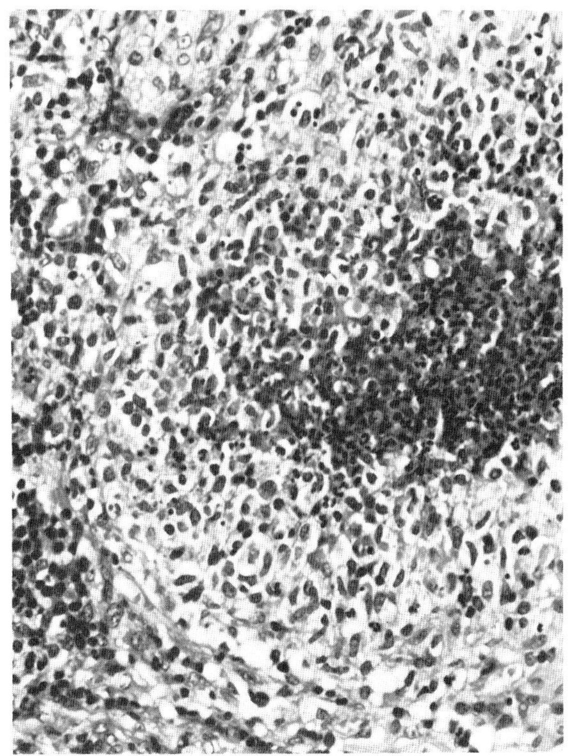

Fig. 6.23 Fully developed microabscess in Yersinial lymphadenitis (same node as Fig. 6.21). Closely packed neutrophil polymorphs are enclosed by a zone of macrophages. (H E × 300)

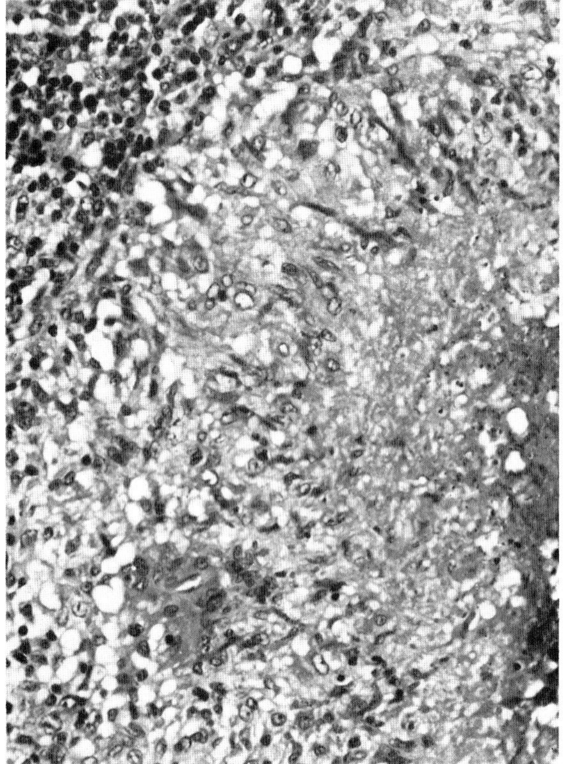

Fig. 6.24 Focal lesion of Yersinial lymphadenitis at a later stage (same node as Figs 6.21 and 6.23). The polymorphs at the centre have degenerated leaving an area of amorphous necrotic debris enclosed by palisaded macrophages. (H E × 300)

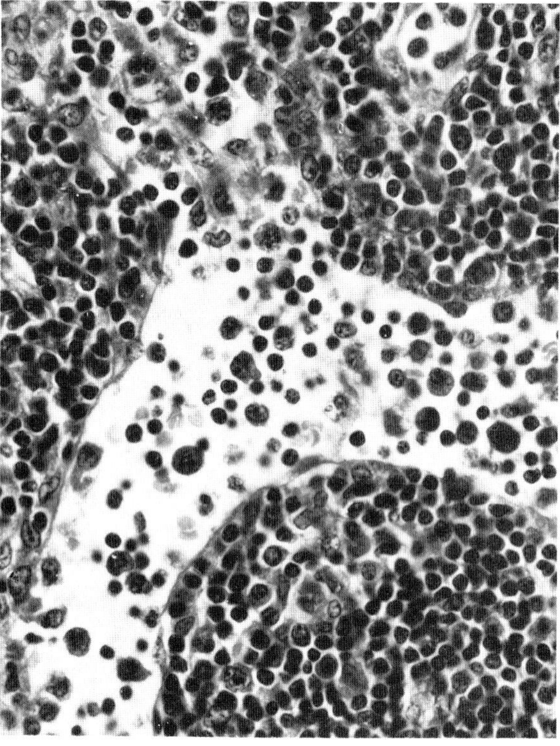

Fig. 6.25 Medullary sinuses from another case of Yersinial lymphadenitis showing large basophilic immunoblasts lying free in the sinuses. A similar picture may be seen in 'non-specific' mesenteric lymphadenitis. (H E × 470)

almost the entire node. In surviving areas there is often evidence of a vigorous immune response and besides follicular hyperplasia, large basophilic immunoblasts may be seen in the pulp and sinuses of the node (Fig. 6.25).

Although the clinical presentation of 'acute mesenteric adenitis' in children is similar, whatever the cause, the histological changes described above serve to distinguish those cases due to *Yersinia* infection from those described merely as 'non-specific'. Even when a mesenteric node biopsy discloses these distinctive changes, however, bacteriological confirmation of the diagnosis should always be attempted by culture of the organism or by serological means. It is probable, though seldom proven, that many cases of non-specific mesenteric adenitis in childhood are due to viruses.

Typhoid fever

The lymph node lesions in typhoid fever are as characteristic of the disease as the lesions in the intestinal lymphoid tissue, although the diagnosis is rarely made on lymph node biopsy. Laparotomy is only likely to be undertaken when perforation of the intestine has occurred. It is, of course, the mesenteric nodes that are primarily involved and, at the height of the disease, these are swollen with punctate areas of necrosis visible on the cut surface. Microscopy shows widespread infiltration of affected nodes, as of the Peyer's patches, by characteristic mononuclear macrophages which progressively replace the normal lymphocyte population. Within the macrophage infiltrate there are ill-defined foci of necrosis, accompanied by nuclear karyorrhexis, which become confluent as

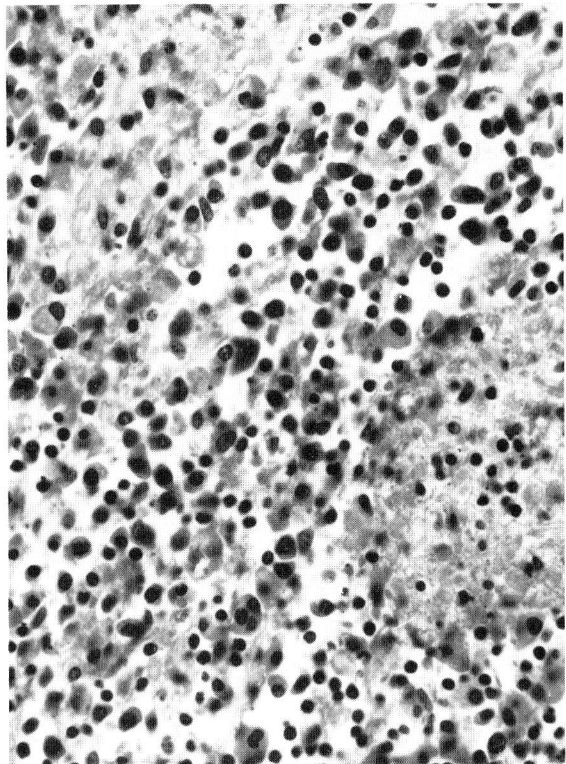

Fig. 6.26 Mesenteric lymph node in typhoid fever (post-mortem specimen) showing characteristic rounded macrophages and foci of necrosis (H E × 470)

the disease advances. In the fully developed lesion the histological appearances are sufficiently distinctive to be virtually diagnostic (Fig. 6.26). Granuloma formation does not occur.

Brucellosis (undulant fever)

Significant peripheral lymphadenopathy is not a common feature of human infection by *Brucella abortus*, *Br. melitensis* or *Br. suis* and it occurs only in chronic cases. However, despite the fact that the nodes may be clinically unimpressive, lymph node biopsy may be resorted to, nevertheless, in a patient with an obscure febrile illness, sometimes associated with splenomegaly as well. The pathological features are similar in each of these infections. The changes may amount to no more than a non-specific reactive hyperplasia, but generally there are clusters of epithelioid histiocytes in the pulp. These may be small and scanty or they may form large non-caseating granulomas associated with a mixed infiltrate of eosinophils and plasma cells. The presence of scattered, large, and sometimes binucleate, cells (probably immunoblasts) in this mixed infiltrate has at times caused confusion with Hodgkin's disease, but typical Sternberg-Reed cells are lacking. Although the granulomatous aspect of the biopsy may suggest the diagnosis of brucellosis, the picture is not diagnostic and the diagnosis should be confirmed by recovery of the organism or by serological means.

Tuberculosis

The dramatic decline in the incidence of pulmonary tuberculosis in Britain in the present century is reflected in a similar decline in the incidence of tuberculous lymphadenitis. The disease is still rife, however, in parts of Asia and elsewhere and most cases seen in the UK today are in Asian immigrants.

Lymph node tuberculosis is particularly characteristic of primary infections and is then seen in the regional nodes draining the portal of entry of *Mycobacterium tuberculosis* or *M. bovis*. Thus, the cervical nodes are involved in the case of tonsillar infection, the bronchopulmonary and tracheobronchial nodes in the case of lung infection and the mesenteric nodes in the case of intestinal (Peyer's patches) infection. Less frequently, primary infections in the eye, ear, skin or mouth may affect the appropriate lymph nodes draining these sites. Widespread nodal tuberculosis is much less frequent in man and its occurrence generally implies an unusual degree of susceptibility to the disease in that individual. It is sometimes seen in old age.

Clinically, tuberculous cervical nodes may be soft or firm in consistency, mobile or fixed and matted. In advanced cases a sinus may have formed to the skin surface. Even when the diagnosis is obvious or strongly suspected, biopsy is still justified by the desirability of removing diseased nodes and culturing the organism to determine its sensitivity to anti-tuberculous drugs. If, at the time of biopsy, tuberculosis is suspected, it is important to ensure that at least a part of the biopsy tissue is put into a sterile dry container for microbiological examination and culture. By the same token, care should be taken in handling fresh tissue to prevent the possible spread of infection and sectioning the fresh tissue in the cryostat should not be undertaken.

The macroscopic features of tuberculous nodes have already been mentioned in Chapter 5 (p. 68). They are often sufficiently distinctive for the diagnosis to be made at this stage and thus the necessary precautions taken. Caseous necrosis, which is such a common feature of nodal tuberculosis, shows up on the cut surface of the node as opaque, chalky, or creamy-white patches. At times, the whole node or the greater part of it may be destroyed by caseation or the white caseous centre may be surrounded by a zone of translucent grey fibrous tissue. In arrested disease, the caseous areas commonly undergo calcification and then the centre of the node may be converted into a dense, radio-opaque, rock-hard mass. Such nodes are still a common finding at post-mortem in the ileocolic mesentery of elderly subjects, where they almost certainly represent the result of drinking milk infected by *M. bovis* in the days before the general introduction of pasteurisation. On other occasions, the occurrence of caseous necrosis in a node may be concealed by secondary suppuration and 'cold abscess' formation. In these circumstances, the diagnosis of tuberculous lymphadenitis may not be suspected at this stage, and the condition may be mistaken for a simple suppurative lymphadenitis or a breaking down neoplasm.

The histological features of typical fibrocaseous tuberculosis of lymph nodes are too well known to require lengthy description. The diagnostic feature is the presence of 'tubercles' — epithelioid cell granulomata of varying size, often containing multinucleate giant-cells of Langhans type, and generally displaying central necrosis if the lesion is of sufficient size (Fig. 6.27). The same description might equally well be applied to several other 'tuberculoid' diseases, which have these histological features in common, but the bare words are inadequate to convey the very distinctive character of tuberculous lesions under the microscope, which often allows a confident diagnosis of tuberculosis to be made even without the demonstration of acid-alcohol-fast *Mycobacteria*. Two points require stressing: (1) The characteristic giant-cells, with their horseshoe-shaped arrangement of nuclei, often lie at the centre of a focal aggregate of epithelioid cells to form a 'giant-cell system' (Fig. 6.28). It is these giant-cell systems and not just the giant-cells themselves, which are so typical of tuberculosis. Even without the presence of giant-cells, the epithelioid cells of tuberculosis often form these same distinctive aggregates. (2) The caseous necrosis of tuberculosis is qualitatively different in appearance from necrosis in general. The structural outlines of the dead tissue are quickly lost and the latter is 'melted down' into a finely granular, eosinophilic, amorphous mass, which is rarely mimicked by other diseases (Fig. 6.29).

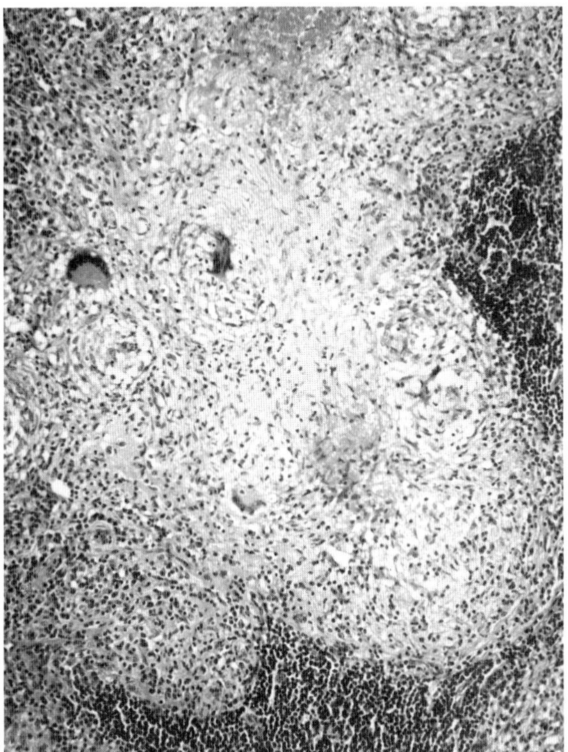

Fig. 6.27 Cervical lymph node showing typical features of active tuberculous lymphadenitis with early caseous necrosis at the centres of the conglomerate tubercles (H E × 120)

The details of the histological picture of course vary from case to case, depending on the duration and activity of the disease, as well as the host response. In early lymph node involvement, as may be seen for example in lymph nodes draining a tuberculous joint, there may merely be small, scattered epithelioid cell granulomata, without giant-

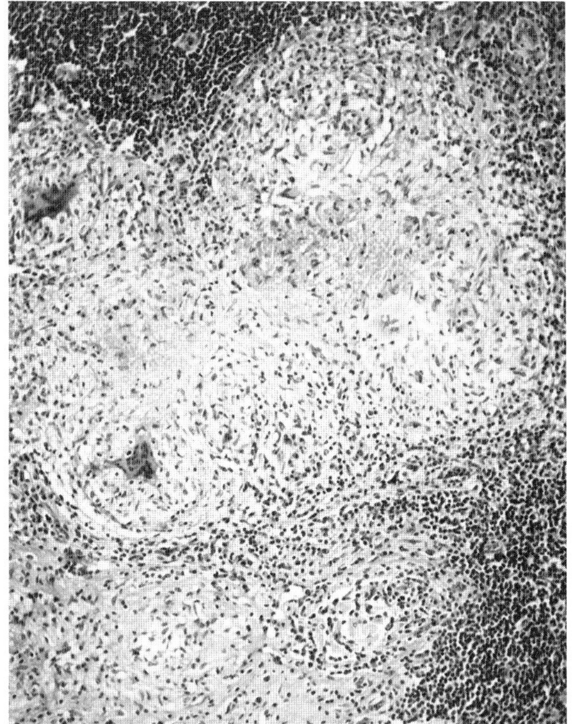

Fig. 6.28 Tuberculous lymphadenitis showing two typical 'giant-cell systems' (left) and early caseous necrosis. Note hyaline fibrosis in lower part of field. (H E × 120)

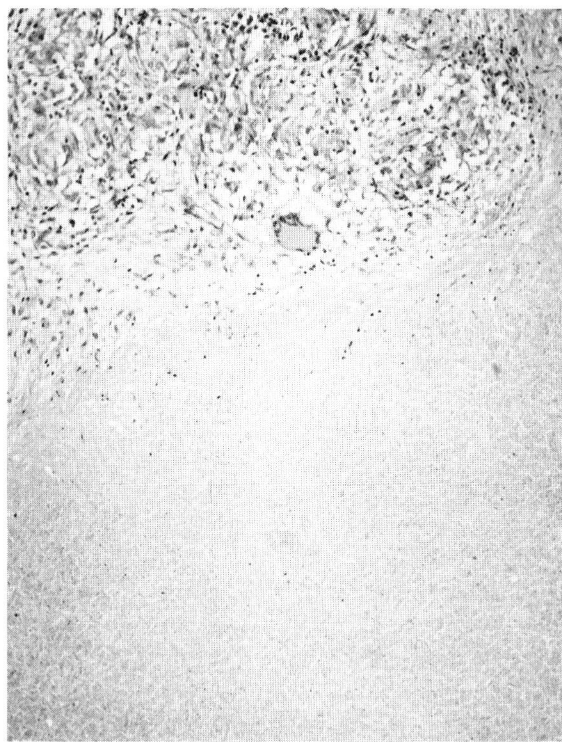

Fig. 6.29 More advanced tuberculous lymphadenitis showing tubercles bordering an extensive area of caseation (H E × 120)

cells or caseation. In such instances the diagnosis is heavily dependent on the demonstration of acid-alcohol-fast organisms in the lesions, or on culture of the node. At the opposite extreme, the whole node may have been destroyed by the spread of caseous necrosis, with little cellular reaction remaining. The rate of progression of the lesion is again very variable. In active lesions, early 'satellite' tubercles are often to be seen at the margin of larger and obviously older, caseating lesions. When the caseous necrosis is extending, fresh necrosis may be identified in the surrounding granulomatous zone, so that the margin of the caseous centre is blurred. In more stable lesions, the caseous material may sometimes be surrounded by a 'palisade' of radially arranged epithelioid histiocytes, such as may be seen in cat-scratch disease and many other similar, necrotising lesions. Occasionally breakdown and liquefaction of the caseous material may ensue, with or without polymorph infiltration. Arrest or healing of the process is marked by 'walling off' of the necrotic foci by dense fibrous tissue, diminution of the granulomatous reaction and deposition of calcium salts in the caseous material. The extent of surrounding fibrosis varies and is sometimes considerable. On rare occasions, spreading, invasive fibrosis has been reported in the mediastinum with envelopment of neighbouring structures, such as is apparently more commonly seen as a sequel of histoplasmosis (Goodwin et al, 1972).

In tuberculous lymphadenitis, as in other granulomatous diseases of lymph nodes, the pathologist's attention is naturally drawn to the granulomatous lesions themselves, often to the neglect of the background immunological response. It is, however, important to note the changes in those parts of the node which remain uninvolved. As might be anticipated in a disease without a striking antibody response to the causative organism, follicular hyperplasia is lacking and plasma cells are generally scanty. On the other hand, there is an abundance of small lymphocytes, many of which are probably T-cells.

The above account relates to the normal form of tuberculosis, whether seen in lymph nodes or other tissues. Apart from the modifications of this process resulting from coincident pneumoconiosis, which need not concern us here, there are two main variant patterns in nodal tuberculosis. These are: (1) non-reactive tuberculosis and (2) tuberculosis without hypersensitivity (endothelial tuberculosis)

1. Non-reactive tuberculosis. In general, tuberculosis is a chronic disorder of slow progression, but at times the disease may present as an acute, febrile illness with rapid loss of weight. This type of presentation may occur either with generalised miliary dissemination of the disease or with the absence or loss of natural defence against *M. tuberculosis.* In the latter circumstance, the organisms may multiply unchecked and whilst, in chronic tuberculosis, acid-alcohol-fast *Mycobacteria* are often difficult to find in sections stained by the Ziehl-Neelsen method, in this non-reactive form of the disease, huge numbers of *Mycobacteria* may be found (Fig, 6.30), identifiable as red masses on the slide under the low power of the microscope. Disseminated nodal tuberculosis is often of this non-reactive type. Various factors may predispose to the development of non-reactive tuberculosis, amongst which may be named — total lack of previous exposure to infection with *M. tuberculosis* in an adult subject, malnutrition, other debilitating disease and chronic myeloid leukaemia.

Macroscopically, the nodes may show extensive ill-defined, pale, lustreless, yellowish-grey areas on the cut surface but they lack the typical, opaque, white caseous foci associated with chronic tuberculosis. Histologically, large areas of necrosis, not typical of caseation but often containing fibrin and red cells as well as nuclear debris, merge with a poorly defined surrounding zone of macrophages (Fig. 6.31). There is little or no granuloma formation, giant cells and at times even macrophages are absent, in which case the term 'non-reactive'

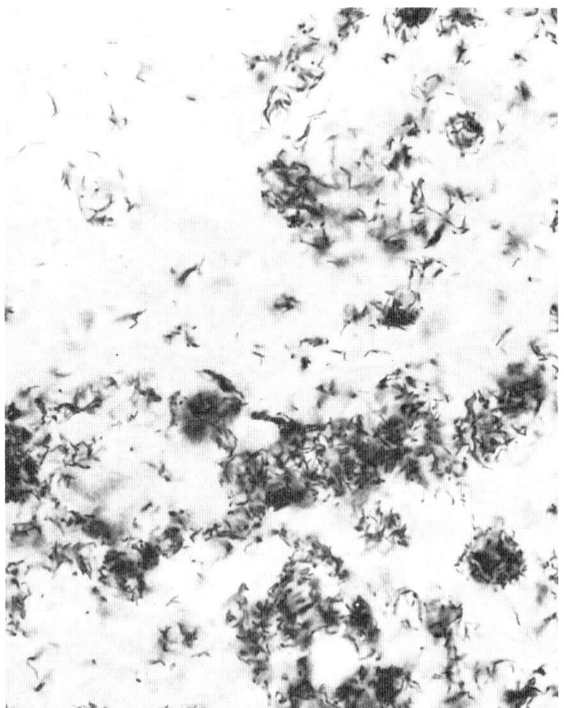

Fig. 6.30 Acute tuberculous lymphadenitis showing masses of *Myco. tuberculosis*, many contained within macrophages (Ziehl Neelsen × 940)

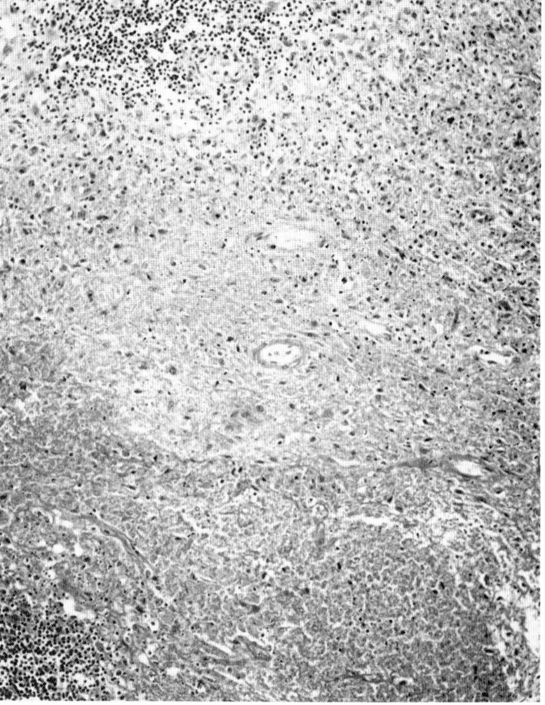

Fig. 6.31 Lymph node showing acute, non-reactive tuberculous lymphadenitis. Spreading caseation with minimal cellular reaction. (Same node as Fig. 6.30.) (H E × 120)

is indeed correctly applied. It is of course of the highest importance to recognise this picture for what it is, not merely for the sake of the patient, but for the sake of all those who might be exposed to infection. In any lymph node biopsies showing unexplained areas of necrosis with little or no cellular reaction, urgent examination for *M. tuberculosis* is mandatory.

2. *Tuberculosis without hypersensitivity.* In the absence of hypersensitivity to tuberculo-protein, which we now know to be mediated by a specific sub-set of T lymphocytes — K (= killer) cells, caseous necrosis does not occur and, in these circumstances, the reaction to tuberculosis in the tissues consists in the development of uniformly sized, non-caseating, epithelioid cell granulomata, sometimes containing multinucleate giant-cells (Fig. 6.32). In lymph nodes, the picture may be indistinguishable from that of sarcoidosis (p. 356) and only the demonstration of an occasional acid-alcohol-fast bacillus in the lesions or the subsequent development of overt tuberculosis in the patient may differentiate those cases which are tuberculous from those which are not. The tuberculin reaction is, of course, negative in either case, but becomes positive if conventional tuberculous disease develops. The apparent identity of the histological picture of 'endothelial tuberculosis' with that of sarcoidosis has for long led to debate as to the true nature of the latter (see p. 355).

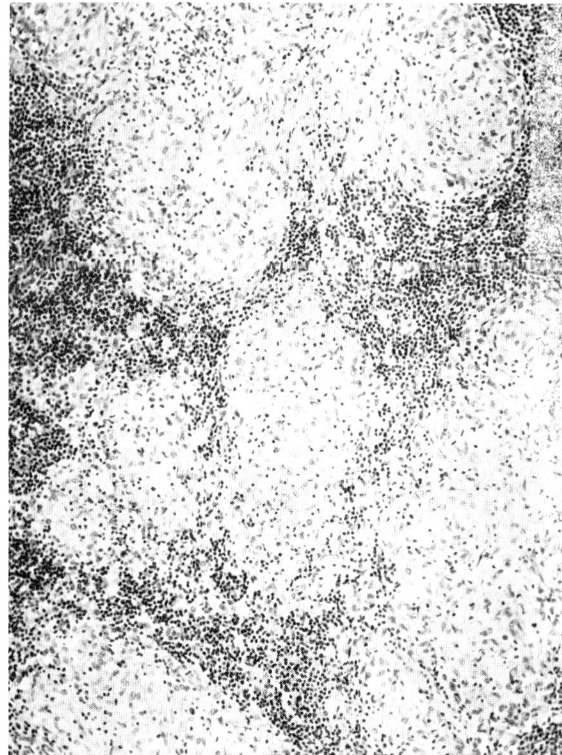

Fig. 6.32 Lymph node showing 'endothelial' tuberculous lymphadenitis. The node was filled with discrete non-caseating granulomata resembling the lesions of sarcoidosis. Occasional acid-alcohol-fast organisms were found. (H E × 120)

Mycobacterial histiocytosis — lymphadenitis due to BCG

The attenuated form of *M. tuberculosis* — the *Bacille Calmette-Guérin* (BCG), which has been very widely used in Britain and continental Europe for prophylactic immunisation against tuberculosis, may at times provoke significant enlargement of the lymph nodes (generally axillary) draining the inoculation site. Biopsy is rarely undertaken for in most instances the cause of the lymphadenopathy is obvious, but occasionally such nodes have been removed for examination. Sometimes the nodes have broken down and formed sinuses and in such instances there is obvious necrosis on biopsy, but at other times the node presents a massive infiltration of histiocytes, without focal granuloma formation, giant-cells, or necrosis and the picture may closely resemble that of lepromatous leprosy (Symmers, 1978, p. 605). In either event, acid-alcohol-fast bacilli are generally present in large numbers in the node.

Lymphadenitis due to 'atypical' Mycobacteria

With the decline in frequency of infections caused by *M. tuberculosis* and *M. bovis*, clinicians and pathologists have become more aware of the existence of other mycobacterial diseases in man. Their true incidence has yet to be defined. The degree to which these infections mimic tuberculosis varies, but in general the clinical illness produced is of a less serious nature than tuberculosis. Whilst lymphadenitis can probably be caused by a variety of these 'atypical' *Mycobacteria*, the most important organism from this point of view appears to be *M. scrofulaceum*, which, as its name implies, may

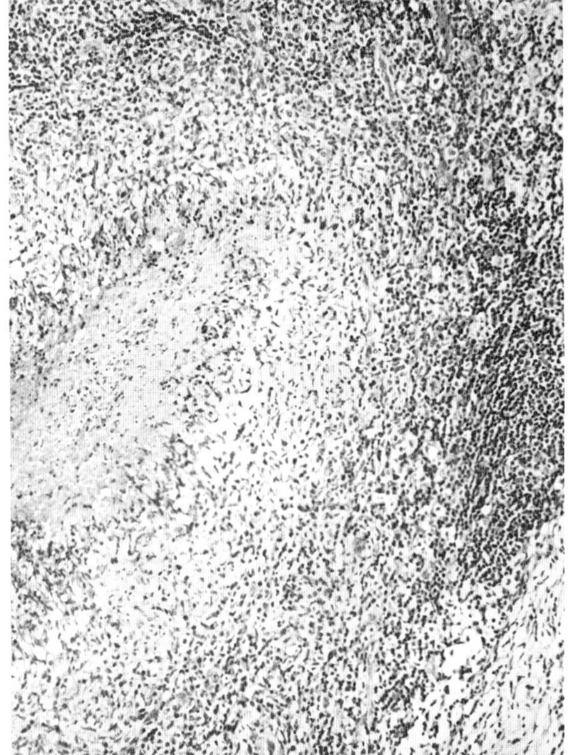

Fig. 6.33 Cervical lymph node from a boy of 9 showing focal granulomatous inflammation with central caseous necrosis due to *Myco. scrofulaceum*. The palisaded histiocytes are characteristic, but a similar picture may be seen in tuberculosis. (H E × 120)

cause cervical lymphadenopathy, especially in children. The histological picture is 'tuberculoid' in character with caseation and granuloma formation indistinguishable from that of tuberculosis (Fig. 6.33). No doubt many cases of 'tuberculous' cervical lymphadenitis in childhood, formerly attributed to *M. bovis* infection, have in fact been instances of *M. scrofulaceum* infection.

Leprosy

Mycobacterium leprae commonly gives rise to lymph node enlargement, more particularly in the lepromatous form of the disease, but lymph node biopsy will only be performed in a small minority of cases, since the diagnosis of leprosy is likely to have been confirmed from nasal scrapings or skin biopsy if the patient is picked up in an endemic area. Lymph node biopsy is most likely to be carried out in circumstances where leprosy is unsuspected and the pathologist should always be on the look out for it. The node is often from the axilla or groin. Unlike tuberculosis, the naked-eye features of the node are not distinctive. On the other hand, the histological picture is highly characteristic. In the early stages, the follicles persist although they do not show significant hyperplasia, whilst the paracortical areas are infiltrated by large, pale, rounded mononuclear histiocytes, often forming small clusters (Fig. 6.34). In conventionally stained sections the largest of these 'lepra cells' have clear, empty-looking vacuoles in the cytoplasm (globi) (Fig. 6.35), but with a modified Ziehl-Neelsen stain (e.g. the Wade-Fite method) the cytoplasm can be seen to be packed with acid-fast organisms (Fig. 6.36). As the disease advances, the number of these lepra cells steadily increases until the whole node is packed with them, the follicles having disappeared and most of the lymphocyte population too. There is

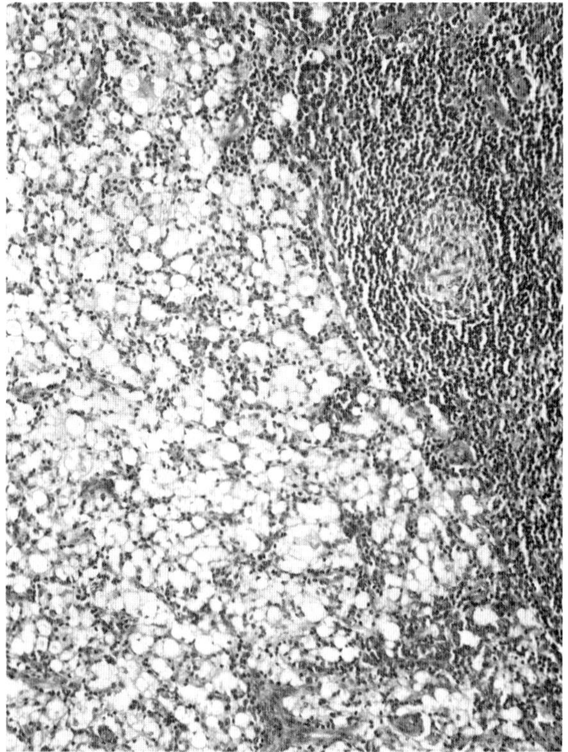

Fig. 6.34 Axillary lymph node from a case of lepromatous leprosy showing preservation of a follicle (upper right) and numerous lepra cells in paracortex (H E × 120)

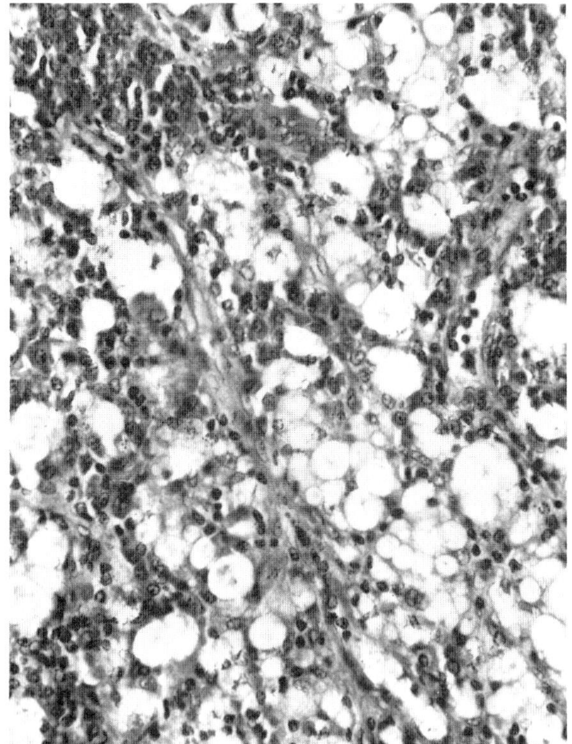

Fig. 6.35 Higher magnification of the same node as Fig. 6.34. There are numerous plasma cells between the often empty-looking lepra cells. (H E × 300)

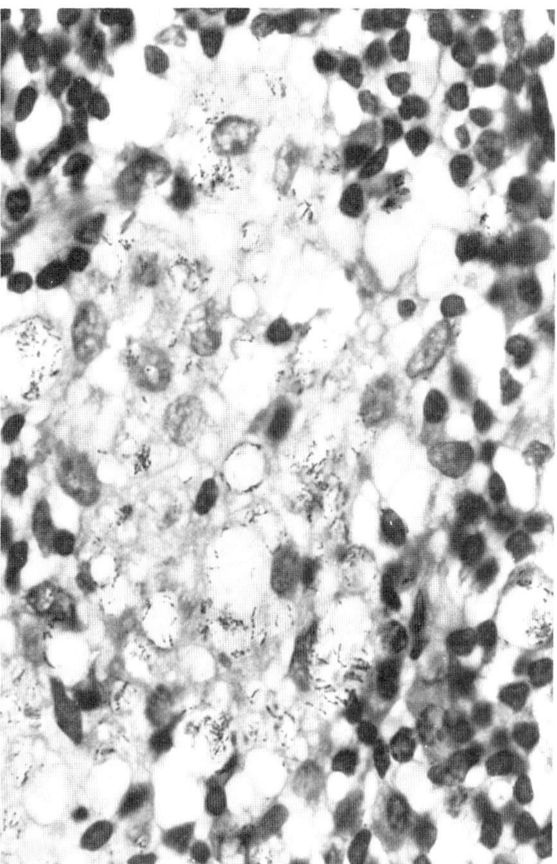

Fig. 6.36 Acid-fast *Myco. leprae* are present in large numbers within the characteristic macrophages. (Same lymph node as Figs 6.34 and 6.35.) (Wade-Fite × 750)

no granuloma formation and necrosis is rarely seen.

There are few conditions which closely mimic this picture. Similar clusters of large, vacuolated macrophages may be seen in silicone lymphadenopathy (Symmers, 1978, p. 569), resulting from the injection into the tissues of silicone preparations for cosmetic purposes. Likewise, the parenteral injection of polyvinylpyrrolidone (PVP) may result in somewhat similar changes in draining lymph nodes (see p. 359). The lepra cells could possibly be confused with 'signet-ring' cells from metastatic gastric carcinoma, but a negative stain for mucin will quickly eliminate that possibility.

Lymph node enlargement is less frequently seen in the tuberculoid and borderline types of leprosy. In the former, the node may show multiple, small, discrete non-caseating focal granulomata, closely resembling the lesion of sarcoidosis. *M. leprae* are difficult to demonstrate in these lesions. In borderline cases, the picture is generally similar to that of tuberculoid leprosy but may indeed be 'borderline' in showing the presence of some lepra cells.

Listeriosis

Listeriosis is caused by a small Gram-positive bacillus — *Listeria monocytogenes*, which infects a variety of animal hosts, from which transmission to man may occur. The disease is of world-wide distribution, but is uncommon in Britain. Human infections have been predominantly in newborn infants, due to placental transmission, and in the elderly, or in immune-compromised individuals. *L. monocytogenes* is thus properly regarded as an opportunistic organism. Whilst the disease is commonly a fulminating septicaemic infection, examples of localised lymphadenitis, usually cervical, are also documented. The involved lymph nodes may suppurate and lead to sinus formation. Macroscopically, affected tissues are reported as showing greyish-white spots which correspond to focal areas of necrosis seen under the microscope. In acute lesions the necrotic foci may be crowded with polymorphs and nuclear debris, but show little cellular reaction at the margin. Later the focus is replaced by macrophages which move in from the periphery (Ishak, 1976).

Melioidosis

Essentially a tropical disease, although cases have been reported from a number of countries, melioidosis is principally endemic in S E Asia. The disease is caused by a small motile, Gram-negative bacillus — *Pseudomonas pseudomallei* — which apparently lives in the soil and water in endemic areas. As with listeriosis, acute infections are generally septicaemic and often fatal, with severe pneumonia and lung abscesses developing. Chronic lesions are often localised to lungs, bones or lymph nodes. Histologically, these show focal areas of necrosis or suppuration with surrounding granulomatous reaction and an occasional giant-cell. In areas where melioidosis is endemic, the chronic form thus enters into the differential diagnosis of several other infectious diseases of lymph nodes, especially tuberculosis, *Yersinia* lymphadenitis, cat scratch disease and lymphogranuloma venereum. The diagnosis may be established by a specific haemagglutination test.

Centrally necrotic and suppurative granulomatous lesions of much the same kind are found in the lymph node lesions of chronic *Glanders*, which is rarely seen in man and has most often been acquired by those working with the organism — *Malleomyces mallei* — in the laboratory.

SPIROCHAETAL INFECTIONS

Syphilitic lymphadenitis

Syphilis is the most important spirochaetal infection to give rise to lymphadenopathy. Nodal involvement is principally a feature of primary and secondary syphilis; it is very rare in the tertiary stage, although a gummatous lymphadenitis can occur. Lymph node biopsy is only likely to be performed for diagnostic purposes in those cases where lymphadenopathy is the most obvious presenting feature and other lesions are either deliberately concealed by the patient or overlooked by both patient and doctor. This is in fact a more frequent occurrence than might be supposed. In the case of primary syphilis, the nodes most usually involved are in the inguinal group, and sometimes the femoral. It is fallacious to suppose that primary syphilitic lymphadenitis is always painless, as commonly stated, and an acutely painful femoral node may sometimes be mistaken for a strangulated femoral hernia and emergency surgery undertaken. The pain in such cases is attributable to ischaemic necrosis, presumably due to acute swelling of the node in the restricted space of the femoral canal (see Ch. 7, p. 145) (Fig. 6.37). The possibility of primary syphilis elsewhere than on the genitalia and in the perineum should not be

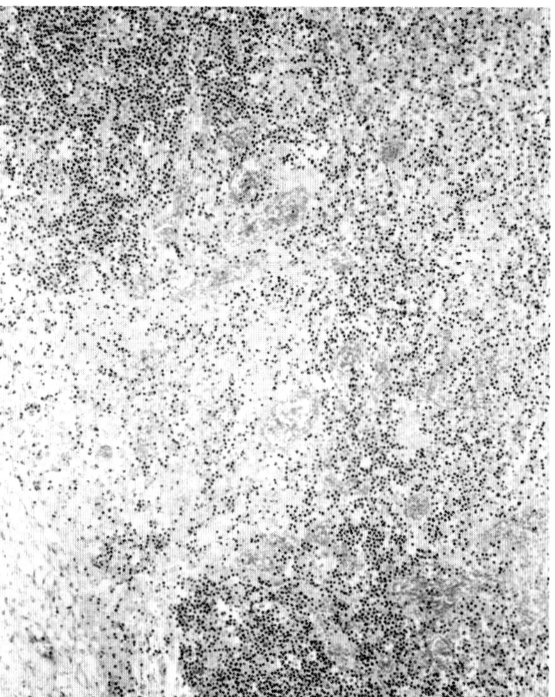

Fig. 6.37 Infarcted femoral lymph node in primary syphilis. Many of the lymphoid cells are necrotic and the node capsule (lower left) is oedematous and thickened. (H E × 120)

forgotten, when lymphadenitis presents in some other region. In secondary syphilis, the lymphadenopathy may be widespread, involving even the epitrochlear nodes, and lymph node enlargement may be the dominant sign, when the rash is fleeting or absent.

Many of the same changes are to be seen in the lymph nodes, whether in the primary or secondary stages of syphilis, and, since the stages often overlap, this account will include both stages. The nodes are generally rubbery in consistency and necrosis is only rarely apparent macroscopically, except in the special instance cited above. Histological examination reveals a node which is generally obviously inflamed and immunologically reactive (Fig. 6.38). Follicular hyperplasia may or may 5 not be a significant feature and only rarely is it of such a degree as to be confused with follicular lymphoma. The capsule is often thickened

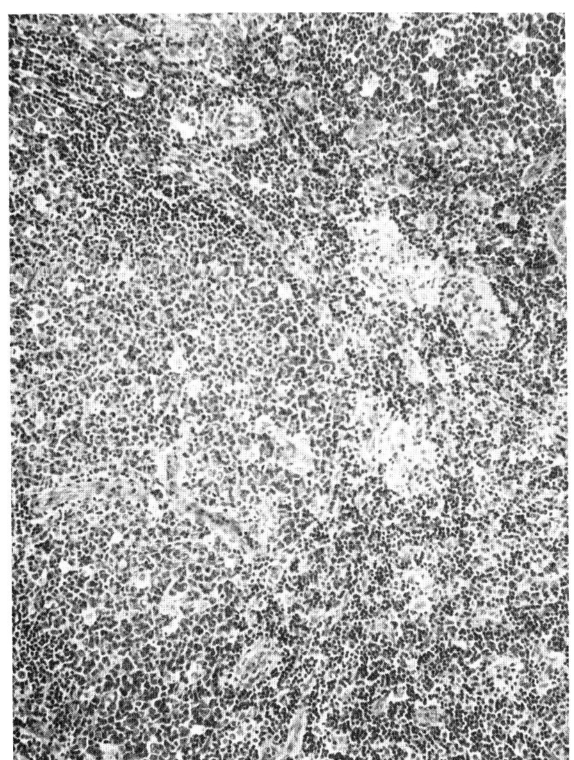

Fig. 6.38 Inguinal lymph node in early secondary syphilis showing ill-defined hyperplastic follicles (lower left and top right) and prominent reactive changes in the T-zone which contains small clusters of epithelioid cells and some immunoblasts (H E × 120)

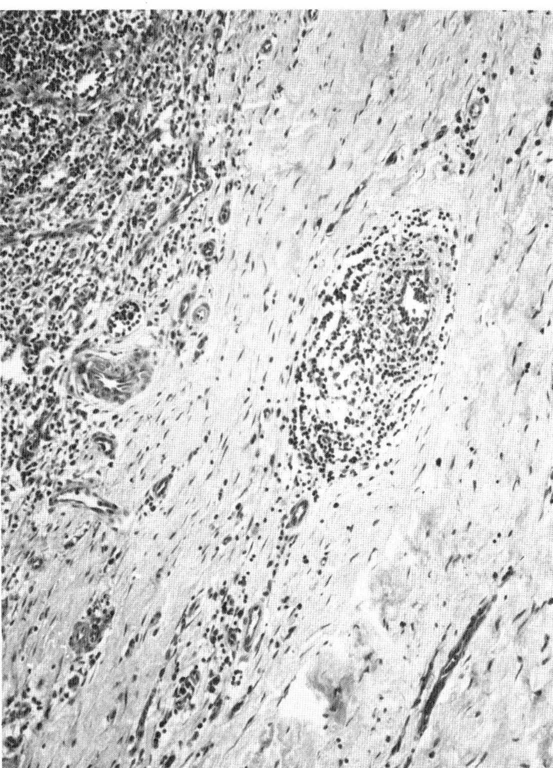

Fig. 6.39 Fibrous thickening of node capsule and perivascular 'cuffing' by lymphocytes and plasma cells (same case as Fig. 6.38) (H E × 120)

and oedematous and both capsule and trabeculae may show some infiltration by lymphocytes and plasma cells which tend to congregate around small blood vessels (Fig. 6.39). Perivascular 'cuffing' may also be a notable feature, both in the fat surrounding the node and in that of the hilar region. The 'cuffed' vessels are not merely surrounded by a collar of lymphocytes and plasma cells, but the walls of these small vessels (mainly venules) are expanded by oedema, so that they stand out with unusual clarity (Figs 6.40, 6.41). At a later stage, the oedema may be succeeded by concentric perivascular fibrosis.

More conspicuous, as a rule, than the follicular hyperplasia, is the expansion of the T-zones which show prominent blood vessels and a mixed cellular infiltration, often including large isolated immunoblasts which impart a 'peppered' appearance to the node similar to that seen in the lymph nodes of some viral diseases (Hartsock et al, 1970). Ma-

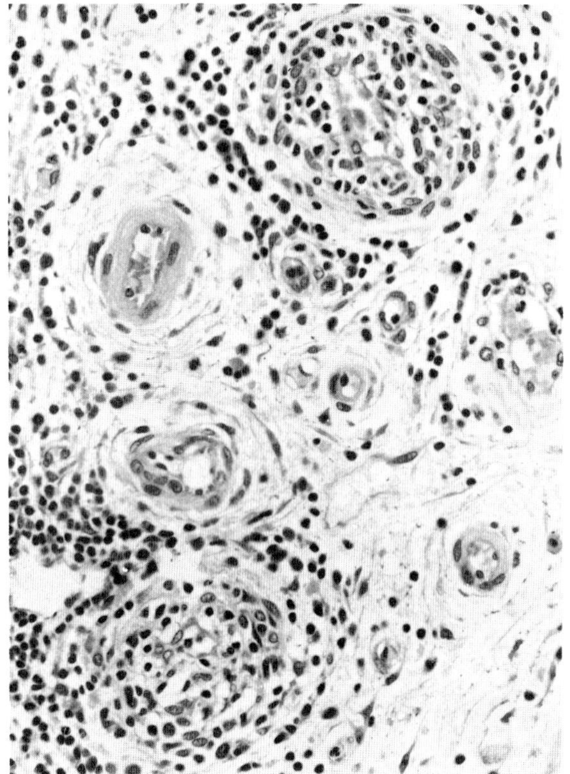

Fig. 6.40 Inguinal lymph node from a case of primary syphilis showing conspicuous 'cuffing' of venules in the hilar region by lymphocytes and plasma cells (H E × 300)

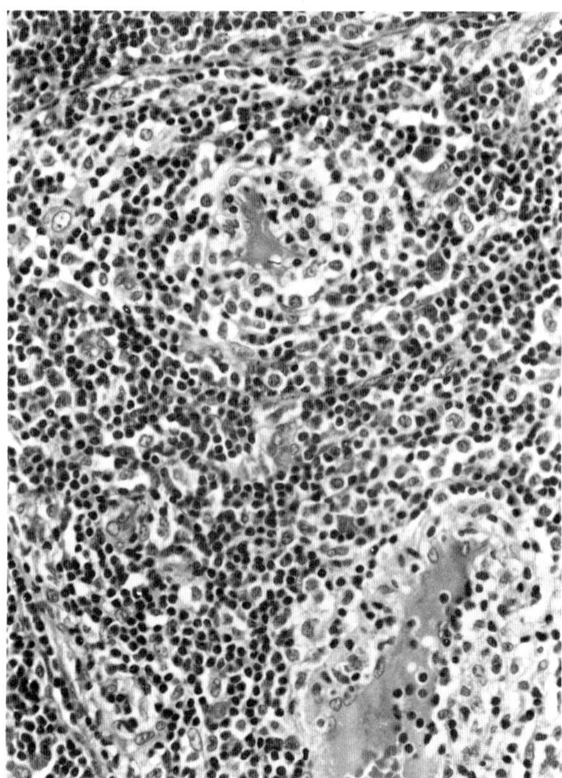

Fig. 6.41 Venules in the node pulp also show angiitis, but are less obvious than hilar or capsular vessels (same node as Fig. 6.40) (H E × 300)

ture and immature plasma cells may be plentiful, as well as plasmacytoid T cells (see Fig. 5.14, p. 78). Small groups of neutrophil and occasionally eosinophil polymorphs may be found, even in the absence of overt secondary infection. Although frank granuloma formation is seldom seen, small clusters of epithelioid histiocytes are generally present (Fig. 6.42) and they may be a very prominent feature. There may also be microscopic foci of necrosis. More obviously acute inflammatory changes with massive polymorph and plasma cell infiltration may result from secondary infection of a chancre.

If the diagnosis is suspected before biopsy is attempted, it may sometimes be confirmed by fine needle aspiration of an enlarged node and examination of the fluid obtained under dark field illumination. *Treponema pallidum* may also be demonstrated, especially in the primary stage, in lymph node sections stained by one of the available silver methods, although this can scarcely be regarded as a diagnostic procedure. Failing the demonstration of live *T. pallidum*, the diagnosis is of course generally confirmed by serological tests.

Fusospirochaetosis (*Vincent's angina*)

Marked swelling of the submandibular lymph nodes may accompany the oral infection caused by the two anaerobic organisms — *Fusobacterium fusiforme* and *Borrelia vincentii*. The lymph nodes in this condition will rarely be excised for biopsy, since the diagnosis is generally obvious from the offensive smell of the swollen and inflamed gums or throat. Further, the diagnosis of Vincent's infection is readily confirmed by the demonstration of the characteristic micro-organisms in a Gram film. Where the swollen lymph nodes are subjected

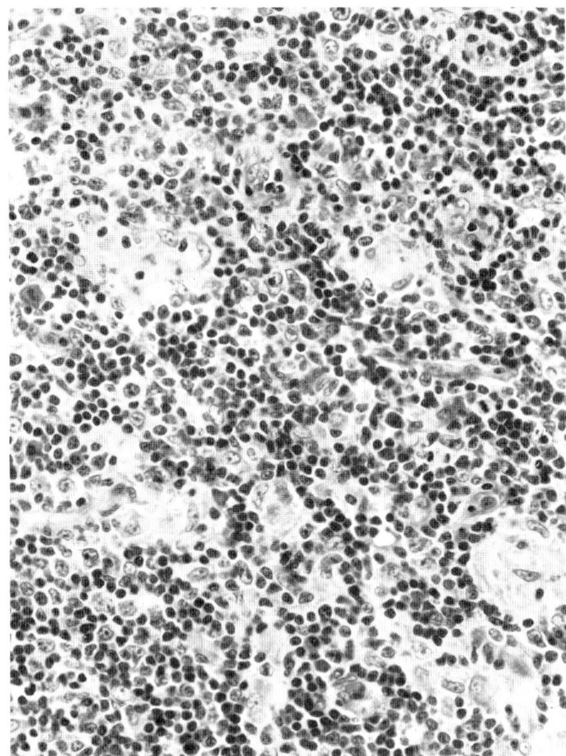

Fig. 6.42 Inguinal lymph node in early secondary syphilis showing mixed infiltrate in the paracortex with groups of epithelioid cells and scattered immunoblasts (same case as Figs 6.38 and 6.39) (H E × 300)

to examination, they may show non-specific inflammatory changes, but may occasionally show widespread necrosis due to the spread of the specific organisms to the nodes (Symmers, 1978, p. 582).

FUNGAL INFECTIONS

A number of different fungal infections may present with lymph node involvement. Many of these are tropical or subtropical infections, but with present day facilities for travel, it is to be expected that isolated cases of most of these will crop up from time to time in Britain. In general, it may be stated that fungal infections tend to present either with chronic suppurative lesions or with granulomatous lesions which often contain multinucleate giant-cells, or with combinations of the two. The differential diagnosis is thus chiefly with tuberculosis and those bacterial infections which mimic tuberculosis. The ease with which the causative organism can be demonstrated varies considerably — even in infections with the same organism.

Actinomycosis

The *Actinomycetes* are no longer classified by taxonomists as true fungi, but are sufficiently closely related to be considered under this heading.

Actinomycosis seldom involves lymph nodes, unless by direct extension of the primary lesion, and presentation of the disease with lymphadenopathy must be extremely rare. *Actinomyces israelii* excites a chronic suppurative reaction with multiple small 'honeycomb' abscesses, surrounded and subdivided by fibrous tissue septa. There is seldom a true granulomatous reaction, although foamy macrophages may congregate in large numbers around the abscesses. Sometimes skin sinuses develop and the characteristic 'sulphur granules', which are colonies of the organism, may be seen with the naked eye in the purulent discharge from such sinuses. If chronic abscesses with surrounding plasma cell reaction lead to a suspicion of actinomycosis, a careful search for colonies of *A. israelii* is warranted, if necessary with examination of interval sections through the block. The organism is Gram-positive and, when present, is easily identified at the centres of the abscess loculi. Confusion may occur with *Actinobacillus actinomycetemcomitans* which may, as its name implies, be present in association with *A. israelii* but which can produce identical lesions on its own. Although the *Actinobacillus* colonies look very similar in a H & E stained section, the organism is Gram-negative. The other principal differential diagnosis, when a long, branching, filamentous organism is found in a suppurative lesion, is some form of *nocardiosis*, but peripheral lymph node involvement is exceptional in infections due to *Nocardia* sp.

True fungal infections causing lymphadenitis

These have been subdivided into two classes, namely, opportunistic infections and primary infections (Symmers, 1978, p. 619). The true 'opportunistic' mycoses are those in which the organism does not attack healthy tissues of healthy individuals and is only able to produce an established infection when the normal bodily defence mechanisms are impaired or suppressed. By contrast, the primary mycoses are caused by pathogenic fungi which may cause infection in previously healthy individuals. The distinction between these classes is relative rather than absolute and probably most deep fungal infections require some depression of immunity before they can give rise to serious systemic infections. An analogous situation is seen with mycobacterial infections (see p. 104). Some of the opportunistic fungi, e.g. *Candida*, may reside on the surface of the skin or juxtacutaneous mucous membranes in individuals who are otherwise healthy or only mildly debilitated, but may give rise to deep, spreading infections when immunity is severely impaired.

The most important mycoses from the point of view of lymph node involvement are summarised in Table 6.2. It is noteworthy that the common opportunistic mycoses (*aspergillosis, mucormycosis* and *candidosis*) are of worldwide distribution, whilst the primary mycoses are of much more re-

Table 6.2 Systemic fungal infections

Country	Disease	Fungus	Portal of entry and spread	Lymph node involvement	Histology of lesion in systemic infections
Worldwide	Aspergillosis	*Aspergillus fumigatus*	Airways → lungs → GIT → Blood stream	–	Necrosis
	Mucormycosis	*Rhizopus* *Absidia* sp. *Mucor*	Nasal passages, airways → lungs → Blood stream	–	Necrosis
	Candidosis	*Candida albicans*	Moist skin, oral mucosa → Airways and lungs → Gastro-intestinal tract → Blood stream	±	Necrosis ± suppuration
Tropics	Chromomycosis	*Phialophora* sp.	Skin and subcutis	±	Suppuration + granulomas
Tropics	Sporotrichosis	*Sporothrix schenkii*	Skin and subcutis	±	Suppuration + granulomas
Europe Tropics Australia	Cryptococcosis	*Cryptococcus neoformans*	Skin, airways → lungs	+	Negligible reaction (cryptococci ++) or granuloma (cryptococci ±)
N America S Asia Africa	Histoplasmosis	*Histoplasma capsulatum*	Lungs, rarely skin Lymphatics → LN Blood stream	++	Histiocytosis → Tuberculoid granulomas ± caseation → calcification
Africa		*H. duboisii*	Skin ? Lungs Blood stream	+	Histiocytosis
N America	Coccidioido- mycosis	*Coccidioides immitis*	Lungs Skin → Blood stream	+	Tuberculoid granulomas ± central suppuration → caseation and calcification
Southern N America Africa	Blastomycosis (N. American)	*Blastomyces dermatitidis*	Lungs Skin → Blood stream (microscopical)	+	Granulomas + suppuration, rarely caseation
S America	Paracoccidi- oidomycosis (S. American Blastomycosis)	*Paracoccidioides brasiliensis*	Upper airways Lungs Skin (microscopical) → Blood stream	+	Granuloma

stricted distribution, being mainly tropical or subtropical diseases. Furthermore, the strictly opportunistic mycoses tend not to spread by lymphatics to involve lymph nodes, but infiltrating diffusely through the tissues, gain access to the blood stream and become disseminated by that route. If lymph nodes are involved at all, this is purely incidental and often terminal.

Cryptococcosis (torulosis) occupies an intermediate position between the strictly opportunistic and the primary mycoses and the organism certainly behaves as an opportunist in temperate climes, in patients with Hodgkin's disease and in other forms of immune depression. Lymph node involvement is quite common, especially involvement of mediastinal nodes, secondary to a lung infection. A confusing picture may arise when nodes already involved by Hodgkin's disease become infected by *C. neoformans* (Fig. 6.43). The degree of histiocytic or granulomatous response to the presence of the organism is very variable but, in the immunodefective patient, the round, yeast-like bodies are often very numerous and are generally easily identified. They appear as somewhat refractile, unstained bodies of varying size in a H & E stained section, with a clear halo around the cell wall. The halo is due to the mucopolysaccharide capsule, which is well shown in sections stained by the PAS or Grocott methods (Fig. 6.44).

The causative fungus is generally readily demonstrable in most of these fungal infections with the exception of *sporotrichosis* in which fungal bodies are notoriously difficult to find and generally require culture for their demonstration.

In *chromomycosis (chromoblastomycosis)*, the brown colour of the organisms renders them particularly conspicuous. In suppurative lesions of this kind, the organisms often lie free in the centres of small abscesses, surrounded by polymorph leucocytes. On the other hand, in granulomatous lesions, the organism should be sought within the cytoplasm of macrophages and es-

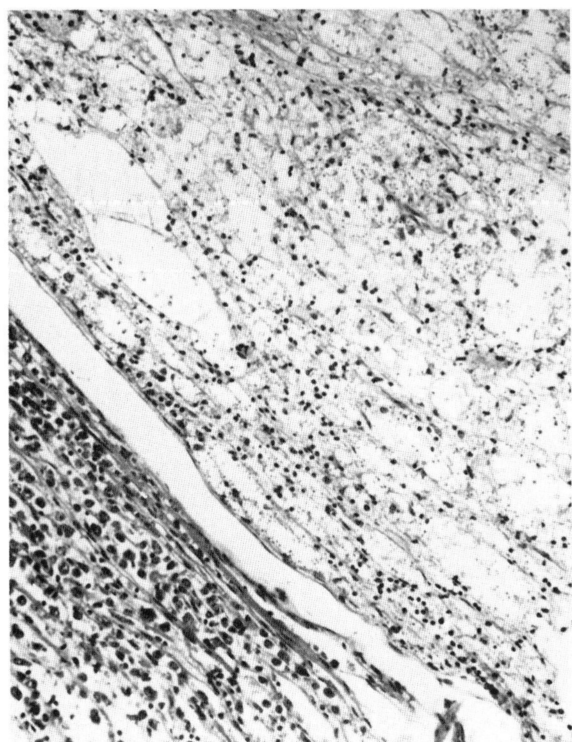

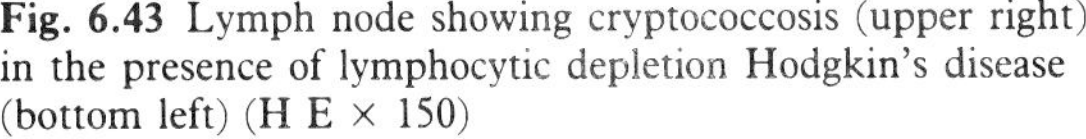

Fig. 6.43 Lymph node showing cryptococcosis (upper right) in the presence of lymphocytic depletion Hodgkin's disease (bottom left) (H E × 150)

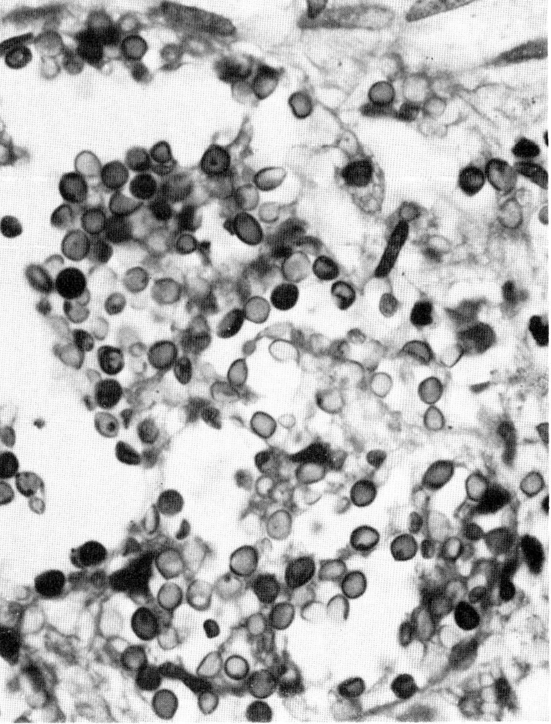

Fig. 6.44 *Cryptococcus neoformans* in lymph node. Note lack of cellular reaction. (Same case as Fig. 6.43.) (PAS × 940)

pecially in the multinucleate giant-cells which are commonly found in the primary mycoses. In *blastomycosis* the fungus propagates by budding and *North American blastomycosis* is distinguished by the production of a solitary bud, whilst in *South American blastomycosis* (*paracoccidioidomycosis*), buds are produced all round the perimeter of the organism.

Histoplasmosis

Histoplasma capsulatum is the most important and most widely distributed pathogenic fungus to give rise to lymph node lesions and lymphadenopathy is a prominent feature at various stages of infection by this organism. *H. capsulatum* is found throughout much of North America, especially in the Southern United States where infection is very common. It is also prevalent in much of Africa and India, but is rare in other parts of the world and does not seem to occur spontaneously in Europe. Histoplasmosis of this type shows, in its pathological features, a striking similarity to tuberculosis. The primary lesion is generally in the lungs and from the primary focus, whether in the lung or elsewhere, there is usually spread to the regional lymph nodes which enlarge and often undergo caseous necrosis (Fig. 6.45). The caseous foci frequently become walled off by fibrous tissue and may calcify in time (Fig. 6.46). The tuberculoid granulomas characteristic of this chronic form of histoplasmosis are sometimes very similar to the 'tubercles' of tuberculosis and the distinction may rely on the demonstration of *H. capsulatum* within occasional giant-cells or in caseous foci. When the organisms are scanty they are much more readily found with the aid of the Grocott hexamine silver stain (Fig. 6.47). This procedure is unnecessary in the more acute forms of histoplasmosis, which are liable to occur in the presence of immune paresis.

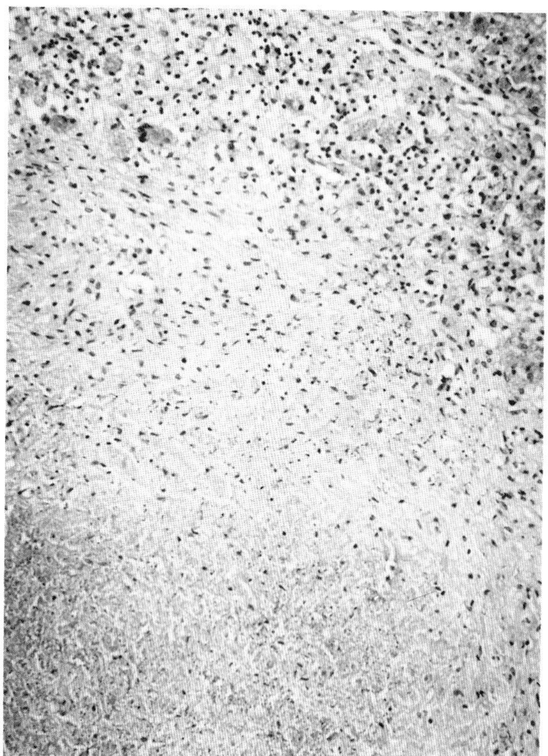

Fig. 6.45 Lymph node in active histoplasmosis due to *H.capsulatum*, showing spreading necrosis and macrophage reaction at the periphery (H E × 120)

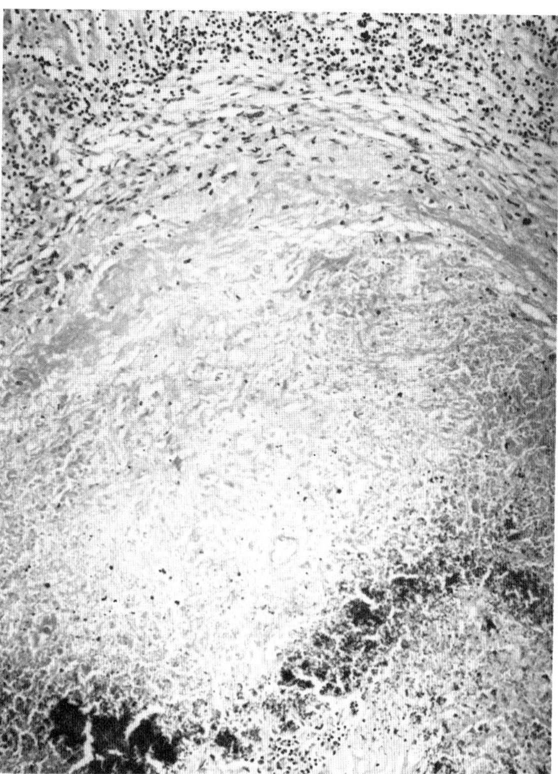

Fig. 6.46 Focus of chronic histoplasmosis in a lymph node showing calcific impregnation of necrotic centre (below) and surrounding 'wall' of fibrous tissue. Structural outlines are more clearly discernible in the necrotic tissue than they are in the caseation of tuberculosis. (H E × 120)

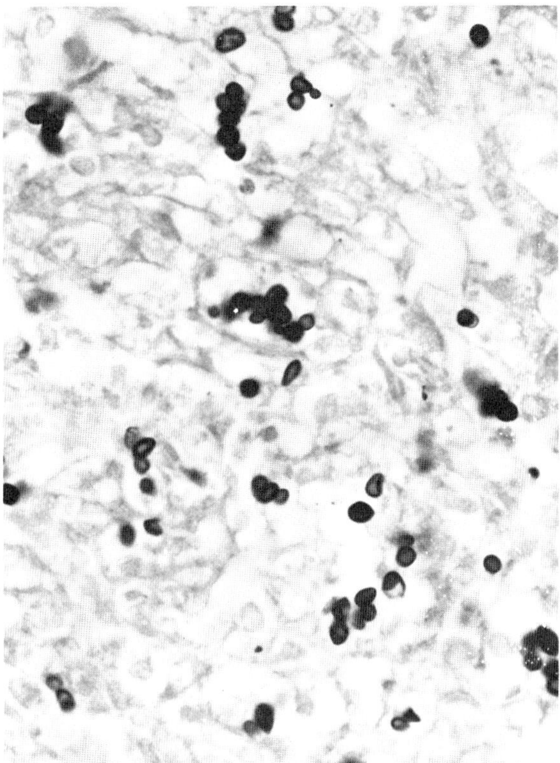

Fig. 6.47 Histoplasma capsulatum in a lymph node. Note budding of the yeasts. (Grocott's hexamine silver × 940)

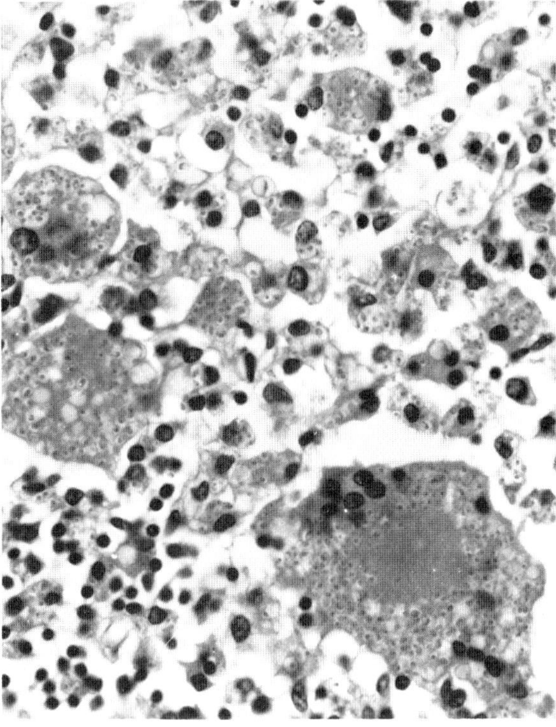

Fig. 6.48 Lymph node from a boy aged 14 showing huge numbers of *H.capsulatum* within macrophages and giant cells. Note clear halo around yeasts. (Post-mortem specimen.) (H E × 470)

Then there is often widespread lymphadenopathy and the encapsulated organisms are found in huge numbers dispersed through the nodes within macrophages and giant cells, (Fig. 6.48). As in acute tuberculosis, there is necrosis but no granuloma formation in this type of case.

H. duboisii has a much more restricted range than *H. capsulatum*, being limited to tropical Africa. Less is known about the natural history and epidemiology of '*African histoplasmosis*' but the organism itself is considerably larger than *H. capsulatum*. Lymph node involvement may occur in the course of the disease and the organism may be found within macrophages and multinucleate giant-cells in the affected nodes.

Other fungal infections

The fungal infections included in Table 6.2, some of which are dicussed above, by no means exhaust the list of recorded mycotic infections of lymph nodes. Most of the mycoses which have been omitted are either very rare, or very restricted in their distribution. Some commoner mycoses have been excluded because lymph node involvement is very uncommon. It should be borne in mind that lymphadenopathy in the presence of an ulcerated fungal infection, (e.g. enlarged inguinal nodes in a patient with *mycetoma* of the foot), seldom implies the spread of infection to the nodes. More often, such nodes will show only non-specific reactive changes on histological examination.

Differential diagnosis of mycoses

As indicated at the beginning of this section, fungal infections enter into the differential diagnosis of all chronic suppurative and granulomatous lesions, especially where suppuration and granuloma formation are found together. In particular, tuberculosis and 'pseudotuberculosis' (p. 98) should be excluded. Chlamydial and protozoal infections are less likely to present difficulties.

Although many fungi are readily visible in sections stained with H & E, they are much more clearly shown by the use of the Periodic-Acid Schiff (PAS) or Grocott Hexamine Silver stains and such stains should always be employed where a fungal infection is suspected, but no organism is visible with routine staining.

When fungal bodies have been found, in a setting which clearly indicates that they are significant (i.e. not extraneous or artefactual), the nature of the fungus may often be deduced from the geographical origin of the patient, the type of reaction and the morphology of the organism. If a fungal infection has been suspected in advance, culture of the fungus will of course establish the species with greater certainty. Exceptionally, multiple fungal infections have been found in a single patient (Symmers, 1978, p. 630). The detailed morphology of the various pathogenic fungi is beyond the scope of this book and for this the reader is referred to works on mycology.

PROTOZOAL INFECTIONS

Lymphadenopathy is a prominent feature of some protozoal infections of man, but is insignificant or absent in some others (e.g. malaria and amoebiasis). In Britain and most of Europe, toxoplasmosis is the most likely protozoal disease to be encountered, but, with modern facilities for air travel, the possibility of exotic infections has always to be borne in mind.

Toxoplasmic lymphadenitis

Toxoplasma gondii is a very widespread, and common protozoal parasite which includes a variety of mammalian and avian species amongst its hosts. Human infections are probably due in most instances to contamination of food by cat faeces (Hutchison et al, 1971), but undoubtedly other sources of infection are responsible from time to time and transplacental transmission of the organism accounts for cases of congenital toxoplasmosis. Whilst toxoplasmosis is commonly seen in otherwise healthy individuals, opportunistic infection also occurs in conditions of depressed immunity.

Lymphadenopathy is the commonest mode of presentation of acquired toxoplasmosis in man and, in most instances, the illness is quite mild, sometimes with malaise and slight pyrexia, but not infrequently without symptoms or signs of constitutional disturbance. A severe illness is quite exceptional. The patients are commonly children or young adults and the presentation is often with a single enlarged node or group of nodes, generally in the cervical, post-auricular, occipital or parotid regions. Occasionally the presenting nodes may be in the axilla, but rarely elsewhere. The nodes may be slightly tender or painless. A feature of the lymphadenopathy is its persistence, often for weeks and sometimes for months, and it is this that generally leads to nodes being excised for biopsy.

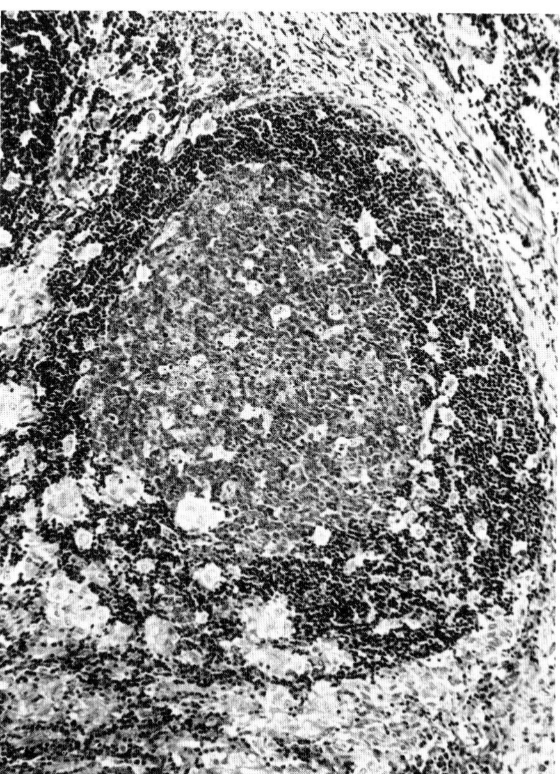

Fig. 6.49 Cervical lymph node showing typical changes of toxoplasmic lymphadenitis. Note capsular thickening and infiltration with periadenitis, follicular hyperplasia and small clusters of epithelioid cells. (H E × 120)

Macroscopically the nodes are unremarkable: they seldom exceed 3 cm and are more often less than 2 cm in diameter.

Histologically, the picture is distinctive and in many instances the diagnosis can be confidently predicted, although confirmation should always be obtained by serological tests (see under differential diagnosis). Three main features contribute to the characteristic histological picture — follicular hyperplasia, epithelioid cell clusters and 'immature sinus histiocytosis' (see p. 347) In distinguishing this picture from that of Hodgkin's disease, it cannot be emphasised too strongly that the lymph nodes of toxoplasmic lymphadenitis present clear evidence of an *inflammatory* process (Fig. 6.49). There is often evidence of periadenitis, neutrophil polymorphs are sometimes present in significant numbers, along with macrophages and transformed lymphocytes in the marginal sinus, and there is always follicular hyperplasia with the development of large germinal centres (see Fig. 6.7). The latter often shown many tingible body macrophages, which may be crammed with haematoxyphil fragments (Fig. 6.50).

The small epithelioid cell clusters, although a rather variable feature, are yet so conspicuous when present that they have come to be regarded by many as the 'hallmark' of toxoplasmic lymphadenitis. In a H & E stained section, the pink-staining clusters stand out very clearly against the dark blue background of lymphocytes (Fig. 6.49, 6.50, 6.51). The clusters may be numerous or scanty, widely distributed or confined to a small area of the node. They are often dotted through the cortex, frequently invading the germinal centres (Figs. 6.49, 6.50). The individual clusters remain small in size even when, as sometimes happens, they become confluent in the marginal sinus and capsular region of the node. Microscopic foci of necrosis may be seen in these circumstances,

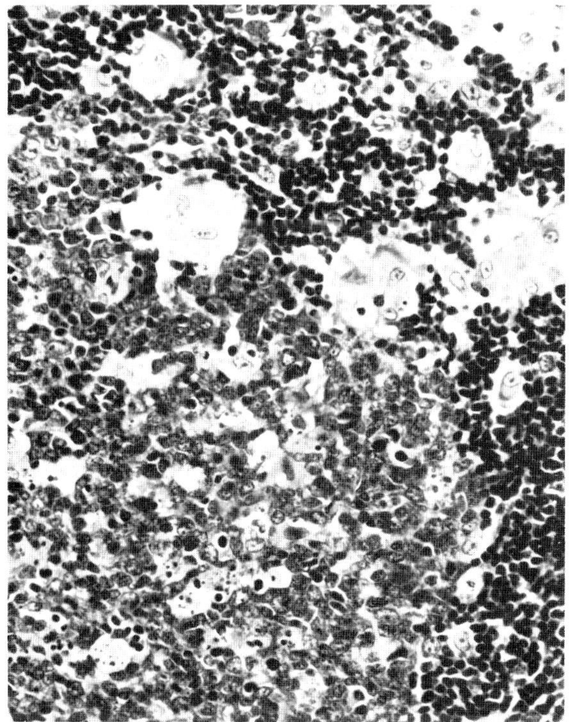

Fig. 6.50 Toxoplasmic lymphadenitis showing part of a hyperplastic germinal centre, penetrated at its upper edge by epithelioid cells. Note tingible-body macrophages containing haematoxyphil fragments (same case as Fig. 6.49). (H E × 300)

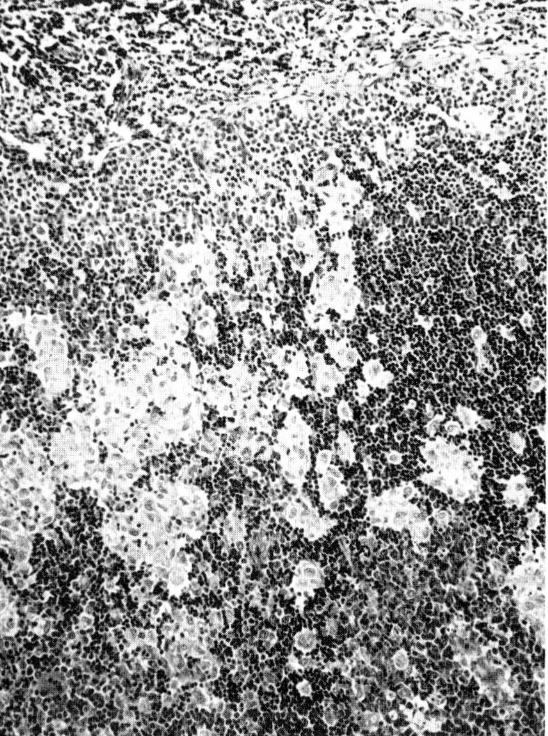

Fig. 6.51 Toxoplasmic lymphadenitis showing partially confluent epithelioid cell clusters and 'immature sinus histiocytosis' in marginal sinus with extracapsular infiltration above. (Same case as Figs 6.49 and 6.50) (H E × 120)

but caseation does not occur and giant-cell formation is exceptional.

'Immature sinus histiocytosis' is not of course unique to toxoplasmosis and this feature is found in a variety of infections (see p. 350), it is, however, particularly commonly found in toxoplasmic lymphadenitis. Focally, the expanded lymph sinuses, both peripheral and central, become choked with rather pale-staining 'monocyte-like' cells, which were originally thought to be immature histiocytes, but which are now recognised as being lymphoid cells which have acquired this distinctive morphology (Fig. 6.52). The precise significance of the phenomenon is unknown.

Very occasionally confirmation of the diagnosis is obtained by the discovery in the lymph node of a *toxoplasma* cyst filled with the merozoites of the parasite (Fig. 6.53) (Stansfeld, 1961). The individual trophozoites cannot be distinguished reliably from nuclear fragments by light microscopy but might, theoretically, be shown up by specific immunostaining.

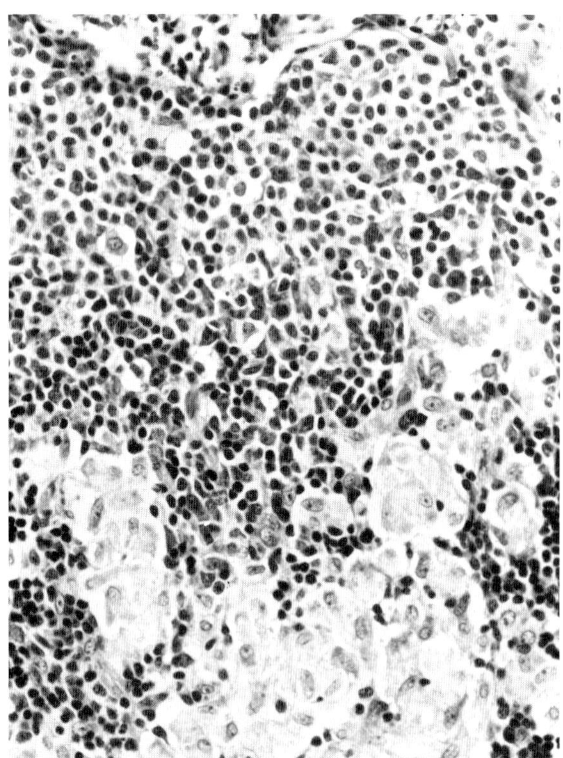

Fig. 6.52 Higher magnification of left half of field of Fig. 6.51 to show details of epithelioid cells and partially transformed lymphocytes in marginal sinus (H·E × 300)

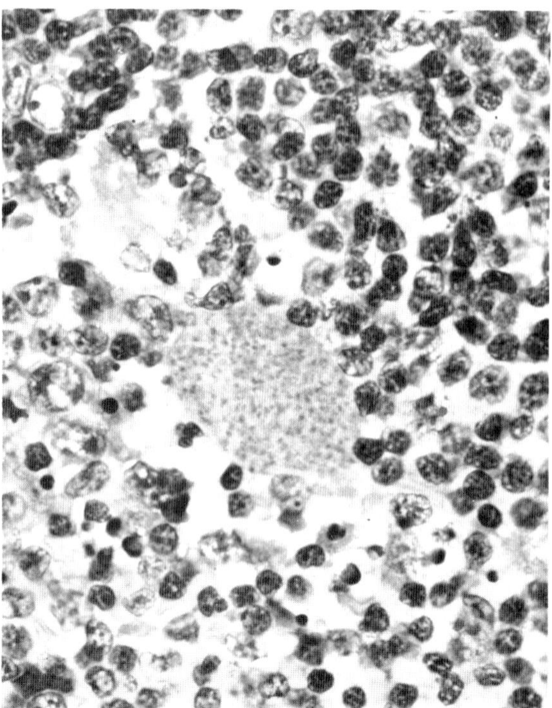

Fig. 6.53 Toxoplasma cyst in a lymph node. The thin-walled cyst is filled with merozoites of the parasite. (H E × 750)

Differential diagnosis

A very similar histological picture may rarely be seen in infectious mononucleosis and for this reason it is important to confirm the diagnosis by other means. The Sabin-Feldman dye test and the complement fixation test are the serological tests most frequently employed.

The epithelioid cell clusters in toxoplasmosis are much smaller than the granulomas of sarcoidosis and tuberculosis and neither of these conditions is associated with follicular hyperplasia of lymph nodes. Small epithelioid cell clusters may of course be found in nodes in other infections, notably, early syphilis, brucellosis and leishmaniasis (kala-azar), each of which may have to be considered in the differential diagnosis.

Hodgkin's disease (HD) is surprisingly often confused with toxoplasmic lymphadenitis, no doubt because small clusters of epithelioid cells are common to both conditions; the background is, however, quite different and it is important to look carefully at this. Even when reactive follicles are still present in the nodes of HD, as they frequently are, these follicles do not show the degree of hyperplasia found in toxoplasmosis and there is always evidence of some architectural disturbance in HD, which is lacking in toxoplasmosis.

Leishmaniasis

There are two different leishmanial diseases of the Old World, due to related, but evidently distinct species — visceral leishmaniasis (kala-azar) caused by *Leishmania donovani*, and cutaneous leishmaniasis (tropical sore), caused by *L. tropica*. In the Americas and especially in the tropical regions of South America, visceral leishmaniasis has a restricted distribution, but cutaneous leishmaniasis is common and widespread. Here it is due to a related species, *L. brasiliensis*. Lymph node involvement is uncommon in cutaneous leishmaniasis and, when it does occur, it is generally confined to the regional nodes draining the cutaneous sore, so that lymph node biopsy is seldom indicated, the cause of the nodal enlargement being obvious.

In contrast, visceral leishmaniasis is often accompanied by lymphadenopathy which may even overshadow the other visceral manifestations of the disease — hepatosplenomegaly and anaemia. Kala-azar is widely distributed, occurring in the Mediterranean region, much of East Africa, the Middle East and India, as well as in Brazil. The infection is transmitted by the bite of sandflies of various species and different animal reservoirs of the parasite have been recorded from different areas — dogs and foxes constituting the principal source in many areas where the disease is endemic. Children and adolescents are most often the victims of this disease, but adult visitors to endemic areas may also acquire kala-azar, so pathologists in any part of the world should be on the look out for the disease, even when it does not occur naturally in their own country. *L. donovani* is carried by the blood stream throughout the body and the parasite is taken up by macrophages, particularly in the liver, spleen and bone marrow, as well as in the lymph nodes, so lymphadenopathy is often generalised although the involved nodes may be quite small. If kala-azar is suspected, the diagnosis is most easily confirmed by means of bone marrow or splenic puncture, although the latter procedure is not without risk. Lymph node puncture is less likely to prove positive unless the nodes are large. The intracellular parasites are much more easily recognised in smears or imprints than they are in sections, but they are found readily enough in a node biopsy, provided that the sections are reasonably thin.

The histological appearances vary. With H & E staining, a small node may appear on low power examination to show little more than a mild sinus histiocytosis with a few macrophages scattered through the pulp, yet, under the high power, *L. donovani* may be seen in large numbers as tiny blue dots in the cytoplasm of histiocytes, the presence of which had not been suspected at a low magnification (Figs. 6.54, 6.55). At other times, there may be a more obvious pulp histiocytosis, ranging from scattered, small clusters of epithelioid cells, like those seen in toxoplasmosis, to large, confluent tuberculoid granulomata with necrosis (Figs. 6.56, 6.57). In such cases the organisms

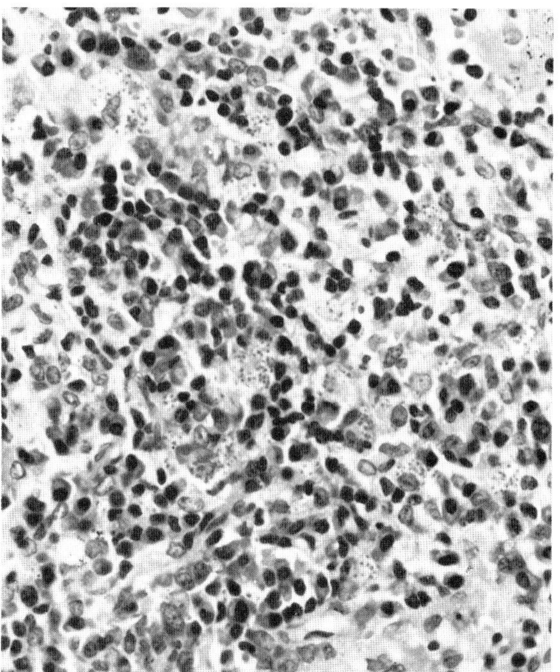

Fig. 6.54 Lymph node from a child with visceral leishmaniasis showing numerous macrophages containing Leishman-Donovan bodies. There are no focal lesions. (H E × 470)

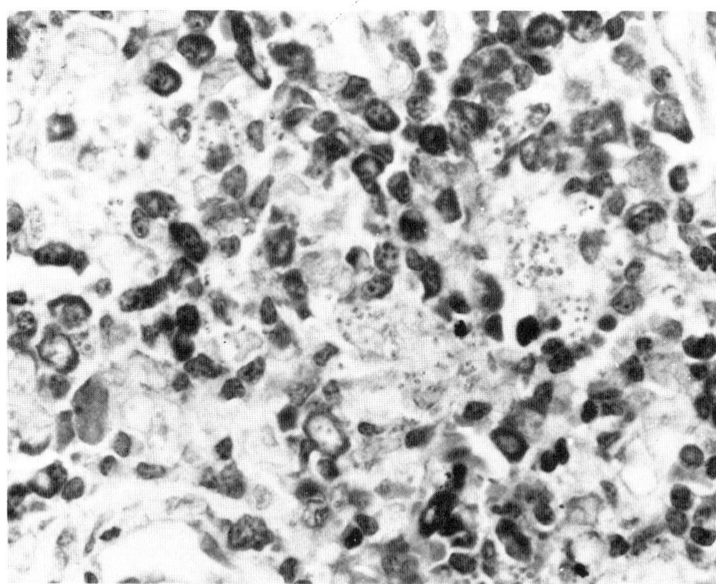

Fig. 6.55 Same lymph node as Fig. 6.54 at a higher magnification. The L -D bodies are clearly visible. Note the abundance of plasma cells. (Giemsa × 750)

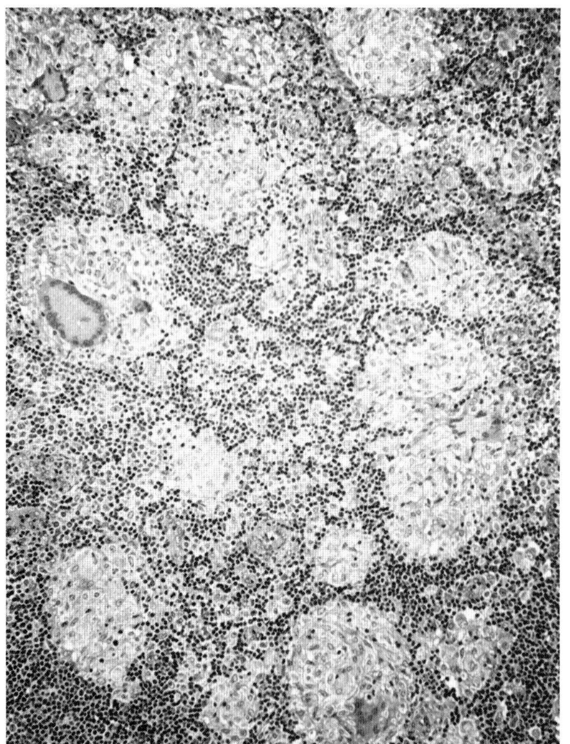

Fig. 6.56 Axillary node from a young adult who had spent 2 weeks in Malta a few months previously and who presented with fever and axillary lymphadenopathy. Much of the node was filled with small granulomata, some containing Langhans' type giant-cells. (H E × 120)

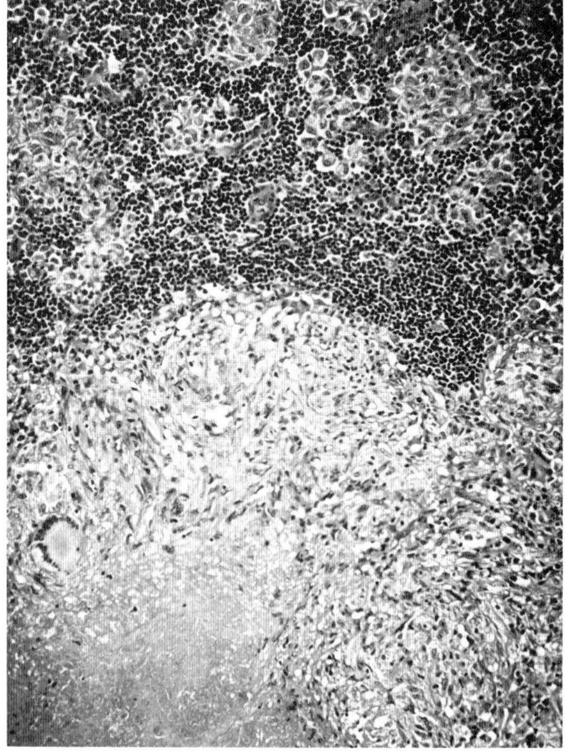

Fig. 6.57 Same lymph node as Fig. 6.56 showing a larger area of confluent granulomatous inflammation with central caseous necrosis. The resemblance to tuberculosis is quite close. (H E × 120)

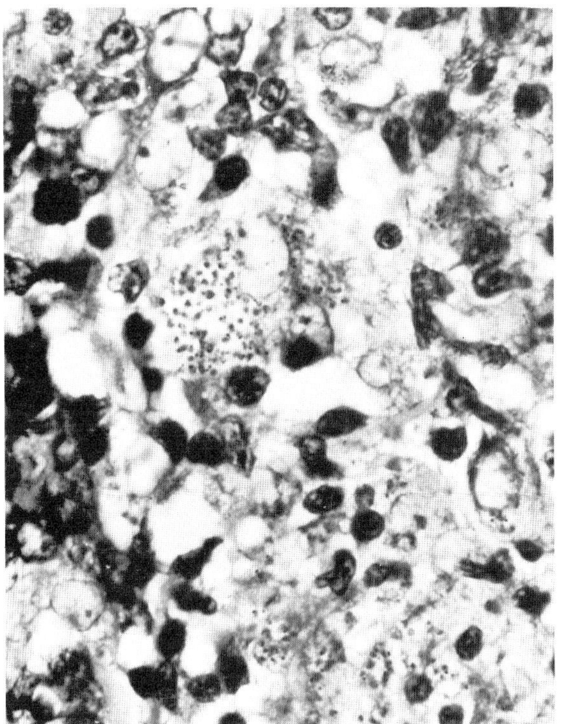

Fig. 6.58 Same lymph node as Figs 6.56 and 6.57. In one or two small foci in the node typical L-D bodies were found within macrophages, confirming the diagnosis of visceral leishmaniasis. Kinetoplasts are just visible in the L-D bodies in the cell at the centre. (Giemsa × 940)

may be less numerous and limited to small foci of histiocytes (Fig. 6.58). There is nearly always a conspicuous plasmacytosis which distinguishes the picture from that of tuberculosis. The intracellular organisms may be mistaken for *Histoplasma capsulatum*, but the latter are more variable in size and are PAS positive, whilst *L. donovani* is PAS negative. There may also be confusion with the leishmanial form of *Trypanosoma cruzi*, the protozoon which causes S. American trypanosomiasis (qv).

Trypanosomiasis

African trypanosomiasis (sleeping sickness) in man is caused by two different protozoa — *Trypanosoma gambiense* and *Trypanosoma rhodesiense*, which have a different geographical distribution, although the organisms are morphologically indistinguishable and both diseases are transmitted by the bites of tse-tse flies (*Glossina* sp). Lymphadenopathy is a conspicuous feature of the early stages of infection, the nodes involved being those draining the site of the tse-tse fly bite. With most species of tse-tse fly, the bite is on the head with consequent enlargement of the post-auricular or occipital nodes (Winterbottom's sign). However, one vector of *Tr. rhodesiense* bites on the legs and the inguinal nodes then become enlarged. At this stage, the diagnosis may be confirmed in a large proportion of cases by fine needle puncture of an enlarged node and immediate examination of a wet film of the aspirate in which the actively motile trypanosomes can be readily seen. Smears can be stained by Giemsa to show the characteristic morphology of the organisms. Lymph node aspiration is generally more reliable than lymph node biopsy, in which the trypanosomes are harder to find and the histological picture is otherwise that of a non-specific acute or subacute lymphadenitis. The lymph node enlargement is remarkably persistent and biopsy at a later stage frequently shows widespread fibrosis in the nodes and capsular thickening.

South American trypanosomiasis (Chagas' disease) is caused by *Trypanosoma cruzi*. The disease is transmitted by blood-sucking reduviid bugs of several species. The disease is particularly prevalent in Brazil, in parts of which it is extremely common. As with African trypanosomiasis, lymphadenopathy in the nodes regional to the portal of entry is the rule in the early stages. Not infrequently the conjunctiva may be the site of entry of infection, when ipsilateral parotid lymphadenopathy accompanies an acute conjunctivitis as the initial manifestation of the disease (Romaña's sign). Phagocytosis of trypanosomes by macrophages occurs in the infected nodes and the organisms then lose their flagellae, becoming transmuted into the leishmanial form of the parasite, in which stage they closely resemble intracellular *L. donovani*. As with visceral leishmaniasis, large numbers of organisms may be seen within the cytoplasm of macrophages in the node.

METAZOAL PARASITES

Lymph node biopsy is not regularly undertaken in the investigation of patients who have infestation by helminths, nevertheless the presence of remnants of worms or, more often, their ova or larvae, may rarely be a chance finding in a lymph node removed with some other diagnosis in mind.

Filariasis, due to one or other of the filarial worms, is naturally the commonest helminthic disease to involve lymph nodes, since the adult worms reside in the lymphatics (Fig. 6.59). The nodal changes in filariasis are discussed in Chapter 7 (p. 155).

In *schistosomiasis* the schistosomules, which develop from the cercariae after these have penetrated through the skin, migrate by superficial lymphatics and may be found in superficial lymph nodes. At a later stage schistosome ova may be found in abdominal lymph nodes, as in many other abdominal or pelvic tissues. Sometimes the ova are clearly distinguishable, even to the identification of a terminal or lateral spine; on the other hand, their structure may be obscured by calcification. In the latter state the ova are often surrounded by fibrosis, whilst, at an earlier stage, each ovum lies at the centre of a small granuloma in which eosinophils mingle with the histiocytes. A variable degree of eosinophilia may be present throughout the node.

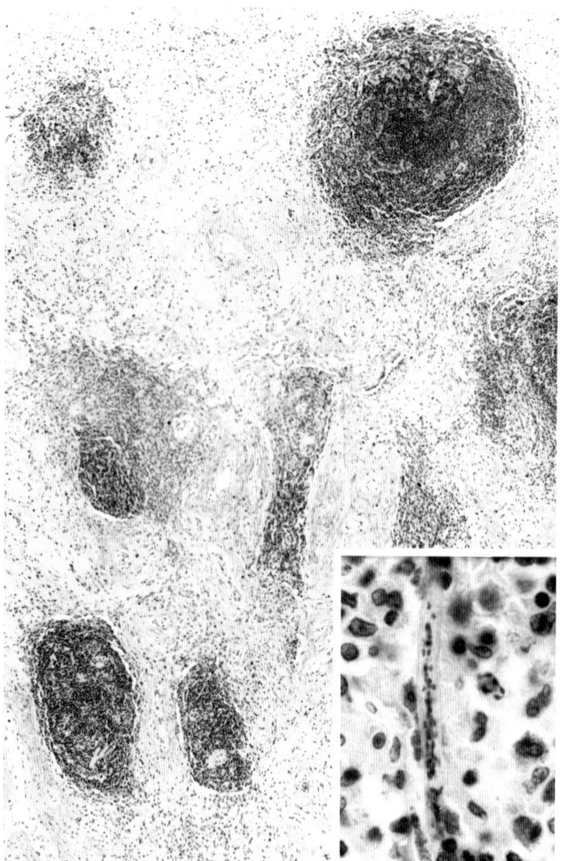

Fig. 6.59 Inguinal lymph node from an African subject with filariasis. Broad tracts of fibrous tissue containing thickened, hyalinised vessels separate residual islands of lymphoid tissue. Inset: a single microfilaria, surrounded by many eosinophils was found after diligent search. (H E main figure × 47, inset × 940)

In other examples of helminthic infestation, lymph node involvement is generally a chance finding and it is impossible to estimate how frequently, for example, larvae of parasitic nematodes (larva migrans) find their way to lymph nodes. In areas of heavy infestation it may be a not uncommon phenomenon. Many pathologists will have had the experience of suspecting a helminth parasite as the cause of an unexplained lymphadenitis, in which focal granulomatous areas are associated with heavy eosinophilia or 'eosinophilic abscesses'. The suspicion is heightened by the discovery of brightly eosinophilic fragments of refractile material at the centres of the granulomatous foci, but such fragments can seldom be positively identified as the remains of a worm. A similar reaction is of course commonly evoked by helminths when they die in the tissues. The foreign body may then be coated with a thick deposit of brilliantly eosinophilic, amorphous material showing, at its periphery, radiating, 'flame-like' formations. The fibrinoid deposit is surrounded by histiocytes, often in palisaded arrangement with a heavy eosinophilia in the surrounding tissues. This distinctive reaction is known as the Splendore-Hoeppli phenomenon after the two authors who independently described it (see Symmers, 1978, pp 672, 750).

RICKETTSIAL AND CHLAMYDIAL DISEASES

Rickettsial diseases

Diseases caused by a variety of *Rickettsial* species are of world-wide distribution and are transmitted to man mainly by the bites of a variety of insect vectors — lice, fleas, ticks and mites. Although obligate intracellular parasites, the organisms are classed as bacteria and the formerly grave prognosis of several varieties of 'typhus' has been dramatically changed since the introduction of antibiotics effective against Gram-negative organisms. The rickettsial diseases of man fall into five separate classes (Pinkerton & Strano, 1976), but all the diseases are characterised by rapid blood-borne dissemination of the organism which colonises vascular endothelial cells throughout the body, setting up a 'microvasculitis', often accompanied by thrombosis in more severely affected vessels. No doubt lymph nodes are often involved by such lesions, but lymphadenopathy is a conspicuous feature only in *Tsutsugamushi disease* (scrub typhus) and in some instances of the relatively mild, Old World forms of tick-borne typhus (*R. rickettsii*). In each of the latter disorders a small necrotic ulcer develops at the site of the mite or tick bite, which may be anywhere on the skin. Enlargement of the regional nodes follows, which may be dramatic in the case of *R. tsutsugamushi* infection. Later, generalised lymphadenopathy may develop, The diagnosis has seldom been made by lymph node biopsy in any of these diseases. It is often suggested, especially in endemic areas or in the course of an epidemic, by the acute febrile illness with characteristic rash, even when no ulcer or scab is present at the site of the vector bite. Confirmation can often be obtained by the Weil-Felix test.

Histology. A broadly similar picture may be seen in the lymph nodes in any of the rickettsial diseases (Symmers, 1978, p. 633). A striking immunoblastic reaction may be found in the sinuses and pulp, recalling the appearances of infectious mononucleosis (see p. 129). There is an accompanying increase of plasma cells, especially around small blood vessels in which the specific changes may be sought. These consist in perivascular oedema and swelling of the vascular endothelium due to cytoplasmic colonisation by *Rickettsiae*. Recognition of the organisms by light microscopy requires good quality sections and Giemsa staining. Microvascular thrombi may be responsible for the patchy and sometimes quite extensive necrosis and haemorrhage in the nodes.

Chlamydial diseases

Like the *Rickettsiae*, the *Chlamydiae* are obligate intracellular parasites, but are now regarded as minute bacteria, rather than viruses. The organisms show two developmental stages in the cell (1) the small, infectious, *elementary bodies* which develop into (2) the somewhat larger, *initial bodies*, which are capable of subdivision by binary fission. There are two currently recognised species of *Chlamydia* pathogenic to man, namely, *Chlamydia trachomatis* (Group A) and *Chlamydia psittaci* (Group B).Infections caused by organisms of Group A are practically confined to man, whilst the organisms of Group B cause ornithosis (psittacosis) in a much wider range of hosts. Infection is usually transmitted by direct contact. Lymph nodal involvement can develop in any of this group of diseases, but it is not of primary importance in either trachoma or ornithosis and it is a quite separate disease, lymphogranuloma venereum (LGV), in which lymphadenopathy is an important feature. Because of the similarity of the lesions of LGV to those of cat scratch disease, that condition will also be considered here, although its aetiology is still unknown.

Lymphogranuloma venereum

Synonyms:
Lymphogranuloma inguinale.
Climatic bubo.
Durand-Nicolas-Favre disease.

This sexually transmitted disease is caused by a *Chlamydia* of Group A (see above). Although of world-wide distribution the disease is most common in tropical countries. The pattern of involvement differs in the two sexes. In males, the primary lesion, a small vesicle or ulcer, generally develops on the external génitalia and is often quite transitory. This may have healed by the time the nodes in one or both groins enlarge, commonly producing prominent 'buboes'. The nodes often become matted and fixed to the skin and breakdown with sinus formation frequently follows. Discharging skin sinuses eventually heal spontaneously but may result in much scarring.

In females, the primary lesion is often on the cervix, but is seldom observed. However, infectivity persists much longer in women than in men. The pelvic and iliac nodes enlarge and there develops a chronic pelvic lymphangitis which may culminate in lymphatic obstruction, leading to chronic vulval oedema and extensive scarring with rectal stricture as a late complication.

In both sexes, fever and constitutional upset may accompany the early, acute stage of the infection.

Macroscopically, the affected nodes (generally inguinal) are often matted and sectioning may reveal multiple small abscesses or larger cavities filled with pus.

Histology. In the early stages the picture may be largely that of a non-specific acute lymphadenitis but showing focal collections of histiocytes in the pulp. These foci soon coalesce, undergo central necrosis and develop into microabscesses (Fig. 6.60). The centres of the lesions are occupied by amorphous debris containing numerous nuclear fragments but often relatively few polymorph leucocytes. However, frank suppuration and softening of the whole centre of the lesion frequently does occur, due to coalescence of the necrotic foci, a characteristically 'stellate' abscess developing (Figs. 6.61, 6.62). The abscesses are surrounded often by a well defined 'wall' of histiocytes, sometimes with a palisaded lining layer and occasional small giant-cells. In the node pulp around the abscesses there is often marked plasma cell infiltration (Fig. 6.63). In time, healing occurs with gross scarring in the node and thickening of the capsule.

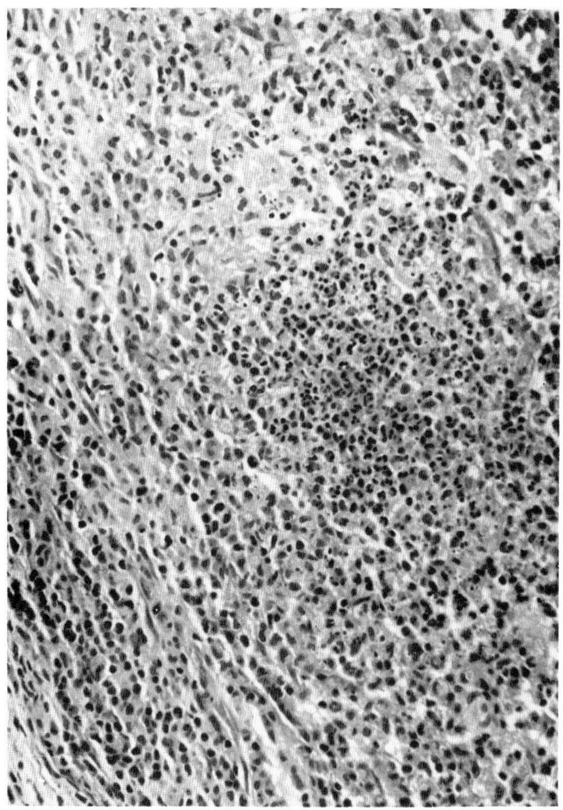

Fig. 6.60 Inguinal lymph node showing early abscess formation in the cortex due to lymphogranuloma venereum. There is much nuclear debris at the centre with histiocytic reaction around. (H E × 300)

Differential diagnosis. The nodal lesions of LGV may be indistinguishable from those of cat scratch disease and the diagnosis made may then be influenced by the age and sex of the patient, the site of the biopsy and the weight of probability in favour of one or other infection. Differentiation of the two diseases can often be achieved by skin testing (intradermal injection of the appropriate test antigen). In the Frei test for LGV the inoculum is derived from *Chlamydia* cultured on yolk sacs of chick embryos: in cat scratch disease (CSD) the test antigen is prepared from the contents of an abscess from a known case of CSD. There is no cross reactivity with these two reagents. If facilities are available, the organism itself may be recovered by culture of infected material on chick embryo yolk sacs, in the case of LGV.

The differential diagnosis also includes other infections characterised by focal necrotising and suppurating granulomas (see under cat scratch disease).

Cat scratch disease

(Cat scratch fever)

This common disease is widespread in Europe and North America and may perhaps be found anywhere where cats are kept as domestic pets. Although it has all the features of an infectious disease and the lesions bear a close resemblance to those of LGV, no infectious agent has yet been isolated and the disease is discussed at this point for convenience, rather than implying that it is due to a *Chlamydia*. Cat scratch disease (CSD) is generally found in households where cats are kept as

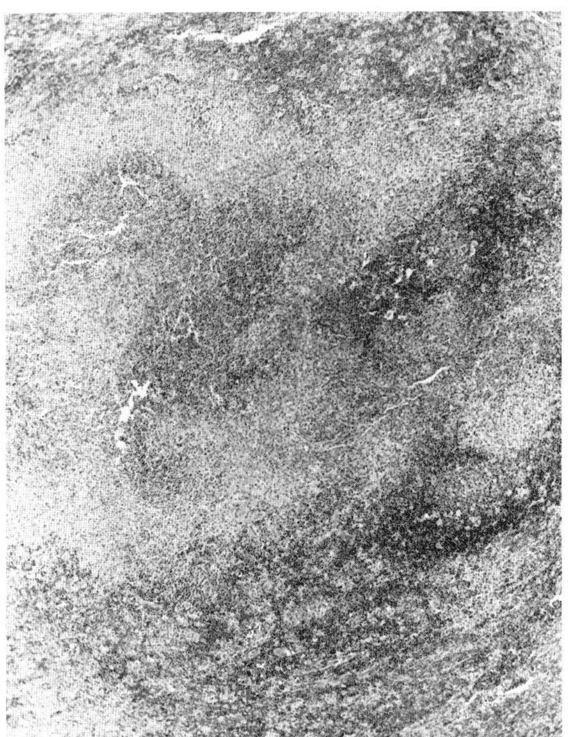

Fig. 6.61 Inguinal lymph node in lymphogranuloma venereum showing characteristic stellate abscess formation. (Same case as Fig. 6.60.) (H E × 47)

Fig. 6.62 Lymphogranuloma venereum. 'Stellate' abscess at higher magnification. (Same case as Figs 6.60 and 6.61.) (H E × 150)

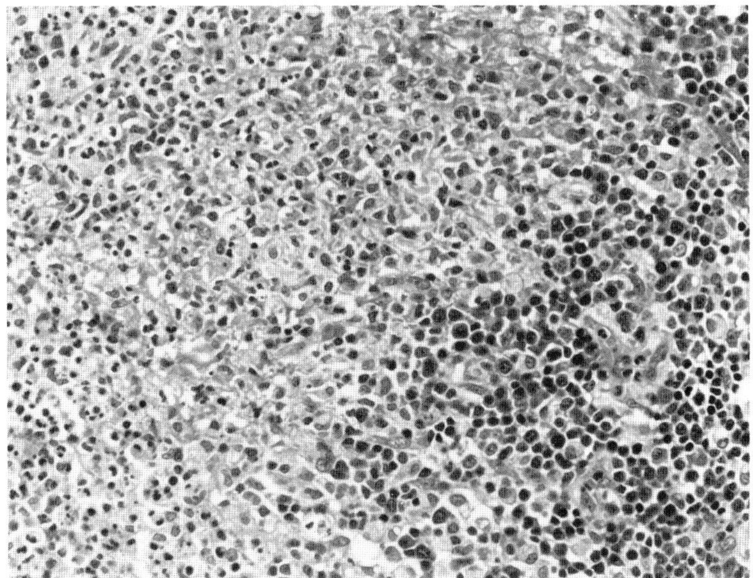

Fig. 6.63 Detail of cellular reaction in lymphogranuloma venereum. Some polymorphs and many nuclear fragments are seen in the abscess centre (left). Around this is a zone of pale-staining histiocytes (middle of field) outside which there are many plasma cells (right). (Same case as Figs 6.60, 6.61 and 6.62) (H E × 300)

pets and the condition often develops following a scratch or bite from a cat. This is not, however, invariable and sometimes it has followed a prick from a thorn or other minor injury in persons who have not handled cats. The disease is commonest in children and young adults. A small blister or papule may develop at the presumed portal of entry through the skin, but such lesions are generally transitory if noticed at all and the presentation is often with enlargement of a lymph node draining the site. The nodes involved are most often from the parotid, cervical or axillary groups, less often inguinal. Lymphadenopathy follows a few days to several weeks after the primary lesion. It often affects only a single node or a small group of nodes which may be tender on palpation. There may be slight fever and constitutional disturbance, but more serious symptoms indicative of pneumonitis or encephalitis are very rare and very few fatalities have been recorded. Although the affected node may break down and become fluctuant with subsequent development of a skin sinus, the disease is generally self-limiting and the lesions heal spontaneously after a few weeks or months. There are no sequelae.

Macroscopically, the node is only moderately enlarged as a rule. The cut surface may be unremarkable, or may show punctate or larger foci of necrosis or actual suppuration. These foci are rarely of large size and may not even be detectable with the naked-eye. Adhesion to surrounding tissue may be evident in the biopsy specimen which is sometimes removed piecemeal.

Histology. As indicated above, there is often a striking similarity between the histological appearances in CSD and those in LGV. Against a background of non-specific immunological reaction (large follicles with prominent germinal centres, immunoblastic reaction and plasmacytosis in the pulp) there is a striking inflammatory component with focal histiocytic aggregates, mainly in the cortex (Fig. 6.64). As in LGV, the latter tend to coalesce, necrosis develops at the centres of the histiocytic foci and small 'microabscesses' may result. In the early stages the necrotic centres are filled with haematoxyphil nuclear fragments and polymorph leucocytes may actually be far fewer than appears at first sight. True suppuration is comparatively uncommon although it may occur.

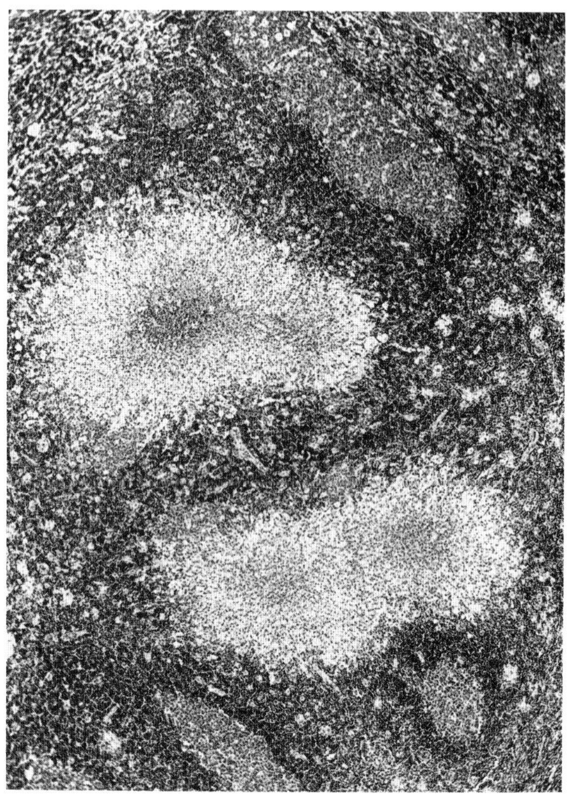

Fig. 6.64 Axillary lymph node showing early lesion of cat scratch disease. Note pronounced follicular hyperplasia. (H E × 47)

The central necrotic area of the lesion is surrounded by a palisaded zone of histiocytes with sometimes a few small multinucleate giant-cells (Fig. 6.65). At a later stage the necrotic foci may become condensed, polymorphs disappear and the lesions then take on a tuberculoid appearance (Fig. 6.66). Small tuberculoid granulomas may also be seen (Fig. 6.67)

In addition to these characteristic focal lesions in CSD, histiocytes may be scattered through the node pulp, sometimes in considerable numbers and eosinophils too are occasionally numerous. 'Immature sinus histiocytosis' (see p. 347) may be present although this is seldom a prominent feature.

Particularly characteristic of cat scratch disease is a well marked periadenitis, with capsular thickening, endolymphangitis of neighbouring lymphatic vessels and often inflammatory cell infiltration of surrounding fat (Fig. 6.68). At a

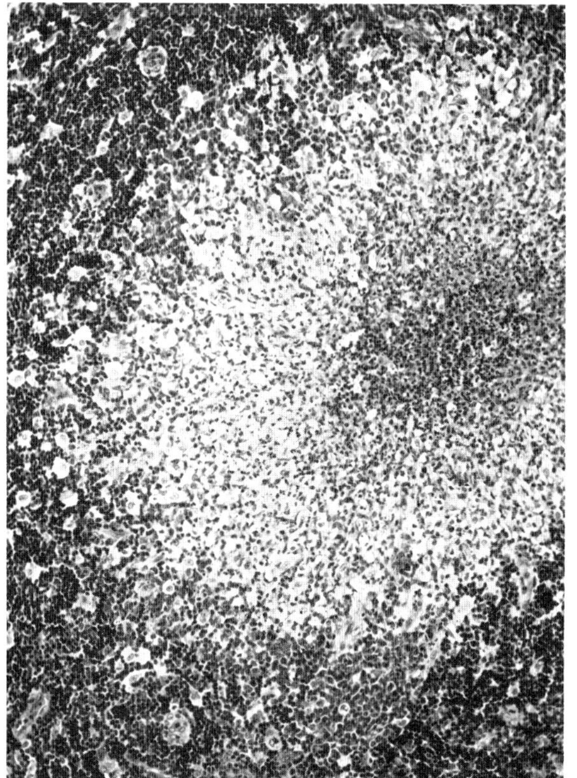

Fig. 6.65 Small focus of histiocytic infiltration with central necrosis ('microabscess') in cat scratch disease (same case as Fig. 6.64) (H E × 120)

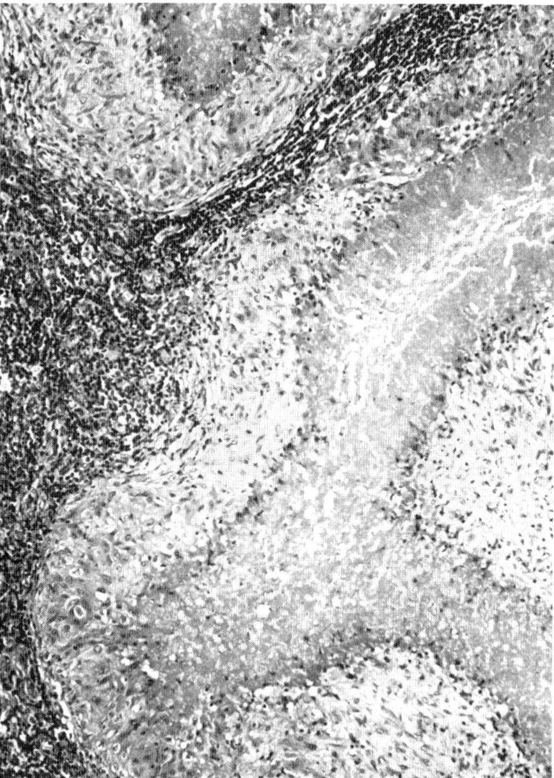

Fig. 6.66 Axillary lymph node showing lesions of cat scratch disease at a later stage. Sharply defined 'geographical' areas of necrosis are surrounded by palisaded histiocytes with early fibrosis of the periphery (compare with Fig. 6.24). (H E × 120)

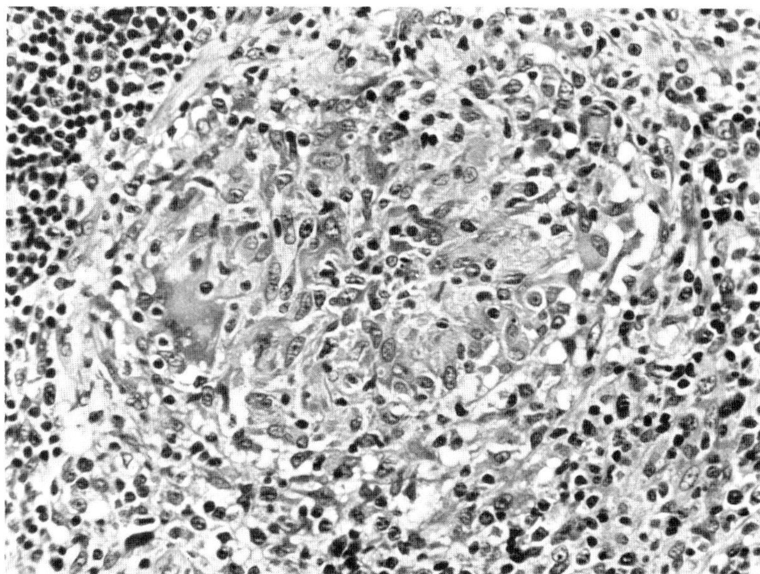

Fig. 6.67 Focal tuberculoid granuloma in lymph node from another case of cat scratch disease. Some plasma cells are present in the surrounding infiltrate. (H E × 300)

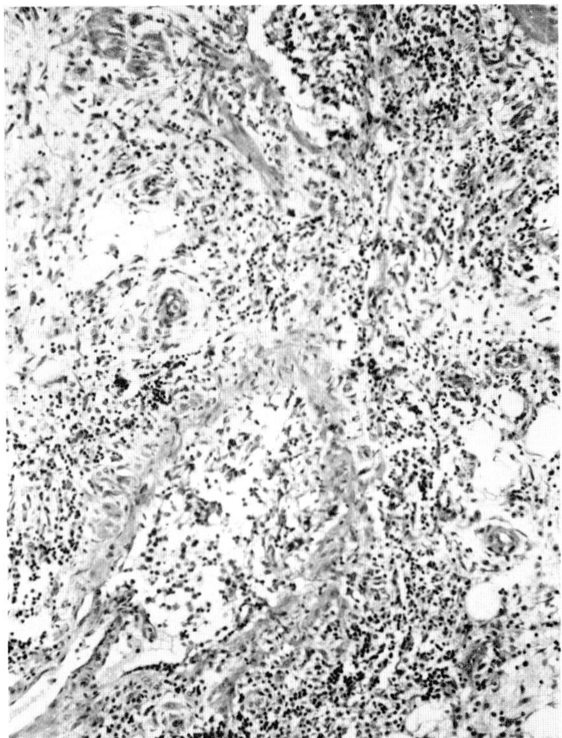

Fig. 6.68 Periadenitis and endolymphangitis of afferent lymphatics in cat scratch disease (H E × 120)

more advanced stage, fibrous scarring in the node may be accompanied by fibrosis in the surrounding tissues.

Organisms are not demonstrable by conventional stains and, as stated above, the cause of CSD remains unknown.

Differential diagnosis. The resemblance of the lymph node lesions to those of LGV has already been pointed out and the differential diagnosis of these two diseases is thus the same. Specific skin tests may help to distinguish CSD and LGV where necessary (see p. 124).

The differential diagnosis also embraces all those types of lymphadenitis in which focal necrosis and/or suppuration is accompanied by a tuberculoid or palisaded histiocytic reaction. These include tuberculosis, some other mycobacterial infections, yersinial lymphadenitis, listeriosis, melioidosis, chronic tularemia and some fungal infections. Most of these can be separated without difficulty on other grounds.

VIRAL DISEASES

There is no doubt that lymph nodes are commonly involved in a great variety of viral infections and lymphadenopathy is an observable feature in many of these, including, for example, the acute haemorrhagic fevers. There is, however, a relatively restricted number of viral diseases in which lymph node biopsy is likely to be performed or is of diagnostic value and these alone will be considered here.

Broadly speaking, viral colonisation of a cell may have one of three effects: (1) the cell may undergo necrosis, (2) the cell may be stimulated to divide, or (3) the virus may inhabit the cell without effecting any visible change in the cell's appearance or function. When necrosis results, the death of many cells in an acute viral infection may then excite an inflammatory reaction and this is seen, for example, in the anterior horn cells in acute poliomyelitis. The proliferative effect is often limited or temporary; on the other hand, it may, in the case of the Epstein-Barr virus and in certain circumstances, lead to perpetuation of the change and to the production of a malignant tumour (Burkitt's lymphoma) or to the 'immortalisation' of a cell line in culture. The known or hypothetical participation of viruses in neoplasms of lymphoid cells is dealt with elsewhere in this book (pp 283, p. 324) and will not be further discussed here.

Infectious mononucleosis (glandular fever)

Although the term 'glandular fever' is still often used as a synonym for infectious mononucleosis, there are many who regard glandular fever as a less specific term, embracing several different infections which may give rise to the syndrome of fever, widespread lymph node enlargement and abnormal lymphocytes in the peripheral blood. In this sense 'glandular fever' covers also several entities discussed under differential diagnosis below, especially lymphadenitis caused by cytomegalovirus, listeriosis and toxoplasmic lymphadenitis. Since 'abnormal' mononuclear cells in the peripheral blood are not the prerogative of infectious mononucleosis, but occur to a lesser degree in other viral infections, it may be objected that the term 'infectious mononucleosis' is no more specific than 'glandular fever' for the disease in question. Be that as it may, infectious mononucleosis (IM) will be used here as implying the disease now known to be caused by a small herpes-type virus — the Epstein Barr virus (EBV).

IM is a common disease of the young throughout the Western world, indeed the virus is ubiquitous and the high incidence of EBV antibodies in the adult population indicates that subclinical infections are common. The sexes are equally affected and the common mode of transmission, by passionate kissing, probably accounts for the high frequency of the disease in adolescents and young adults.

Clinically the typical presenting features are fever, sore throat and widespread lymphadenopathy. Splenomegaly may be found on examination. The occurrence of a rash is usually attributable to the administration of ampicillin for the sore throat. The illness varies greatly in severity and although in the great majority of instances IM is a benign, self-limiting disease, patients may at times be severely ill, even in the absence of overt complications. The latter include hepatitis and jaundice, thrombocytopenia, 'spontaneous' splenic rupture and CNS complications — particularly encephalomyelitis and Guillain-Barré syndrome. Fatalities are rare, but deaths have occurred from asphyxia due to tonsillar swelling, as well as from the complications enumerated above. The disease also appears to carry a very grave prognosis in immunodeficient boys who may develop "X-linked lymphoproliferative disease" (Purtilo's syndrome).

Blood changes. One of the most distinctive features of the disease is the presence in the circulating blood of abnormal mononuclear cells. These vary in number but often constitute up to 60% or even more of the nucleated cells in the peripheral blood at the height of the disease. Originally thought to be monocytes, the abnormal cells are now known to be transformed lymphocytes and, as remarked above, similar cells may be found in smaller numbers in other viral diseases. An incautious diagnosis of acute leukaemia has frequently been made from the examination of a blood film in IM and Damashek (1969) has not inaptly described the changes as those of a 'reversible leukaemia'.

The other characteristic haematological finding in IM is the appearance of antibodies in the serum. These include a variety of 'heterophil' antibodies, as well as antibodies to EBV, and the diagnostic test for the disease — the Paul-Bunnell test — is based on the presence of antibodies which agglutinate sheep erythrocytes after absorption with guinea pig serum.

Lymph node changes. Lymph node biopsy is unlikely to be undertaken when a diagnosis of IM is suspected, unless the presentation is atypical. This means that the pathologist may have no advance warning, when confronted with a lymph node section showing apparent architectural effacement and proliferation of atypical lymphoid cells and may be led into making a wrong diagnosis of malignant lymphoma. Pathologists should be constantly on their guard against making this potentially serious mistake and it should be remembered that abdominal as well as superficial node groups may be involved — indeed the presentation may be abdominal.

Macroscopically the nodes are seldom more than 2–3 cm in diameter. They are generally soft, and the cut surface is pink and featureless, though it may be blotched with haemorrhage.

Histologically the changes vary a good deal, perhaps depending upon the stage at which the biopsy is taken (Gowing, 1975). In some instances, probably early in the disease, *follicles* are preserved and may indeed be hyperplastic, with prominent germinal centres. Later the follicles are inconspicuous and are overrun by proliferating lymphoid cells, so that the normal pattern becomes obscured. The *paracortex* is the site of the initial transformation and proliferation of lymphoid cells (Fig. 6.69). Early on, scattered immunoblasts are seen in the expanded T-zones, just as in some other DNA virus diseases (herpes zoster, vaccinia, CMV). These large, pale cells, sometimes in mitosis, stand out against the background of small lymphocytes, imparting a spotty effect at low magnification. Further expansion of the T-zones probably develops rapidly (Fig. 6.70) and generally, by the time the node is removed for biopsy, the follicles have all but disappeared and the pulp is filled with actively dividing immunoblasts which have

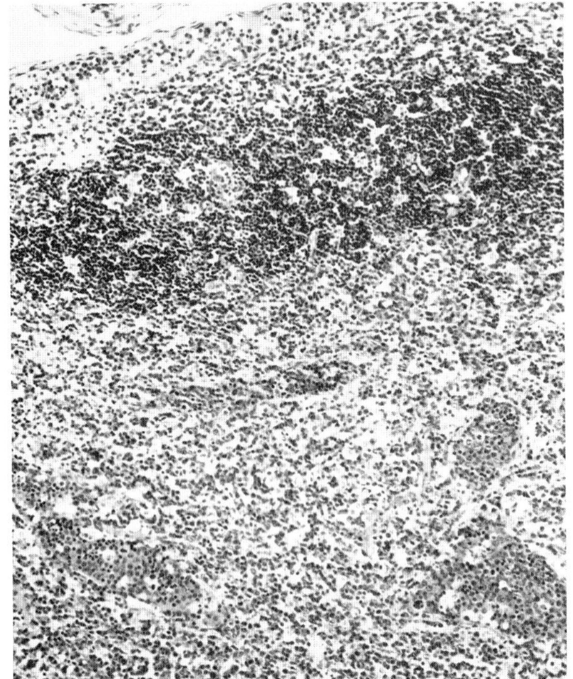

Fig. 6.69 Mesenteric lymph node removed at laparotomy from a girl of 11 who presented with acute abdominal symptoms. The changes are typical of infectious mononucleosis and this diagnosis was subsequently confirmed. The paracortex is expanded and the cortex reduced showing an inactive follicle (left). Note the dilated sinuses packed with cells. (H E × 120)

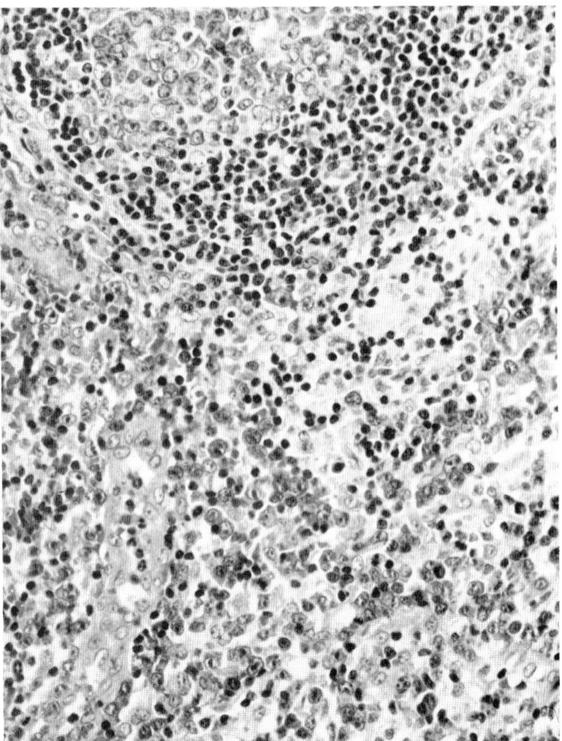

Fig. 6.70 Inguinal lymph node from a young man with infectious mononucleosis, showing a small germinal follicle (above) and proliferating immunoblasts in the paracortex (H E × 300)

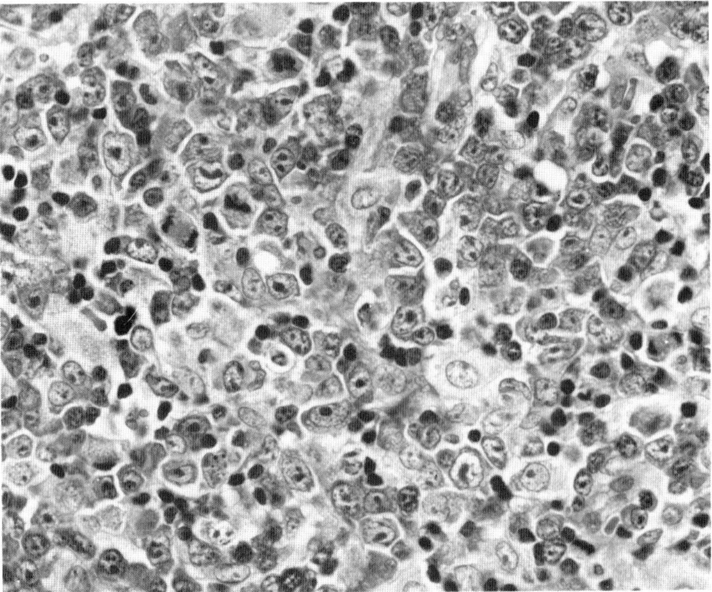

Fig. 6.71 Detail of paracortical infiltrate in infectious mononucleosis showing large immunoblasts, some in mitosis (same case as Fig. 6.70) (H E × 470)

replaced in varying degree the small lymphocyte population (Fig. 6.71). Although the blast cells are mainly mononuclear (corresponding to the cells which appear in the peripheral blood), binucleate and atypical giant forms are sometimes found and these may closely resemble Sternberg-Reed cells (Fig. 6.72) (Lukes & Tindle, 1969; Tindle et al, 1972).

The wholesale blastic transformation, with many mitoses and perhaps atypical cells may immediately suggest a diagnosis of malignant lymphoma, but on careful inspection several features may be seen which militate against a malignant proliferation. First, although the immunoblasts may be in solid clumps, these are interspersed with other cells (Fig. 6.73); they are rarely in diffuse, uninterrupted sheets covering large areas of the node, as is usual in a high grade malignant lymphoma. Secondly, the immunoblasts of IM are not uniform, they often vary in respect of the degree of cytoplasmic basophilia. Many of the blast cells at this stage have a strongly basophilic and pyroninophilic cytoplasm, of an intensity seldom rivalled by malignant cells. Thirdly, these large pyroninophilic cells are found not only in the dense pulp of the node but, as in other infections, they are regularly to be seen in large numbers in the *sinuses*. (Figs. 6.69, 6.73). The sinuses may have appeared at first sight to be obliterated, but on close inspection they are found to be dilated and stuffed with immunoblasts (Fig. 6.74). At this time, many of the pyroninophilic cells begin to exhibit features of plasmacytoid differentiation and then plasma cells of all degrees of maturity mingle with the still proliferating immunoblasts (Fig. 6.75). The thickened capsule of the node is often infiltrated by lymphoid cells including some mature plasma cells.

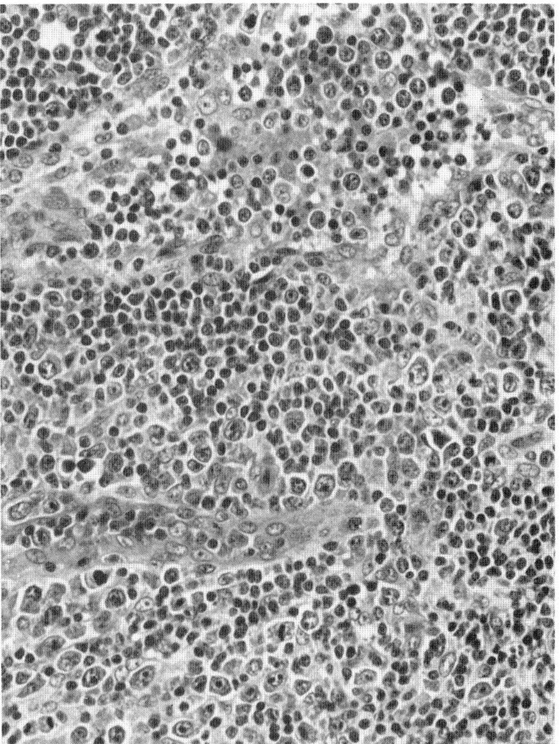

Fig. 6.73 Another area of the same node as Figs 6.70 and 6.71 showing immunoblasts interspersed with lymphocytes. Note dilated sinus filled with blast cells (top). (H E × 300)

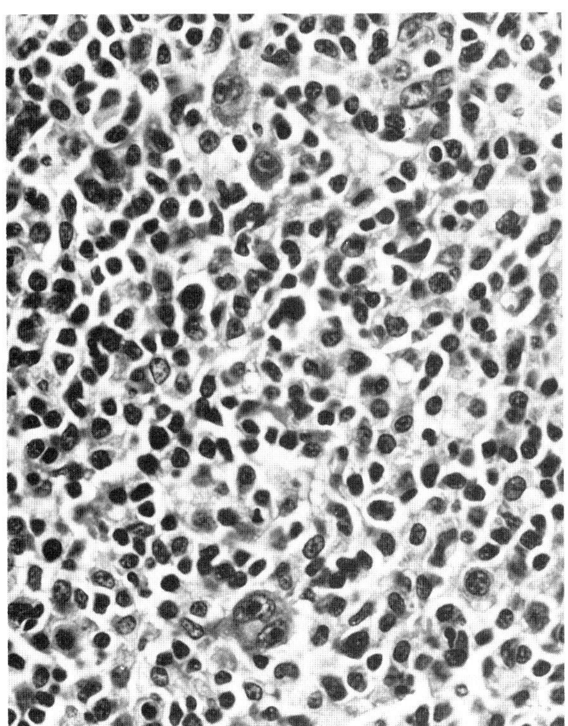

Fig. 6.72 Tonsil from a boy of 17 with infectious mononucleosis showing Sternberg-Reed like cells (H E × 470)

In place of the sinus change described above the sinuses may show 'immature sinus histiocytosis' (p. 347) — a phenomenon which is generally indicative of a reactive process. Epithelioid cell clusters may be seen in the pulp. These are often

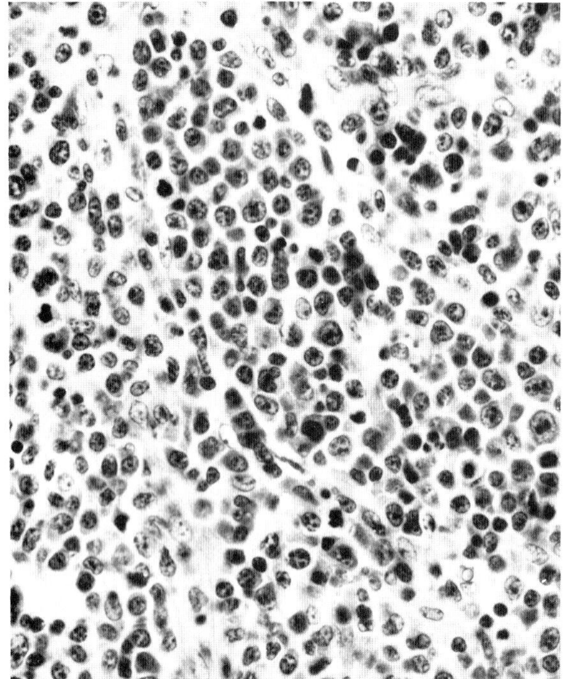

Fig. 6.74 Dilated sinus filled with large lymphoid cells many showing evidence of plasmacytoid differentiation (same case as Fig. 6.69) (H E × 470)

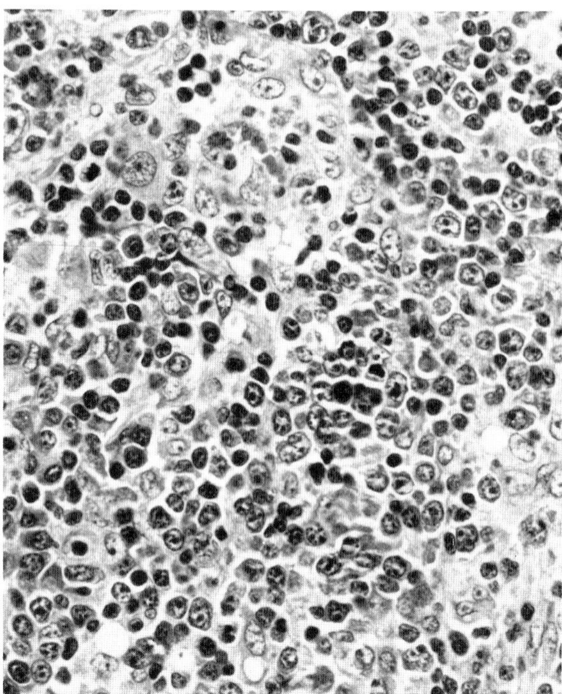

Fig. 6.75 Immunoblasts mingled with immature plasma cells and macrophages (top). (Same case as Figs 6.70, 6.71 and 6.73.) (H E × 470)

scanty and not a conspicuous feature, but occasionally they are numerous and then the histological picture may closely resemble that of toxoplasmosis. Small foci of necrosis are not uncommon in lymph nodes in IM, but extensive necrosis is more commonly seen in the tonsils than in the nodes. Polymorphs are seldom seen except in the presence of necrosis.

Differential diagnosis. Infectious mononucleosis has first, and most importantly, to be distinguished from a malignant lymphoproliferative disorder — lymphoma or leukaemia. In making this distinction, the age of the patient and the clinical history may help, as well, of course, as the result of a Paul-Bunnell or 'monospot' test. The points enumerated above will help to distinguish the histological picture from that of a high grade non-Hodgkin's lymphoma. The resemblance to Hodgkin's disease may sometimes be close, but generally only in small areas of the node, and Sternberg-Reed-like cells are only diagnostic of Hodgkin's disease when seen in an appropriate setting.

Differentiation of IM from other infections which may cause 'glandular fever', e.g. cytomegalovirus lymphadenitis, toxoplasmosis and listeriosis, is seldom a problem, although occasionally IM may produce changes resembling those of toxoplasmosis. The distinction may be made by serological tests. Finally some instances of drug hypersensitivity may produce a clinical and pathological picture with a resemblance to infectious mononucleosis. The clinical history and result of a Paul-Bunnell test will help to resolve the issue.

Cytomegalovirus lymphadenitis

The virus of cytomegalic disease is again a herpes type virus (CMV), probably of world-wide distribution. Although formerly regarded as an opportunistic infection, causing intrauterine and neonatal deaths and only liable to attack adults rendered susceptible by immune deficiency or suppression, CMV disease is now recognised as occurring sporadically in previously healthy individuals. The commonest form for the disease to take is a 'glandular fever' type illness resembling infectious mononucleosis but differing from the latter in the absence of sore throat (Klemola & Kääriäinen, 1965). 'Cytomegalovirus mononucleosis' is also distinguished by a negative Paul-Bunnell reaction and a sharply rising titre of complement fixing antibodies for CMV. There is significant lymphadenopathy in only a minority of cases (Jordan et al, 1973) and the histological features in lymph nodes have seldom been recorded. In a personally observed case, sections of the node showed both large reactive germinal follicles and a prominent immunoblastic reaction in the paracortical areas. The histological features were not specific in that cells showing cytomegalic change were not found and the diagnosis was based on the observation of a dramatic rise in the CMV complement-fixing antibody titre coinciding with the patient's illness. The histological picture was, however, very similar to that present in a lymph node section shown to the author by Professor Lennert, in which isolated large lymphoid cells in both germinal centres and pulp showed typical CMV inclusions. It seems that CMV inclusions are seldom found in the lymph node sections in this disease and the diagnosis must generally be based, therefore, on isolation of the virus from fresh tissue or on serological evidence. When CMV inclusions are present their appearance is pathognomonic, even when, as is usual, only scattered cells are affected. The affected cells, which may be of almost any type, are very large, with a very large round or ovoid inclusion body in the centre of the large nucleus. The inclusion body stands out sharply, by virtue of its intense staining and because it is surrounded by a clear halo. The expanded cytoplasm contains granular appearing basophilic material to one side of the nucleus. Such cells may be picked out with the low power of the microscope.

Lymphadenitis caused by Herpes viruses

The three Herpes group viruses associated with exanthematous eruptions — *Herpesvirus varicella-zoster (HVZ)*, *Herpesvirus hominis (HVH)* and *Herpesvirus simiae (Herpes B virus — HVB)* — are all liable to produce lymphadenitis, regionally or sometimes more generally. However, lymph node biopsy is unlikely to be undertaken, except in occasional cases of zoster (HVZ). Although specific inclusion bodies have very rarely been found in lymph node sections in this disease, the nodes frequently show a characteristic picture of immunoblastic proliferation in the T-zones, giving the latter a spotty or 'peppered' appearance under the low power of the microscope (Figs. 6.76, 6.77). There may be some follicular hyperplasia, although this is not a striking feature.

In disseminated disease caused by HVH or HVB, focal necroses have been found in lymph nodes, as in other tissues.

Post-vaccinial lymphadenitis

With the eradication of smallpox and thus removal of the necessity for vaccination, this condition is likely to be of academic rather than practical importance in the future. At the time of writing, cases may yet be observed, since some countries are still insisting upon vaccination. The local cutaneous lesion caused by the *Vaccinia* virus (*Poxvirus officinale*) at the site of the vaccination, is commonly accompanied by enlargement of the regional lymph nodes, which may be painful. As a rule the nodes subside spontaneously with healing of the skin lesion, but occasionally the nodal swelling recurs later. If the patient presenting to the doctor fails to report the fact of a recent vaccination in the vicinity of the nodal swelling, a biopsy may be taken of the latter to establish the diagnosis.

Histologically the reaction is similar to that seen in other viral infections previously discussed, namely a proliferation of immunoblasts in the T-zones, generally with suppression of the follicles. The presence of clumps of large, transformed cells with frequent mitoses and disturbance of the normal architecture may lead to an erroneous diagnosis of malignancy, but the same remarks apply here as have been advanced in the discussion on infectious mononucleosis (see p. 131).

Measles

Unlike the viral diseases discussed hitherto, measles is caused by a RNA virus — more specifically a *paramyxovirus*. Swelling of the lymphoid tissues throughout the body occurs in the prodromal stage of measles and this may sometimes lead to a biopsy

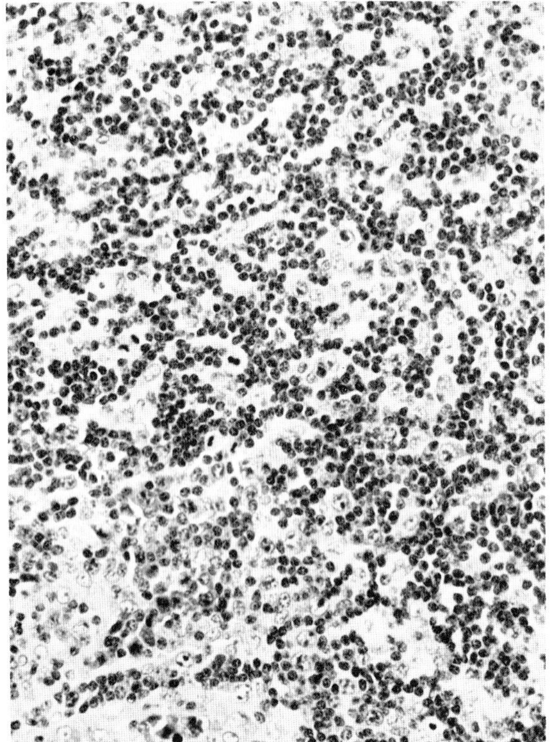

Fig. 6.76 Lymph node in Herpes zoster showing 'peppered' appearance of paracortex due to scattered immunoblasts, some in mitosis (H E × 300)

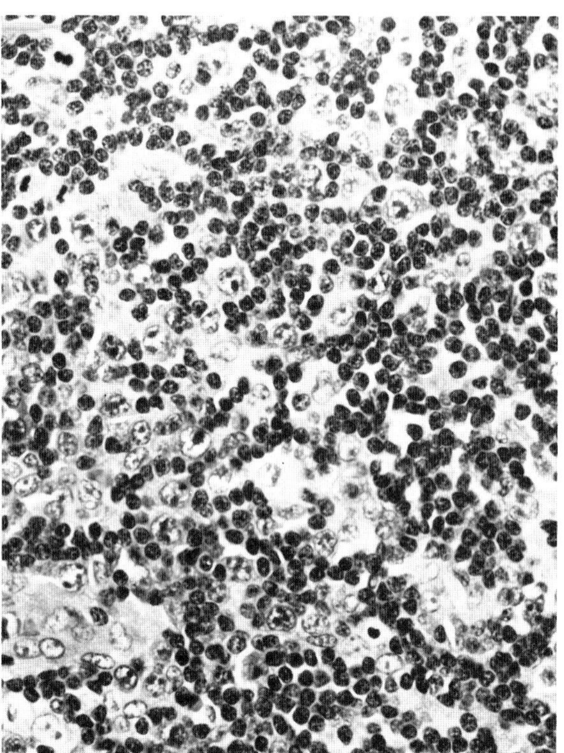

Fig. 6.77 Higher power of same node as Fig. 6.76 to show immunoblasts. A similar picture is seen in many viral infections. (H E × 470)

being taken from a lymph node or tonsil, or even to appendicectomy, since swelling of the appendicular lymphoid tissue may obstruct the lumen and clinically simulate acute appendicitis.

The histological changes in the lymphoid tissues from any of these sites are specific for measles, but the pathologist seldom has the satisfaction of coming first with the diagnosis, since the rash has generally appeared by the time the sections are through.

Histologically, there is follicular hyperplasia with the formation of large germinal centres and, within these, highly distinctive, multinucleate giant-cells may be seen (Warthin-Finkeldey giant-cells) (Figs. 6.78, 6.79). The crowded, hyperchromatic nuclei of these cells render them very conspicuous and they are readily identified on low-power examination of the section. Not every germinal centre is involved, but some centres may contain several such cells. Warthin-Finkeldey giant-cells presumably result from a process of cell fusion, such as is seen with cells in culture when infected with certain viruses. Cells of this type are not, however, entirely specific for measles and occasional syncitial lymphoid cells may be seen in malignant lymphomas (especially centroblastic-centrocytic lymphoma) and in a variety of reactive states (Kjeldsberg & Kim, 1981). Warthin-Finkeldey giant-cells do not contain viral inclusion bodies and are morphologically quite different from the giant-cells found in the lung in measles pneumonia.

Other viral infections

Lymphadenopathy is at times a notable clinical feature of some virus diseases other than those already discussed, but either because the diagnosis is obvious without recourse to lymph node biopsy (e.g. rubella), or because the histological changes in the nodes are apparently non-specific (rubella and adenovirus infections), these do not call for further discussion here.

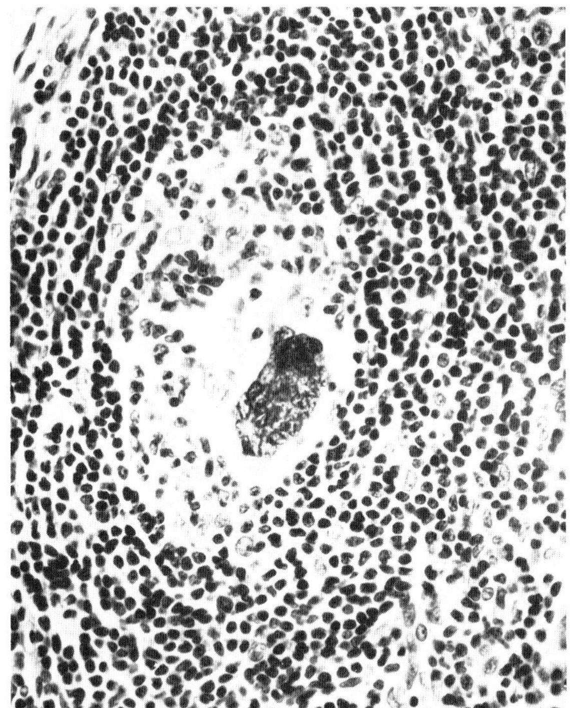

Fig. 6.78 Mesenteric lymph node from a child with measles showing a Warthin-Finkeldey giant-cell in a small germinal centre (H E × 375)

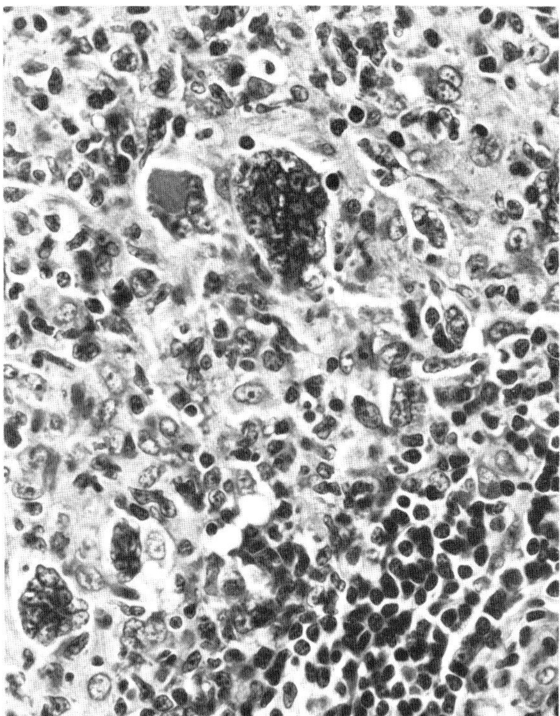

Fig. 6.79 Tonsil from another case of measles showing several Warthin-Finkeldey giant-cells in a hyperplastic germinal centre (H E × 470)

One is often tempted to speculate whether the changes seen in a lymph node biopsy section may be due to a 'viral infection'. This applies particularly in those instances where an immunoblastic reaction is seen in the interfollicular pulp and sinuses, with or without other features, such as focal necrosis or epithelioid cell clusters. No doubt many such cases are of viral aetiology, but proof is lacking and the nature of the 'virus' remains undetermined, since all the available tissue has already been fixed and the patient recovers.

DRUG REACTIONS

Introduction

The lymphoreticular tissues may produce an immune response to inanimate chemical antigens or haptens, just as they do to living organisms and their products. Certain classes of drugs are notoriously liable to induce a reaction in the subjects to which they are administered, but it is equally clear that individuals differ greatly in their susceptibility to sensitisation in this way. There is obviously involvement of the immune system in the production of all kinds of hypersensitivity to chemical compounds, but lymphadenopathy in the course of the sensitisation process is relatively uncommon. It is seen most often in hypersensitivity of serum sickness type, lymph node enlargement being a feature of serum sickness itself. However, although different patterns of clinical presentation have been described in association with this form of hypersensitivity, it appears that there is a continuous spectrum of pathological changes in the lymphoreticular tissues, ranging from a perfectly banal lymphoid hyperplasia at one end of the spectrum, through varying degrees of lymphoid dysplasia, to the very rare development of a true malignant lymphoma at the other. The real importance of this subject lies in the fact that many patients with a simple drug hypersensitivity reaction have been wrongly diagnosed as having a malignant lymphoma on misinterpretation of a lymph node biopsy. This is not to deny that drug hypersensitivity may itself be a dangerous condition especially if the offending drug is not withdrawn.

Types of drug and mode of action

Although this type of hypersensitivity has been reported with a variety of unrelated chemical compounds, certain classes of drug known to produce hypersensitivity also have common configurations in their molecular structure which may help to explain the tendency to provoke an immune response. Some drugs (e.g. sulphonamides) are known to act as haptens, readily becoming attached to serum albumin (Davis, 1942) In other instances the mode of action is less clear.

The principal classes of drug provoking sensitisation of this type are: sulphonamides, thiouracil and related compounds, penicillins, phenylbutazone and some other antipyretics (e.g. indomethacin), some antimalarials (Cullen et al, 1979) and anticonvulsants — notoriously the hydantoins.

The frequency with which hypersensitivity reactions arise varies greatly with different drugs. They are uncommon, for instance, with penicillins, having regard to the widespread use of antibiotics. On the other hand lymphadenopathy is very common in individuals undergoing anticonvulsant therapy with hydantoin compounds. This may be partly a reflection of the duration of administration of the drug in question. Signs of hypersensitivity may appear within a few weeks from the first administration of a drug or may not appear for many months and patients on anticonvulsants are generally on long term therapy.

Clinical presentation

The classical presentation of serum sickness type hypersensitivity is with fever, urticarial skin rashes and lymphadenopathy, generally widespread. The rashes may be fleeting and are sometimes more erythematous than urticarial. If a lymph node biopsy is suspected of showing a drug reaction, a history of a skin rash is valuable confirmatory evidence. Joint pains are also a common feature, sometimes with effusions into the joints.

Some patients present with fever and a 'mononucleosis' type of blood picture, with or without lymphadenopathy, and drug hypersensitivity is thus a differential diagnosis of infectious mononucleosis and the other infections which mimic it (p. 132). More serious symptoms may develop in a minority of cases or if the drug is not stopped: jaundice due to a hepatotoxic reaction, which may even prove fatal, and agranulocytosis, due to marrow toxicity. Liver and bone marrow damage may also result from a direct toxic action of some drugs, which has nothing to do with hypersensitivity.

The lymphadenopathy which is associated with hydantoin medication is somewhat different in that it frequently appears without associated fever or skin rashes, though it is commonly associated with hypertrophy of the gums. Furthermore, as already stated, it is extremely common in epileptics on long term therapy with anticonvulsant drugs. It is in this group too that cellular atypia may be most marked in the hyperplastic lymphoid tissues (see below).

Pathological features

Macroscopically the lymph nodes may be quite large, measuring up to 3 cm or more in diameter. They are discrete and of variable consistency. Sometimes small foci of necrosis may be visible on the cut surface.

Histology. Although there is a common thread running through all these cases, the picture varies considerably from case to case and no doubt varies too with the timing of the biopsy. As with many viral infections, the immunoblastic reaction, which is the dominant theme, affects the T-zones of the node, often partly sparing the follicles which generally appear unreactive and lack germinal centres (Fig. 6.80). By contrast, the expanded T-zones contain a polymorphic infiltrate with many transformed cells, often atypical in varying degree, cells in mitosis, plasma cells, histiocytes and eosinophils. The relative proportions of the different cellular ingredients vary — in one case there may be a preponderance of blast-type cells, in another, plasma cells, in a third, eosinophils, and in a fourth, macrophages. There is variation too within

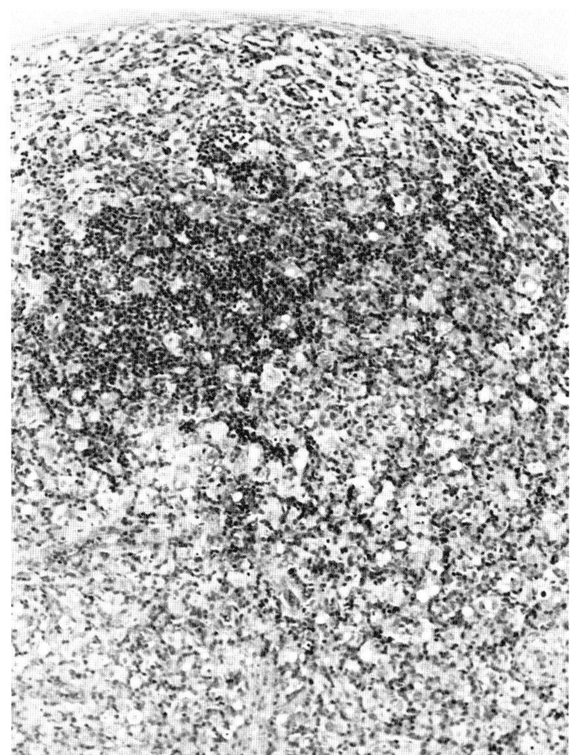

Fig. 6.80 Lymph node biopsy from a two and a half year old girl who was inadvertently given sulphadimidine for a urinary infection after she had previously shown evidence of sensitivity to sulpha drugs. The paracortex shows wholesale transformation of lymphocytes into immunoblasts and there is infiltration of eosinophils and macrophages. A non-reactive follicle remains (top left). (H E × 120)

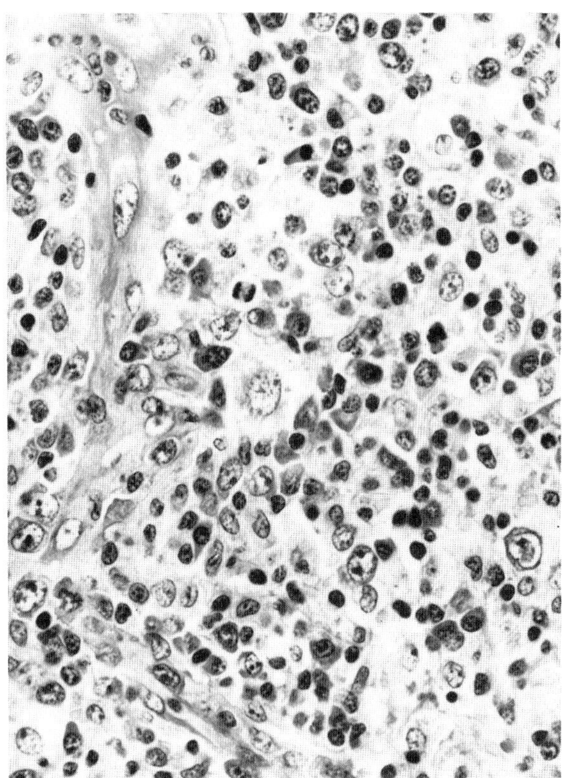

Fig. 6.81 Lymph node biopsy from a case of hydantoin hypersensitivity. Proliferating venules and a mixed infiltrate, including many immunoblasts and plasma cells, combine to produce an exact mimicry of angiommunoblastic lymphadenopathy. (H E × 470)

a single node, though the whole node is affected by changes in some degree.

As is the rule with T-zone reactions, the post-capillary venules tend to stand out, due to endothelial swelling and there may on occasion be a marked proliferation of small blood vessels in the paracortex (Fig. 6.81). When this is combined with extinction of the follicles and a polymorphic infiltrate as described above, it will readily be appreciated that the picture may be indistinguishable from that of angioimmunoblastic lymphadenopathy (AIL) (p. 176). Indeed a proportion of patients in whom a diagnosis of AIL is made on a lymph node biopsy, give a history of drug administration prior to the onset of their disease (Lukes, 1975). In some patients presenting with this picture the lymphadenopathy and other symptoms have regressed completely on witholding the drug (Cullen et al, 1979) (Figs 6.82, 6.83).

Necrosis is another variable feature in the nodes in drug hypersensitivity. In some instances, there is little or none — on the other hand, there may be very extensive necrosis, which can be either a wholesale necrosis of transformed cells in the paracortex (sparing the follicles), or actual infarction of the whole or parts of the node (Fig. 6.84). In the latter instance there may be a demonstrable necrotising arteritis, as part of the hypersensitivity picture, with arterial thrombosis to account for the infarction. At other times, venular thrombi are found within small, peripheral infarcts. A finding of definite angiitis is a strong pointer to a diagnosis of drug reaction (Krasznai & Szegedi, 1969) (Fig. 6.85). In those instances cited above, where

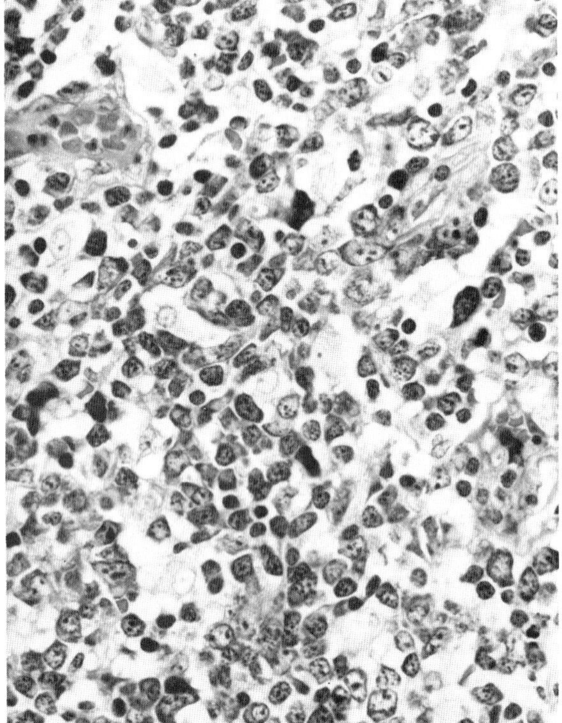

Fig. 6.82 Lymphadenopathy due to hypersensitivity to an antimalarial drug. The histological picture was not distinguishable from that of angioimmunoblastic lymphadenopathy, but the nodes subsided and the patient got better when the drug was withheld. The field shows large numbers of immunoblasts and plasma cells with many macrophages. (Giemsa × 470)

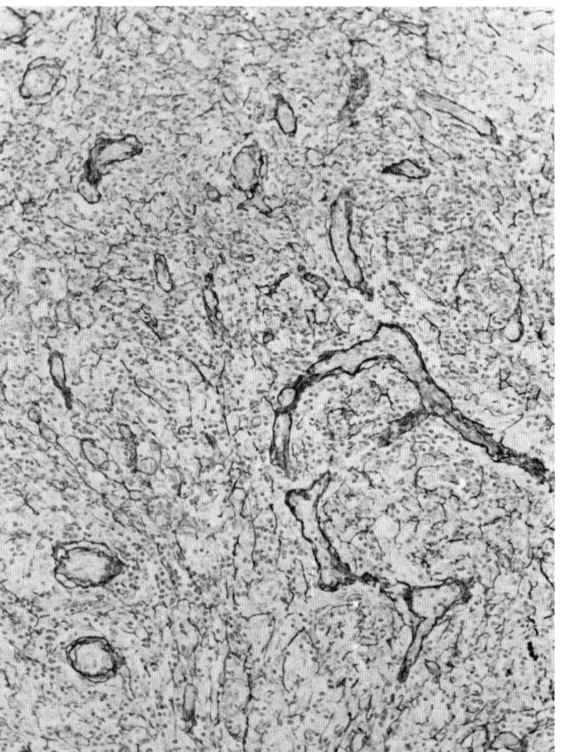

Fig. 6.83 Same node as Fig. 6.82 showing striking proliferation of venules in the paracortical areas. The vascular changes are identical to those found in angioimmunoblastic lymphadenopathy. (Compare Fig. 8.23, p. 178) (Gordon and Sweets reticulin × 120)

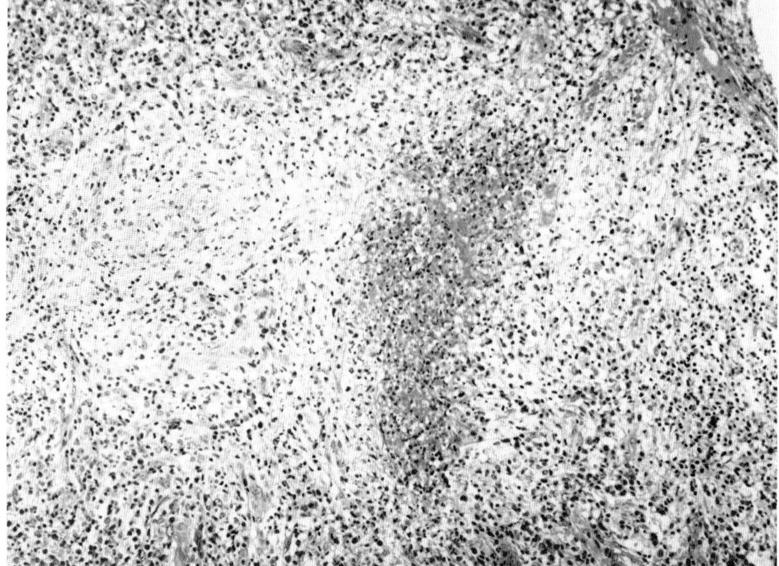

Fig. 6.84 In this case of hydantoin hypersensitivity there was widespread peripheral infarction of the node — a common finding in drug hypersensitivity. The figure shows a small focus of infarction. (Same case as Fig. 6.81.) (H E × 120)

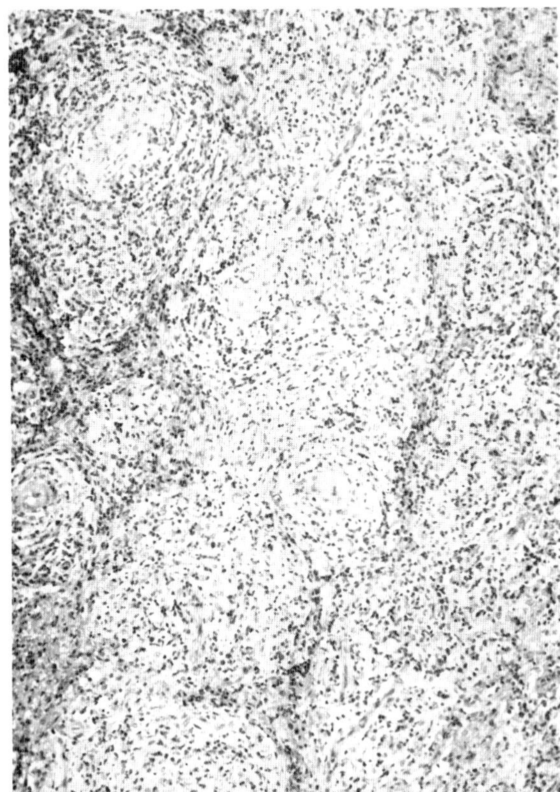

Fig. 6.85 Lymph node biopsy from a case of penicillin hypersensitivity in a boy of 8. The node shows evidence of widespread angiitis in the striking perivascular oedema, accompanied by concentric perivascular inflammatory cell infiltration. There is severe lymphocyte depletion. (H E × 120)

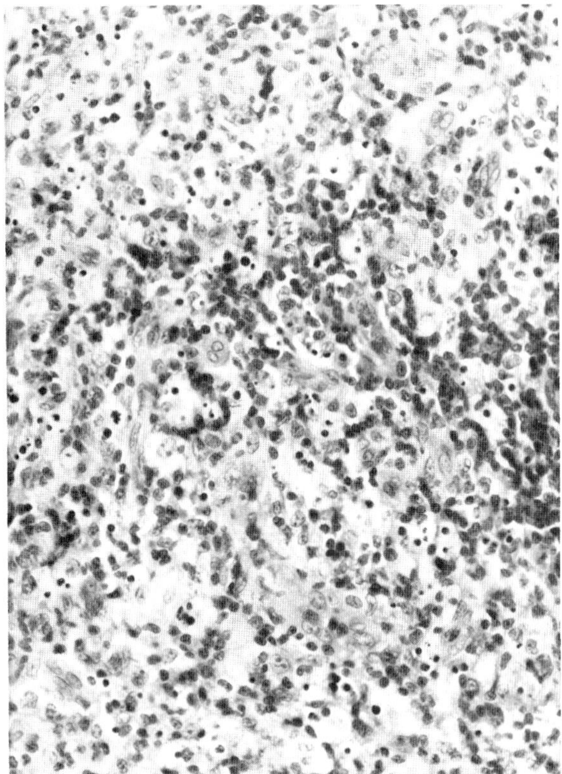

Fig. 6.86 Same node as Fig. 6.85. Remnants of a follicle persist (right), but within the T-cell areas there is wholesale lymphocyte destruction and the field is littered with nuclear fragments, many contained within macrophages which are abundant. (H E × 300)

widespread necrosis of transformed cells occurs, massive infiltration by macrophages follows and at that stage, the node shows a remarkable picture of lymphocyte depletion with many macrophages phagocytosing nuclear debris (Fig. 6.86).

The totally unfamiliar histological picture, with apparent deletion of normal landmarks may incline the pathologist to suspect malignancy in such cases and the suspicion may be heightened, not only by the degree of mitotic activity, but by the presence of bizarre blast-type cells, sometimes of binucleate or multinucleate type. These cells may have very prominent nucleoli and may indeed be indistinguishable from Hodgkin and Sternberg-Reed cells (p. 202). In this respect too, there may be a close resemblance between a drug reaction and the picture of infectious mononucleosis (p. 131). Such bizarre blast cells may be found in small numbers in the reactions to a variety of drugs, but they have been noted particularly frequently in hydantoin reactions and it is in association with this group of drugs that cases of malignant lymphoma have been reported (Hyman & Sommers, 1966) There can be no doubt that some of the reported cases of malignant lymphoma following hydantoin lymphadenopathy are genuine enough and a progression of histological changes has been observed in successive lymph node biopsies in a few instances (Gams et al, 1968).

However, the frequent lack of follow-up information in published reports of malignant lymphoma in hydantoin lymphadenopathy, the high proportion of cases which have been diagnosed as Hodgkin's disease and the observation of changes closely resembling those of Hodgkin's disease in cases of hydantoin reaction which have subsequently regressed spontaneously, all incline one to believe that true malignant lymphomas developing in these circumstances are probably much rarer than the number of published cases might suggest.

Prognosis

In the great majority of instances of drug-induced lymphadenopathy, the lymph node swellings, like the other features of the reaction, subside spontaneously when the drug is stopped. Symptoms may, however, recur if, at any time, the same or an allied drug is given again. If the patient continues to take the offending drug, the lymphadenopathy may increase and there is a risk of the patient developing more serious complications like hepatitis or agranulocytosis. With the hydantoins, there is a very small risk of malignant lymphoma supervening, but, it seems, a much greater risk of the patient's condition being misdiagnosed as malignant lymphoma and the patient then subjected to potentially dangerous treatment.

Differential diagnosis

If a good history is available the diagnosis may be suspected before recourse to lymph node biopsy. The presence of widespread, symmetrical lymphadenopathy, associated with skin rashes, joint pains and fever strongly favour a drug reaction. The patient may, however, deliberately or otherwise, fail to mention the taking of a drug and it may then be left to the pathologist to suggest the diagnosis. As indicated in the discussion above, the main differential diagnoses to be considered are (1) a viral lymphadenitis, especially infectious mononucleosis, (2) immunoblastic lymphadenopathy (p. 175), and (3) malignant lymphoma — particularly Hodgkin's disease. In regard to the last, it needs to be emphasised that a diagnosis of Hodgkin's disease should always be based on sounder evidence than the finding of a few cells resembling Sternberg-Reed and Hodgkin cells, but it must be admitted that the differential diagnosis may at times be extraordinarily difficult.

REFERENCES

Cullen M H, Stansfeld A G, Oliver R T D, Lister T A, Malpas J S 1979 Angio-immunoblastic lymphadenopathy: report of ten cases and review of the literature. Quarterly Journal of Medicine 48: 151–177

Damashek W 1969 Speculations on the nature of infectious mononucleosis. In: Carter R L, Penman H G (eds) Infectious mononucleosis, Blackwell Scientific Publications, Oxford, p 255

Davis B D 1942 Binding of sulphonamides by plasma proteins. Science 95:78

Eimoto I, Kikuchi M, Mitsui I 1983 Histiocytic necrotizing lymphadenitis: an ultrastructural study in comparison with other types of lymphadenitis. Acta Pathologica of Japan 33 (5): 863–879 (in English)

Feller A C, Lennert K, Stein H, Bruhn H-D, Wuthe H-H 1983 Immunohistology and aetiology of histiocytic necrotizing lymphadenitis. Report of three instructive cases. Histopathology 7: 825–839

Gams R A, Neal J A, Conrad F G 1968 Hydantoin-induced pseudo-pseudolymphoma. Annals of Internal Medicine 69: 557–568

Goodwin R A Jr, Des Prez R M 1973 Pathogenesis and clinical spectrum of histoplasmosis. Southern Medical Journal 66: 13–25

Gowing N F C 1975 Infectious mononucleosis: histopathologic aspects. In: Sommers S C (ed) Pathology Annual, Appleton-Century-Crofts, New York, p 1–20

Hartsock R J, Halling W, King F M 1970 Luetic lymphadenitis — a clinical and histologic study of 20 cases. American Journal of Clinical Pathology 53: 304–314

Hutchison W M, Dunachie J F, Work K, Siim J Chr 1971 The life cycle of the Coccidian parasite, *Toxoplasma gondii*, in the domestic cat. Transactions of the Royal Society of Tropical Medicine and Hygiene 65: 380–399

Hyman G A, Sommers S C 1966 The development of Hodgkin's disease and lymphoma during anticonvulsant therapy. Blood 28: 416–427

Ishak K G 1976 Listeriosis. In: Binford C H, Connor D H (eds) Pathology of Tropical and Extraordinary Diseases. Armed Forces Institute, Washington D C Section 5, Ch 7, p 178–186

Jordan M C, Rousseau W E, Stewart J A, Noble G R, Chin I D Y 1973 Spontaneous cytomegalovirus mononucleosis. Annals of Internal Medicine 79: 153–160

Kikuchi M 1972 Lymphadenitis showing focal reticulum cell hyperplasia with nuclear debris and phagocytes. Acta Haematologica of Japan 35: 379–380 (in Japanese)

Kjeldsberg C R, Kim H 1981 Polykaryocytes resembling Warthin-Finkeldey giant-cells in reactive and neoplastic lymphoid disorders. Human Pathology 12: 267–272

Klemola E, Kääriäinen L 1965 Cytomegalovirus as a possible cause of a disease resembling infectious mononucleosis. British Medical Journal 2: 1099–1102

Krasznai G, Szegedi G 1969 Lymphadenopathie, verursacht

durch arzneimittel. Acta morphologica Academiae Scientiarum Hungaricae 17 (2): 175–185

Lennert K, Müller-Hermelink H K 1975 Lymphocyten und ihre funktionsformen — morphologie, organisation und immunologische bedeutung. Verhandlungen der Anatomischen Gesellschaft 69: 19–62

Lukes R J, Tindle B H 1975 Immunoblastic lymphadenopathy: a hyperimmune entity resembling Hodgkin's disease. The New England Journal of Medicine 292: 1–8

Lukes R J, Tindle B H, Parker J W 1969 Reed-Sternberg-like cells in infectious mononucleosis. (letter) Lancet 2: 1003–1004

Pileri S, Kikuchi M, Helbron D, Lennert K 1982 Histiocytic necrotizing lymphadenitis without granulocytic infiltration. Virchows Archiv A (Pathol Anat) 395: 257–271

Pinkerton H, Strano A J 1976 Rickettsial Diseases. In: Binford C H, Connor D H (eds) Pathology of Tropical and Extraordinary Diseases. Armed Forces Institute, Washington D C, Section 3, Ch 1, p 87–100

Poppema S, Kaiserling E, Lennert K 1979 Hodgkin's disease with lymphocytic predominance, nodular type (nodular paragranuloma) and progressively transformed germinal centres — a cytohistological study. Histopathology 3: 295–308

Stansfeld A G 1961 The histological diagnosis of toxoplasmic lymphadenitis. Journal of Clinical Pathology 14: 565–573

Symmers W St C 1978 The Lymphoreticular System. In: Systemic Pathology, Vol 2, 2nd edn. Churchill Livingstone, Edinburgh, p 504–891

Tindle B H, Parker J W, Lukes R J 1972 'Reed-Sternberg Cells' in infectious mononucleosis? American Journal of Clinical Pathology 58: 607–617

Wood J B, Valteris K, Hardy R H, Pearson A D 1976 Imported tularaemia. British Medical Journal 1: 811–812

J.D. Davies

Vascular disturbances

INTRODUCTION

Disorders primarily affecting the vasculature of lymph nodes are uncommon in comparison with disorders involving the lymphoid tissue. Nevertheless, a lymph node biopsy may, from time to time, show lesions which are of vascular origin or in which vascular changes are a prominent feature. Many such lesions are manifest either in ischaemic changes in the node parenchyma, or in vascular proliferation. The former are associated with vascular obstruction, and the latter include reactive vascular hyperplasia, malformations and neoplasms. However, since ischaemia itself may lead to local vascular proliferation, the exact pathogenesis of vasoformative lesions cannot always be inferred from the morphological appearances seen in a single section. Both local and systemic disease may affect lymph nodal vessels, the microanatomy of which is briefly described below.

Vascular supply of lymph nodes

Reference has been made in Chapter 1 to the anatomy of blood and lymph vessels supplying lymph nodes (p. 10). Injection studies of the microanatomy of these vessels have mostly been performed in animals. Human investigations (Calvert, 1901) have been few. In general, the principal arteries and veins pass through the hilum of superficial lymph nodes and radiate to the medulla, paracortex and the inner part of the cortex. The remaining vessels penetrate the capsule to supply the superficial cortex and a limited zone around the trabeculae. In some deeply situated lymph nodes in man the trabecular vessels are more prominent than they are in superficial nodes. This variation in vascular supply may be related to the more complex arrangement of the lymphoid architecture of deep lymph nodes (Denz, 1947), both in animals and man (Bélisle & Sainte-Marie, 1981; Semeraro & Davies, 1984).

Afferent lymphatic vessels penetrate the lymph node capsule to open into the marginal sinus as already described in Chapter 1. The endothelial lining of the outer, subcapsular side of the marginal sinus resembles that of the afferent and efferent lymphatic vessels. Its cells are non-phagocytic, unlike those lining the intranodal sinuses. There is some evidence that lymph nodes may possess their own intrinsic lymphatic vessels (Steinmann et al, 1982). These are normally inconspicuous, but become more prominent in the trabeculae of intensely reactive lymph nodes.

Experimental vascular extirpation

Experimental extirpation of the arterial, venous and lymphatic vessels of lymph nodes, either alone or in combination, has been performed in several animal species. Although there are differences, depending upon the lymph node site, animal species and the experimental procedure, a general pattern appears evident. Combined arterial and venous ligation led to infarction of most of the nodal tissue, leaving a viable rim of subcapsular cortical tissue intact (Osogoe & Courtice, 1968). Ligation of the arteries, veins *and* lymphatic vessels produced more rapid and complete necrosis of the entire lymphoid tissue of the nodes. Similarly, totally devascularised nodal autografts exhibited complete infarction with subsequent fibrous replacement (Tilak &Howard, 1975). Deprivation of the afferent lymphatic vessels resulted in depletion of lymphoid cells and macrophages in the lymph nodes, a decrease in density of the post-capillary venules and a reduction of the height of their endothelium (Hendriks et al, 1980). Partial or complete occlusion of veins combined with complete ligation of efferent lymphatics produced, in rabbit lymph nodes, capsular thickening, depletion of nodal lymphocytes or actual infarction (Steinmann et al, 1982). The same authors found that complete occlusion of the efferent lymphatics *with or without* venous occlusion resulted in vascular proliferation which resembled vascular sinus transformation (VST) in the human lymph node (see p. 149).

In general, ligation of more than one type of vessel is necessary to produce infarction of lymph nodes. This reflects the dual vascular supply of nodes from blood vessels and lymphatic channels. Occlusion of supplying or draining vessels may, in combination with reduced flow in the other system, render a lymph node liable to infarction.

Significance of blood in lymph sinuses (so-called 'vascularisation of sinuses')

The presence of red blood cells in the sinuses of lymph nodes is a commonly observed change which usually results from rupture of small blood vessels into the sinusoidal system. It is, by itself, of no clinical significance. Local trauma appears to be the most common cause of this phenomenon, but it may also result from reversal of flow in the lymphatico-venous communications which occur in lymph nodes (Lancet, 1961). Under the microscope, the walls of the lymph sinuses appear to retain their structural integrity and there are no specific accompanying changes in the node. Unlike vascular transformation of sinuses (see below), there is no loss of lymphoid tissue. Phagocytosis of extravasated red cells by sinus-lining histiocytes quickly follows, with conversion of haemoglobin into haemosiderin. In cases of long standing this may lead to reactive endothelial proliferation and sinusoidal fibrosis (Dorfman & Warnke, 1974). Apart from trauma, other conditions associated with extravasation of blood into lymph sinuses include passive venous congestion, diffuse nodal vasodilatation (see below) and nodal 'haemangiomatoids'.

In this context, it must be pointed out that haemal nodes (haemolymph nodes) do not occur in man. They are found in ungulates, rodents and possibly in primitive primates. True haemal nodes are lymph-node-like structures equipped with blood-filled sinuses. Afferent lymphatic channels are either absent (Turner, 1969), or scanty (Kazeem et al, 1982; Kazeem & Scothorne, 1982). The term haemolymph node is best avoided, since it has been uncritically applied in the past to both haemal nodes and human lymph nodes with blood in the lymph sinuses.

BLOOD VESSELS

The small blood vessels in a lymph node section may be abnormally conspicuous for one of two reasons, either because they are dilated, or because they have undergone proliferation, i.e. there are more vessels than normal. We shall consider first the subject of simple vasodilatation and, subsequently, situations in which vasoproliferation occurs. As intimated in the introduction to this chapter, ischaemia, resulting from vascular occlusion, is itself an important trigger for vasoproliferation and for this reason ischaemic changes in lymph nodes will be discussed before vasoproliferative disorders. The latter are predominantly benign and self-limiting conditions, although their pathogenesis in many instances is ill-understood and their terminology is confusing.

Vasodilatation in lymph nodes

Diffuse vasodilatation, of either passive or active type, leads to prominence of small veins throughout the lymph node and in the perinodal connective tissue. In the former, local or general venous stasis produces the change. Pulmonary hilar lymph nodes from patients in congestive cardiac failure commonly display marked vasodilatation. Venous occlusion and trauma in the course of surgical excision may also be responsible for vascular distension in lymph nodes, when fresh red blood cell extravasation into the perinodal tissue may give a clue to the origin of the lesion.

Active vasodilatation in lymph nodes is seen as a component of an inflammatory reaction in the nodes (Lott & Davies, 1983). Lymph nodes draining the colon in ulcerative colitis are especially prone to this reaction, and usually display an accompanying low-grade periadenitis.

Lymph node infarction

Whilst infarction in any site usually implies vascular occlusion, in infarcted lymph nodes, as elsewhere, a random section often fails to show the blocked vessel or vessels responsible for the lesion. Conversely, vasculitis may be found without infarction. It is important to try to distinguish lymph node infarction from necrosis due to other causes (e.g. infection or hypersensitivity), although, in practice, this is not always easy. A distinction is drawn here between total and subtotal infarction of a lymph node, on the one hand, and segmental or focal infarction, on the other, for the causation and differential diagnoses of these two lesions are often different.

Total or subtotal infarction

Much the commonest cause of massive infarction of a lymph node is the presence within that node of an expanding neoplasm whether primary (lymphoma) or metastatic (usually carcinoma). When, as is frequently the case, the tumour in the node is totally necrotic, this may pose diagnostic problems. The size of the residual ghost-like cells, their microanatomical disposition, and the use of connective-tissue (especially reticulin) stains may help to reveal the true nature of the necrotic tissue and at least confirm that one is dealing with a neoplasm. Examination of sections from different levels of such nodes is always worthwhile in an attempt to detect any residue of viable and morphologically recognisable tumour.

A superficially similar, subtotal, coagulative necrosis involving non-neoplastic human lymph nodes, was first reported in 1972 (Davies & Stansfeld) when five cases of 'spontaneous' lymph node infarction were traced in the biopsy material submitted to a single hospital laboratory over a period of 16 years. Four similar cases were subsequently described (Schwartz et al, 1976) in a Czechoslovakian centre in a 3-year period. Subsequent comparison of the numbers of surgical biopsies received by the two centres (Schwartz, 1982, personal communication) suggests that the lesions were comparable in frequency, one being seen in 12 to 20 thousand surgical specimens. None the less only 13 cases of the phenomenon had been reported by early in 1982 (Elie et al, 1982). It is thus clear that this is an uncommon lesion. Even 2 years later, when the phenomenon had excited more general interest, Kiesler and Dirschmid (1984) were able only to add a further 20 cases culled from the subsequent literature.

Such necrosis of benign lymph nodes is accompanied by characteristic clinical manifestations. Pain and moderate enlargement of nodes in the axilla or groin may be prominent in the early stage. Pyrexia may accompany necrosis of superficial (Benisch & Howard, 1975) or deep (Watts et al, 1980) lymph nodes. Although the pathogenesis of this lesion is often unclear, in some cases pre-

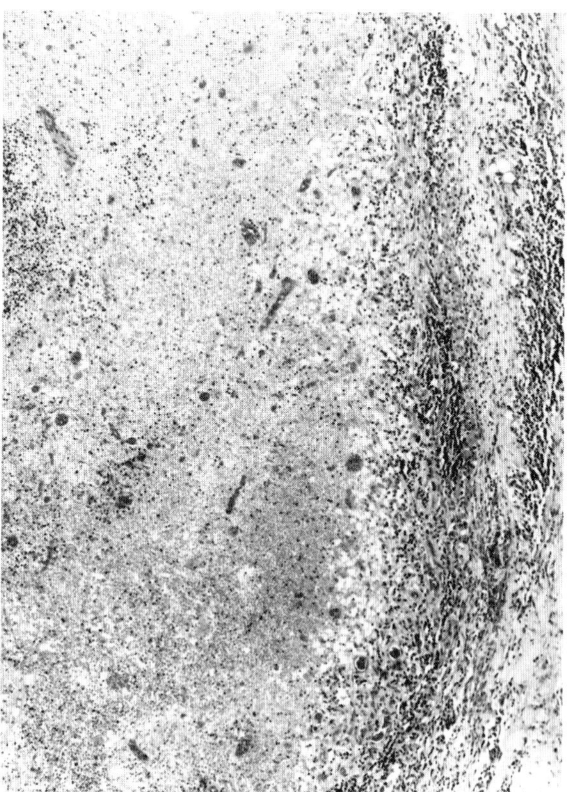

Fig. 7.1 'Spontaneous' infarction of lymph node. The greater part of the node is totally necrotic with a few lymphocytes persisting in the granulation tissue which has formed beneath the capsule (right) and in isolated pockets in the interior of the node (left). (H E × 60)

disposing local vascular stasis is suggested by a history of tight bandaging, thrombophlebitis or vascular surgery in the region of the affected node. A similar mechanism may explain infarction occurring in inflamed nodes which are confined within restricted anatomical compartments, notably the femoral nodes in primary syphilis (Symmers, 1978) (see p. 108). The morphological similarities between the changes in these necrotic human lymph nodes and experimental nodal lesions induced by vascular ligation are also indicative of an ischaemic origin.

The sequence of changes observed in affected nodes is typical of infarction. A few days after onset, most of the node contains ghost-like necrotic lymphoid cells with only a narrow subcapsular margin of surviving lymphoid tissue (Fig. 7.1) which may include an occasional cortical follicle. The periphery of the node becomes heavily infiltrated by polymorphonuclear leucocytes and fibrin. A fortnight after the acute onset of necrosis, the initial reaction around the node becomes replaced by granulation tissue (Fig. 7.1), with an increased proportion of small round cells, macrophages, eosinophils and some plasma cells. Lesions examined in succeeding weeks show increasing fibrosis in the maturing granulation tissue until, months after the onset of acute pain, the necrotic material is replaced by fibrous tissue. In the first few weeks the connective tissue framework, which is most readily demonstrated by reticulin staining, is preserved intact in the necrotic areas. A variable degree of dilatation of the deep nodal sinuses is demonstrable at this stage (Fig. 7.2). In many cases occlusive thrombi are visible in nodal and hilar veins or lymphatic vessels. In the late stage some recanalisation of veins becomes apparent.

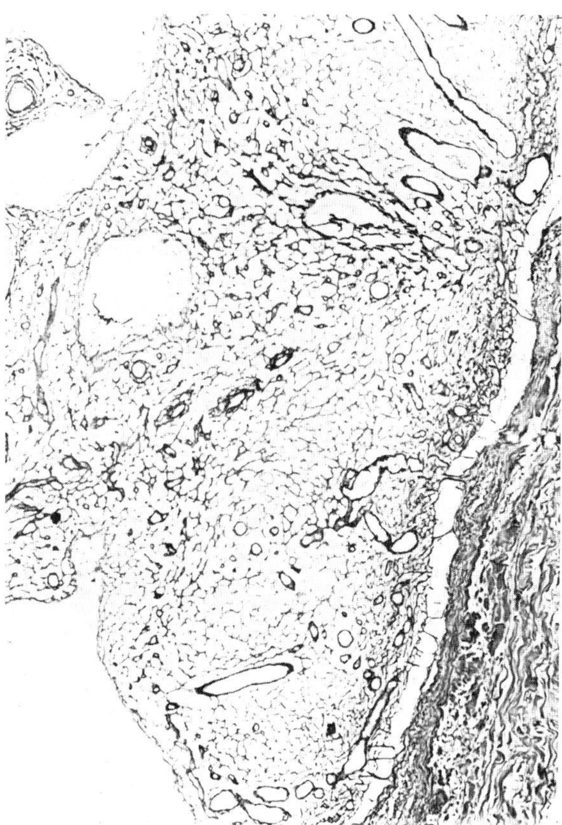

Fig. 7.2 'Spontaneous' lymph node infarction. There is condensation of reticulin beneath the still patent marginal sinus and the deep sinuses are dilated — a common finding several weeks after the onset. Otherwise the reticulin pattern shows little alteration from the normal (compare with Fig. 7.3b). (Gordon and Sweets reticulin × 60)

The *differential diagnosis* of spontaneous infarction of lymph nodes is important. The condition is uncommon, and should not be overdiagnosed. Necrosis of tumours in lymph nodes is much more frequent, and this possibility must be carefully considered in every case. Malignant lymphomas occasionally show extensive, or even total necrosis in lymph nodes (Fig. 7.3a). Although nodular sclerosing Hodgkin's disease and malignant lymphomas of centroblastic-centrocytic type (Lennert, 1978) are well known to show extensive or total necrosis, we have encountered examples of the phenomenon in most types of malignant lymphoma. Metastatic carcinoma in lymph nodes may also be subject to extensive necrosis. A warning sign that one is not dealing with 'spontaneous' infarction is pronounced enlargement of the nodes. In such circumstances a diagnosis of spontaneous infarction can only be made with great caution. As mentioned above, the use of reticulin stains is especially useful in distinguishing extensive necrosis of nodal tumour from spontaneous necrosis of previously normal lymph nodes (Fig. 7.3b). If necessary further biopsy of nodes from the same, or possibly another site should be recommended.

There is generally less difficulty in distinguishing spontaneous infarction of lymph nodes from

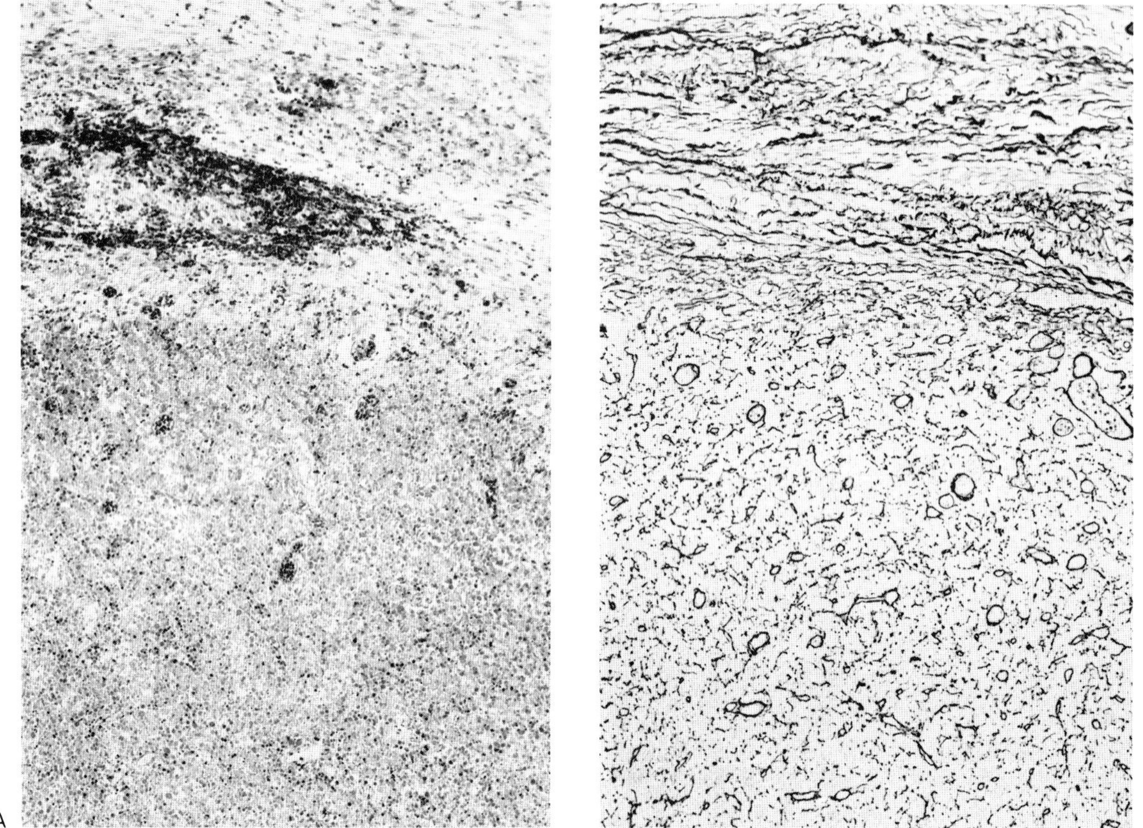

Fig. 7.3 Total infarction of lymph node in malignant lymphoma (diffuse). (a) shows 'ghost' cells in the necrotic node and surrounding granulation tissue (top). (b) same field, illustrating the value of silver impregnation in revealing complete loss of the normal reticulin pattern. ((a) H E, (b) Gordon and Sweets reticulin, both × 80)

infective lesions such as tuberculosis or syphilitic gumma. In the caseous necrosis of tuberculous lymphadenitis, the structural outlines of the necrotic tissue are lost much more rapidly and completely than they are in simple infarction and the necrotic areas are nearly always surrounded by the typical granulomatous reaction (p. 102). In tertiary syphilis also, there is a chronic inflammatory reaction around areas of gummatous necrosis, which is lacking in spontaneous infarction. Haemorrhagic necrosis, which is not characteristic of 'spontaneous' lymph nodal infarction, is a feature of plague, anthrax, acute coccal infections, diphtheria, and has rarely been noted in association with advanced acute appendicitis (Symmers, 1978).

Spontaneous infarction of non-neoplastic lymph nodes does not always imply a benign prognosis. Indeed, in the author's personal experience, subtotal necrosis of apparently normal lymph nodes has been associated with, or has heralded, malignant disease elsewhere, in about 30% of such cases. Malignant lymphomas or carcinomas, including primaries in the breast and pancreas, have followed apparently simple nodal infarction within months. Few cases of this sequence had been documented until recently (Gorelkin & Majmudar, 1978), but a cautious warning to the clinician in charge of such patients would seem prudent. Although there seems to be a risk that spontaneous infarction of vascular lymph nodes may herald malignant lymphoma, the quantitation of the risk is difficult to establish. A reported risk rate of later malignant lymphoma of 81% (Cleary et al, 1982) may reflect the nature of the material examined. Further data on carefully followed-up cases are required to assess the overall risk of lymphoma.

Segmental infarction

Segmental or focal infarction may, of course, occur in malignant lymphomas and metastatic carcinoma, but necrosis of this pattern may also be seen in a much wider range of conditions. Thrombotic occlusion of vessels in polyarteritis nodosa may produce focal (Lennert, 1961), or massive (Symmers, 1978) infarction of a lymph node. Similarly, embolism of atheromatous material may produce nodal infarction with a marked histiocytic palisading around the necrotic foci (Shah & Kisilevsky, 1978). Such histiocytic reaction requires distinction from the macrophage and granulomatous infiltrates which may accompany abscesses in lymph nodes, particularly lymphogranuloma venereum and the suppurating tuberculoid lesions of cat scratch disease (p. 124). Primary vascular lesions in systemic lupus erythematosus (p. 165), drug hypersensitivity (p. 137) and Kawasaki's disease are also associated with focal necrosis of lymph nodes. The infarcts in these conditions are often more conspicuous than the underlying vascular lesions which frequently require multiple sections to reveal their presence. Incomplete nodal necrosis is also a feature of 'histiocytic necrotising lymphadenitis without granulocytic infiltration' (Pileri et al, 1982; Kikuchi et al, 1977). In this disease of young women, the node shows focal necrosis with much karyorrhexis and a predominantly histiocytic reaction, but with a striking absence of polymorphs (see p. 87). The lesion is essentially inflammatory and the absence of associated thrombosis (Kikuchi et al, 1977) makes it unlikely that the necrotic foci are true infarcts.

Rarely, localised trauma from fine needle aspiration biopsy of lymph nodes may produce segmental infarction of lymph nodes (Davies & Webb, 1982). Isolated venous thrombosis and haemosiderin deposits serve to distinguish this type of lesion from other types of nodal necrosis.

Vasculitis in lymph nodes

Primary vasculitic lesions are infrequently observed in lymph node biopsy material, but this may not necessarily reflect the true incidence of such lesions. Lymphadenopathy is not a common accompaniment of *polyarteritis nodosa* in the adult and therefore lymph node biopsy is rarely performed in patients with this disease. It is only when arteritic lesions lead to extensive infarction of a node and consequent pain, that biopsy of the node may be contemplated. Much more frequently, small vasculitic lesions in lymph nodes occur as part of a widespread polyarteritis (Fig. 7.4) and such lesions are either asymptomatic or overshadowed by other, more dramatic, manifestations of the disease. The true incidence of arteritic lesions in lymph nodes is unknown.

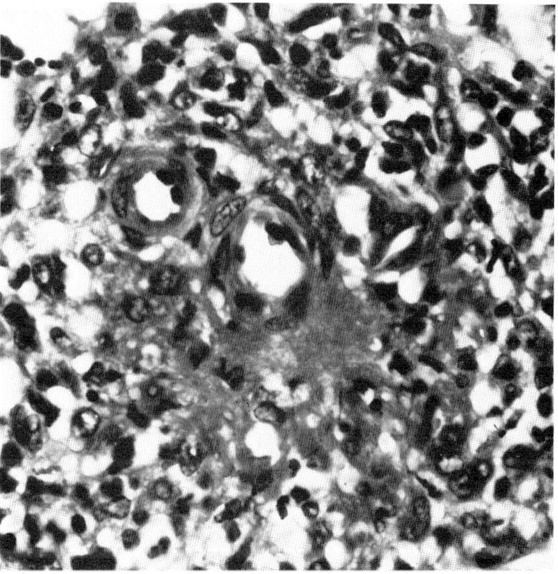

Fig. 7.4 Necrotising arteritis in a mesenteric lymph node from a child with Henoch-Schönlein disease. Similar vasculitic lesions were present in the intestinal wall. There is fibrinoid material around the vessel but no thrombosis and the node was not infarcted. (H E × 470)

From time to time, however, *necrotising arteritis* is seen in lymph nodes, either as a chance and unexpected finding in a patient with some other disease, when the likelihoood is that the vasculitis is an unimportant epiphenomenon, or as a manifestation of the primary disease process in that patient. As an example of the first situation, we have seen focal necrotising arteritis in a colic node in a patient with active ulcerative colitis. There was no evidence of nodal infarction or of arteritis in the bowel itself. In acute polyarteritis nodosa (as opposed to benign focal arteritis and the more indolent forms of systemic arteritis), fibrinoid necrosis of the vessel wall is generally accompanied by a much more florid inflammatory reaction, a greater tendency to thrombosis and hence to infarction of the node. As mentioned above, such infarction may be extensive or very limited. It may, indeed, be altogether absent, even in the presence of significant arteritic lesions (Fig. 7.4). In *Wegener's granulomatosis*, on the other hand, infarction of a lymph node may be very extensive and accompanied by a distinctive giant-cell reaction, although this type of lesion is more likely to be seen in autopsy material than in a lymph node biopsy. Lymph node involvement has not been a conspicuous feature of the rare angiocentric, lymphoma-like 'lymphomatoid granulomatosis' (Liebow et al, 1972). The disease principally affects the lungs and in those cases where lymph nodes have been examined there have not been any constant histological changes (Liebow et al, 1972).

On occasions, a lymph node biopsy may disclose a diffuse vasculitis affecting many small vessels, both arteries and veins, without necrosis, but accompanied by significant inflammatory cell infiltration of the thickened vessels which are thereby rendered very conspicuous. Usually the infiltrating cells include a large proportion of eosinophils and there may, at times, be a massive eosinophilia, so that the picture merges into that of eosinophilic lymphadenitis (see p. 88). Whilst the histological picture in such cases strongly suggests a hypersensitivity angiitis (Zeek, 1953), a history of food or drug allergy may be lacking. The lymph nodes in these uncommon cases may be significantly enlarged.

There are three other disorders in which vasculitic changes may be associated with significant lymphadenopathy, calling for lymph node biopsy. These are: systemic lupus erythematosus (SLE) (see p. 165), drug hypersensitivity (see p. 137) and Kawasaki's disease in childhood. In SLE, the vasculitic changes are seldom the central feature of the histological picture and since this disease is dealt with in Chapter 8, it will not be further discussed here.

Vasculitis in drug hypersensitivity

Vasculitic lesions and lymphadenopathy are both, at times, features of a drug hypersensitivity reaction and the vasculitic lesions may be present in a lymph node biopsy, as well as occurring in other tissues. Skin rashes are a common accompaniment of this form of hypersensitivity and their presence in association with a widespread lymphadenopathy should lead one to suspect the diagnosis. The vasculitic lesions may take one of two forms: either a widespread involvement of small vessels, often with thrombosis and micro-infarcts in the node cortex (see Fig. 6.84) or, less commonly, a focal necrotising arteritis like that of classical polyarteritis nodosa. We have encountered the latter type of lesion in the lymph node biopsy of a patient who was found to have sensitivity to iodine and who had been on iodine medication.

Kawasaki's disease

Synonym:
Mucocutaneous lymph-node syndrome.

First described in Japan in 1967, this acute, febrile, exanthematous disease of childhood has, in recent years, been increasingly recognised in Europe and the USA. The aetiology is unknown, although it is presumably due to an infectious agent. The disease is characterised by fever, erythematous skin rashes, oedema, especially of the extremities, lesions of the conjunctiva and oral mucosa, cervical lymphadenopathy and coronary arteritis, which may lead to fatal complications. The arteritis in this disease seems to be confined to the larger coronary vessels but there is evidence of a microscopic vasculitis within the lymph nodes, attended by the formation of fibrin thrombi in the smaller vessels and patchy infarction of the nodes (Marsh et al, 1980; Giesker et al, 1982). The latter authors believe the histological picture to be sufficiently distinctive to warrant biopsy of an enlarged cervical node to establish the diagnosis.

Thrombotic microangiopathy

Synonyms:
Thrombotic thrombocytopenia
Mosehcowitz's disease

The distinctive microscopic thrombi of this rare disease may be encountered in the small vessels of

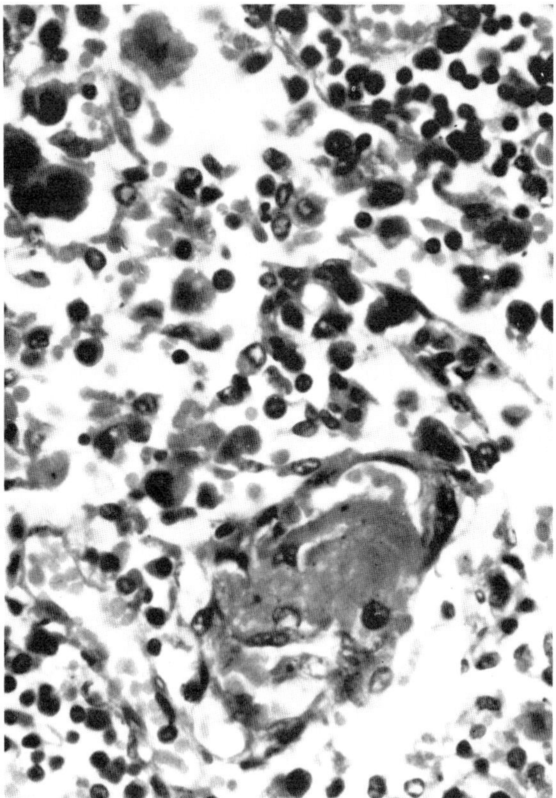

Fig. 7.5 Lymph node in thrombotic microangiopathy (Moschcowitz's disease) showing a small vessel plugged with platelet thrombus. The lymph sinuses contained many macrophages filled with ingested erythrocytes (top left). (H E × 300)

lymph nodes, as in a great variety of other sites, but it is unlikely that a lymph node biopsy will be expressly taken with this diagnosis in mind. It only requires that the pathologist should spot the homogeneous microvascular thrombi, when they do occur, and appreciate their significance, for a rapid diagnosis may be life-saving. There is no histological evidence of an accompanying vasculitis (Fig. 7.5).

Congestive vasoproliferation — vascular transformation of sinuses (VST)

This uncommon but distinctive lesion of lymph nodes was first described by Haferkamp et al (1971). It is characterised by a proliferation of capillary sized vessels which form a vascular network in the marginal sinus of the node, sometimes extending into the deeper sinuses (Figs 7.6, 7.7). The new formed vessels are surrounded by fibrous tissue, which effectively obliterates the original lumen of the sinuses, and the vascular proliferation may extend also into the adjacent perinodal tissues. There is usually an associated atrophy of lymphoid tissue, together with local haemosiderosis. VST has been found in lymph nodes in the vicinity of large thrombosed veins and the presence of thrombosis also in the local hilar veins suggests that interference with the venous drainage of the node might be responsible for the lesion. It appears, however, from experimental work, that the underlying mechanism is probably obstruction of the efferent lymphatic vessel of the node, with or without associated venous occlusion (Steinmann

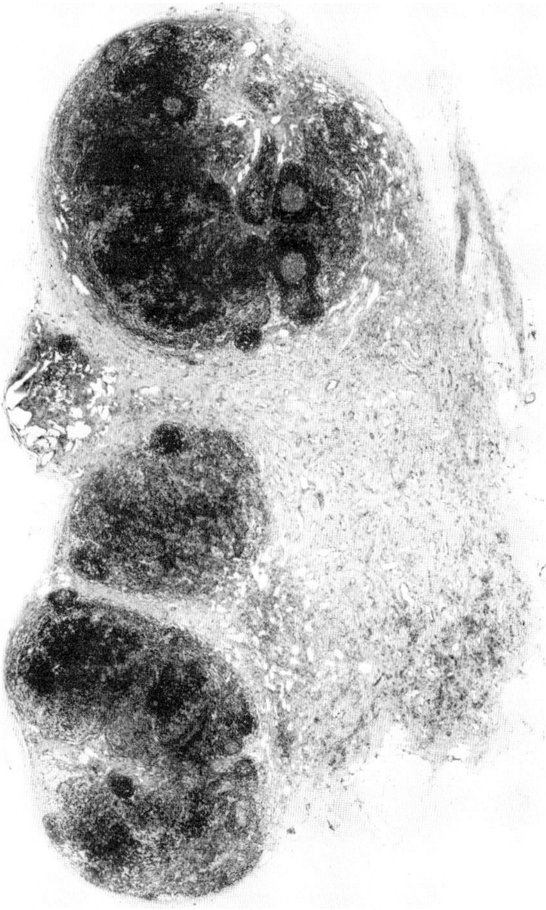

Fig. 7.6 Lymph node showing vascular tranformation of sinuses. A network of vascular channels extends round the marginal sinus of the upper part of the node and out into the surrounding connective tissue. (H E × 6)

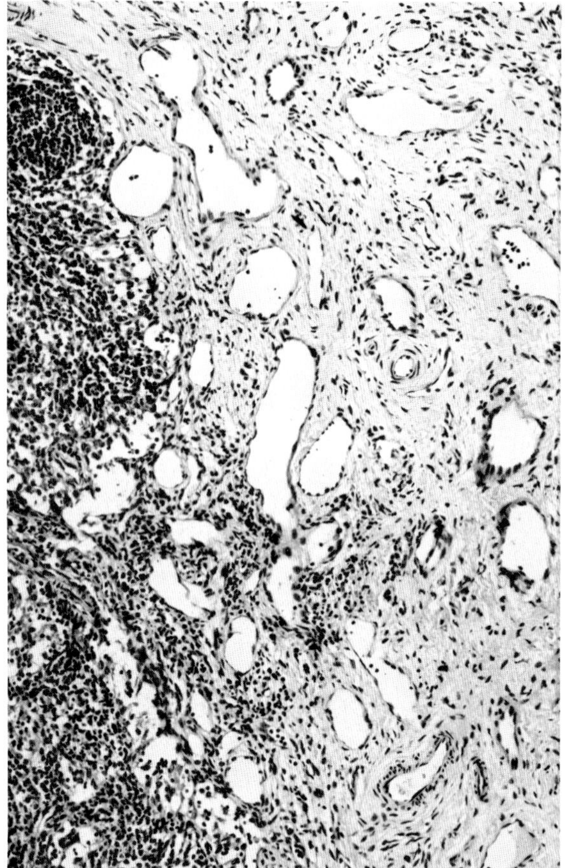

Fig. 7.7 Higher power view of part of Fig. 7.6 showing detail of vascular proliferation (H E × 100)

et al, 1982) (see p. 143). Originally described in cervical nodes, VST has also been found in axillary nodes and abdominal nodes (Dorfman & Warnke, 1974; Symmers, 1978).

Clinically, such cases have presented as painful lymph nodes swellings or as an incidental finding in the course of surgical exploration of the neck or abdomen, in which case the affected nodes are picked out by their congested appearance.

The lesion is distinguishable from Kaposi's sarcoma by the stricter localisation of the vasoformative tissue to the marginal sinus, the lack of plump spindle cells and the presence of hilar venous thrombosis.

Vasoproliferation in reactive states

Proliferation of blood vessels is one of the central features of granulation tissue formation and is an accompaniment of the inflammatory reaction in any part of the body, including the lymph nodes. Sometimes in chronic inflammation there is a striking increase of small vessels in a lymph node, which may be further accentuated by persistent vasodilatation to produce a haemangiomatous appearance in the node. Unlike the spleen, lymph nodes probably never show true haemangiomas (Rappaport, 1966). This reactive type of vasoproliferation is often accompanied by a marked reactive plasmacytosis in the node and it is interesting to note that lymphoplasmacytic and plasmacytic lymphomas are the two types of malignant lymphoma which are sometimes associated with a pseudo-angiomatous appearance in the involved lymph nodes (Lennert, 1978).

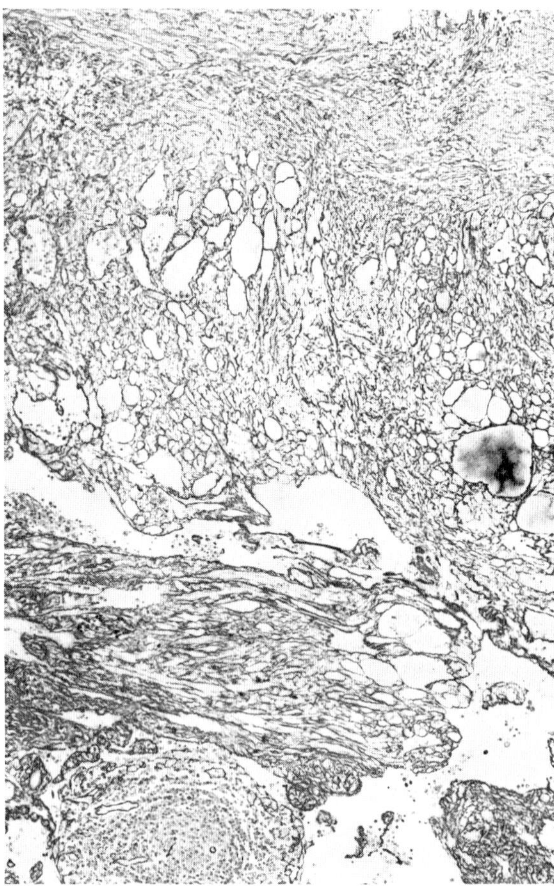

Fig. 7.8 Margin of lymph node showing reactive angiomatous vascular proliferation. The upper half of the field shows a network of vessels in the capsular and perinodal tissue. The marginal and cortical sinuses (below) are dilated. (Gordon and Sweets reticulin × 60)

Under the title of 'hyperimmune angiofollicular and plasmacytic polyadenopathy', Diebold et al (1980) described two patients with a widespread lymphadenopathy, characterised by a massive plasma cell reaction and focal capillary proliferation with vasodilatation. The vascular lesions (Fig. 7.8) involved the hilum, capsule, pericapsular tissue and medulla. The aetiology of the disorder in these two patients was obscure, as it was in a similar, personally observed case, with more restricted lymph node involvement. The pattern of vascular proliferation in such cases is quite different from that seen in angioimmunoblastic lymphadenopathy (AIL) (p. 178) and there should, therefore, be no difficulty in distinguishing the two lesions. Furthermore, the blood vessels in the condition under discussion, may show hyaline thickening of their walls, which is never seen in AIL.

A marked proliferation of small blood vessels is also a feature of giant lymph node hyperplasia (angiofollicular hyperplasia, Castleman's disease) (p. 186) — another condition of unknown aetiology. The histological picture is again quite distinctive and it is unlikely that the two conditions are closely related.

A quite different proliferative lesion of lymph node blood vessels is one which is provoked by the presence of a malignant neoplasm in their vicinity. These lesions, which have been called 'angiomatosis' of lymph nodes, (Fayemi & Toker, 1975) or 'haemangiomatoids' (Lott & Davies, 1983), are usually found in axillary lymph nodes draining breast carcinoma, but have also been described in

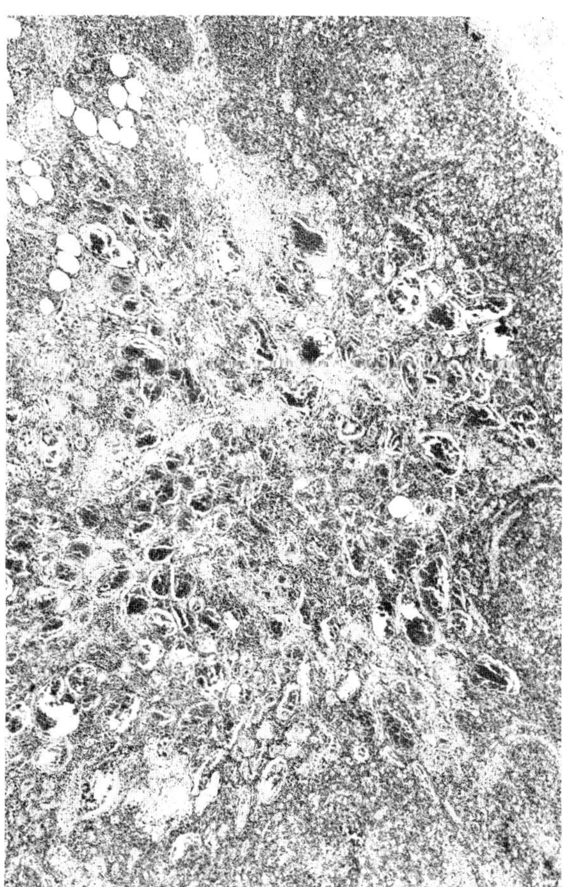

Fig. 7.9 Lymph node 'haemangiomatoid' lesion. A radially arranged collection of dilated venules occupy the medullary region of the node and encroach upon the cortex. (H E × 30)

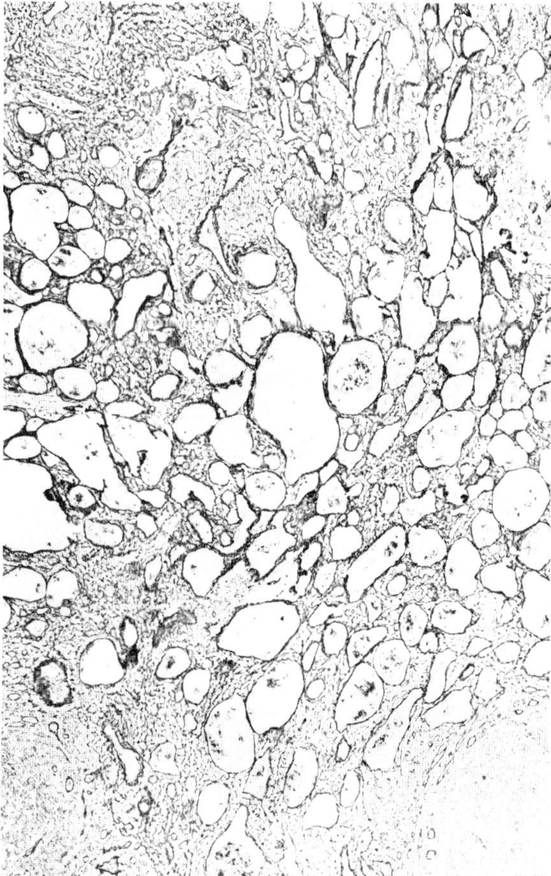

Fig. 7.10 'Haemangiomatoid' lesion in lymph node showing thin-walled venules (Gordon and Sweets reticulin × 40)

association with Hodgkin's disease. Lymph node 'haemangiomatoids' affect single lymph nodes in a chain draining the neoplasm (Lott & Davies, 1983). They consist of a radially arranged proliferation of dilated small vessels, which are filled with blood (Figs 7.9, 7.10). The vessels are found in the medulla, paracortex or cortex and replace the lymphoid structure. They appear to arise from arteries in the core of the lesion but show no direct communication with adjacent post-capillary venules.

Vasoproliferation in malignant disease

The presence of a malignant neoplasm in almost any site may induce the local blood vessels to proliferate and one commonly sees evidence of this phenomenon in malignant lymph nodes, whether occupied by malignant lymphomas or metastatic tumours.

The occurrence of pseudo-angiomatous lesions in plasma cell tumours has been alluded to earlier. Hairy cell leukaemia is well known to produce angiomatoid lesions in the spleen and liver (Nanba et al, 1977), but similar vascular changes have not apparently been noted in affected lymph nodes in this disease. Hodgkin's disease is commonly accompanied by marked vascular proliferation, which is one reason why it may be confused with angio-immunoblastic lymphadenopathy. The blood vessels in nodular sclerosing Hodgkin's disease may be conspicuous for other reasons too. Arteries in the node itself and in its vicinity often show thickening of their walls and obliterative endarteritis, whilst trabecular arteries are frequently thrown into relief by concentric perivascular sclerosis (see p. 209).

Proliferation of post-capillary venules

The types of nodal vascular proliferation described above mainly involve arteries, veins and capillary vessels, rather than the specialised post-capillary, or high endothelial, venules which are a unique anatomical feature of lymphoid tissues (see p. 10). These vessels, as already noted, are characteristic of the paracortical areas of lymph nodes and stimulation of T-cell activity in nodes results in an expansion of the paracortex and an increase of post-capillary venules in these regions. This is true, not only of benign reactive situations (see p. 95), but also of several T-cell malignant lymphomas (see ch. 12).

Vasoproliferation with lymphoid hyperplasia in soft tissues — angiolymphoid hyperplasia with eosinophilia

This unusual lesion deserves mention here, since the localised, subcutaneous swellings may be mistaken for lymph nodes, not only by the surgeon taking the biopsy, but also by the pathologist who examines the specimen. Subcutaneous angiolymphoid hyperplasia with eosinophilia (Wells & Whimster, 1969), eosinophilic folliculosis of the skin or Kimura's disease (Kawada et al, 1965), eosinophilic granuloma of soft tissues (Takenaka et al, 1976) and eosinophilic granuloma of lymph nodes and soft tissue (Chang & Che'n, 1962) are amongst the names applied to lesions which, if not identical, at least appear to be closely related to one another. It is only the more deeply situated lesions in this group, and those in which the vascular proliferation is attended by a particularly heavy lymphoid infiltration, that are likely to be mistaken for lymph nodes. The subject has been well reviewed by Wright et al (1981), who reported a case in which lymphadenopathy was simulated. The mimicry of a lymph node may be very close in the more compact nodules, since the central area of abnormal vascular and endothelial proliferation may be surrounded by a wide zone of lymphoid tissue containing well formed germinal follicles and intervening T-zones with post-capillary venules. The absence of lymph sinuses may be the only distinguishing feature (Wright et al, 1981). The aetiology of the condition is unknown, but the associated eosinophilia, a finding of IgE in the follicles (Wright et al, 1981) and sometimes a suggestive history, point to a possible allergic basis for the lesions.

Malignant vasoformative tumours in lymph nodes

Kaposi's sarcoma

This is without doubt the most frequently encountered vasoformative neoplasm in lymph nodes, although it is still a rarity in most parts of the world. In much of Africa, South of the Sahara, Kaposi's sarcoma is quite a common lesion. In African adults the presentation is usually with skin lesions, as it is in Caucasians of a generally older age group. Bhana et al (1970) found lymph node involvement in 16 out of 48 adult African patients and these included the only 4 females in the series. In patients under 30 years of age, there tended to be widespread lymphadenopathy and a poor prognosis, whilst, in older subjects, solitary lymph node deposits were found in the drainage area of a fungating skin lesion. Slavin et al (1970) in reporting a series of 51 cases of Kaposi's sarcoma in East African children, found lymph node involvement in 26, and 19 of these were in children under 6 years of age, in whom the disease tended to run a more rapid and aggressive course. In young children the presentation of the disease was often with widespread lymphadenopathy in the absence of skin lesions.

Outside Africa, Kaposi's sarcoma has, until recently, been regarded as a rare disease, generally occurring in elderly subjects and presenting with multiple skin nodules on the extremities. Lymph node involvement occurred late, if at all, in such subjects. Recently, however, there have been reports of a more aggressive form of Kaposi's sarcoma arising among white, male homosexuals with 'Acquired Immunodeficiency Syndrome' (Lancet, 1983) (see p. 162) in New York and in California (Gottlieb & Ackerman, 1982). Some cases of this kind have been reported in Europe too (Thomsen & Jacobsen, 1981; Brunet et al, 1983). Nodal lesions with Kaposi's sarcoma in the capsule or subcapsular tissue have occurred in these relatively young men (Finkbeiner et al, 1982), although whether the lymph node lesions are metastatic or multicentric is uncertain (Costa & Rabson, 1983).

The more frequent occurrence and more aggressive behaviour of Kaposi's sarcoma in immunodeficient subjects has been underlined by these recent reports and the disease has been found alongside opportunistic infections such as pneumocystis pneumonia and cytomegalovirus infection (Urmacher et al, 1982). In this light, it is not surprising that Kaposi's sarcoma has been reported on a number of occasions in association with malignant lymphomas. The association is most frequent with Hodgkin's disease, but other types of malignant lymphoma have been found with Kaposi's sarcoma from time to time (Reynolds et al, 1965; Safai et al, 1980).

Macroscopically, nodes involved by Kaposi's sarcoma may sometimes be grossly enlarged, especially in young African patients. They have a red or reddish brown, haemorrhagic appearance on section.

Histologically, the picture is usually unmistakeable. The lymphoid tissue is infiltrated and replaced by a disorderly mass of spindle cells, of varying compactness, containing slits filled with red cells (Fig. 7.11). More clearly defined, thin-walled, sinusoidal vessels are seen at the periphery of the tumour, where haemosiderin deposits may

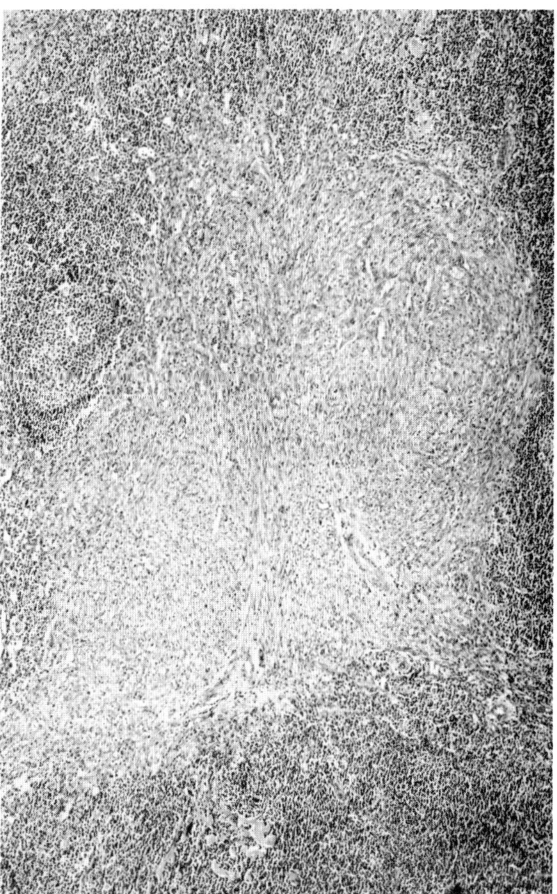

Fig. 7.11 Inguinal lymph node from a three and a half year old African boy showing a central focus of Kaposi's sarcoma. Vascular slits can be seen in a haphazardly arranged mass of spindle cells. (H E × 40)

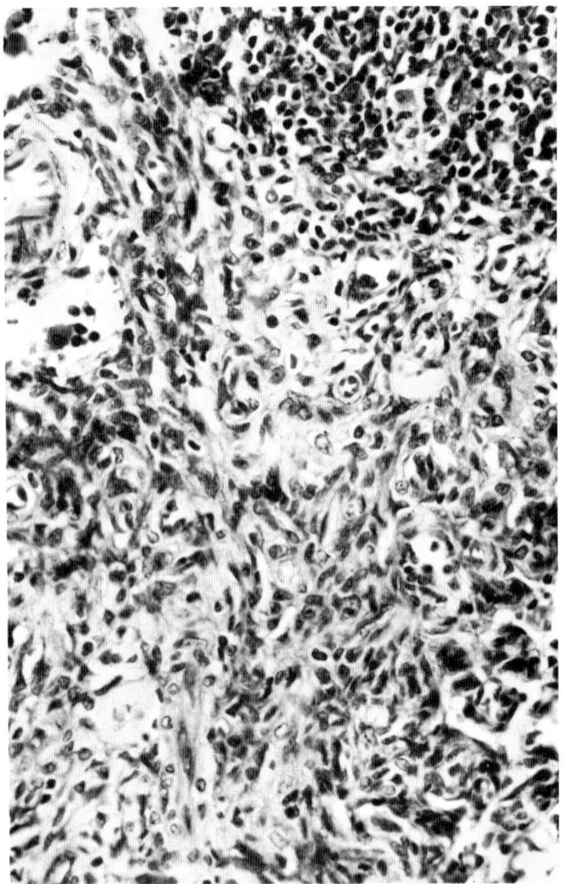

Fig. 7.12 Kaposi's sarcoma in a lymph node showing the margin of the lesion (H E × 300)

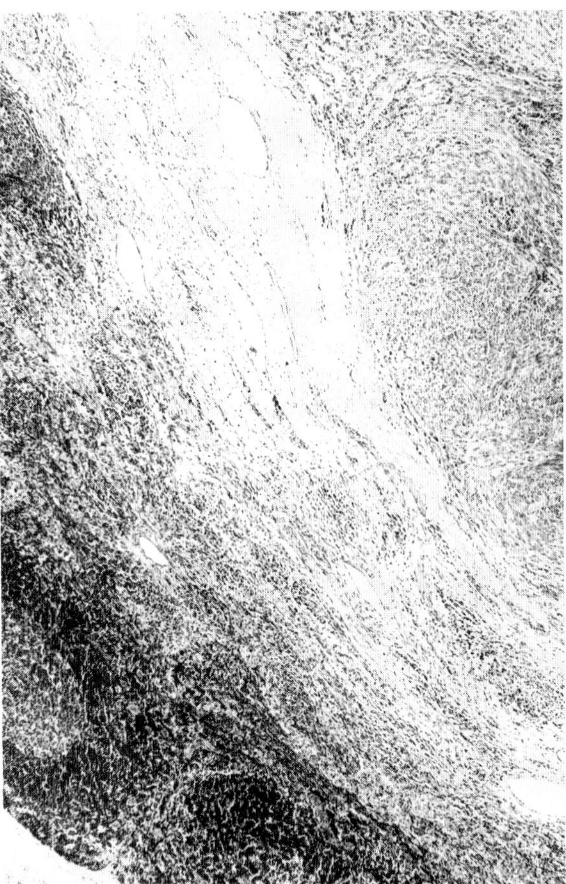

Fig. 7.13 Another lymph node biopsy showing a central, encapsulated mass of Kaposi's sarcoma (H E × 40)

be seen (Fig. 7.12). Mitoses are readily found and may be numerous. A peripheral mononuclear cell reaction is much less clearly seen in lymph nodes than in the skin tumours. In those cases where the process appears to arise primarily in lymph nodes, it often begins centrally in the nodes and spreads outwards, so that the expanding tumour is surrounded by a compressed rim of lymphoid tissue and may even be enclosed by a fibrous capsule (Fig. 7.13). However, when the nodal disease is secondary to cutaneous involvement, it starts at the periphery in the region of the marginal sinus (Bhana et al, 1970). When Kaposi's sarcoma occurs in association with malignant lymphomas, the two conditions may be intermingled (Massarelli et al, 1982) or may affect different sites. In fact, the Kaposi's sarcoma is usually limited to skin lesions in the presence of nodal lymphoma. It is important not to mistake reactive follicular hyperplasia, which is sometimes striking in lymph nodes draining ulcerated cutaneous lesions, for follicular lymphoma. Likewise, a reactive plasmacytosis should not be mistaken for a plasmacytoma (Lubin & Rywlin, 1971).

The *differential diagnosis* includes not only other vasoformative neoplasms, notably angiosarcoma (qv) but also other vascular or haemorrhagic spindle cell neoplasms metastasising to lymph nodes. These may include leiomyosarcoma and malignant fibrous histiocytoma in particular.

Other vasoformative neoplasms

True angiosarcoma occurring in lymph nodes is generally metastatic from a primary growth elsewhere. Cutaneous angiosarcomas, arising in the head and neck region, not uncommonly metastasise to cervical nodes (Rosai et al, 1976), but it is uncommon for angiosarcomas of the breast to involve axillary nodes. Macroscopically, angiosarcoma produces soft, haemorrhagic and sometimes cystic deposits which are generally easily diagnosed on microscopic examination, being composed of thin-walled, anastomosing vascular channels, lined sometimes by plump endothelium but lacking the spindle-cell background of Kaposi's sarcoma.

Whilst nodal metastasis in angiosarcoma has an unfavourable prognostic significance, it seems that the presence of nodal metastasis in the curious 'malignant endovascular papillary angioendothelioma of the skin in childhood' (Dabska, 1969) does not worsen the prognosis. Another rare tumour of childhood and young adults — the angiomatoid variant of malignant fibrous histiocytoma (Enzinger, 1979), although not, in fact, a vasoformative tumour, may look like one, since these tumours frequently contain blood-filled cysts. Furthermore the presence of much lymphoid tissue, including germinal follicles, around the primary tumour may create the impression of a lymph node metastasis. True metastases do occur but are rare (Enzinger, 1979).

LYMPH VESSELS

As indicated in the section on the vascular supply of lymph nodes, the lymphatic and blood vessels are not totally independent of one another. Lesions affecting one system may affect the other, and the effect upon the lymph node is often dependent upon the degree of involvement of the two sets of vessels.

Lymphoedema and lymph nodes

Secondary lymphoedema may arise as a result of obstruction of lymphatic vessels outside lymph nodes, or as a consequence of intranodal lesions. Carcinomatous obstruction is the best known cause of lymphatic obstruction in this country and is usually readily detectable histologically. Filariasis of long standing is the most frequent cause of lymphoedema of the lower limbs in some tropical areas. At this stage of the disease, the inguinal nodes show lymphoid atrophy, scarring and eosinophil infiltration whilst the lymph sinuses are generally dilated and sometimes grossly so. Close search may reveal the presence of microfilariae in the scar tissue (see Fig. 6.59, p. 122). At an earlier stage, adult worms may be found in these nodes.

The relation between '*primary*' lymphoedema and lymph node changes has until recently been less obvious. However, lymphangiography has often shown lymph nodal abnormalities in primary hypoplastic lymphoedema. Histologically the lymph nodes show a variable degree of capsular and trabecular fibrosis and in some cases fibrosis of the hilum, and medullary and marginal sinuses (Kinmonth & Wolfe, 1980). Over one-third of the lymph node surface area may be replaced by fibrosis. Lymphoid atrophy and encirclement by fibrosis may complete the picture. Similar lymph node fibrosis can affect mesenteric lymph nodes in intestinal lymphangiectasis (Belaiche et al, 1980). That such lymph node changes may at least contribute to the lymphoedema is supported by the less marked nodal fibrosis of bilateral hyperplastic lymphoedema, in which lymphatic obstruction beyond the regional lymph nodes is suspected (Kinmonth & Wolfe, 1980).

Lymphatic hygromas and lymphangiectasis

Hygromas of the lymphatic vessels in the neck may also involve the cervical lymph nodes (Figs 7.14, 7.15). The hilar vessels become distended and filled with lymph and mononuclear cells (Goetsch, 1938). Enlarged blood vessels and haemorrhage into the dilated sinuses are also common and may lead to possible misinterpretation of the lesion as a haemangioma.

Several cases of small intestinal lymphangiectasis have been reported in association with macroglobulinaemia. The mesenteric lymph nodes have shown distension of their sinuses by coagulated lymph rich in IgM (Harris et al, 1983). Gross dilatation of lymph sinuses is also rarely found in association with low grade malignant lymphomas (see Fig. 10.49, p. 261).

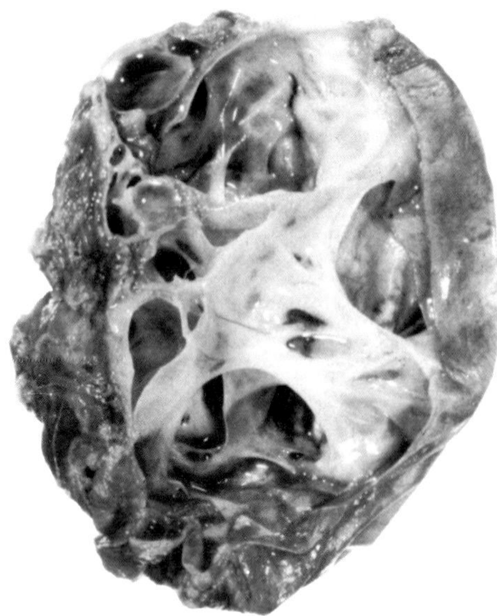

Fig. 7.14 Cystic hygromatous lymph node from the mediastinum of a 37 year old man

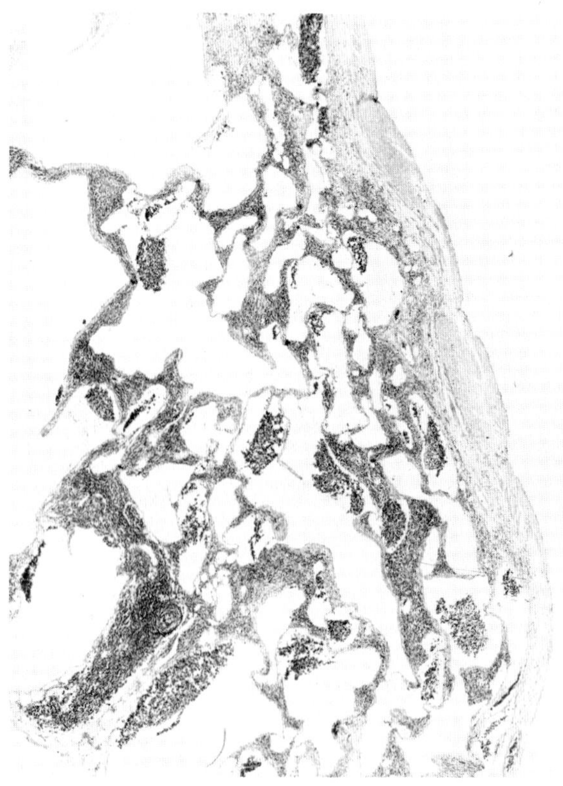

Fig. 7.15 Section of the lymph node shown in Fig. 7.14 showing gross distension of lymph sinuses and thin intervening strands of lymphoid tissue (H E × 20)

Lymphangiomyomatosis

In this uncommon disorder, which is confined to women and which may be related to tuberous sclerosis, proliferation of smooth muscle cells occurs chiefly in the lymphatics of the lungs, culminating in the production of one form of 'honeycomb lung'. In addition to involvement of lymphatic trunks, including the thoracic duct, lymph nodes may be involved in the myoproliferative process (Corrin et al, 1975). In a series of 28 cases of pulmonary lymphangiomyomatosis reported by these authors, lymph nodes were known to be affected in 9 patients. These included axillary, cervical, subclavian, mediastinal, para-aortic and pelvic nodes. Grossly the involved nodes were described as 'spongy, resilient and pale tan or white' in colour (Corrin et al, 1975). The smooth muscle proliferation was associated with lymph channels which became subdivided in a plexiform manner. In cases where much of the node was replaced by a meshwork of smooth muscle the resultant obstruction was probably responsible for the associated chylous effusions in serous cavities (Corrin et al, 1975).

REFERENCES

Belaiche J, Vesin P, Chaumette M T, Julien M, Cattan D 1980 Lymphangiectasis intestinales et fibrose des ganglions mesentériques. Gastroentérologie clinique et biologique 4: 52–58

Bélisle C, Sainte-Marie G 1981 Topography of the deep cortex of the lymph nodes of various mammalian species. Anatomical Record 201: 553–561

Benisch B M, Howard R G 1975 Lymph-node infarction in two young men. American Journal of Clinical Pathology 63: 818–823

Bhana D, Templeton A C, Master S P, Kyalwazi S K 1970 Kaposi sarcoma of lymph nodes. British Journal of Cancer 24: 464–470

Brunet J B et al 1983 Acquired immunodeficiency syndrome in France. Lancet 1: 700–701 (Letter)

Calvert W J 1901 On the blood vessels of human lymphatic gland. Johns Hopkins Hospital Bulletin 12: 177–178

Chang T, Che'n C 1962 Eosinophilic granuloma of lymph nodes and soft tissues. Report of 21 cases. Chinese Medical Journal 81: 384–387

Cleary K R, Osborne B M, Butler J J 1982 Lymph node infarction foreshadowing malignant lymphoma. American Journal of Surgical Pathology 6: 435–442
Corrin B, Liebow A A, Friedman P J 1975 Pulmonary lymphangiomyomatosis. American Journal of Pathology 79: 348–382
Costa J, Rabson A S 1983 Generalised Kaposi's sarcoma is not a neoplasm. Lancet 1:58
Dabska M 1969 Malignant endovascular papillary angioendothelioma of the skin in childhood. Cancer 24: 503–510
Davies J D, Stansfeld A G 1972 Spontaneous infarction of superficial lymph nodes. Journal of Clinical Pathology 25: 689–696
Davies J D, Webb A J 1982 Segmental lymph-node infarction following fine-needle aspiration. Journal of Clinical Pathology 35: 855–857
Denz F A 1947 Age changes in lymph nodes. Journal of Pathology and Bacteriology 59: 575–591
Diebold J, Tulliez M, Bernadou A, Audouin J, Tricot G, Reynes M, Bilski-Pasquier G 1980 Angio-follicular and plasmacytic polyadenopathy: a pseudotumourous syndrome with dysimmunity. Journal of Clinical Pathology 33: 1068–1076
Dorfman R F, Warnke R 1974 Lymphadenopathy simulating the malignant lymphomas. Human Pathology 5: 519–550
Elie H, Joubert B, Mandard J C 1982 Infarctus ischémique spontané massif d'un ganglion lymphatique cervical. Annales de pathologie 2: 240–242
Enzinger F M 1979 Angiomatoid malignant fibrous histiocytoma. Cancer 44: 2147–2157
Fayemi A O, Toker C 1975 Nodal angiomatosis. Archives of Pathology 99: 170–172
Finkbeiner W E, Egbert B M, Groundwater J R, Sagebiel R W 1982 Kaposi's sarcoma in young homosexual men: a histopathologic study with particular reference to lymph node involvement. Archives of Pathology and Laboratory Medicine 106: 261–264
Giesker D W, Krause P J, Pastuszak W T, Hine P, Forouhar F A 1982 Lymph node biopsy for early diagnosis in Kawasaki disease. American Journal of Surgical Pathology 6: 493–501
Goetsch E 1938 Hygroma colli cysticum and hygroma axillae. Pathologic and clinical study and report of twelve cases. Archives of Surgery 36: 394–479
Gorelkin L, Majmudar B 1978 Spontaneous primary lymph node infarction in a patient with lymphoma. Southern Medical Journal 71: 1451–1452
Gottlieb G J, Ackerman A B 1982 Kaposi's sarcoma — an extensively disseminated form in young homosexual men. Human Pathology 13: 882–892
Haferkamp O, Rosenau W, Lennert K 1971 Vascular transformation of lymph node sinuses due to venous obstruction. Archives of Pathology 92: 81–83
Harris M, Burton I E, Scarffe J H 1983 Macroglobulinaemia and intestinal lymphangiectasia. Journal of Clinical Pathology 36: 30–36
Hendriks H R, Eestermans I L, Hoefsmit E C M 1980 Depletion of macrophages and disappearance of postcapillary high endothelial venules in lymph nodes deprived of afferent lymphatic vessels. Cell and Tissue Research 211: 375–389
Kawada A, Takahashi H, Anzai T 1965 Eosinophilic lymphofolliculosis of the skin (Kimura's disease). Japanese Journal of Dermatology 76: 61–72
Kazeem A A, Reid O, Scothorne R J 1982 Studies on hemolymph nodes I. Histology of the renal haemolymph node of the rat. Journal of Anatomy 134: 677–683
Kazeem A A, Scothorne R J 1982 Studies on hemolymph nodes II. The regional origin of the afferent lymphatics. Journal of Anatomy 135: 1–4
Kiesler J, Dirschmid K 1984 Der Lymphknoteninfarkt. Pathologe 5: 33–36
Kikuchi M, Yoshizumi T, Nakamura H 1977 Necrotizing lymphadenitis. Virchows Archiv A. Pathological Anatomy and Histology 376: 247–253
Kinmonth J B, Wolfe J H 1980 Fibrosis in the lymph nodes in a primary lymphoedema. Annals of the Royal College of Surgeons of England. 62: 344–354
Lancet 1961 Barrier function of lymph glands. 2:1442
Lancet 1983 Acquired immunodeficiency syndrome. Lancet I: 162–164
Lennert K 1961 Lymphknoten — Diagnostik in Schnitt und Ausstrich. Bandteil A: Cytologie und lymphadenitis. In: Lubarsch O, Henke F, Rössle R, Uehlinger E (eds) Handbuch d spez path Anat u histol. Vol 1/3A. Springer-Verlag, Berlin, p 379–380
Lennert K, Mohri N 1978 Histopathology and diagnosis of non-Hodgkin's lymphoma. In: Malignant lymphomas other than Hodgkin's disease. Lennert K (ed) Springer-Verlag, Berlin, p 111–469
Liebow A A, Carrington C R, Friedman P J 1972 Lymphomatoid granulomatosis. Human Pathology 3: 457–558
Lott M F, Davies J D 1983 Lymph node hypervascularity: haemangiomatoid lesions and pan-nodal vasodilatation. Journal of Pathology 140: 209–219
Lubin J, Rywlin A M 1971 Lymphoma-like lymph node changes in Kaposi's sarcoma. Archives of Pathology 92: 338–341
Marsh W L, Bishop J W, Koenig H M 1980 Bone marrow and lymph node findings in a fatal case of Kawasaki's disease. Archives of Pathology and Laboratory Medicine 104: 563–567
Massarelli G, Tanda F, Denti S 1982 Primary Kaposi's sarcoma and Hodgkin's disease in the same lymph node. American Journal of Clinical Pathology 78: 107 111
Mattila J, Alavaikko M, Järventie G, Lehtinen M, Pitkänen R 1980 Macroglobulinaemia with abdominal symptoms caused by intestinal extracellular macroglobulin. Virchows Archiv A Pathological Anatomy and Histology 389: 241–251
Nanba K, Soban E J, Bowlings M C, Berard C W 1977 Splenic pseudosinuses and hepatic angiomatous lesions: distinctive features of hairy cell leukaemia. American Journal of Clinical Pathology 67: 415–426
Osogoe B, Courtice F C 1968 The effects of occlusion of the blood supply to the popliteal lymph node of the rabbit on the cell and protein content of the lymph and on the histology of the node. Australian Journal of Experimental Biology and Medical Science 46: 515–524
Pileri S, Kikuchi M, Helbron D, Lennert K 1982 Histiocytic necrotizing lymphadenitis without granulocytic infiltration. Virchows Archiv A. Pathological Anatomy and Histology 395: 257–271
Pressman J J, Simon M B 1961 Experimental evidence of direct communications between lymph nodes and veins. Surgery, Gynecology and Obstetrics 113: 537–541
Rappaport H 1966 Tumors of the hematopoietic system. Armed Forces Institute of Pathology, Washington D C, p 357

Reynolds W A, Winkelmann R K, Soule E H 1965 Kaposi's sarcoma — a clinico-pathological study with particular reference to its relationship to the reticuloendothelial system. Medicine 44: 419–443

Rosai J, Sumner H W, Kostianovsky M, Perez-Mesa C 1976 Angiosarcoma of the skin. Human Pathology 7: 83–109

Safai B, Mike V, Giraldo G, Beth E, Good R A 1980 Association of Kaposi's sarcoma with second primary malignancies — possible etiopathogenic implications. Cancer 45: 1472–1479

Salzstein S L, Ackerman L V 1959 Lymphadenopathy induced by anticonvulsant drugs and mimicking clinically and pathologically malignant lymphoma. Cancer 12: 164–182

Schwartz A, Horáček J, Štěrba K 1976 Infarckt minzi uzliny neznámé etiologie. Casopis lékaru čezkych 115: 524–526

Semeraro D, Davies J D 1984 The arterial supply of human lymph nodes. Bristol Medico-Chirurgical Journal 99:31

Shah K H, Kisilevsky R 1978 Infarction of lymph nodes: a cause of palisading macrophage reaction mimicking necrotising granulomas. Human Pathology 9: 597–599

Slavin G, Cameron H McD, Forbes C, Mitchell R M 1970 Kaposi's sarcoma in East African children. Journal of Pathology 100: 187–199

Steinmann G, Földi E, Földi M, Rácz P, Lennert K 1982 Morphologic findings in lymph nodes after occlusion of their efferent lymphatic vessels and veins. Laboratory Investigation 47: 43–50

Symmers W StC 1978 The lymphoreticular system. In: Systemic Pathology, Vol 2, 2nd edn. Churchill Livingstone, Edinburgh, p 504–891

Takenaka T, Okuda M, Usami A, Kawabori S, Ogami Y, Kubo K, Hirotsugu U 1976 Histological and immunological studies on eosinophilic granuloma of soft tissue, so-called Kimura's disease. Clinical Allergy 6: 27–39

Thomsen H K, Jacobsen M 1981 Kaposi sarcoma among homosexual men in Europe. Lancet 2:688

Tilak S P, Howard J M 1965 Regeneration and autotransplantation of lymph nodes. Annals of Surgery 161: 441–446

Turner D R 1966 The vascular tree of the haemal node in the rat. Journal of Anatomy 104: 481–493

Urmacher C, Myskowski P, Ochoa M, Kris M, Safai B 1982 Outbreak of Kaposi's sarcoma with cytomegalovirus infection in young homosexual men. American Journal of Medicine 72: 569–575

Watts J C, Sebek B A, McHenry M C, Esselstyn C B 1980 Idiopathic infarction of intraabdominal lymph nodes. American Journal of Clinical Pathology 74: 687–690

Wells G C, Whimster I W 1969 Subcutaneous angiolymphoid hyperplasia with eosinophilia. British Journal of Dermatology 81: 1–15

Wright D H, Padley N R, Judd M A 1981 Angiolymphoid hyperplasia with eosinophilia simulating lymphadenopathy. Histopathology 5: 127–140

Zeek P M 1953 Periarteritis nodosa and other forms of necrotizing angiitis. New England Journal of Medicine 248: 764–772

Primary and secondary immune disorders

INTRODUCTION

Lymph nodes play an important part in the immune response and any pathological alterations of their structure are likely to result in, or reflect concurrent alterations in immune responsiveness. In this sense, some conditions described in other chapters, such as sarcoidosis and lymphoid neoplasms, are often associated with characteristic alterations of the patient's humoral or cellular immunity. The aim of this chapter is to describe the lymph node pathology of a group of disorders many of which are at present better characterised by clinical or immunological criteria than by specific morphological changes in the nodes. We shall discuss first the group of immune deficiencies, congenital and acquired, then the changes due to immunosuppression, before passing on to autoimmune disorders and allied forms of immune disturbance, including amyloidosis of lymph nodes. Finally we shall consider two groups of conditions of unknown aetiology, which may be broadly considered as immunological disorders, namely, angioimmunoblastic lymphadenopathy and Castleman's disease.

IMMUNOLOGICAL DEFICIENCIES

Immunological deficiency may be suspected when a patient displays undue susceptibility to infections, but it must always be remembered that there may be other reasons for such increased susceptibility. Suspected immune deficiencies are usually investigated by immunoglobulin estimations and lymphocyte function studies. Lymph node biopsy is not indicated in most cases, but if carried out it should be done after stimulation by injection of diphtheria or tetanus toxoid in the drainage area a week before biopsy (Fudenberg et al, 1971; WHO Scientific Group 1979). A notable exception is the rapid enlargement of lymph nodes in a patient known to be immunodeficient, since this may represent development of a lymphoma, to which these patients are particularly prone. Material obtained at necropsy may be helpful in the understanding of the pathogenesis of particular types of immune deficiency.

In recent years a large number of different syndromes have been described, but because of their rarity or relative lack of histological information we will restrict this account to those which are more common and those in which the nature of the defect is better understood. For practical purposes immunological deficiencies can be classified into three groups: defects affecting mainly humoral immunity, defects affecting mainly cell mediated immunity, and combined defects.

Defects in humoral immunity

Congenital sex-linked recessive agammaglobulinaemia (Bruton's type)

First described by Bruton (1952) in boys, this type is thought to have an X-linked recessive mode of inheritance. Some immunoglobulin can be detected in the serum, but this is negligible and patients are particularly susceptible to bacterial infections from which they die if untreated. The disease is usually noticed at about 6 months of age, when maternal antibodies disappear. Cellular immunity may also be slightly impaired (Cooperband et al, 1968) but the children can usually cope with

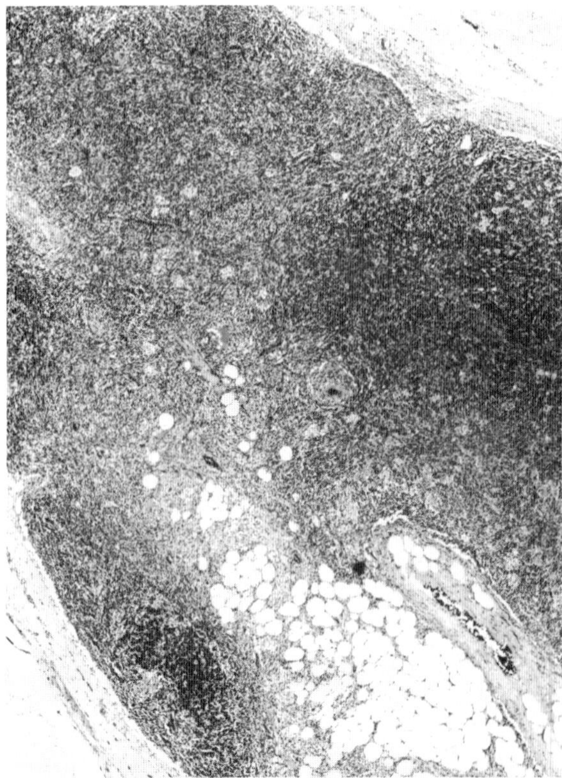

Fig. 8.1 Lymph node from a boy with Bruton's type agammaglobulinaemia. No well formed follicles with germinal centres are present. (H E × 20)

viral and fungal infections, although deaths due to hepatitis and *Pneumocystis carinii* pneumonia have been recorded (Peterson et al, 1965.)

Histologically the lymph nodes show a lack of lymphoid follicles with germinal centres (Fig. 8.1). Plasma cells are absent, but small lymphocytes and scattered pyroninophilic cells, some large and with prominent nucleoli, are present in the paracortex. It is not unusual to see also increased numbers of histiocytes and aggregates of epithelioid cells, but this finding is not restricted to a single type of immunological defect.

In the peripheral blood, lymphocyte numbers are normal, but the children are deficient in all immunoglobulin types. The late development of acute lymphoblastic leukaemia has been described.

Similar antibody deficiencies can occur in girls and boys without a family history. These are thought to represent a non-sex linked form of congenital agammaglobulinaemia. The lymph nodes show appearances similar to those described above.

Acquired primary hypogammaglobulinaemia

In this condition the deficiency appears later in life without being preceded by a neoplasm or a specific disease of the immune system. Most patients are between 30 and 50 years of age and females are affected as often as males. As a rule, some immunoglobulin can be detected in the serum (Henry & Goldman, 1974) and not uncommonly the disease may be accompanied by other disorders of the immune system such as malabsorption (Hughes et al, 1971) and thymoma. Extirpation of the thymoma does not alter the immune deficiency (Peterson et al, 1965). Lympho-reticular neoplasms have been described late in the course of the disease. Amyloidosis, probably secondary to recurrent infections, can also complicate the picture (Gaffney & Lee, 1978).

The lymph nodes may be of normal size or very small. As a rule lymph follicles are absent or very atrophic (Fig. 8.2) lacking germinal centres, although the follicular arterioles are often discernible. If germinal centres are present, they usually contain few phagocytes with tingible bodies and it is common to find epithelioid cells within them. Epithelioid cell clusters are also common in paracortical areas (Fig. 8.3).

Acquired hypogammaglobulinaemia has been described in families. Relatives of patients may suffer from other immune disorders such as hypergammaglobulinaemia, multiple myeloma, rheumatoid arthritis and lupus erythematosus (Peterson et al, 1965), so that a genetic abnormality of late expression is possible.

Variable immune deficiency

This term comprises a variety of immunoglobulin deficiencies in which individuals may lack some but not all immunoglobulin types (Hobbs, 1968). One of the commonest partial deficiencies is IgA and IgG deficiency with normal or raised IgM. Patients with this disorder may have lymph nodes with few plasma cells, but sometimes there is follicular hyperplasia and many lymphoid cells within the follicles contain IgM. The abnormality is com-

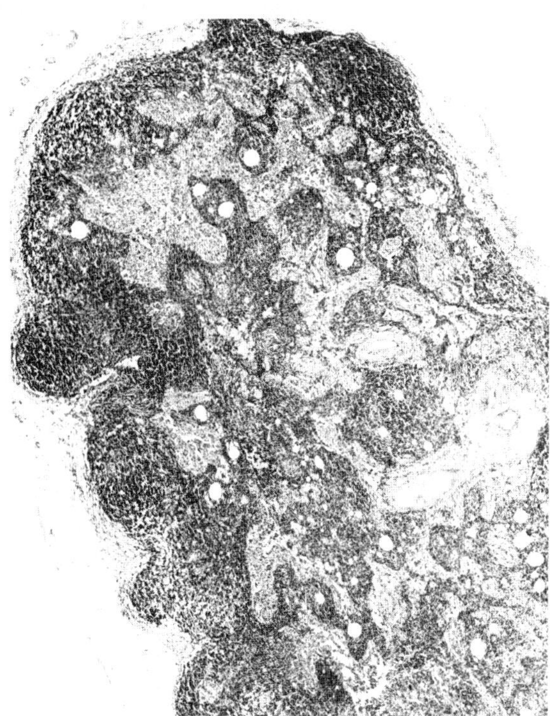

Fig. 8.2 Lymph node from a 56 year old woman with acquired hypogammaglobulinaemia. The follicular cortex is atrophic and no well-developed germinal centres are seen. (H E × 20)

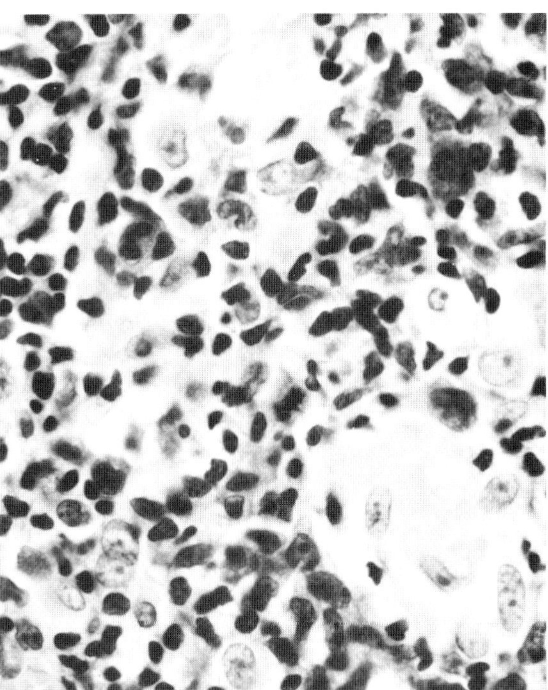

Fig. 8.3 Same lymph node as that in Fig. 8.2. There are groups of epithelioid histiocytes in the paracortex. Other cells are lymphocytes of various sizes. No plasma cells are seen. This patient developed a high grade malignant lymphoma 2 years later. (H E × 350)

monest in the gut-associated lymphoid tissue, when IgM has been shown to be polyclonal in type (Nagura et al, 1979).

Secondary acquired hypogammaglobulinaemia

This can be due to defective production or excessive loss. The former mechanism is by far the commonest and can result from treatment with immunosuppressive drugs, infections, malnutrition and neoplasms of the immune system and other sites. Excessive loss can occur through the urine in the nephrotic syndrome, through the intestine in intestinal lymphangiectasia and through the skin in exfoliative dermatitis.

Defects in cellular immunity

Congenital defects are rare and some immunoglobulin deficiency is often present as well. The better defined conditions are the Wiskott-Aldrich syndrome, ataxia-telangiectasia, Di Giorge's syndrome and Nézelof's syndrome. Acquired defects are best represented by the recently described 'acquired immunodeficiency syndrome' (AIDS).

Wiskott-Aldrich syndrome

This comprises eczema, thrombocytopenia and increased susceptibility to infections (Aldrich et al 1954). It is thought to be X-linked. Affected boys suffer from fungal, viral and bacterial infections and have a high incidence of lymphoreticular neoplasms. Patients seldom survive beyond the first decade. Cell-mediated immunity deteriorates as the child gets older and the lymph nodes show a progressive depletion of lymphoid cells from the paracortical areas (compare Fig. 8.6). The thymus is usually normal and the defect is thought to be in the afferent limb of the cellular immune system, either in the processing or the recognition of certain antigens (Levin et al, 1970).

Ataxia-Telangiectasia

This disease is defined by the neurological deficit and telangiectases which appear from the age of 3 years in the conjunctiva and exposed areas of the skin. Patients are particularly susceptible to respiratory tract infections from which they die in the second or third decades. They also have an unusually high incidence of malignant lymphomas.

The defect is predominantly one of cellular immunity but affected children often lack serum and secretory IgA and IgE. The lymph nodes usually have lymphoid follicles with poorly developed lymphocytic mantles and a reduction of plasma cells (Peterson et al, 1965). Others have noticed a depletion of lymphocytes in the paracortex.

The thymus of these patients is hypoplastic, lacking lymphoid tissue. The nature of the genetic defect is not known, but a hypothetical mesenchymal abnormality has been postulated to account for the thymic, vascular and neural defects.

Di Giorge and Nézelof syndromes

In both these conditions the thymus is hypoplastic. In Di Giorge's syndrome there is a characteristic facial appearance with hypertelorism, low-set, notched pinnae and nasal clefts; the parathyroids are hypoplastic and there are frequently cardiovascular congenital malformations. In Nézelof's syndrome the parathyroids are normal. In both cases there is a defect of cellular immunity and the lymph nodes have germinal centres, but depleted paracortical areas. The cause of the defect is thought to be a congenital lack of development of the thymus and other structures of the 3rd and 4th pharyngeal pouches.

Acquired immunodeficiency syndrome (AIDS)

This syndrome was first highlighted by the clustering of opportunistic infections and Kaposi's sarcoma in male homosexual communities in California and New York but has since been described in non-homosexuals, including females and haemophilia sufferers. Clinically the patients may present with *Pneumocystis carinii* pneumonia, *Cryptococcus* infection, candidiasis, herpes virus infections, Kaposi's sarcoma or autoimmune phenomena such as SLE or thrombocytopenic purpura. Immunologically there is a defect of cellular immunity with inversion of the helper/suppressor T-lymphocyte ratio in peripheral blood, lymphopenia, defective skin reactivity to antigens and, in some cases, polyclonal hyperglobulinaemia. The disease is probably communicable* and the clinical, epidemiological and aetiological considerations are well reviewed by Waterson (1983).

In some patients, opportunistic infections may be preceded by generalised lymphadenopathy, fever, loss of weight and diarrhoea. We have examined lymph nodes from 16 patients with this syndrome, all of which showed follicular hyperplasia with polyclonal increase in plasma cells (particularly IgG and IgM). In some cases there were also conspicuous polymorphs in the sinuses. These findings are similar to those reported by Guarda et al (1983) who found follicular hyperplasia in 10 of 11 cases, the exception being a patient with depleted nodes, absent germinal centres and prominent vessels. The only patient with normal cellular immunity in that series also had granulomas in lymph nodes. The possibility of AIDS should therefore be considered in the differential diagnosis of follicular hyperplasia in adults (see Ch. 6, p. 89) particularly when the germinal centres are large or irregular in shape with a 'geographical' or 'confluent' pattern (Fig. 8.4).

Others have commented upon the disappearance of follicles in lymph node biopsies from AIDS patients, with varying degrees of vascular proliferation and lymphocytic depletion, culminating in nodal atrophy with fibrosis. Marche et al (1984) have suggested a progressive evolution of the lesions from the initial stage of lymphadenopathy with follicular hyperplasia, through a stage resembling angioimmunoblastic lymphadenopathy to lymph node atrophy with cell depletion and fibrosis. Fully developed immunodeficiency was not found by these authors in the initial stage. Kaposi's sarcoma of lymph nodes and malignant lymphomas have also been described in AIDS patients (Ziegler et al, 1982; Doll & List, 1982; Stern et al, 1982) and the development of Kaposi's sarcoma in nodes has been noted to succeed earlier changes of AIDS (Marche et al, 1984).

* See footnote on p. 324

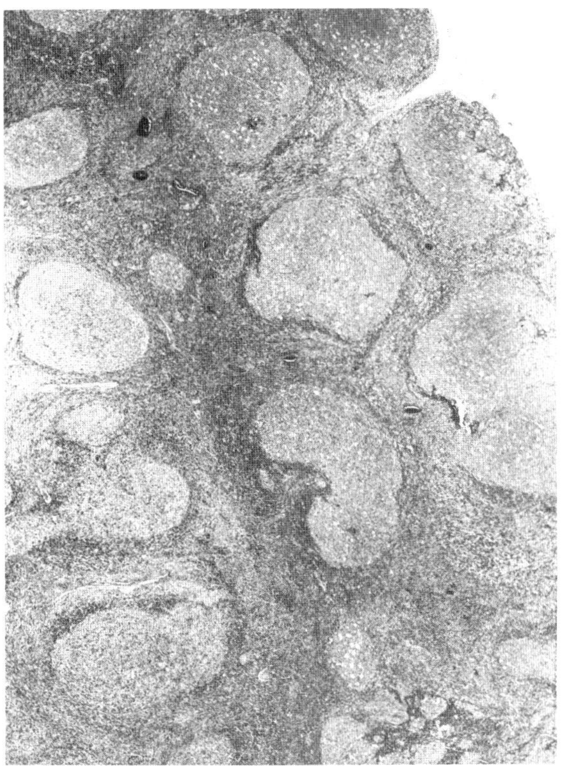

Fig. 8.4 Inguinal lymph node biopsy from a male homosexual aged 29, who presented with fever, diarrhoea and generalised lymphadenopathy. An axillary lymph node biopsy showed similar features. Immunological studies were typical of AIDS with reversal of the normal ratio of T-helper and T-suppressor cells. (H E × 16)

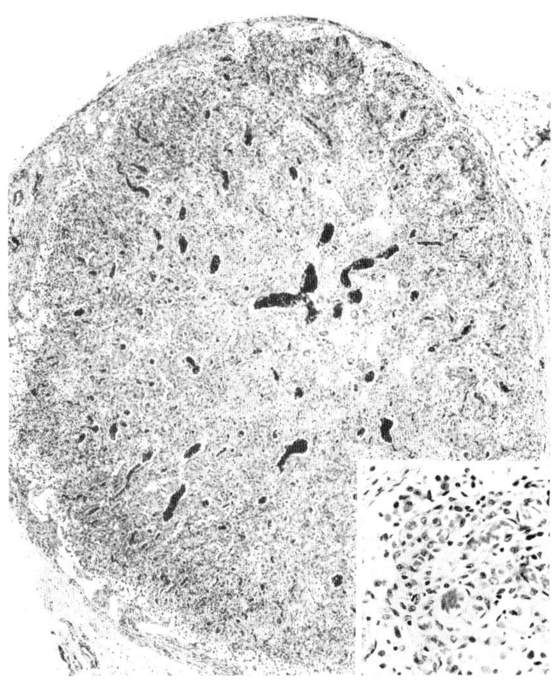

Fig. 8.5 Lymph node from a male infant who died due to severe congenital combined immunodeficiency (Swiss type agammaglobulinaemia). Vessels and sinuses are present but lymphocytes are almost totally absent. (H E × 21 × 250)

Combined immunodeficiencies

Swiss-type agammaglobulinaemia

This is so named because it was first discovered and studied by Swiss workers. Patients seldom survive the first months of life and are deficient in immunoglobulins and lymphocytes in the peripheral blood. It is inherited in an autosomal recessive way and is thought to be due to a defect of the stem cells which populate the primary lymphoid organs. The thymus is rudimentary and the lymph nodes, although having sinuses and blood vessels, lack development of any lymphoid tissue (Fig. 8.5).

Thymic alymphoplasia and dysplasia

These are less severe disorders belonging to the same group.

Reticular dysgenesis

This is a combined defect of the immune and haemopoietic systems. Children seldom survive even a few days. Lymph nodes are said to be absent (Peterson et al, 1965).

IMMUNOSUPPRESSION

The effects of radiotherapy on lymph nodes

Both irradiation of a localised area and total body irradiation have profound effects on the numbers of circulating lymphoid cells but recovery is the rule within a variable period of time dependent on the total dose administered (Grosch & Hopwood, 1979). Repopulation of B-lymphocyte areas in lymph nodes may occur at different rates from repopulation of the paracortex and appearances such as that seen in Figure 8.6 may result. Lymph nodes from areas irradiated for the eradication of neoplasms may show obliterative endarteritis, in-

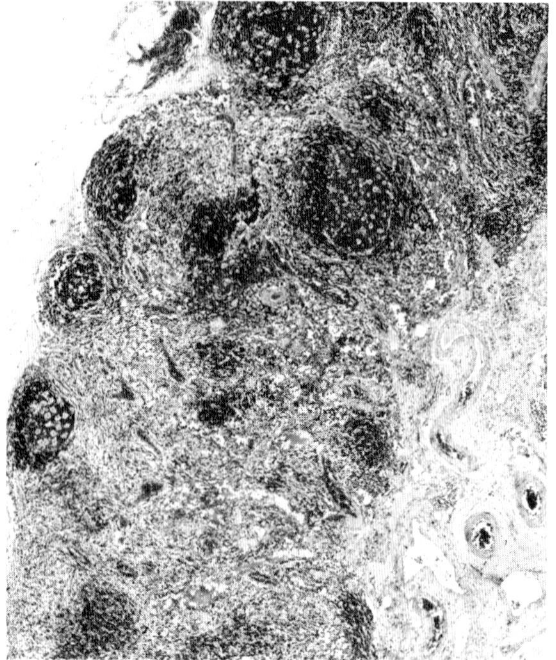

Fig. 8.6 Axillary lymph node from a boy of 14 who had received radiotherapy for an osteosarcoma of the upper humerus on that side. The paracortex is severely depleted of lymphocytes, but the follicles are relatively preserved. The picture is similar to that seen in the Wiskott-Aldrich syndrome. (H E × 20)

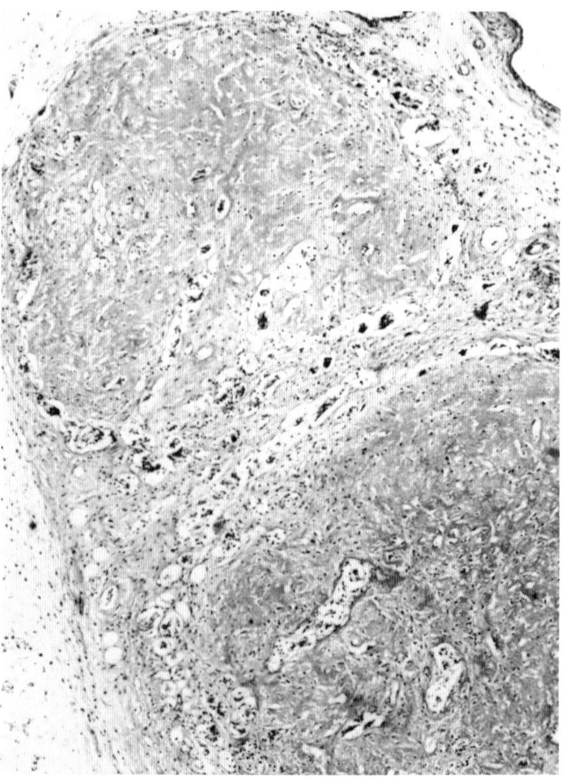

Fig. 8.7 Post-mortem lymph node from a woman of 60 who had received intensive chemotherapy for acute leukaemia. Previously infiltrated areas of the node are replaced by amorphous hyaline material — a picture similar to that seen following irradiation of tumourous areas in nodes. Death was due to overwhelming infection. (H E × 36)

creased fibrous tissue in capsule and trabeculae and focal calcification within the trabeculae. Parts of the node formerly occupied by tumour are commonly replaced by necrotic debris or hyaline material.

The effects of chemotherapy on lymph nodes

Most agents used for the therapy of cancer or for immunosuppression have an effect on both T and B lymphocytes (Harris et al, 1976). Short courses of combination chemotherapy have a profound immunosuppressive effect with recovery in about 18 days. Prolonged treatment with a single drug has less significant effect. Little is known of the effects of chemotherapy on the structure of normal lymph nodes in the human, although vigorous treatment for leukaemias or other tumours may result in replacement of neoplastic tissue by hyaline material and cell debris (Fig. 8.7) presumably the result of vascular damage and cell death. Enlargement of lymph nodes in immunosuppressed individuals may occasionally be due to the development of a malignant tumour. Of 166 patients with second neoplasms after immunosuppression, reviewed by Penn (1976), 31 were lymphoreticular and 75 haemopoietic.

LYMPHADENOPATHY IN AUTOIMMUNE DISORDERS

Systemic lupus erythematosus

Introduction

Systemic lupus erythematosus (SLE) is characterised by well defined clinical criteria (Cohen & Canoso, 1972) and by the presence of various autoantibodies in the serum, of which those against double stranded DNA are most useful for diagnostic confirmation. Production of autoantibodies and subsequent immune complex deposition explain some of the pathological features of the disease, particularly the renal and vascular lesions, but little is known of the causes of this production. Defective B-lymphocyte regulation by T-lymphocytes has been postulated and in active phases of SLE there may be lymphocytotoxic antibodies, lymphopenia and defective type IV immune reactions (Hughes & Lachmann 1975; Paty et al, 1975). Lymph node enlargement is also common in active SLE, nevertheless lymph node biopsy is seldom performed and to our knowledge no studies with modern immunohistochemical methods have been carried out to correlate the morphological changes in the nodes with information derived from studies of peripheral blood and thoracic duct lymphocytes.

Frequency of lymph node enlargement in SLE

Localised or generalised involvement of lymph nodes is recorded at some stage in the evolution of the disease in about half the patients (Fox & Rosahn, 1943; Estes & Christian, 1971; Dubois 1974a). Superficial lymph nodes, particularly those in the neck, are commonly affected (Fox & Rosahn 1943) and occasionally, cervical lymphadenopathy leading to a biopsy may be the presenting clinical sign (Dubois, 1974a). Deep nodes may appear enlarged on lymphangiography (Ricken et al, 1971). At necropsy, mesenteric, tracheobronchial and retroperitoneal nodes are often enlarged. Exceptionally, hilar lymphadenopathy on chest X-ray may be prominent (Kassan et al, 1976; Taryle & Ellis, 1979).

Histopathology

Lymph node enlargement is usually discrete, single nodes seldom exceeding 3 cm in maximum dimension. No naked-eye abnormalities are seen in most cases, but in a few there may be yellow areas of necrosis. Occasionally, necrosis is so extensive that the lymph node fragments during removal. Before steroids were introduced in the treatment of SLE, necrosis was found in about a quarter of enlarged nodes and more often at autopsy (Klemperer et al, 1941). In more recent accounts, necrosis was either absent or present only at autopsy (Gold & Gowing 1953; Moore et al, 1956; Cruickshank, 1958) and has been regarded as a terminal phenomenon. It is possible that steroids may have altered the natural course of lupus lymphadenopathy. Harvey et al (1954) comment on the disappearance of lymph node enlargement within weeks or months of treatment, but on occasions this may persist (Kassan et al, 1976) and a diagnosis of SLE based on histological criteria is occasionally made (Garrido & Cueva 1972).

Microscopically, in most lymph nodes with necrotising lesions lymph follicles are few or absent (Fig. 8.8). Necrosis in SLE lymph nodes was first described by Short (1907) but our detailed knowledge of these lesions dates from the classic accounts of Ginzler & Fox (1940), Klemperer et al (1941), Fox & Rosahn (1943) and Teilum (1945). Necrosis is often very extensive and involves ir-

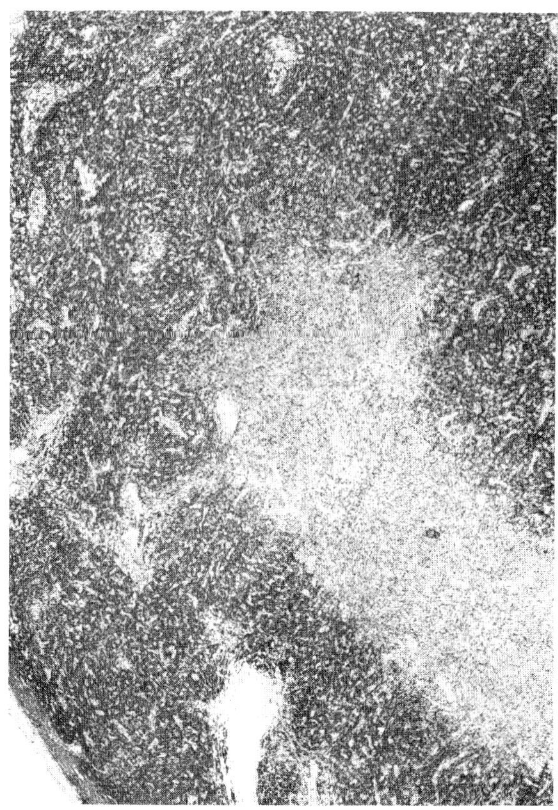

Fig. 8.8 Lymph node in systemic lupus erythematosus. Note absence of follicles and ill-defined necrosis in the middle of the node. (H E × 20)

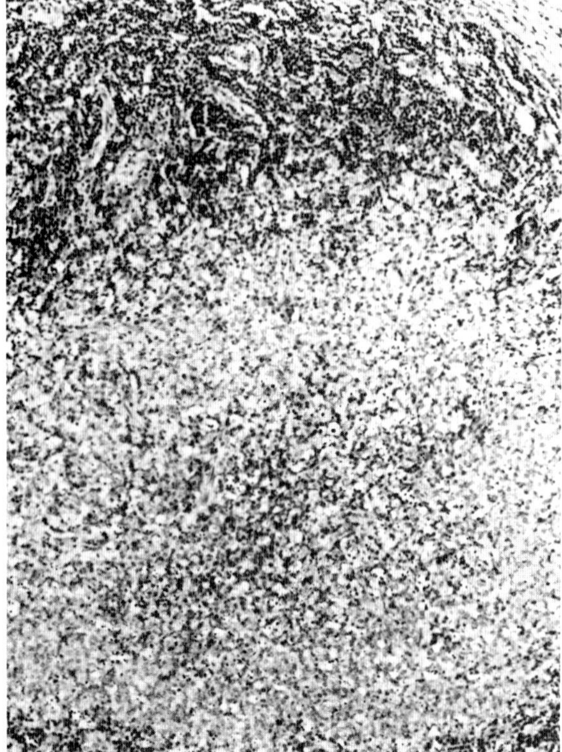

Fig. 8.9 Systemic lupus erythematosus. Well defined focus of blastic transformation with early necrosis. Compare with Fig. 6.3 (p. 87). (H E × 60)

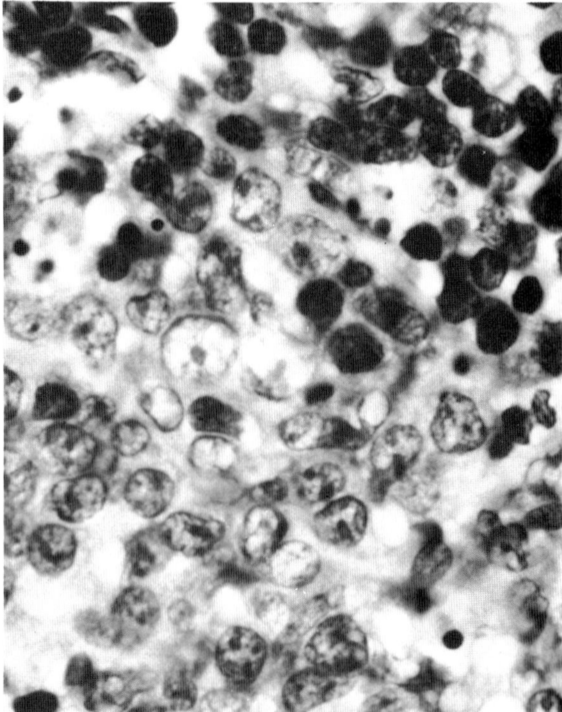

Fig. 8.10 Systemic lupus erythematosus. High magnification of the boundary between dark and pale staining cells of Fig. 8.9. The pale cells are large lymphoid cells with vesicular nuclei and discernible nucleoli. Some nuclear debris due to necrosis of individual cells is present. (H E × 600)

regular areas near the capsule or near the hilum (Fig. 8.8), but when focal, it involves the paracortex rather than such follicles as may remain. In the earliest lesions (Fig. 8.9) necrosis is confined to the centres of focal areas where small lymphocytes have been replaced by larger pyroninophilic lymphoid cells and immunoblasts (Fig. 8.10). Histiocytes and polymorphs may be present in small numbers. In more advanced lesions (Fig. 8.11) there is marked karyorrhexis and coagulative necrosis of individual cells whose outlines are still discernible. Some intercellular eosinophilic material, usually described as fibrinoid in early accounts, may be present and some apparently viable, usually large lymphoid cells are often seen in the necrotic areas. Occasionally haematoxylin bodies (HB) are present in advanced lesions, either scattered (Fig. 8.11 insert) or in the collagen of the lymph node capsule or that surrounding vessels. HB were first described in lymph nodes by Ginzler & Fox (1940). Their homogeneous structure and characteristic violet staining with haematoxylin reflect their content of partially depolymerised DNA, protein, carbohydrate and globulins (Klemperer et al, 1950; Gueft & Laufer, 1954; Moore et al, 1956; Godman et al, 1958). Electron microscopical observations of HB (Grishman et al, 1979) suggest a mixture of nuclear and cytoplasmic material. In the absence of necrosis, the enlarged lymph nodes of patients with SLE often show non-specific changes. Follicular hyperplasia is mentioned in a minority of cases but most authors describe follicular atrophy in the majority (Klemperer et al, 1941; Fox & Rosahn, 1943; Gold & Gowing, 1953; Moore et al, 1957; Cruickshank, 1958). Plasma cells, sometimes containing Russell bodies, are often increased in numbers, even when the follicles are atrophic. The sinuses are usually distended and contain histiocytes, plasma cells and lymphocytes of various sizes. Most authors remark on the presence of large cells, variously described as reticulum cells, histiocytes or immunoblasts. These cells may

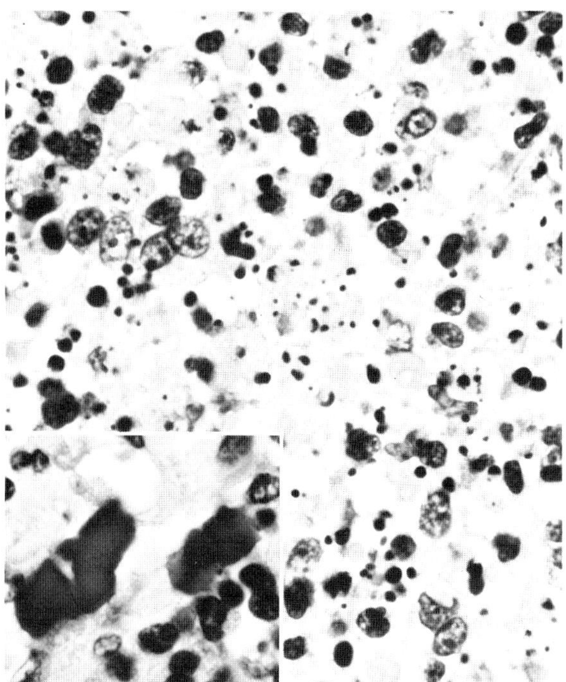

Fig. 8.11 Systemic lupus erythematosus. Necrotic centre of lesion showing nuclear pyknosis and karyorrhexis with eosinophilic homogenisation of cell cytoplasm. Scattered viable lymphoid cells are seen, as well as macrophages. (H E × 400) Inset: haematoxylin bodies in lymph node showing homogeneous structureless appearance. (H E × 580)

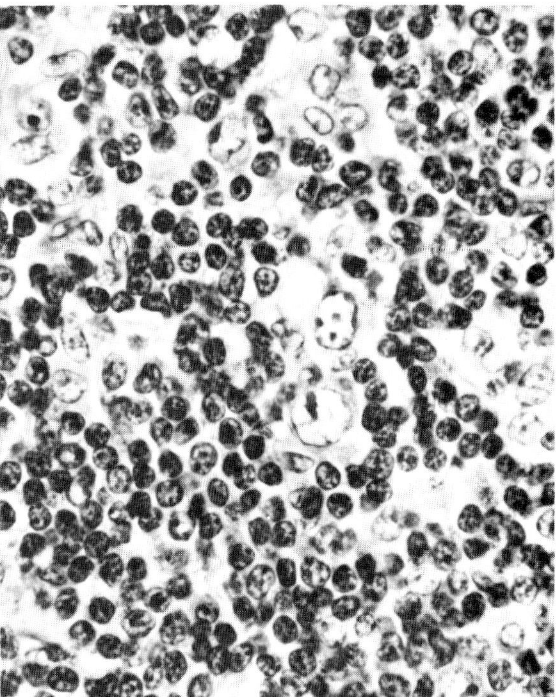

Fig. 8.12 Systemic lupus erythematosus. There is a mixture of small lymphocytes and scattered large immunoblasts with vesicular nuclei and small eccentric nucleoli. These cells can be mistaken for Sternberg-Reed cells leading to an erroneous diagnosis of Hodgkin's disease. (H E × 350)

resemble Sternberg-Reed cells (Foldes, 1946; Emberger et al, 1976) but in our experience can be distinguished by their smaller nucleoli (Fig. 8.12). They are strongly pyroninophilic and apparently represent an immunoblastic proliferation in the paracortex.

Differential diagnosis

The necrotising lesions of SLE, particularly when they contain HB, are so characteristic as to be virtually diagnostic in the context of the other lymph node changes described, but formation of HB is not exclusive to SLE (Worken & Pearson, 1953; Elsner & Iotti, 1973). Unfortunately HB are not present in every case of SLE, although Gueft & Laufer (1954) found them in 10 of their 14 cases after extensive search with high magnification.

Small areas of necrosis accompanied by an exuberant immunoblastic transformation can be seen in salmonellosis, brucellosis, some viral infections and toxoplasmosis. As a rule the necrosis is more focal and complete, lacking 'ghost cells' and haematoxylin bodies. In toxoplasmosis there are usually follicular hyperplasia and presence of epithelioid cell clusters. Both these features are absent in SLE.

Extensive necrosis should be differentiated from that of primary syphilitic lymphadenitis, particularly since patients with SLE may have false positive serological tests for syphilis; as a rule this is not difficult (see p. 108) since the vascular lesions and characteristic periadenitis of primary syphilis are absent in SLE. For similar reasons there is usually no difficulty in distinguishing SLE from infarction of either normal or neoplastic nodes (p. 144–5).

Of greater importance is the differential diagnosis between SLE and the 'histiocytic necrotising lymphadenitis without granulocytic infiltration' first described in Japan in 1972 but seen since in Europe (Pileri et al, 1982) (see p. 87). This condition also affects predominantly young women and is characterised by fever, leucopenia and neck lymphadenopathy in which necrosis is a distinctive feature. However, in SLE the large cells in the necrotic areas are predominantly lymphoid rather than histiocytic and phagocytosis of nuclear debris is less conspicuous. Pileri et al (1982) stress the presence of polymorphs in SLE as a further differentiating feature but polymorphs can be absent in otherwise classical lupus lymphadenitis. As a rule the absence of HB, preservation of follicular architecture and presence of numerous histiocytic cells (thought to be interdigitating reticulum cells) militate in favour of histiocytic necrotising lymphadenitis but in some cases the histological differentiation may be difficult. The differentiation between SLE and Kawasaki's disease (mucocutaneous lymph node syndrome) is unlikely to present many clinical problems and histologically (p. 148) the foci of necrosis in Kawasaki's disease are usually associated with vascular lesions, including microthrombi, swelling of endothelium and infiltration of arterial walls with lymphoid and histiocytic cells (Giesker et al, 1982).

When necrosis is absent the changes in enlarged nodes from SLE patients are not distinctive and may be impossible to distinguish from other conditions in which immunoblastic proliferation unaccompanied by follicular hyperplasia occurs, such as glandular fever, hydantoin lymphadenopathy or immunoblastic lymphadenopathy (Konovalova & Fraik, 1976; Schechter, 1980). Although vascular proliferation is occasionally present in SLE, it seldom reaches the intensity seen in immunoblastic lymphadenopathy (p. 176). Care should be taken not to mistake the sometimes alarming immunoblastic proliferation of SLE for Hodgkin's disease (Harvey et al, 1954) but it should also be remembered that almost every type of lymphoma and leukaemia has been described complicating SLE and this possibility should be considered in these patients, although the contribution of lymphoreticular malignancy as a cause of death in SLE is less than 1% (Dubois, 1974b).

Pathogenesis of SLE lymphadenopathy

Although thrombosis and necrosis of vessels are often seen within advanced necrotic lesions in SLE lymphadenitis, vasculitis is not a feature in early lesions and there is no evidence that the necrosis is due to ischaemia. Whether this necrosis of unknown pathogenesis precedes or follows the blastic transformation is impossible to tell, but it is tempting to postulate an abortive lymphocyte transformation with lymphorrhexis, perhaps mediated by lymphocytotoxic autoantibodies. It is of interest that exaggerated immunoblastic transformation has been described in the lymph nodes of New Zealand B mice with SLE-like syndrome (Haustein & Raetz, 1973) and that interdigitating cells, normally present in the paracortex and thought to have an important function in the regulation of T-lymphocyte responses, have been found lacking both in New Zealand B mice and in 3 cases of human SLE (Klug, 1978).

Lymphadenopathy in other autoimmune and hypersensitivity diseases

Rheumatoid arthritis and related conditions

Prominent enlargement of superficial lymph nodes may be found in up to 75% of patients with rheumatoid arthritis (Motulsky et al, 1952). The axillary, cervical and supraclavicular nodes are most often involved but the inguinal, epitrochlear and preauricular nodes, or even nodes in unusual places, such as in the forearm or thigh, along the course of vessels, have been found enlarged (Motulsky et al, 1952; Cruickshank, 1958; Nosanchuk & Schnitzer, 1969). They can be quite large (up to 5 cm) and histologically show either simple reactive follicular hyperplasia or giant follicular hyperplasia (see p. 90). In some cases there is capsular thickening and pericapsular infiltration with lymphocytes and plasma cells, whilst plasma cells may be prominent in the sinuses and medullary cords. Neutrophil polymorphs may be found in the sinuses where they may undergo necrosis to form small abscesses. None of these features is specific and similar changes can be seen in the lymphadenopathy of secondary syphilis (p. 109) and in the acquired immunodeficiency syndrome (p. 162) in a different clinical context. In the past, rheumatoid lymphadenopathy has been mistaken for follicular lymphoma and many patients have received radiotherapy and chemotherapy. The differential diagnosis from follicular lymphoma is not difficult (p. 264) and it should be remembered that although lymphomas do occur in patients with rheumatoid arthritis (Miller, 1967) their incidence is low.

Similar histological changes are found in lymph nodes in juvenile rheumatoid arthritis (Still's disease) and Felty's syndrome (Pruzanski 1980) where the incidence of lymphadenopathy is between 40 and 50%. In rheumatoid arthritis and allied conditions hyperglobulinaemia and cryoglobulinaemia are common.

Mixed connective tissue disease

These patients have a mixture of symptoms of SLE, scleroderma and polymyositis (Sharp et al, 1972). Lymphadenopathy is present in about 68% of patients but histological information is scant and features non-specific.

Scleroderma and dermatomyositis

Enlargement of superficial lymph nodes is not uncommon in dermatomyositis, but in the few instances in which lymph node biopsy has been carried out, sections have shown non-specific changes, such as reactive follicular hyperplasia (Lennert, 1961). Although occasional instances of fibrosis of lymph nodes have been described in scleroderma (Symmers, 1978) lymphadenopathy is not a feature of this condition and significant pathological alterations have not been found with any consistency in any large series (Leinwand et al, 1954).

Sjögren's syndrome

Enlargement of lymph nodes is very rare in the Sjögren-Mikulicz syndrome except when the sicca complex is associated with extrasalivary signs and symptoms. When lymph node biopsy has been carried out, this has shown follicular hyperplasia and, in one instance, arteritis (Shearn, 1971). In rare cases the regional lymph nodes (preauricular and cervical) may enlarge and show almost complete obliteration of their architecture by plasma cells, small lymphocytes and larger, primitive plasmacytoid cells and immunoblasts. The term 'pseudolymphoma' which has been used for such appearances (Anderson & Talal, 1972) is not perhaps a happy one but it emphasises the tendency of such patients to develop overt lymphoid neoplasia, notably lymphoplasmacytoid lymphoma and immunoblastic sarcoma, in the course of time.

Thyrotoxicosis and Hashimoto's thyroiditis

The presence of superficial lymphadenopathy and even splenomegaly in a small proportion of patients with Graves' disease is well known. Cervical, axillary and epitrochlear nodes may be enlarged and can reach 3 cm in longest dimension. If the characteristic features of hyperthyroidism are not obvious, such patients may undergo lymph node biopsy to exclude a lymphoma (Levy & Levin, 1951). Histologically such nodes show reactive follicular hyperplasia with no unusual features.

Enlargement of lymph nodes adjacent to the thyroid gland is not uncommon in Hashimoto's thyroiditis. The nodes usually show non-specific hyperplasia. In both Graves' disease and Hashimoto's thyroiditis these nodes may contain islands of non-neoplastic thyroid tissue and care should be taken not to diagnose metastatic thyroid carcinoma on that account (see p. 395). As many as one-quarter of malignant lymphomas of the thyroid may occur in patients with thyroiditis but involvement of regional nodes by the lymphoma is a late development (Woolner et al, 1966).

Polyarteritis nodosa

Lymph node hilar arteries can be affected in this condition (Symmers, 1978) which may be a cause of lymph node infarction (see Ch. 7).

AMYLOID LYMPHADENOPATHY

The nature of amyloid

Amyloid is the generic name for a variety of predominantly protein substances deposited extracellularly as structureless material when viewed by light microscopy. It has characteristic tinctorial properties; particularly the ability to bind Congo red dye, after which a green/orange birefringence (dichroism) is obtained with polarised light. This and other properties of amyloid depend on a common structural arrangement of the polypeptide chains which make up amyloid fibrils — the so-called β-pleated sheet structure (Eanes & Glenner, 1968). The chemical composition of the polypeptide chains varies with the type of amyloidosis. Amyloid complicating immunoproliferative disorders is related to immunoglobulins produced by the neoplasm, usually fragments of light chains (AL proteins). It is also becoming evident that, with the exclusion of heredofamilial amyloidosis, cases previously classified as primary systemic amyloidosis are also due to deposition of AL proteins and the frequency of detection of an abnormal serum or urinary paraprotein has increased to over 90% with improved methodology (Cathcart et al, 1972; Glenner, 1980b). In contrast, secondary or reactive amyloidosis is due to deposition of polypeptides whose common denominator is the presence of arginine as the N-terminal aminoacid (AA proteins). An antigenically related serum factor (SAA) may be found in acute phases of the predisposing disease, but the antigen is different in different patients. Its cell of origin is unknown. Amyloid found in some endocrine tumours is probably related to the hormones they manufacture, but this has only been proved in medullary thyroid carcinoma (Glenner, 1980a).

Amyloid in lymph nodes

Involvement of lymph nodes in 'lardaceous disease' is already mentioned by Samuel Wilks (1856). Its frequency and importance varies in different forms of amyloidosis.

In *primary amyloidosis* lymph node enlargement is occasionally a prominent physical sign. Thus Eisen (1946), records it in 17% of patients and Rukavina et al (1956), in a review of 154 cases, give an incidence of 11% with localised or generalised lymphadenopathy. Cases of primary amyloidosis first diagnosed on biopsy of enlarged lymph nodes have been reported by Dillon & Evans (1942), Symmers (1956b) and Mackenzie (1963). Prominent lymphadenopathy later on in the course of the disease is not uncommon (Lindsay & Knorp, 1945) and at necropsy, Briggs (1961) found lymph node amyloid in 69% of patients with primary amyloidosis.

Amyloidosis apparently restricted to lymph nodes is rare and studies of other tissues are not always complete. Scheurlen et al (1973) and Ko et al (1976) have reported 'tumourous' enlargement of lymph nodes due to amyloidosis associated with paraproteinaemia. In one case the lymph node enlargement was present for 13 years and the patient died of unrelated causes. We have found amyloid restricted to cervical, mediastinal and para-aortic lymph nodes in a patient who died of cerebral infarction. Amyloid was not found in any other organ at necropsy. It is possible that these cases represent low grade immunocyte proliferations which are not overtly neoplastic and are comparable to the localised amyloid tumours of the lung.

Systemic amyloidosis associated with lymphoid neoplasms has been described in multiple myeloma, plasmacytoma, Waldenström's macroglobulinaemia, with and without overt malignant lymphoma (Hobbs & Morgan, 1963; Forget et al, 1966; Azzopardi & Lehner, 1966), nodular lymphomas (Cathcart et al, 1972; Tschang, 1976), immunoblastic sarcoma (Knowles & Shevchuk 1978) and non-malignant proliferations of B lymphocytes, such as the plasma cell variant of Castleman's disease (Miralles Garcia et al, 1978) (see p. 188). Amyloid localised to lymph nodes has also been reported in immunoblastic lymphadenopathy (Madri & Fromowitz 1978).

In *secondary amyloidosis* lymph node involvement at necropsy was found in 53% of Briggs' series (1961), but enlargement of nodes leading to diagnostic biopsy is usually due to the primary disease and not to amyloid deposition, which is discrete (Tribe, 1966).

Systemic amyloidosis in Hodgkin's disease has always been thought to be of secondary type and in one case amyloid has been confirmed as being of AA type (Glenner, 1980b). Amyloid can occur in association with mixed cellularity Hodgkin's disease, when it is rarely found in the nodes (Wallace et al, 1950; Razis et al, 1959) and in lymphocyte predominant Hodgkin's disease (Azzopardi & Lehner, 1966) in a proportionately higher number of cases and with occasional formation of amyloid tumours in the nodes (Short & Castleman, 1949). This could be related to the longer clinical course of lymphocyte predominant Hodgkin's disease, but it is of interest that the nodular variant of the latter has been regarded as a B-cell neoplasm by Poppema et al (1979). An association between the treatment of Hodgkin's disease with nitrogen mustards and systemic amyloidosis has been reported (Cardell, 1961) and there is some evidence of a causal relationship in experimental work (Heefner & Sorenson, 1962).

Histopathology

Macroscopically the appearance of the nodes depends on the amounts of amyloid present: when scanty the nodes appear normal in size and consistency, when abundant, they are firm and rubbery with a consistency resembling that of cartilage on sectioning. Amyloid of long standing or that occurring in patients with hypercalcaemia secondary to renal failure may show focal calcification (Bottomley et al, 1974). The nodes show orange-yellow specks on the cut surface (Fig. 8.13) and feel gritty when sliced. Otherwise the surface varies in colour from greyish to slightly reddish (Mackenzie, 1963) and haemorrhages are not uncommon, particularly in cases with paraproteinaemia and purpura. They are seldom longer than 2.5 cm (Symmers, 1956a) but there are exceptional cases in which amyloid tumours have reached 15 cm. Haemorrhage may contribute to the enlargement (Dillon & Evans, 1942). Within a given patient, amyloid may involve all nodes or be restricted to one or several groups. It is not infrequent to find considerable variations in the amounts of amyloid present in the adjacent nodes.

Histologically, discrete deposits of amyloid are usually found in the walls of vessels or along the reticulin framework of the nodes (see Fig. 10.30, p. 248). When abundant, amyloid can involve the whole node or capriciously spare parts of it (Fig. 8.14). Sinuses and follicles are the structures

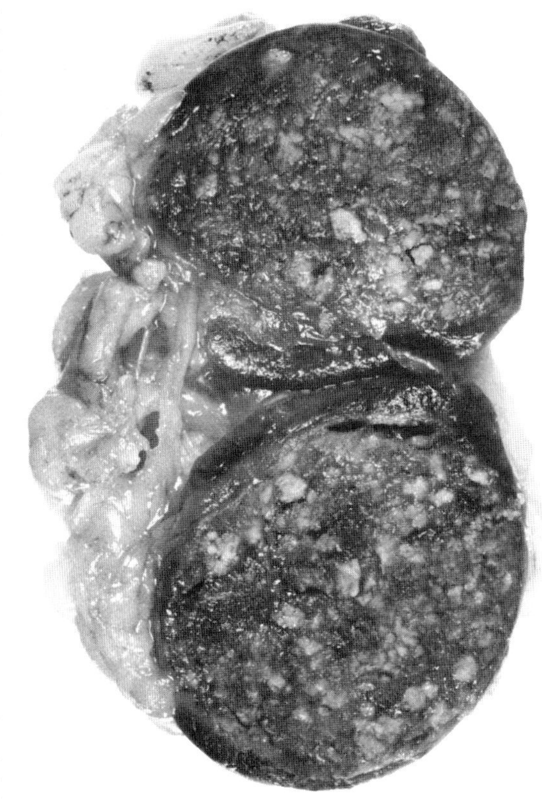

Fig. 8.13 Naked-eye appearance of an axillary lymph node heavily infiltrated by amyloid (primary amyloidosis). Some of the pale areas were yellow and hard due to calcification. (Scale on left is in mm.)

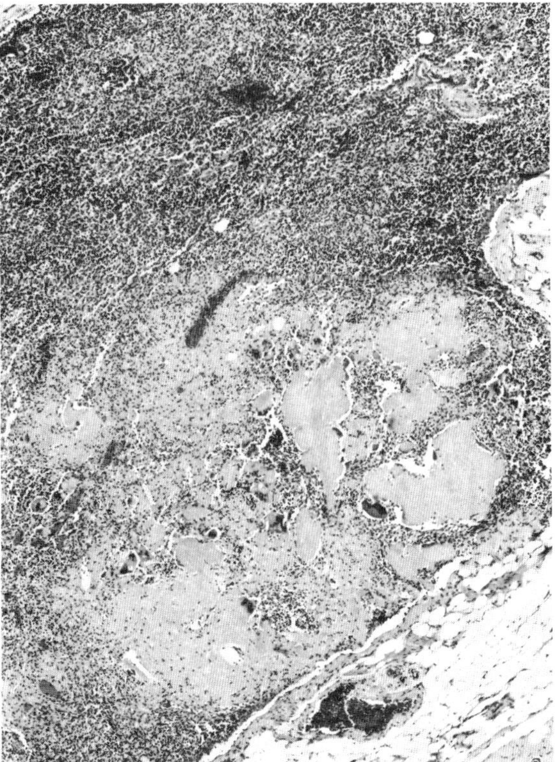

Fig. 8.14 Focal deposits of amyloid replacing part of a small cervical lymph node (primary amyloidosis) (H E × 20)

most often spared (Symmers, 1956a), although nodular deposition has been described (Mackenzie, 1963). Abundant amyloid usually forms irregular masses which may be centrally calcified or ossified and are often surrounded by multinucleated giant-cells of foreign body type (Fig. 8.15).

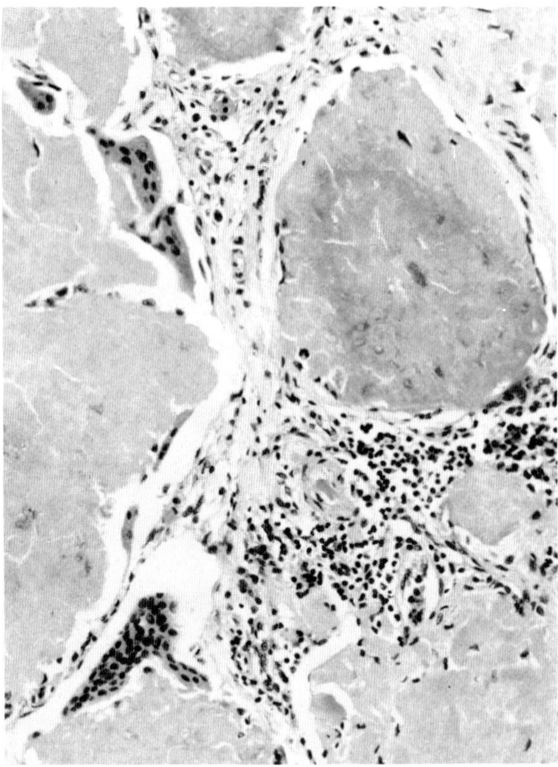

Fig 8.15 Amyloid deposits in lymph node with foreign-body type giant cells on the surface of the deposits (primary amyloidosis) (H E × 100)

In primary systemic amyloidosis it is common to find lymphocytes and plasma cells amongst the amyloid masses. Follicles with reactive centres are not prominent, but the structure of the nodes is preserved in all but the most severely involved nodes.

Histochemical differentiation of AL and AA amyloid can be carried out in paraffin sections by the resistance of AL proteins to trypsin digestion and potassium permanganate oxidation (Wright et al, 1977) and this helps in categorising cases of secondary amyloidosis.

Differential diagnosis

Since the mechanism of amyloid deposition in primary amyloidosis and neoplasms of lymphoid cells is basically similar, it would be anticipated that some cases may be difficult to categorise as either neoplastic or non-neoplastic. This is particularly so if neoplastic cells are few, amongst abundant amyloid (Baker et al, 1949; Bottomley et al, 1974). It is not suprising that some of these inconclusive cases have responded to radiotherapy.

It must not be forgotten that thyroid medullary carcinoma and renal carcinoma can produce amyloid and can present with metastatic lymphadenopathy. The identification of carcinoma cells is usually easy, but in metastases of thyroid medullary carcinoma amyloid can be prominent and the tumour inconspicuous or necrotic. In this situation the presence of necrosis and total disruption of lymph node architecture should be helpful.

Green birefringence after Congo red staining is probably the most reliable method to identify amyloid on light microscopy. Some cases which are negative or weakly positive can give positive metachromatic reactions with methyl violet. This stain and Thioflavine T should be used before concluding that the material present in a lymph node is not amyloid. The condition most likely to be confused with amyloidosis is the so-called lymph node hyalinosis (q.v.). Smaller amounts of hyaline or other proteinaceous material which can be confused with amyloid may be found in a variety of neoplasms and non-neoplastic conditions.

OTHER LYMPHADENOPATHIES ASSOCIATED WITH IMMUNOLOGICAL ABNORMALITIES

Lymph node 'hyalinosis'

(Para-amyloidosis)

Sclerosis or hyalinisation is a common finding in advanced stages of inflammatory or neoplastic lymphadenopathy. As a rule, both collagen and hyaline — the latter possibly resulting from the deposition of as yet unidentified blood proteins — can be found in these nodes. In most cases of lymph node 'hyalinosis' there is residual inflammation (such as sarcoid granulomata) or residual neoplasia (such as Hodgkin's disease), which allows us to categorise the hyalinisation as secondary to another recognisable pathological process. Occasionally, extensive hyalinisation occurs without easily identifiable primary cause; the architecture of the nodes may be still discernible or may be completely obliterated and the hyaline material may be arranged in solid or concentric masses or show a lace-like pattern with abundant lymphocytes and plasma cells in non-hyalinised areas (Fig. 8.16). In a few cases hyalinisation has been found in association with transient hyperglobulinaemia, particularly increase in IgM (Osborne et al, 1979). In other instances there is evidence of a low-grade lymphoplasmacytoid lymphoma in the nodes (see p. 248 and Fig. 10.30). It is possible that in these cases the hyaline may represent immunoglobulin fractions which do not have a β-pleated structure when deposited in tissues and do not therefore have the properties of amyloid. The role of other biologically active substances, such as lymphokines, which could stimulate fibrogenesis, is still to be determined.

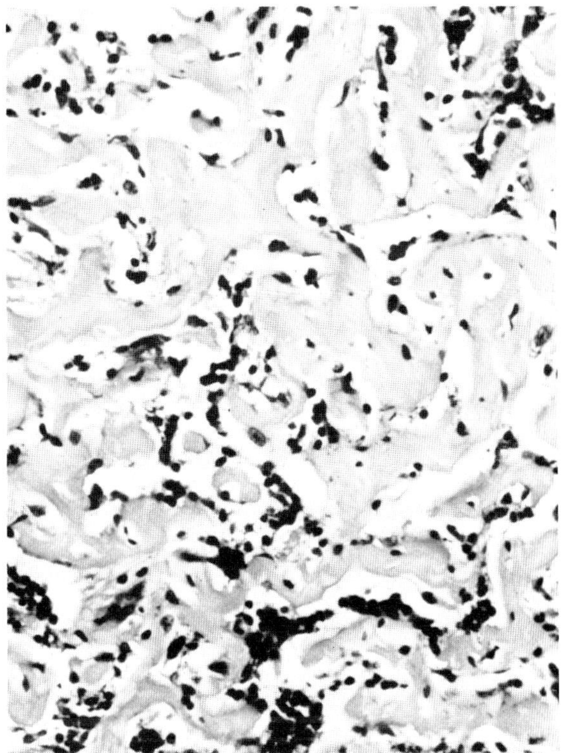

Fig. 8.16 'Hyalinosis' of lymph node. Incidental finding in axillary lymph nodes from 70 year old patient who died of cerebrovascular disease. (H E × 160)

Sinus histiocytosis with massive lymphadenopathy (SHML)

Polyclonal hypergammaglobulinaemia with particularly high levels of IgG has been noted in about 80% of patients with this condition which is fully reviewed in Chapter 14 (p. 350). In some cases there have been transient reduction of skin reactivity to a variety of antigens and reduced lymphocyte responses to non-specific mitogens in vitro (Becroft et al, 1973; Pruzanski, 1980).

Chronic benign lymphadenopathy in childhood

Recurrent enlargement of lymph nodes which, on biopsy, show non-specific reactive follicular hyperplasia has been described in young children. Its cause is unknown and immunological studies have shown high IgG and IgA with apparently normal T cell function (Kissane & Gephardt, 1974; Pruzanski, 1980).

The 'constipated' plasma cell syndrome

Intracytoplasmic PAS positive inclusions of Russell body type are occasionally very prominent in lymphoplasmacytoid and other lymphomas (see Ch. 10) and can rarely occur in large numbers in lymphadenopathies which are not overtly neoplastic. We have seen one case in which the lymph node architecture was preserved but sinuses and medullary cords were filled with plasma cells containing such inclusions. The patient had a peripheral neuropathy from which he died 2 years later. Lough & Shuster (1975) have reported a similar case in which a patient with SLE showed this picture in lymph nodes and had monomeric IgM in the serum. They postulated an acquired defect of macroglobulin polymerisation resulting in its cytoplasmic accumulation. From the practical point of view it is important not to mistake these cells for histiocytes containing phagocytosed red cells. Equally, care should be taken not to diagnose the 'constipated' plasma cell syndrome until the possibility of a true lymphoma has been excluded.

Epithelioid germinal centres in lymph nodes

Germinal centres composed almost exclusively of epithelioid cells and presumed dendritic reticulum cells have been seen in angioimmunoblastic lymphadenopathy and the multicentric variant of Castleman's disease, where they have been thought to represent exhaustion of the B-lymphocyte response to an unknown stimulus (Frizzera et al, 1983). Similar appearances (Figs. 8.17, 8.18) can sometimes be seen in lymph nodes from young children dying with fulminating infections, Reye's syndrome and sudden infant death syndrome (Millikin, 1977). No detailed immunological studies have been carried out in these patients and it is not known whether these striking histological changes are due to a pre-existing immune defect or are the result of overwhelming infection.

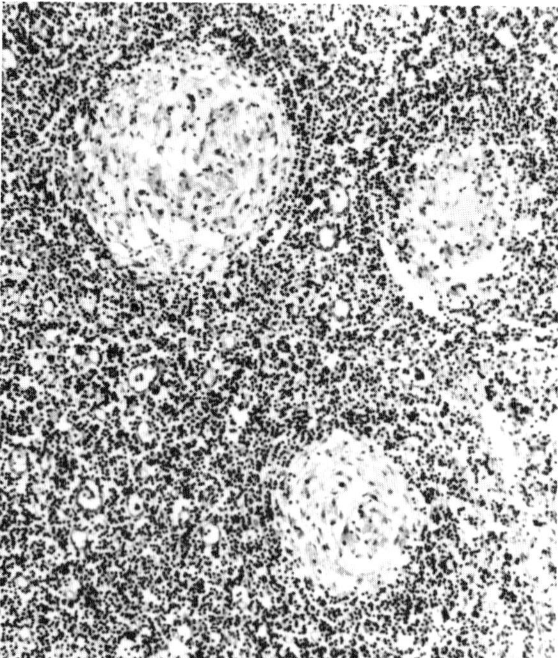

Fig. 8.17 Post-mortem cervical lymph node from a boy of 6 who was found dead after a brief history of respiratory disease. The germinal centres of the follicles are replaced by epithelioid cells. (H E × 100)

Sarcoidosis

The incidence or hyperglobulinaemia in sarcoidosis has been variously reported to be between 25 and 50%. Defects in cellular immunity are often present and are ill-understood (see Ch. 14).

The lymph nodes in graft rejection and the graft versus host reaction

There is little published information about lymph node changes in non-immunosuppressed human graft recipients, but experiments in animals suggest that the type of reaction depends on the nature of the graft (Baldwin et al, 1979). Skin grafts elicit a predominantly T-lymphocyte response, whereas well vascularised grafts, such as the heart, also elicit an intense B-lymphocyte response, characterised morphologically by a marked increase in lymph node size and the presence of many plasma cells in the sinuses and medullary cords. This is accompanied by the presence of cytotoxic antibodies in the serum which could play a part in graft rejection. It is to avoid graft rejection that most human recipients are treated with immunosuppressants. When bone marrow transplantation is contemplated, prior treatment with high doses of cyclophosphamide and/or whole body irradiation are necessary for success. Unfortunately donor lymphoid cells in the graft can provoke a graft-versus-host reaction (GVHR) with acute or

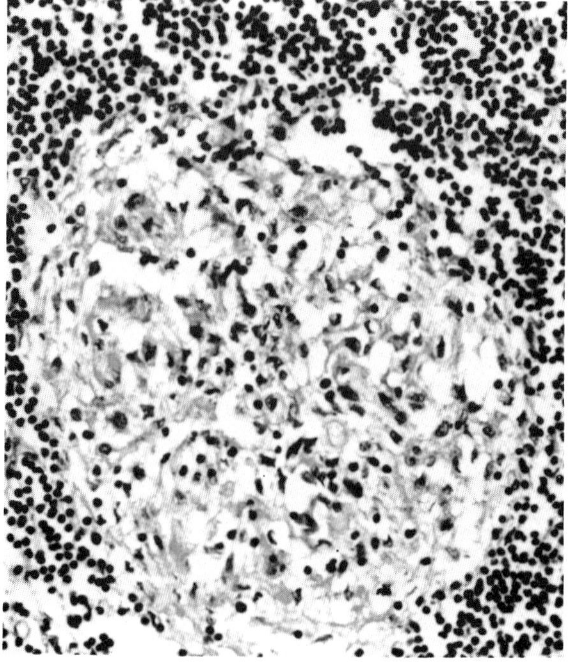

Fig. 8.18 Higher magnification of the same node as Fig. 8.17 to show detail of epithelioid germinal centre (H E × 250)

chronic damage of skin, gastrointestinal tract mucosae, liver and, less often, heart and kidney (Mathé et al, 1960; Kersey et al, 1971). Prior treatment with cyclophosphamide causes atrophy of lymphoid tissue which is maximal after 7 to 10 days and which recovers after 20 to 25 days. When GVHR develops in these previously treated patients, changes occur in lymph nodes and other lymphoid organs. These have been well studied by Slavin & Santos (1973) and Woodruff et al (1976) who recognise three phases: early lymphoid proliferation, developing lymphoid atrophy and lymphoid reconstitution.

In the phase of lymphoid proliferation small numbers of small lymphocytes appear in the previously depleted nodes. Later on, the cells found are larger, have intense cytoplasmic pyroninophilia and frequent mitoses. A variable number of non-lymphoid cells, particularly histiocytes, is always present. This phase lasts for about 8 to 10 days. From about the 10th to the 30th day post-transplant, there is a reduction in total numbers of lymphoid cells accompanied by lymphocytorrhexis and aggregation of lymphocytes in the cortex. These changes have been interpreted as a sign of aggression by donor lymphocytes and may result in almost total depletion which is maximal between 30 and 78 days post-transplant. Lymphoid reconstitution starts in B-lymphocyte dependent areas and may not be complete as late as 215 days post-transplant. As a rule, some degree of both antibody and cell mediated immune deficiency remains. These lymph node changes are thought to be due to the multiplication of donor lymphocytes in the host's lymph nodes, providing a population of 'aggressor' lymphocytes which are responsible for the damage to other organs. The phase of lymphoid atrophy might be a result either of loss of donor lymphocytes, due to their death and migration to target organs, or of exhaustion of host histocompatibility stimulation.

ANGIO-IMMUNOBLASTIC LYMPHADENOPATHY (IMMUNOBLASTIC LYMPHADENOPATHY)

Introduction

Angio-immunoblastic lymphadenopathy (AIL) was characterised as a clinico-pathological entity by the parallel work of Lukes & Tindle (1973, 1975) and Frizzera et al (1974, 1975). The latter authors introduced the term 'angio-immunoblastic lymphadenopathy with dysproteinaemia' but many writers have since dropped dysproteinaemia from the title. Earlier descriptions of entities sharing some clinical and pathological features with AIL exist both in the German and French literature (Westerhausen & Oehlert, 1972; Flandrin et al, 1972). Lennert (Radaszkiewicz & Lennert, 1975) coined the term 'lymphogranulomatosis X' for the same disorder, but also widened the definition of the disease, (Schnaidt et al, 1980a). Although AIL commonly involves the spleen, bone marrow, liver, lung, skin and gastrointestinal tract, this account will be restricted to the pathology of the lymph nodes.

Clinical picture

The disease affects mainly elderly individuals, most patients being between the ages of 40 and 90, but a few cases have been described in young people (see review by Cullen et al, 1979) and in children (Fiorillo et al, 1981). The development of lymphadenopathy may be preceded by skin rashes and some patients have a previous history of auto-immune disease, such as Sjögren's syndrome, hypothyroidism and pernicious anaemia, but in most cases the disease appears *de novo*. An association with the administration of drugs, particularly antibiotics and antimalarials, has been noted in about 20% of cases and at least one reported case was preceded by a glandular fever-like process (Seigneurin et al, 1981). Men and women are affected in about equal numbers.

The commonest presentation is one of sudden onset of malaise, fever and tender, generalised lymphadenopathy, but in about 15% of cases lymph node enlargement may be localised. Hepatosplenomegaly is present in about two-thirds of patients and other symptoms, such as weight loss, skin rashes, pruritus and night sweats in about half. More rarely there are respiratory symptoms (Bradley et al, 1981), arthralgias (Raskin et al, 1982), pleural and peritoneal effusions (Cullen et al, 1979) and neurological symptoms, including the Guillain-Barré syndrome (O'Donnell et al,

1980; Schober, 1982). The patients are manifestly ill people and the clinical picture is often so distinctive that the diagnosis is suspected by those familiar with the disease before biopsy is carried out.

Laboratory investigations disclose anaemia, which is often haemolytic with a positive Coombs test. Leucocytosis is common and eosinophilia is present in a few patients. There may be an absolute lymphopenia and plasma cells, plasmacytoid lymphocytes and 'atypical mononuclear' cells are commonly found in the peripheral blood. Bone marrow investigations show an excess of plasma cells and plasmacytoid blasts in the aspirate and although trephine biopsies show characteristic changes, these are usually not diagnostic (Pangalis et al, 1978; Brearley et al, 1979; Schnaidt et al, 1980b). The sedimentation rate is markedly elevated and there is polyclonal hypergammaglobulinaemia with particularly high levels of IgG, but hypogammaglobulinaemia can develop in the course of the disease. It is not unusual to find hypoalbuminaemia, hyponatremia and laboratory evidence of hypothyroid function, although patients do not present clinical hypothyroidism (Cullen et al, 1979).

Since some of the symptoms resemble those seen in autoimmune diseases, the patients are often investigated for such, and rheumatoid factor, antinuclear factors, thyroid autoantibodies and antimitochondrial antibodies are occasionally found (Cullen et al, 1979). On the other hand, skin testing for delayed hypersensitivity with various antigens shows a high incidence of cutaneous anergy (Neiman et al, 1978). Hypocomplementaemia, immune complexes and cryoglobulinaemia are also common and hypercalcaemia in severe disease has been reported (Gan & Van der Weyden, 1981).

Pathology of the lymph nodes

These are usually moderately enlarged (2–3 cm), often tender and occasionally painful. Larger nodes and even a mass of matted nodes 16 cm in diameter have been described (Nathwani et al, 1978). Superficial and deep nodes can be involved and in 85% of cases lymphadenopathy is generalised.

Macroscopically the nodes are discrete, as a rule, but they show no distinctive features.

Histologically there are three major abnormalities: a diffuse effacement of nodal architecture, a striking proliferation of 'arborising' blood vessels and a mixed cell infiltrate which includes many plasma cells and immunoblasts. The loss of architecture may be total, but not infrequently the peripheral sinus or other sinuses may be discernible as slits. Despite the patency of the peripheral sinus, the capsule is usually thickened and infiltrated by the same cells as are present in the node, especially plasma cells. Commonly this infiltrate extends into the pericapsular and hilar adipose tissue (Fig. 8.19). At low magnification, the pulp of the node often appears rather depleted of cells, due to a gross reduction of the small lymphocyte population and this makes the vascular proliferation all the more obvious (Fig. 8.20). Rarely a few follicles with reactive centres remain, but more often the follicles have gone or are represented only by ac-

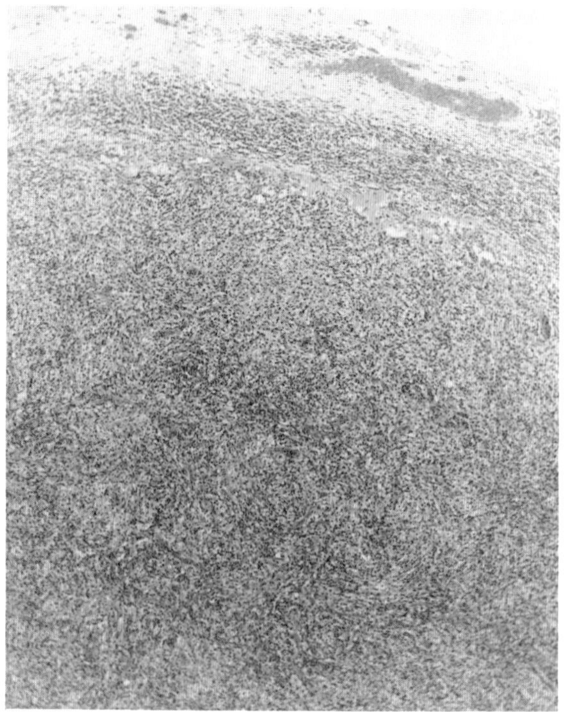

Fig. 8.19 Lymph node in angioimmunoblastic lymphadenopathy. Low power view showing loss of pattern, patent marginal sinus and thickened infiltrated capsule. (H E × 47)

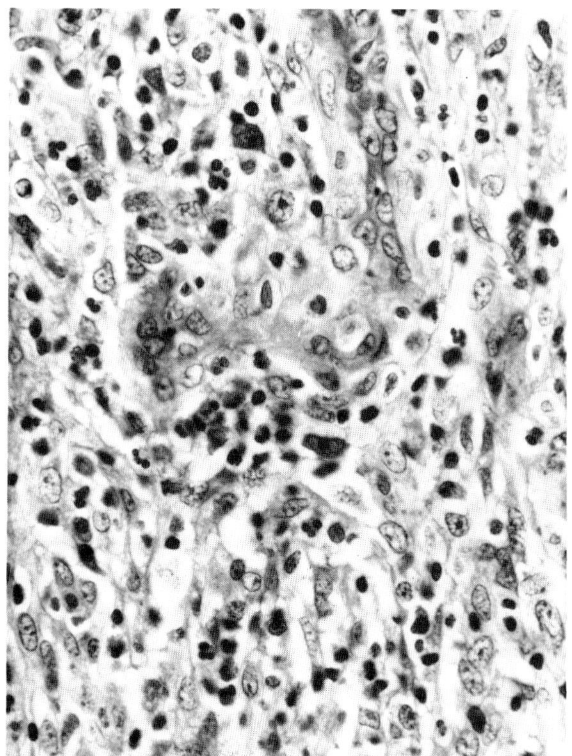

Fig. 8.20 Loss of lymphocytes sometimes makes the node in AIL appear empty, thus further accentuating the vascular prominence (H E × 470)

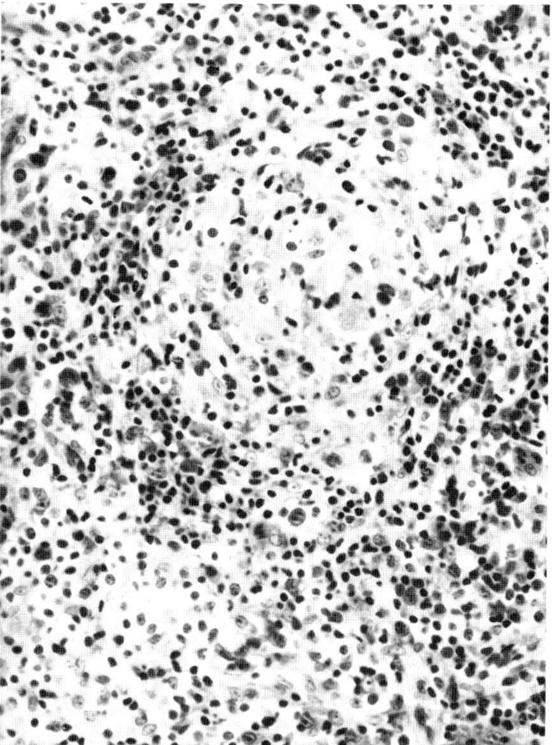

Fig. 8.21 Atrophic germinal follicle in AIL, represented only by concentrically arranged histiocytes. Usually the follicles have disappeared altogether by the time the node is biopsied. (H E × 300)

cumulations of histiocytes arranged in a concentric fashion (Fig. 8.21).

The numerous, branching blood vessels throughout the node are one of the most conspicuous features as a rule and can be readily seen with HE staining (Fig. 8.22), though the widened, 'dissected' walls of these vessels are better revealed with PAS staining or silver impregnation, (Figs. 8.23, 8.24). From the character of their walls and prominence of the lining endothelial cells these vessels are almost certainly derived from post-capillary venules, although from the pattern of branching they may appear to resemble capillaries. The PAS stain may also reveal the presence of amorphous deposits of PAS positive material (eosinophilic with HE staining), lying amongst the cells, around the vessels or within 'burnt-out' follicles (Fig. 8.25). Some authors (e.g. Lukes & Tindle, 1975) have laid stress on this finding, but it is an inconstant and unspecific feature. The material has been variously interpreted as a derivative of cell breakdown or blood protein. Ultrastructurally it consists of basement membrane-like material with long spacing collagen fibres and may also contain immunoglobulins (Neiman et al, 1978; Schnaidt et al, 1980a). Rarely amyloid has been reported in the nodes in AIL (Madri & Fromowitz, 1978).

The cell infiltrate is characteristically polymorphous, often without a clear predominance of any one cell type (Fig. 8.26). Whilst typical small lymphocytes with round nuclei are often severely reduced in numbers, one commonly sees widely dispersed lymphocytes with more irregular nuclei, suggestive of T-cells. Plasma cells are often numerous and frequently include atypical and even giant forms. Immunoblasts are a constant feature, but vary considerably in numbers; they may be diffusely scattered or form solid clusters or even sheets when plentiful (Fig. 8.27). Some show evi-

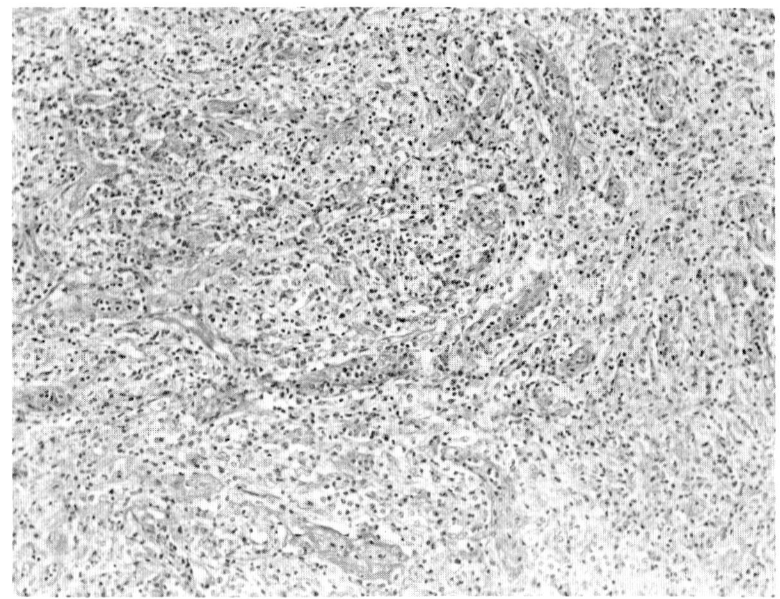

Fig. 8.22 The 'arborising' vascular pattern is one of the most distinctive features of the lymph node in AIL (H E × 120)

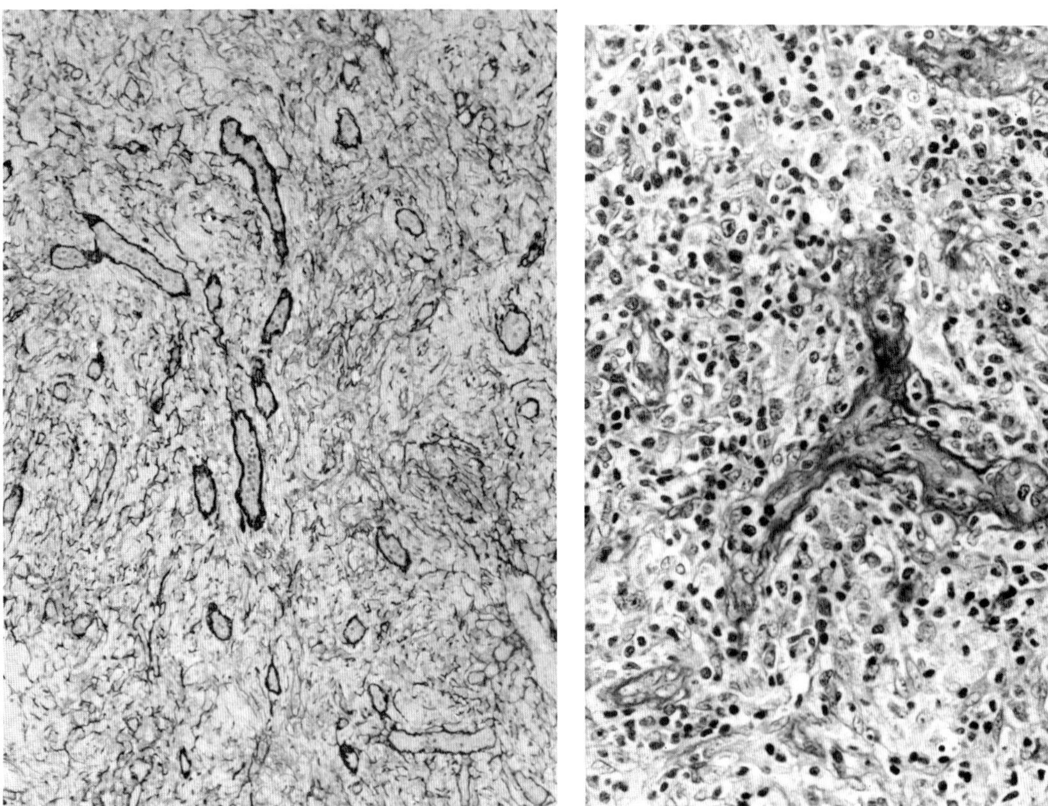

Fig. 8.23 Same lymph node as Fig. 8.22 with the vascular pattern revealed by silver impregnation (compare with Fig. 6.83, p. 138) (Gordon and Sweets reticulin × 120)

Fig. 8.24 Lymph node from another case of AIL showing branching venules clearly outlined by PAS staining (PAS × 300)

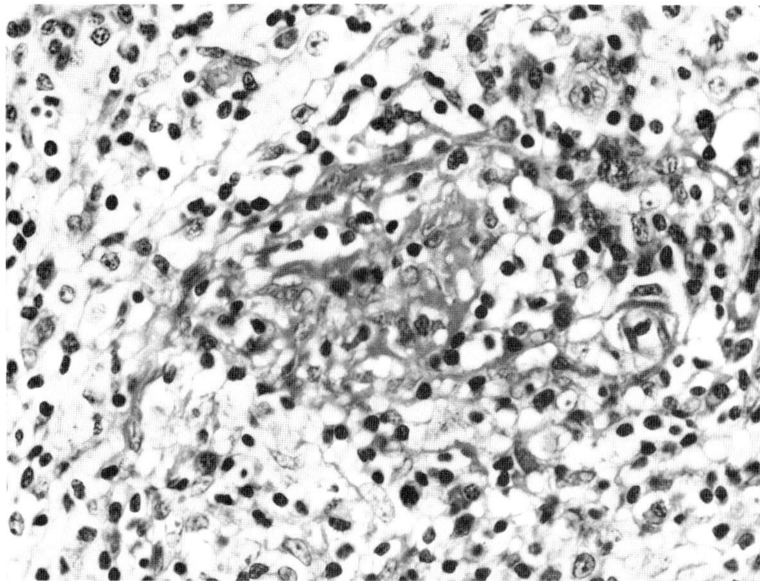

Fig. 8.25 Deposition of PAS-positive amorphous material in the interstitium of lymph node in AIL (same node as Fig. 8.22) (PAS × 470)

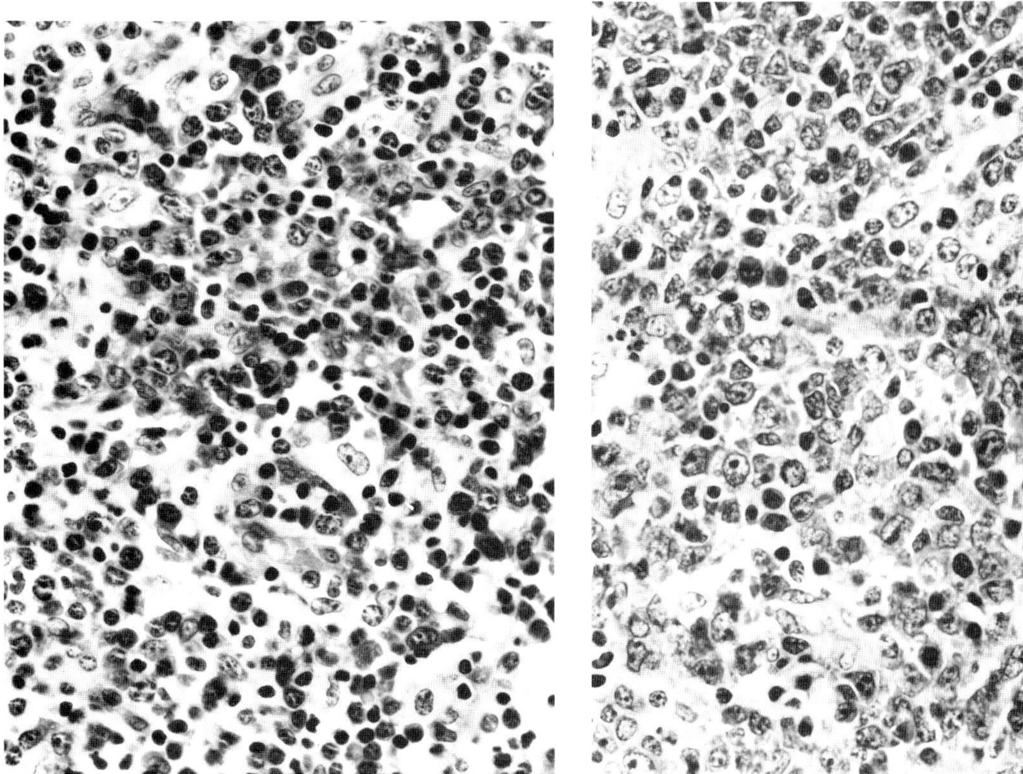

Fig. 8.26 Lymph node in AIL showing many plasma cells, besides immunoblasts, histiocytes and a few eosinophils (H E × 470)

Fig. 8.27 In this lymph node from another patient with AIL, immunoblasts predominated throughout much of the node, but there was still no evidence of sarcomatous transformation (H E × 470)

dence of plasmacytoid differentiation by light microscopy and electron microscopical observations have shown rough endoplasmic reticulum in some of the immunoblasts, confirming their B-lymphocyte derivation (Valdes & Blair, 1976; Neiman et al, 1978; Schnaidt et al, 1980a). By immunostaining it can be shown that the B-cells are polyclonal in type (Moore et al, 1976; Neiman et al, 1978). Mitoses are often numerous, especially when immunoblasts predominate, and abnormal mitoses are sometimes seen. Occasional giant, polyploid, blast cells with a superficial resemblance to Sternberg-Reed cells may also be found.

Other types are more variable in the frequency with which they occur. Eosinophils may be numerous or virtually absent. Clusters of epithelioid histiocytes are conspicuous in some cases and absent in others (Fig. 8.28). Aggregates of distinctive

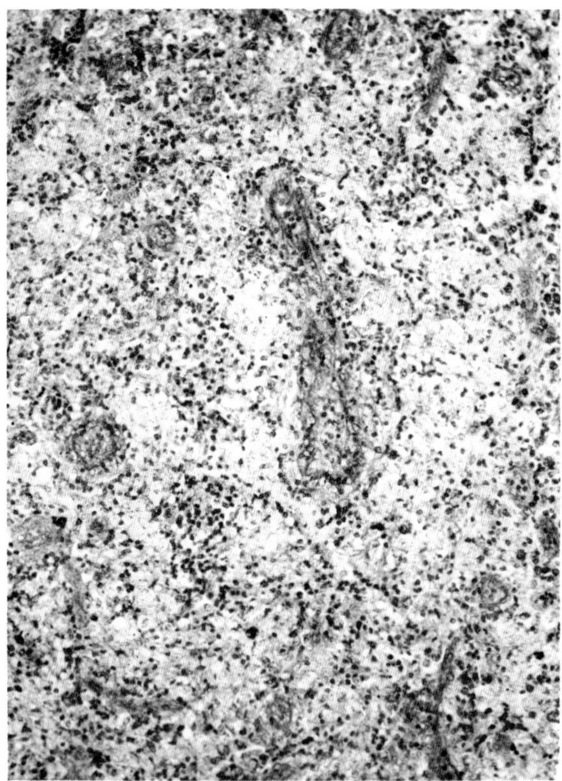

Fig. 8.28 Lymph node biopsy in a case of AIL characterised by prominent epithelioid cell clusters throughout the node (compare with Figs. 9.37 (p. 220), 10.26 (p. 246) and 12.34 (p. 321)). The patient, a man of 69, died from pneumocystis pneumonia and cytomegalovirus infection. (Giemsa × 120)

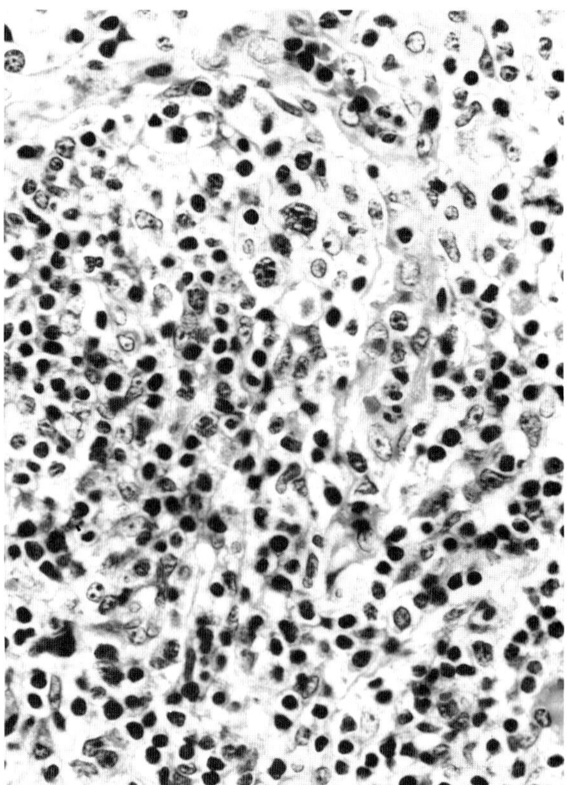

Fig. 8.29 Besides immunoblasts, 'clear' cells were a prominent feature in this case of AIL in a man of 50. Although the presentation and histological features were typical of AIL, a later biopsy showed equally typical changes of T-zone lymphoma. (H E × 470)

lymphoid cells with abundant, pale cytoplasm have often been noted in AIL (Nathwani et al, 1978; Cullen et al, 1979) (Fig. 8.29). These cells are now widely believed to be a form of T-lymphocyte and their presence, sometimes in large numbers, raises the question of whether 'AIL' showing this picture may not in fact be a form of peripheral T-cell lymphoma (see differential diagnosis and p. 318).

Lennert has proposed five subdivisions of 'lymphogranulomatosis X' based on the predominant cell type — plasma cell, lymphocyte, immunoblast, epithelioid cell and mixed cellularity types (Lennert et al, 1979), but there is at present no information on the clinical or prognostic value of this classification. It does, however, seem likely that the presence of solid clusters or sheets of immunoblasts in the node biopsy may signal the transformation of AIL into an immunoblastic sarcoma, as suggested by Nathwani et al (1978).

Nature of angio-immunoblastic lymphadenopathy and its relation to malignant lymphomas

Two main theories have been advanced to account for this strange disease, of which the aetiology is still completely obscure. Neither theory satisfactorily explains all the known facts.

1. A hyperimmune reaction?

According to this theory AIL is believed to be a hyperimmune reactive proliferation of lymphoid cells, provoked by some unknown stimulus, possibly a virus, though none has yet been demonstrated. The original descriptions of AIL stressed the breakdown of normal immune responses and pointed out that patients died from infections rather than as a result of a new growth. Neither the clinical nor the pathological features were held to favour the idea of a neoplasm. On the other hand, the *polyclonal* B-cell proliferation, obvious immunological disturbance, often with overt autoimmune phenomena, and well documented spontaneous remissions, in spite of the generally grave prognosis, have been advanced in support of a primary immunological disturbance. Evidence of both T-cell and B-cell malfunction has been documented in AIL (Rudders & DeLellis, 1977; Klajman et al, 1981).

2. A type of malignant lymphoma?

The alternative hypothesis, that AIL is in fact an unusual type of malignant lymphoma, has received strong backing from some clinicians, who have observed the rapid and sometimes gross enlargement of lymph nodes, spleen and liver in patients with this disease and the shrinkage of the masses with chemotherapy. A parallel has been drawn with Hodgkin's disease, which is now generally agreed to be a neoplasm, despite a long held belief that the process was inflammatory. Hodgkin's disease may present in a similar way with fever and disturbed immunity, and the affected tissues show a polymorphous infiltrate not altogether unlike that seen in AIL. The frequent finding of abnormal karyotypes in AIL is more in keeping with a neoplastic disorder, even in the absence of unequivocal histological proof (Nathwani et al, 1978; Cullen et al, 1979; Kaneko et al, 1982). Some of the objections to this theory — in particular the occurrence of spontaneous remissions — have been mentioned above.

More than one disease?

The failure of either theory to explain fully the observed facts about AIL and the variable behaviour of the disease raise the question of whether AIL, as currently conceived, represents more than one entity. It is of interest that those cases apparently triggered-off by drug hypersensitivity most frequently remit on withdrawal of the offending drug and seem to have a better prognosis (Blanchard et al, 1983) which could reflect a different aetiology, despite the similarity of the histological changes and clinical presentation. At the opposite end of the spectrum are those cases which do progress and behave like a malignant neoplasm.

A premalignant disorder?

It is possible to combine the two theories outlined above and to suggest that an abnormal immune proliferation, intitiated perhaps by more than one different 'trigger' mechanism, could strongly predispose to the development of a malignant lymphoma. Lukes & Tindle (1975) observed the development of immunoblastic sarcoma in two out of 32 patients with immunoblastic lymphadenopathy and many similar cases have been reported subsequently (see Cullen et al, 1979). In 1978 Nathwani et al studied this problem by comparing 48 patients who had the classical histological features of AIL with 36 patients whose nodes showed, in addition, intravascular or extravascular 'clusters' of immunoblasts (Fig. 8.30), or less well defined extravascular 'islands' of blasts and 'primitive lymphoid cells with clear cytoplasm'. The authors interpreted these features as representing incipient immunoblastic lymphomas arising in a background of AIL and showed that AIL and malignant lymphoma could coexist in different nodes in the same patient. The therapeutic failure

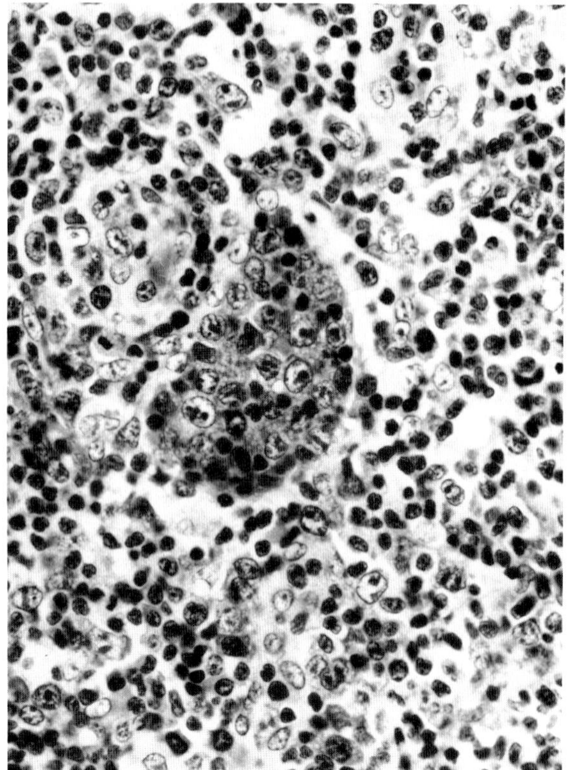

Fig. 8.30 Lymph node biopsy in AIL showing a solid cluster of immunoblasts within a distended venule. Such a finding may signal transformation into an immunoblastic lymphoma. (H E × 470)

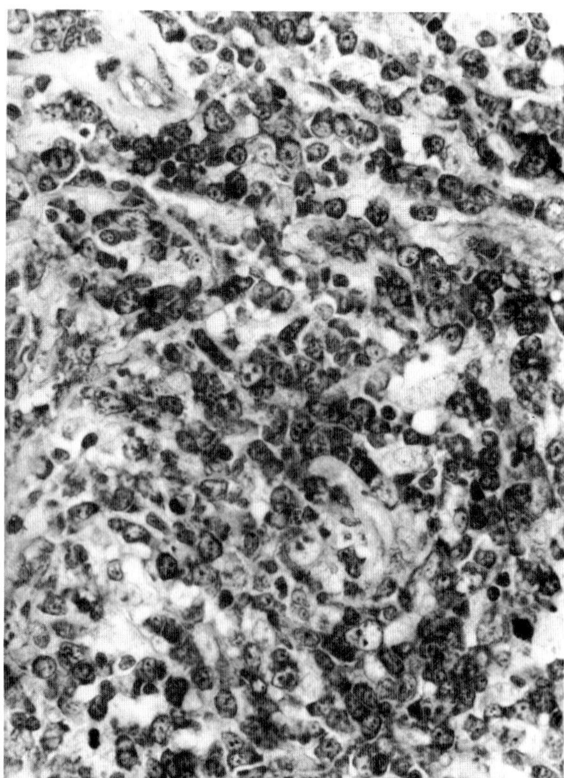

Fig. 8.31 Transformation of AIL into a high-grade malignant lymphoma of B-immunoblastic type. Note the monomorphism of the cells. (Giemsa × 470)

rate and incidence of unequivocal lymphoma at necropsy were considerably higher when these 'clusters' and 'islands' were found in the initial lymph node biopsy (Nathwani et al, 1978).

Nature of derived malignant lymphomas in AIL

In most reported instances of unequivocal malignant lymphoma developing in the course of AIL, the tumour has been described as an immunoblastic sarcoma (ML immunoblastic) (Fig. 8.31). It is natural to assume that such tumours would be of B-cell type, since they arise on a basis of B-cell proliferation and since the great majority of malignant lymphomas arising in patients with suppressed or disordered immunity are of this nature (see p. 295). The B-cell origin of the tumour in some cases has been confirmed by the obvious plasmacytoid features of the neoplastic cells, the demonstration by immunostaining of a monoclonal B-cell population, or detection of a monotypic band in the patient's serum by electrophoresis (Cullen et al, 1979; Boros et al, 1981). However, proof of the B-cell nature of the neoplasm is often lacking in case reports and there are certainly some instances in which AIL has evolved into a T-cell lymphoma (Lennert et al, 1979). Furthermore, there appears to be a type of T-cell lymphoma which may be difficult to distinguish from AIL, either clinically or pathologically (Watanabe et al, 1980) (see p. 318). Specifically, those cases of AIL which are characterised by prominent clusters of pale or clear cells in the node, are those which are under suspicion of being a form of T-cell lymphoma (see Fig. 8.29). This group would appear to include some of the patients described by Nathwani et al (1978) as having a bad prognosis. Evidence has not been adduced as to whether such cases are malignant from the outset or whether malignant transformation occurs in the course of an initial immune disturbance.

Nature of immune defect in AIL

The idea that AIL is a hyperimmune reaction resulting from loss of T-lymphocyte suppressor activity and consequent hyperfunction of B-lymphocytes is appealingly simple, but is not supported by the facts. Phenotypic studies in AIL typically show a high proportion of T-cells in the node with reversal of the T-helper/T-suppressor cell ratio so that T-suppressor cells are the predominant type (Habeshaw, 1983). Interestingly, the same phenotypic abnormality characterises AIDS which shows other similarities to AIL (see p. 162), although the histological picture is quite different, at least in the initial stages. Further studies may shed light on the nature of this mysterious disease.

Differential diagnosis

In the typical case of AIL, both the clinical and pathological features are so distinctive that the diagnosis is seldom in doubt. Great caution should be exercised, however, in making a diagnosis of AIL on a lymph node biopsy when the clinical features of the case do not support this diagnosis. This applies especially when only localised lymphadenopathy is found.

Clinically and histologically AIL may be confused with Hodgkin's disease for which it has doubtless been mistaken in the past (Lukes & Tindle, 1975). However, typical Sternberg-Reed cells are not seen in AIL and Coombs positive haemolytic anaemia is rare in Hodgkin's disease. The presence of intact germinal follicles generally favours Hodgkin's disease (p. 201). The type of AIL characterised by abundant epithelioid cells has to be distinguished from a variety of conditions, both reactive and neoplastic, in which epithelioid cells are a marked feature. Of these, neoplasms present the greater difficulty, notably, Hodgkin's disease, some lymphoplasmacytoid lymphomas (p. 247) and especially so-called Lennert's lymphoma (lymphoepithelioid lymphoma) (p. 320). Some lymphoplasmacytoid lymphomas (immunocytomas) may show a confusingly polymorphous cell picture and marked vascularity, but eosinophils are generally absent. If necessary, immunostaining may help by demonstrating whether the B-cells are monoclonal (immunocytoma) or polyclonal (AIL).

Lennert's lymphoma is now widely regarded as a type of peripheral T-cell lymphoma and the distinction of AIL from this lesion, as from some other types of T-cell lymphoma may present great difficulty (see p. 322). As discussed above (p. 180) it seems possible, indeed likely, that some cases which have been diagnosed as AIL in the past were in reality cases of T-cell lymphoma of this type (p. 318).

At the other end of the spectrum are reactive lymphadenopathies in which vascular proliferation may be prominent and follicles inconspicuous and in which immunoblasts may be present, such as postvaccinial lymphadenitis, glandular fever and lymphadenopathy due to anticonvulsants and other types of drug hypersensitivity. The clinical history and some histological features discussed elsewhere (Ch. 6) should make the distinction easy. Since patients with AIL can develop a lupus-like syndrome and anti-DNA antibodies (Schechter, 1980) the different lymph node biopsy findings may be essential in reaching the correct diagnosis. There should be no difficulty differentiating AIL from other autoimmune diseases but it must be remembered that patients with other autoimmune syndromes can develop AIL (Pruzanski, 1980).

Prognosis

Aside from the generally better prognosis of drug-induced AIL, mentioned above (p. 181), (Blanchard et al, 1983), the prognosis is rather unpredictable and does not appear to depend on the type of treatment (Cullen et al, 1979; Blanchard et al, 1983). There are spontaneous remissions and there are rapid progressions with involvement of many organs by either cellular infiltrates characteristic of AIL or by unequivocal immunoblastic lymphoma (Nathwani et al, 1978) which may involve spleen, liver, lung, gastrointestinal tract (Bauer et al, 1982; Moreb et al, 1983) and skin, although it must be stressed that the majority of skin rashes in AIL are non-neoplastic and unspecific (Bernengo et al, 1981). Well over 60% of patients die and the commonest cause of death is infection complicating the state of depressed immunity associated with this condition or its present methods of treatment.

CASTLEMAN'S DISEASE

Introduction

Castleman was the first to study in detail lymphoid tumours of the mediastinum with characteristic histological features which had until then been mistaken for thymomas grossly, radiologically and histologically (Castleman & Towne, 1954; Castleman, 1955; Castleman et al, 1956). Similar tumours had been previously described under a variety of other names, such as giant haemolymph nodes, giant mediastinal nodes etc (see Lee et al, 1965; Tung & McCormack, 1967). Subsequently the condition has received many other names, including lymph nodal hamartoma (Abell, 1957; Lattes & Pachter, 1962), follicular lymphoreticuloma (Zettergren, 1961), angiofollicular lymph node hyperplasia (Harrison & Bernatz, 1963), angiomatous lymphoid hamartoma (Tung & McCormack, 1967), benign giant lymphoma (Flendrig, 1970) and giant lymph node hyperplasia (Keller et al, 1972; Couch, 1980). Since such names imply a pathogenesis which is at present unproven, or are similar to names used for other, totally different conditions, we prefer to use the eponymous term Castleman's disease.

It was soon evident that the condition occurred in regions other than the mediastinum and even in places where lymph nodes are not normally present (Cohen, 1957; Zettergren, 1961) and in 1970 Flendrig first pointed out the association between the presence of abundant plasma cells in some cases of Castleman's disease and the presence of systemic abnormalities. This observation was later confirmed by Keller et al (1972) who reviewed their extensive material and subdivided the disease into 'hyaline-vascular' and 'plasma cell' types. More recently Leibetseder & Thurner (1973), Gaba et al (1978) and others described a form of multicentric lymphadenopathy with histological similarities to Castleman's disease which was also associated with systemic and immunological abnormalities. These three types will be described separately.

Localised hyaline-vascular type

This is the commonest type, comprising about 90% of cases. It has been described in all races and at all ages (between 8 and 66 years in the series of Keller et al, 1972), but most patients are between 30 and 40 at presentation (Castleman et al, 1956; Tung & McCormack, 1967). In some cases the existence of a mass, relatively stable in size, was known for many years prior to its removal and in a 14 year old girl who had a mediastinal mass removed, there was noticeable widening of the mediastinal shadow in X-rays taken at the age of 6 weeks (Abell, 1957). In 75% of cases the tumours are intrathoracic (Tung & McCormack, 1967; Keller et al, 1972) the commonest locations being the anterior mediastinum, hila of the lungs, posterior mediastinum and carinal region. They are occasionally found between the lung fissures, simulating lung neoplasms, and in one instance the bulk of the mass was intrapericardial (Virmani et al, 1982). Outside the thorax, common sites are the neck and retroperitoneum and rare sites include the pelvis, axilla, muscles — particularly those of the shoulder girdle — the thigh and the larynx (Cohen, 1957; Lattes & Pachter, 1962; Climie et al, 1964; Daley & Cornog, 1967; Tung & McCormack, 1967; Keller et al, 1972). Intrathoracic masses are usually found incidentally when a chest X-ray is done for other reasons, but sometimes they cause compression of the airways and symptoms such as cough, recurrent infections, dyspnoea and haemoptysis. Extrathoracically, pressure symptoms or an obvious lump are the presenting signs. Anaemia, thrombocytopenia (Krasznai & Juhász, 1969) or myasthenia gravis in association with a retroperitoneal mass (Emson, 1973) have been reported, but there was no proof that these were related to the presence of the lymphoid masses.

Macroscopically the lesions are round or ovoid (Fig. 8.32) varying in size between 2 and 16 cm in largest dimension. Usually a single mass is present but rarely this is lobulated, suggesting coalescence of several masses. The tumours are well

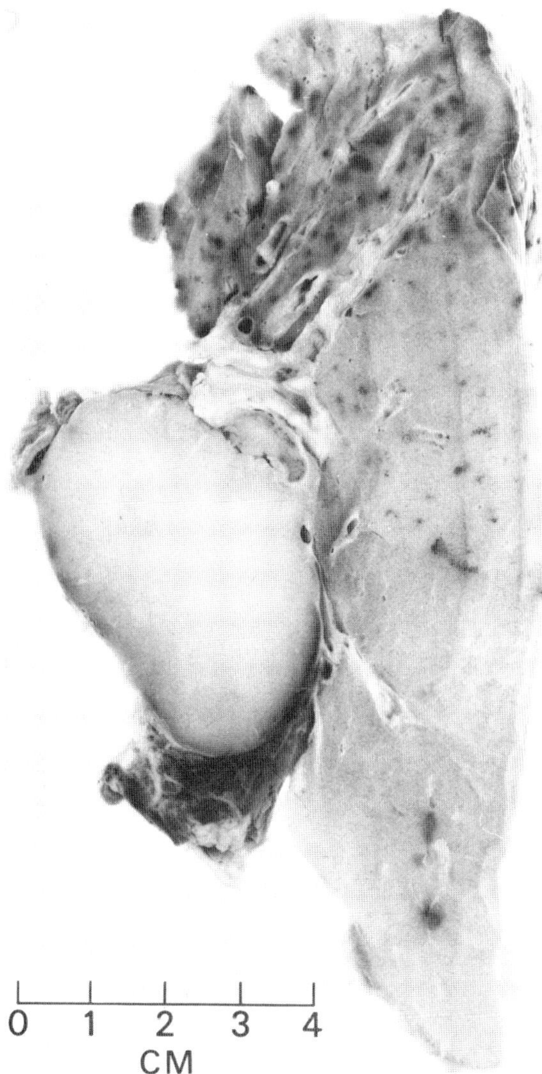

Fig. 8.32 Castleman's disease. Encapsulated, ovoid mass at the hilum of the upper lobe of the left lung. The patient, a woman aged 27, had suffered from migrainous attacks for 11 years. Chest X-ray showed an apparent lung tumour and lobectomy was performed.

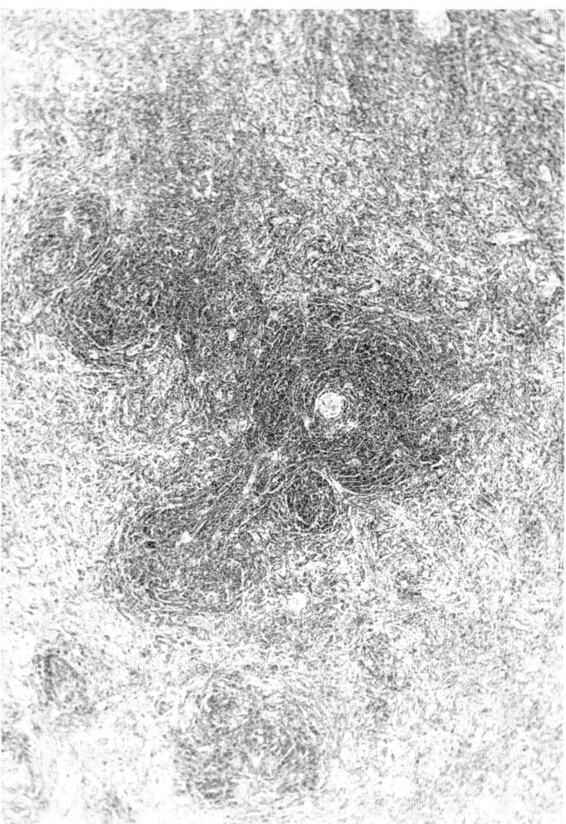

Fig. 8.33 Castleman's disease, hyaline vascular type. A mediastinal mass from a youth aged 16. Low power view showing follicle-like structures and intervening vascular tissue. (H E × 47)

circumscribed or even encapsulated. The cut surface is homogeneous and grey-pink, but a distinct nodular pattern may be seen on close examination. They may be very vascular and bleed profusely on removal.

Histologically the structure of these tumour-like masses differs from that of a lymph node chiefly in the absence of lymph sinuses (Fig. 8.33). Commonly they are at least partially enclosed by a well defined fibrous capsule and the internal organisation of the mass shows a certain resemblance to that of a lymph node, since it is composed of numerous follicle-like structures and a richly vascular interfollicular tissue. The network of rather sinusoidal vessels is sometimes very obvious, recalling the appearances of the splenic red pulp, but at other times the vessels are partly concealed by closely packed small lymphocytes and the vascularity is only appreciated in reticulin preparations (Fig. 8.34). The lymphocytes are often disposed in long rows and parallel arrays — a pattern no doubt partly determined by the underlying vascular structure (Fig. 8.35). At first sight the 'follicles' which are characteristic of this lesion may be mistaken for reactive follicles with small germinal centres and a wide lymphocyte mantle. On closer inspection the centre is seen to be composed

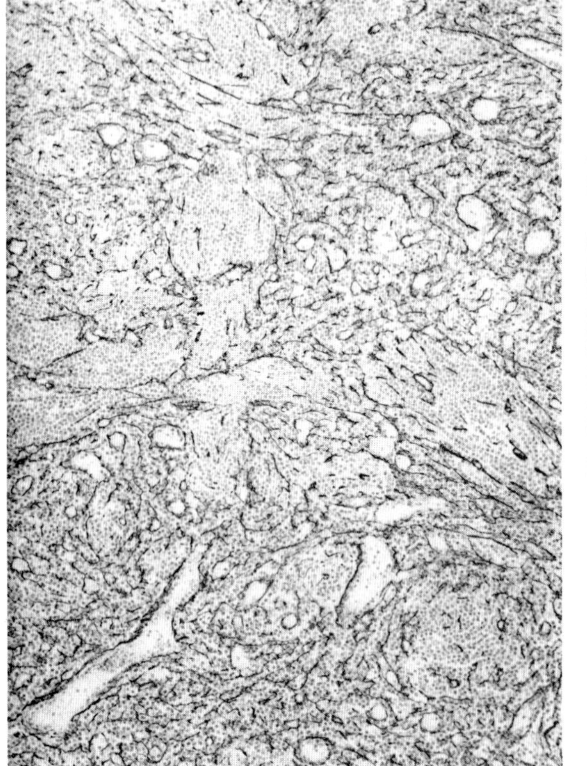

Fig. 8.34 Castleman's disease, hyaline vascular type (same case as Fig. 8.33), showing rich network of vessels between the lymphocytic aggregates (Gordon and Sweets reticulin × 120)

Fig. 8.35 Castleman's disease, hyaline vascular type (same case as Figs. 8.33 and 8.34). Parallel arrays of uniform small lymphocytes give a distinctive pattern to the 'tumour'. A pseudofollicle is seen (top left). (H E × 120)

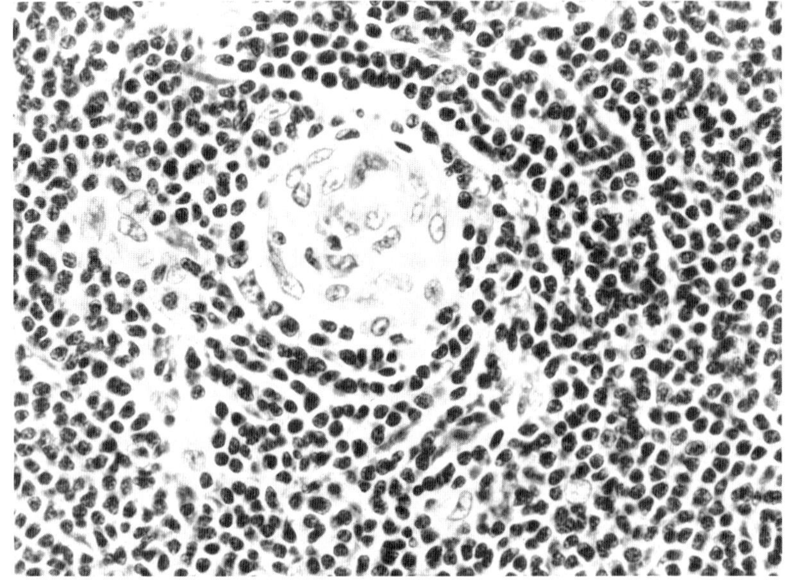

Fig. 8.36 Castleman's disease, hyaline vascular type (same case as Figs. 8.33, 8.34 and 8.35). Centre of pseudofollicle showing a thickened vessel with concentric layers of proliferated endothelium, surrounded by concentrically packed small lymphocytes. (H E × 470)

of a blood vessel with swollen, often proliferated, endothelial cells in concentric arrangement and interposed hyaline material — the whole structure bearing a superficial resemblance to a Hassall's corpuscle (Fig. 8.36). This feature and the mediastinal location of the masses gave rise to the earlier designation of 'pseudo-thymoma'. The remainder of the 'follicle' is made up of closely packed and often concentrically arranged small lymphocytes. Other 'follicles' consist merely of a closely packed aggregate of small lymphocytes without a central vessel, whilst others again may be true secondary follicles with a small germinal centre, usually of inactive appearance.

The predominant cells in these lesions are small lymphocytes, showing no evidence of mitotic activity, but sometimes a few plasma cells and large, transformed cells are found. The latter have sometimes been interpreted as Sternberg-Reed cells (Tung & McCormack, 1967; Fisher et al, 1970) and even transition to malignant lymphoma suggested, however, the illustrations are unconvincing and Case 2 of Fisher et al (1970) had no features diagnostic of Castleman's disease. The rarely encountered, intramuscular lymphoid masses ('pseudo lymphomas') have often been regarded as variants of Castleman's disease, but although often circumscribed, generally do not show encapsulation and they may be unrelated. These too consist predominantly of small lymphocytes of uniform appearance. Secondary changes, such as extensive areas of hyalinisation, and even calcification, are commonly found in long-standing lesions. In some instances remnants of lymph node structure may be discernible within the mass (Keller et al, 1972) and adjacent lymph nodes may contain hyaline-vascular 'follicles', suggesting that the masses have originated in lymph nodes (Figs. 8.37, 8.38).

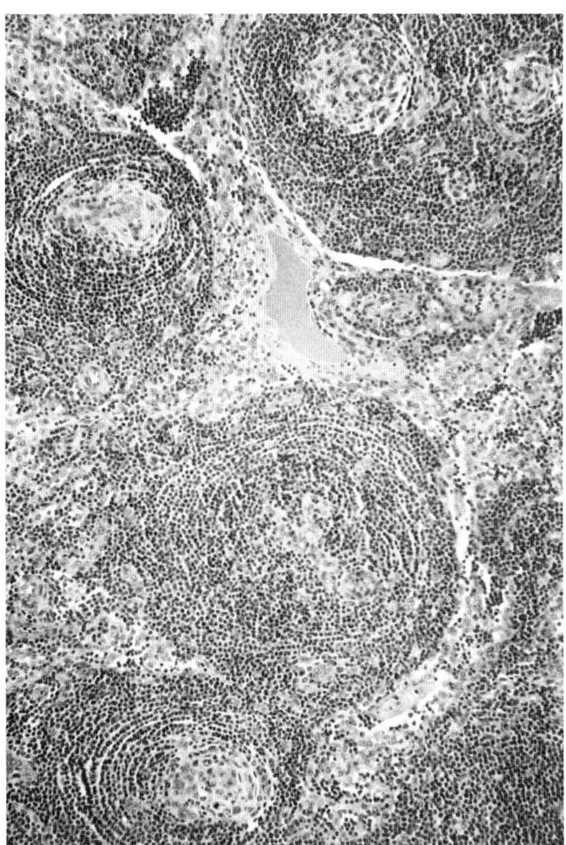

Fig. 8.37 Biopsy of an enlarged cervical lymph node (note lymph sinuses) from another patient, showing hyaline vascular follicles identical with those of Castleman's disease (H E × 120)

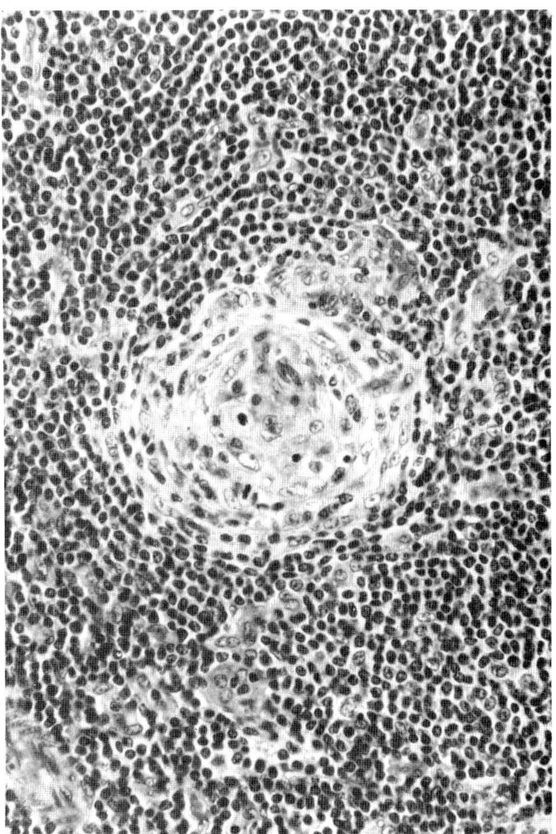

Fig. 8.38 Centre of one of the hyaline vascular 'follicles' from the same node as Fig. 8.37 (H E × 300)

Localised plasma cell type

This rare variant of Castleman's disease is seen in 10% of cases only and can occur at any age. Of 12 patients reviewed by Keller et al (1972), 9 were male and 3 female, between the ages of 8 and 45 (mean 26) but it has been described in older people (Mallory & Spink, 1968; Yu & Carson, 1976). The mediastinum, mesentery and retroperitoneum are the commonest sites. Most patients present with general malaise or unexplained fever. Investigations disclose refractory anaemia, elevated sedimentation rate, polyclonal hyperglobulinaemia with particularly high levels of IgG, and sometimes hypoalbuminaemia. Retardation of growth may be noticeable in children (Lee et al, 1965; Neerhout et al, 1965; Burgert et al, 1975; Van Vliet et al, 1978). Peripheral neuropathy (Mallory & Spink, 1968; Yu & Carson, 1976) and the nephrotic syndrome with minimal change nephropathy (Humpherys et al, 1975) have been reported. It is remarkable that all these signs and symptoms remit soon after the excision of the mass, so that evidence for a causal relationship is very strong. Indeed, in one case (Burgert et al, 1975) anti-erythropoietic activity was demonstrated in the patient's serum but this disappeared 6 days after the operation. In a 62 year old man the liver contained deposits of amyloid (Miralles Garcia et al, 1977) but amyloid has not been described within the lymphoid masses.

Macroscopically the lesions do not differ significantly from those of the hyaline-vascular type, but in some cases the masses were lobulated, giving the impression of several lymph nodes matted together (Moir et al, 1982).

Histologically the appearances differ from those of the hyaline-vascular type in three main respects: first, the majority of cells in the interfollicular areas are plasma cells rather than small lymphocytes (Fig. 8.39); secondly, although some follicles possess the characteristic concentric, hyaline-vascular structures, others (sometimes a majority) have reaction centres which only differ from the

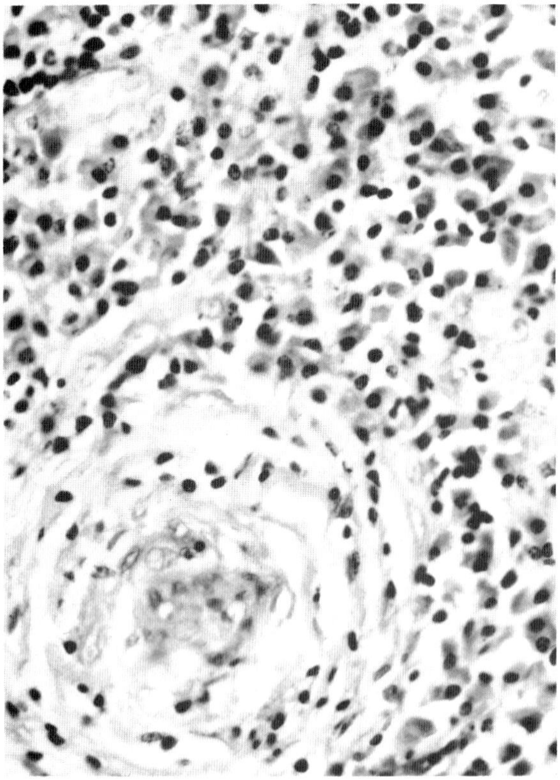

Fig. 8.39 Castleman's disease, localised plasma cell type. A hyaline vascular structure is seen (lower left), but the surrounding cells are all plasma cells. (H E × 375)

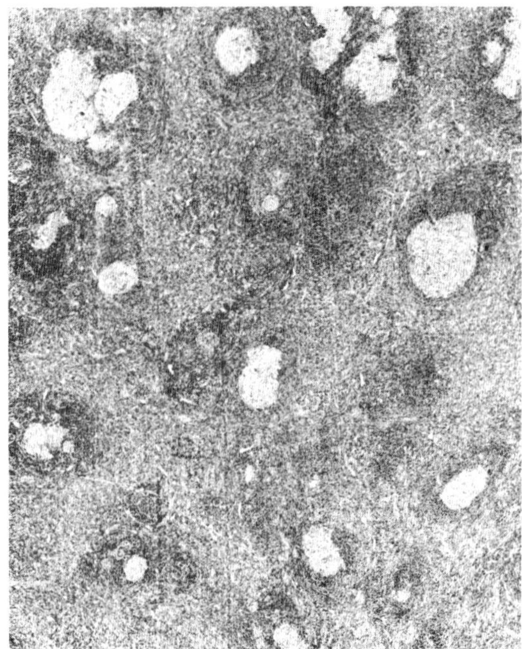

Fig. 8.40 Castleman's disease, localised plasma cell type (same case as Fig. 8.39). A few hyaline vascular 'follicles' are present, but other follicular structures are true germinal follicles. (H E × 16)

normal in their undue prominence and irregularity in outline and distribution (Fig. 8.40); finally, it is not uncommon to find areas of preserved lymph node architecture, or for adjacent smaller lymph nodes to show similar changes.

Multicentric Castleman's disease

In recent years, a disease characterised by enlargement of several lymph nodes with clinical and histological similarities to the plasma cell variant of Castleman's disease has been described (Leibetseder & Thurner, 1973; Laurens et al, 1973; Gaba et al, 1978; Weisenburger, 1979; Couch, 1980; Diebold et al, 1980; Bartoli et al, 1980; Al-Jabi & McCaughey, 1981; Hineman et al, 1982; Frizzera et al, 1983). Although there are variations in the presentation and course followed by each patient, there are also remarkable similarities well outlined by Frizzera et al (1983) who had access to histological material from 15 cases. The patients are usually older (41 to 74 years; mean 57) and present with fever, weight loss and night sweats. Less common features are skin rashes, arthralgias, 'sicca syndrome' and pruritus, so that extensive investigations to exclude a 'collagen' disease are often undertaken. Two patients presented with peripheral neuropathy (Gaba et al, 1978; Hineman et al, 1982) and one with the nephrotic syndrome due to immune complex membranous nephropathy (Weisenburger, 1979). Thrombotic thrombocytopenic purpura has also been described (Couch, 1980). On examination the patients often have splenomegaly and hepatomegaly; several groups of superficial lymph nodes may be enlarged but sometimes the enlargement appears mainly in one region, spreading to other regions at a later date. There is invariably anaemia, polyclonal hyperglobulinaemia and on occasions, bone marrow plasmacytosis. A monoclonal IgG paraproteinaemia was also present in one case (Hineman et al, 1982). In a minority of patients the disease progresses rapidly, haemolytic anaemia develops and patients die, usually of intercurrent infections; in other patients the disease follows an indolent course, with exacerbations and remissions and patients are alive 10 and 20 years after the onset of symptoms. In one case Kaposi's sarcoma preceded the onset of the disease and in another it complicated its course. Pulmonary infiltrates of lymphoid cells, apparently non-neoplastic, were present in one patient with respiratory symptoms and another patient developed a malignant lymphoma, confirmed at autopsy (Frizzera et al, 1983). A search for autoantibodies in these patients has been consistently negative.

Macroscopically the lymph nodes removed from these patients are of smaller size seldom exceeding 5 or 6 cm in largest dimension.

Histologically the features that relate this condition to Castleman's disease are the presence of concentric hyaline-vascular structures in some follicles, the increased vascularity of the interfollicular areas and the presence of abundant plasma cells as well as reactive germinal centres of irregular outline, like those of the localised plasma cell variant. However, in some cases plasma cells are sparse and the condition has been compared to the hyaline-vascular type (Gaba et al, 1978). Very often the sinusoidal architecture of the nodes is partly preserved and sinuses may be dilated or 'angiomatoid' (Diebold et al, 1980; Frizzera et al, 1983). Other lymph nodes removed at the same time or at different times from these patients have shown non-specific, predominantly follicular hyperplasia, follicular atrophy with or without accumulation of plasma cells and rarely, the presence of epithelioid germinal centres (see p. 174).

Significance of the different types of Castleman's disease

It is not known whether the three main forms of this condition represent different entities or variants of the same disorder and there is no agreement as to what the nature of this disorder is. Castleman et al (1956) regarded the localised variety as a hyperplasia in lymph nodes draining the lung or the intestine and perhaps an abnormal host reaction to infective agents entering the body at those sites (Keller et al, 1972). They also regarded the hyaline-vascular and plasma cell types as the 'inactive' and 'active' forms of the same process, and both Flendrig (1970) and Keller et al (1972) have remarked on the existence of intermediate forms with both patterns in the same mass. Abell (1957), Lattes & Pachter (1962), Frizzera et al (1983) and others, have favoured the hamartomatous nature of these lumps, stressing the young age of the patients, the absence of lymph node architecture in most cases and the ectopic location of a few. The neoplastic theory (Zettergren, 1961) is not shared by many and immunohistochemical studies support the polyclonal nature of the plasma cell proliferation (Jones et al, 1983). However, monoclonal proliferations have also been described (York et al, 1981) and the plasma cell variant may respond to radiotherapy (Nordstrom et al, 1978).

The multicentric variety is clearly a reactive process occurring in pre-existing superficial lymph nodes and has been interpreted as an abnormal immune response of unknown aetiology but perhaps due to a defect in regulatory mechanisms of the immune system (Diebold et al, 1980; Frizzera et al, 1983). The occurrence in elderly patients, association with Kaposi's sarcoma, known to occur in immunological deficiency states (see p. 153, 162), and predisposition to infections favour that view. The association between the intensity of the histological changes, as measured by the numbers of plasma cells and prominent germinal centres, and the occurrence of systemic manifestations speaks in favour of the latter being attributable to immunoglobulins or other lymphocyte products but little is known of the underlying mechanisms involved.

REFERENCES

Abell M R 1957 Lymph nodal hamartoma versus thymic choristoma of pulmonary hilum. Archives of Pathology and Laboratory Medicine 64: 584–588

Aldrich R A, Steinberg A G, Campbell D C 1954 Pedigree demonstrating a sex-linked recessive condition characterised by draining ears, eczematoid dermatitis and bloody diarrhoea. Pediatrics 13: 133–139

Al-Jabi M, McCaughey W T E 1981 Multicentric angiofollicular hyperplasia. Canadian Medical Association Journal 124: 1023–1025

Anderson L G, Talal N 1972 The spectrum of benign to malignant lymphoproliferation in Sjögren's syndrome. Clinical and Experimental Immunology 10: 199–221

Azzopardi J G, Lehner T 1966 Systemic amyloidosis and malignant disease. Journal of Clinical Pathology 19: 539–548

Baker G P, De Navasquez S, Maclean K S 1949 Primary generalised amyloidosis in a young adult. Guy's Hospital Reports 98: 95–109

Baldwin W M, Hendry W, Birinyi L K, Tilney N L 1979 Immune responses to organ allografts. I — Intense B-cell response to heart allografts in lymphoid tissues of unmodified rats. Laboratory Investigation 40: 695–702

Bartoli E, Massarelli G, Soggia G, Tanda F 1980 Multicentric giant lymph node hyperplasia: a hyperimmune syndrome with a rapidly progressive course. American Journal of Clinical Pathology 73: 423–426

Bauer T W, Mendelsohn G, Humphrey R L, Mann R B 1982 Angioimmunoblastic lymphadenopathy progressing to immunoblastic lymphoma with prominent gastric involvement. Cancer 50: 2089–2098

Becroft D M O, Dix M R, Gillman J C, Beth J L, MacGregor, Shaw R L 1973 Benign sinus histiocytosis with massive lymphadenopathy: transient immunological defects in a child with mediastinal involvement. Journal of Clinical Pathology 26: 463–469

Bernengo M G, Levi L, Zina G 1981 Skin lesions in angioimmunoblastic lymphadenopathy: histological and immunological studies. British Journal of Dermatology 104: 131–139

Blanchard F, Briancon S, Cohen J H M, Bethevenot G, Reyes F 1983 Prognostic factors in angioimmunoblastic lymphadenopathy. Lancet 1: 1449–1450

Boros L, Bhaskar A G, D'Souza J P 1981 Monoclonal evolution of angioimmunoblastic lymphadenopathy. American Journal of Clinical Pathology 75: 856–860

Bottomley J P, Bradley J, Whitehouse G H 1974 Waldenström's macroglobulinaemia and amyloidosis with subcutaneous calcification and lymphographic appearances. British Journal of Radiology 47: 232–235

Bradley S L, Dines D E, Banks P M, Hill R W 1981 The lung in immunoblastic lymphadenopathy. Chest 80: 312–318

Brearley R L, Chapman J, Cullen M H, Horton M A, Stansfeld A G, Waters A H 1979 Haematological features of angioimmunoblastic lymphadenopathy with dysproteinaemia. Journal of Clinical Pathology 32: 356–360

Briggs G W 1961 Amyloidosis. Annals of Internal Medicine 55: 943–957

Bruton O C 1952 Agammaglobulinemia. Pediatrics 9: 722–727

Burgert E O, Gilchrist G S, Fairbanks V F, Lynn H B, Dukes P P, Harrison E G 1975 Intraabdominal angiofollicular lymph node hyperplasia (plasma cell variant) with an antierythropoietic factor. Mayo Clinic Proceedings 50: 542–546

Cardell B S 1961 Role of cytotoxic agents in production of amyloidosis in Hodgkin's disease. British Medical Journal 1: 1145–1148

Castleman B 1955 Tumours of the Thymus Gland. Atlas of Tumour Pathology sect. V, Fasc. 19 A F I P, Washington D C, p 68–75

Castleman B, Iverson L, Pardo Menendez V 1956 Localized mediastinal lymph node hyperplasia resembling thymoma. Cancer 9: 822–830

Castleman B, Towne V W 1954 Case records of the Massachusetts General Hospital, case 40011. New England Journal of Medicine 250: 26–30

Cathcart E S, Ritchie R F, Cohen A S, Brandt K 1972 Immunoglobulins and amyloidosis: an immunologic study

of sixty two patients with biopsy-proven disease. American Journal of Medicine 52: 93–101
Climie A R W, Waggoner L G, Krabbenhoft K L 1964 Lymphoid hamartoma of the larynx. Laryngoscope 74: 1381–1388
Cohen A S, Canoso J J 1972 Criteria for the classification of SLE-status. Arthritis and Rheumatism 15: 540–543
Cohen H 1957 Tumor-like proliferations of lymphoid tissue. Occurrence in deltoid muscle and mediastinum. Journal of the Mount Sinai Hospital 24: 750–760
Cooperband S R, Rosen F S, Kibrick S 1968 Studies on the in vitro behavior of agammaglobulinemic lymphocytes. Journal of Clinical Investigation 47: 836–847
Couch W D 1980 Giant lymph node hyperplasia associated with thrombotic thrombocytopenic purpura. American Journal of Clinical Pathology 74: 340–344
Cruickshank B 1958 Lesions of lymph nodes in rheumatoid disease and in disseminated lupus erythematosus. Scottish Medical Journal 3: 110–117
Cullen M H, Stansfeld A G, Oliver R T D, Lister T A, Malpas J S 1979 Angio-immunoblastic lymphadenopathy: report of ten cases and review of the literature. Quarterly Journal of Medicine 189: 151–177
Daley M, Cornog J L 1957 Pelvic retroperitoneal lymphoid hamartoma. Journal of Urology 97: 235–239
Diebold J, Tulliez M, Bernadou A, Audouin J, Tricot G, Reynes M, Bilski-Pasquier G 1980 Angiofollicular and plasmacytic polyadenopathy: a pseudotumorous syndrome with dysimmunity. Journal of Clinical Pathology 33: 1068–1076
Dillon J A, Evans L R 1942 Primary amyloidosis; a report of three cases. Annals of Internal Medicine 17: 722–731
Doll D C, List A F 1982 Burkitt's lymphoma in homosexuals. Lancet 1: 1026–1027
Dubois E L 1974a The clinical picture of systemic lupus erythematosus; In: 'Lupus Erythematosus' 2nd edn. University of Southern California Press, Los Angeles, p 342–343
Dubois E L 1974b Causes of death in systemic lupus erythematosus; In: 'Lupus Erythematosus' 2nd edn. University of Southern California Press, Los Angeles, p 637
Eanes E D, Glenner G G 1968 X-ray diffraction studies of amyloid filaments. Journal of Histochemistry and Cytochemistry 16: 673–677
Eisen H N 1946 Primary systemic amyloidosis. American Journal of Medicine 1: 144–160
Elsner B, Iotti R M 1973 Lesiones viscerales del lupus eritematoso sistémico; análisis de 60 casos. Revista Clinica Española128: 245–250
Emberger J M, Navarro M, Oules O, Vallat G, Brunel M 1976 Présence de cellules type Sternberg dans une adénopathie lupique. Nouvelle presse Medicale 5: 1994
Emson H E 1973 Extrathoracic angiofollicular lymphoid hyperplasia with coincidental myasthenia gravis. Cancer 31: 241–245
Estes D, Christian C L 1971 The natural history of systemic lupus erythematosus by prospective analysis. Medicine (Baltimore) 50: 85–95
Fiorillo A, Pettinato G, Raia V, Migliorati R, Angrisani P, Buffolano W 1981 Angioimmunoblastic lymphadenopathy with dysproteinemia: report of the first case in childhood evolving towards spontaneous remission. Cancer 48: 1611–1614
Fisher E R, Sieracki J C, Goldenberg D M 1970 Identity and nature of isolated lymphoid tumours (so called nodal hyperplasia, hamartoma and angiomatous hamartoma) as revealed by histologic, electron microscopic and heterotransplantation studies. Cancer 25: 1286–1300
Flandrin G, Daniel M T, El Yafi G, Chelloul N 1972 Sarcomatoses ganglionnaires diffuses à différenciation plasmocytaire avec anémie hémolytique auto-immune. Actualites Hématologiques 6: 25–41
Flendrig J A 1970 Benign giant lymphoma: clinicopathologic correlation. In: Clark R L, Cumley R W (eds) The Year Book of Cancer. Year Book Medical Publishers Chicago, p 296–299
Foldes J 1946 Acute systemic lupus erythematosus. American Journal of Clinical Pathology 16: 160–173
Forget B G, Squires J W, Sheldon H 1966 Waldenström's macroglobulinemia with generalised amyloidosis. Archives of Internal Medicine (Chicago) 118: 363–375
Fox R, Rosahn P 1943 The lymph nodes in disseminated lupus erythematosus. American Journal of Pathology 19: 73–95
Frizzera G, Massarelli G, Banks P M, Rosai J 1983 A systemic lymphoproliferative disorder with morphologic features of Castleman's disease. American Journal of Surgical Pathology 7: 211–231
Frizzera G, Moran E M, Rappaport H 1974 Angio-immunoblastic lymphadenopathy with dysproteinaemia. Lancet 1: 1070–1073
Frizzera G, Moran E M, Rappaport H 1975 Angioimmunoblastic lymphadenopathy. Diagnosis and Clinical course. American Journal of Medicine 59: 803–818
Fudenberg H, Good R A, Goodman H C, Hitzig W, Kunkel H G, Roitt I M, Rosen F S, Rowe D S, Seligmann M, Soothill J R 1971 Primary immunodeficiencies. Report of a WHO committee. Pediatrics 47: 927–946
Gaba A R, Stein R S, Sweet D L, Variakojis D 1978 Multicentric giant lymph node hyperplasia. American Journal of Clinical Pathology 69: 86–90
Gaffney E F, Lee J C K 1978 Systemic amyloidosis and hypogammaglobulinemia. Archives of Pathology and Laboratory Medicine 102: 558–559
Gan E, Van der Weyden M B 1981 Hypercalcaemia and angioimmunoblastic lymphadenopathy. British Medical Journal 282: 437
Garrido C M, Cueva F O 1972 Adenitis necrotizante lúpica. Archivos de la Fundación Roux Ocefa 6: 211–215
Giesker D W, Krause P J, Pastuszak W T, Hine P, Forouhar F A 1982 Lymph node biopsy for early diagnosis in Kawasaki disease. American Journal of Surgical Pathology 6: 493–501
Ginzler A M, Fox T T 1940 Disseminated lupus erythematosus: a cutaneous manifestation of a systemic disease (Libman-Sacks). Report of a case. Archives of Internal Medicine 65: 26–50
Glenner G G 1980a Amyloid deposits and amyloidosis. The β-fibrilloses (first of two parts). New England Journal of Medicine 302: 1283–1292
Glenner G G 1980b Amyloid deposits and amyloidosis. The β-fibrilloses (second of two parts). New England Journal of Medicine 302: 1333–1343
Godman G C. Deitch A D, Klemperer P 1958 The composition of the LE and hematoxylin bodies of systemic lupus erythematosus. American Journal of Pathology 34: 1–23

Gold S C, Gowing N F C 1953 Systemic lupus erythematosus: a clinical and pathological study. Quarterly Journal of Medicine 22: 457–481
Grishman E 1979 Ultrastructure of hematoxylin bodies in SLE. Archives of Pathology and Laboratory Medicine 103: 573–576
Grosch D S, Hopwood L E (eds) 1979 In: Biological Effects of Radiations 2nd edn. Academic Press, New York, p 198–200
Guarda L U, Butler J J, Mansell P, Harsh E M, Reuben J, Newell G R 1983 Lymphadenopathy in homosexual men. Morbid anatomy with clinical and immunologic correlations. American Journal of Clinical Pathology 79: 559–568
Gueft B, Laufer A 1954 Further cytochemical studies in systemic lupus erythematosus. Archives of Pathology and Laboratory Medicine 57: 201–226
Habeshaw J A 1983 Personal communication
Harris J, Sengar D, Stewart T, Hyslop D 1976 The effect of immunosuppressive chemotherapy on immune function in patients with malignant disease. Cancer 37: 1058–1069
Harrison E G, Bernatz P E 1963 Angiofollicular mediastinal lymph node hyperplasia resembling thymoma. Archives of Pathology and Laboratory Medicine 75: 284–292
Harvey A M, Schulman L E, Tumulty P A, Conley C L, Schoenrich E H 1954 Systemic lupus erythematosus: a review of the literature and clinical analysis of 136 cases. Medicine (Baltimore) 33: 291–437
Haustein U F, Raetz H F 1973 Histologische untersuchung der lunge, milz, lymphknoten sowie des thymus bei New Zealand mäusen im zeitlängsschnitt. Allergie Und Immunologie (Leipzig) 19: 9–27
Heefner W A, Sorenson G D 1962 Experimental amyloidosis. I-Light and electronmicroscopic observations of spleen and lymph nodes. Laboratory Investigation 11: 585–593
Henry K, Goldman J M 1975 The Lymphocyte. In: Harrison C V, Weinbren K (eds) Recent Advances in Pathology Vol. 9, Churchill Livingstone, Edinburgh. p 30–72
Hineman V L, Phyliky R L, Banks P M 1982 Angiofollicular lymph node hyperplasia and peripheral neuropathy. Mayo Clinic Proceedings 57: 379–382
Hobbs J R 1968 Immune imbalance in dysgammaglobulinaemia type IV. Lancet 1: 110–114
Hobbs J R, Morgan A D 1963 Fluorescence microscopy with thioflavine-T in the diagnosis of amyloid. Journal of Pathology and Bacteriology 86: 437–442
Hughes G R V, Lachmann P J 1975 Systemic lupus erythematosus. In: Gell P G H, Coombs R P A, Lachman P J (eds) Clinical Aspects of Immunology. Blackwell, Oxford, p 1132
Hughes W S, Cerda J J, Holtzapple P, Brooks F P 1971 Primary hypogammaglobulinemia and malabsorption. Annals of Internal Medicine 74: 903–910
Humpherys S R, Holley K E, Smith L H, McIlrath D C 1975 Mesenteric angiofollicular lymph node hyperplasia (lymphoid hamartoma) with nephrotic syndrome. Mayo Clinic Proceedings 50: 317–321
Jones E L, Crocker J, Gregory J, Guibarra M, Curran R C 1983 Angiofollicular lymphoid hyperplasia: an immunohistochemical and enzyme-histochemical study. Journal of Pathology 140: 167 (abstract)
Kaneko Y, Larson R A, Variakojis D, Haren J M 1982 Nonrandom chromosome abnormalities in angioimmunoblastic lymphadenopathy. Blood 60: 877–887
Kassan S S, Moss M L, Reddick R L 1976 Progressive hilar and mediastinal lymphadenopathy in systemic lupus erythematosus on corticosteroid therapy. New England Journal of Medicine 294: 1382–1383
Keller A R, Hochholzer L, Castleman B 1972 Hyaline-vascular and plasma cell types of giant lymph node hyperplasia of the mediastinum and other locations. Cancer 29: 670–683
Kersey J H, Meuwisen H J, Good R A 1971 Graft versus host reactions following transplantation of allogeneic hematopoietic cells. Human Pathology 2: 389–402
Kissane J M, Gephardt G N 1974 Lymphadenopathy in childhood. Long-term follow-up in patients with non-diagnostic lymph node biopsies. Human Pathology 5: 431–439
Klajman A, Yaretzky A, Schneider M, Holoshitz Y, Shneur A, Griffel B 1981 Angioimmunoblastic lymphadenopathy with paraproteinaemia: a T- and B-cell disorder. Cancer 48: 2433–2437
Klemperer P, Gueft B, Lee S L, Leuchtenberger C, Pollister A W 1950 Cytochemical changes of acute lupus erythematosus. Archives of Pathology and Laboratory Medicine 49: 503–516
Klemperer P, Pollack A D, Baehr C 1941 Pathology of disseminated lupus erythematosus. Archives of Pathology and Laboratory Medicine 32: 569–631
Klug V H 1978 Über interdigitierende zellen in lymphknoten bei sklerodermie und lupus erythematodes. Dermatologie Monatsschrift 164: 889–893
Knowles D M, Schevchuk M 1978 Pleomorphic reticulum cell sarcoma, monoclonal gammopathy and amyloidosis: an immunoperoxidase study. Cancer 41: 1883–1889
Ko M S, Davidson J W, Pruzanski W 1976 Amyloid lymphadenopathy. Annals of Internal Medicine 85: 763–764
Konovalova V I, Fraik T A 1976 Immunoblastic lymphadenitis in systemic lupus erythematosus. Terapevticheskii Arkhiv 48: 113–115
Krasznai G, Juhász I 1969 Angiomatous lymphoid tissue hyperplasia. Journal of Pathology 97: 148–151
Lattes R, Pachter M R 1962 Benign lymphoid masses of probable hamartomatous nature. Analysis of 12 cases. Cancer 15: 197–214
Laurens A, Hiltenbrand C, Antoine H, Durosoir J, Chomette P 1973 La maladie de Castleman. Aspects cliniques évolutifs, anatomo-pathologiques et étiopathogéniques. A propos d'une forme clinique atypique. Annales de Medecine Interne (Paris) 124: 651–656
Lee S L, Rosner F, Rivero I, Feldman F, Hurwitz A 1965 Refractory anemia with abnormal iron metabolism; its remission after resection of hyperplastic mediastinal lymph nodes. New England Journal of Medicine 272: 761–766
Leibetseder F, Thurner J 1973 Angiofollikuläre lymphknotenhyperplasie (Zwiebelschalenlymphom). Medizinische Klinik (Munchen) 68: 817–820
Leinwand I, Duryee A W, Richter M N 1954 Scleroderma (based on a study of over 150 cases). Annals of Internal Medicine 41: 1003–1041
Lennert K 1961 (ed) In: Lymphknoten diagnostik in schnitt und ausstrich bandteil a cytologie und lymphadenitis. Springer Verlag, Berlin, p 379
Lennert K, Knecht H, Burkert M 1979 Vorstadien maligner lymphome. Verhandlungen der Deutschen Gesellschaft fur Pathologie (Stuttgart) 63: 170–196

Levin A S, Spitler L E, Stites D P, Fudenberg H H 1970 Wiskott-Aldrich syndrome, a genetically determined cellular immunologic deficiency: clinical and laboratory responses to therapy with transfer factor. Proceedings of the National Academy of Sciences (USA) 67: 821–828

Levy R C, Levin H G 1951 Thyrotoxicosis simulating features of lymphoma. Annals of Internal Medicine 35: 1371–1373

Lindsay S, Knorp W F 1945 Primary systemic amyloidosis. Archives of Pathology and Laboratory Medicine 39: 315–322

Lough J, Shuster J 1975 Constipated plasma cells associated with monomeric macroglobulinemia. Human Pathology 6: 251–255

Lukes R J, Tindle B H 1973 Immunoblastic lymphadenopathy. Workshop on Classification of non-Hodgkin's lymphomas. University of Chicago.

Lukes R J, Tindle B H 1975 Immunoblastic lymphadenopathy. A hyperimmune entity resembling Hodgkin's disease. New England Journal of Medicine 292: 1–8

Mackenzie D H 1963 Amyloidosis presenting as lymphadenopathy. British Medical Journal 2: 1449–1450

Madri J A, Fromowitz F 1978 Amyloid deposition in immunoblastic lymphadenopathy. Human Pathology 9: 157–162

Mallory A, Spink W W 1968 Angiomatous lymphoid hamartoma in the retroperitoneum presenting with neurologic signs in the legs. Annals of Internal Medicine 69: 305–308

Marohe C, Saimot A G, Diebold J, Kernbaum S 1984 Le syndrome de lymphadénopathie généralisée en relation avec le SIDA. Aspects histopathologiques des ganglions. Bulletin de l'Academie Nationale de Medecine (Paris) 168: 271–277

Mathé G, Bernard J, De Vries M J, Schwarzenberg L, Larrieu M J, Lalanne C M, Dutreix A, Amiel J L, Surmont J 1960 Nouveaux essais de greffe de moelle osseuse homologue après irradiation totale chez des enfants atteints de leucémie aigüe en rémission. Le problème du syndrome secondaire chez l'homme. Revue d'Hématologie 15: 115–161

Miller D G 1967 The association of immune disease and malignant lymphoma. Annals of Internal Medicine 66: 507–521

Millikin P D 1977 Epithelioid germinal centers. An acquired immunologic deficit? American Journal of Clinical Pathology 67: 545–549

Miralles Garcia J M, Garcia Iglesias C, Parra Fragua T, Cuñado Rodriguez A 1978 Linfadenitis gigantofolicular de células plasmáticas y amiloidosis hepática. Revista Clinica Española 150: 205–208

Moir D H, Choy T, Dalton W R 1982 Giant lymph node hyperplasia: persistence of symptoms for 15 years. Cancer 49: 748–750

Moore R D, Weisberger A S, Bowerfind E S 1956 Histochemical studies of lymph nodes in disseminated lupus erythematosus. Archives of Pathology and Laboratory Medicine 62: 472–478

Moore R D, Weisberger A S, Bowerfind E S 1957 An evolution of lymphadenopathy in systemic disease. Archives of Internal Medicine 99: 751–759

Moore S B, Harrison E G, Weiland L H 1976 Angioimmunoblastic lymphadenopathy. Mayo Clinic Proceedings 51: 273–280

Moreb J, Matzner Y, Polliack A 1983 Angioimmunoblastic lymphadenopathy. A case with an unusual clinical course with marked tumorous infiltration of multiple organs and striking intestinal involvement. Cancer 51: 487–491

Motulsky A G, Weinberg S, Saphir O, Rosenberg E 1952 Lymph nodes in rheumatoid arthritis. Archives of Internal Medicine 90: 660–676

Nagura H, Kohler P F, Brown W R 1979 Immunocytochemical characterisation of the lymphocytes in nodular lymphoid hyperplasia of the bowel. Laboratory Investigation 40: 66–73

Nathwani B, Rappaport H, Moran E M, Pangalis G A, Kim H 1978 Malignant lymphoma arising in angioimmunoblastic lymphadenopathy. Cancer 41: 578–606

Neerhout R C, Larson W, Mansur P 1965 Mesenteric lymphoid hamartoma associated with chronic hypoferremia, anemia, growth failure and hyperglobulinemia. New England Journal of Medicine 280: 922–925

Neiman R S, Dervan P, Haudenschild C, Jaffe R 1978 Angioimmunoblastic lymphadenopathy. An ultrastructural and immunologic study with review of the literature. Cancer 41: 507–518

Nordstrom D G, Tewfik H H, Latourette H B 1978 Giant lymph node hyperplasia: a review of the literature and report of two cases of plasma cell variant responding to radiation therapy. Journal of Radiation Oncology, Biology and Physics 4: 1045–1048

Nosanchuk J S, Schnitzer B 1969 Follicular hyperplasia in lymph nodes from patients with rheumatoid arthritis. A clinicopathologic study. Cancer 24: 343–354

O'Donnell P P, Jiji R, Vigorito R, Price T R 1980 Angioimmunoblastic lymphadenopathy. Its occurrence with meningeal involvement. Archives of Neurology 37: 598–599

Osborne B M, Butler J, Mackay B 1979 Proteinaceous lymphadenopathy with hypergammaglobulinemia. American Journal of Surgical Pathology 3: 137–145

Pangalis G A, Moran E M, Rappaport H 1978 Blood and bone marrow findings in angioimmunoblastic lymphadenopathy. Blood 51: 71–83

Paty J C, Sienknecht C W, Townes A S, Hanissian A S, Miller J B, Masi A T 1975 Impaired cell mediated immunity in disseminated lupus erythematosus. A controlled study of 23 untreated patients. American Journal of Medicine 59: 769–779

Penn I 1976 Second malignant neoplasms associated with immunosuppressive medications. Cancer 37: 1024–1032

Peterson R D A, Cooper M D, Good R A 1965 The pathogenesis of immunologic deficiency diseases. American Journal of Medicine 38: 579–604

Pileri S, Kikuchi M, Helbron D, Lennert K 1982 Histiocytic necrotizing lymphadenitis without granulocytic infiltration. Virchows Archiv A (Pathol. Anat.) 395: 257–271

Poppema S, Kaiserling E, Lennert K 1979 Hodgkin's disease with lymphocytic predominance, nodular type (nodular paragranuloma) and progressively transformed germinal centres — a cytohistological study. Histopathology 3: 295–308

Pruzanski W 1980 Lymphadenopathy associated with dysgammaglobulinemia. Seminars in Hematology 17: 44–62

Radaszkiewicz T, Lennert K 1975 Lymphogranulomatosis X. Klinisches Bild, Therapie und Prognose. Deutsche Medizinische Wochenschrift 21: 1157–1163

Raskin R J, Tesar J T, Lawless O J 1982 Polyarthritis in immunoblastic lymphadenopathy. Arthritis and Rheumatism 25: 1481–1485

Razis D V, Diamond H D, Craver L F 1959 Hodgkin's disease associated with other malignant tumours and certain non-neoplastic diseases. American Journal of Medical Sciences 238: 327–335

Ricken D, Beltz L, Marsteller H J, Sennekamp J 1971 Zur frage der miterkrankung der lymphknoten beim lupus erythematodes disseminatus. Verhandlungen Deutschen Gesellschaft 77: 1138–1141

Rudders R A, De Lellis R 1977 Immunoblastic lymphadenopathy. A mixed proliferation of T and B lymphocytes. American Journal of Clinical Pathology 68: 518–521

Rukavina J G, Block W D, Jackson C E, Falls H F, Carey J H, Curtis A C 1956 Primary systemic amyloidosis: a review and experimental, genetic and clinical study of 29 cases with particular emphasis on the familial form. Medicine 35: 239–334

Schechter S L 1980 Differentiating SLE from angioimmunoblastic lymphadenopathy. New England Journal of Medicine 303: 396–397

Scheurlen P G, Haun W, Mäusle E, Wolff G 1973 Generalisierte tumorförmige lymphknotenamyloidose mit polyneuropathie und makroglobulinämie. Deutsche Medicinische Wochenschrift 98: 1947–1951

Schnaidt U, Thiele J, Georgii A 1980a Angioimmunoblastic lymphadenopathy, fine structure of the lymph nodes by correlation of light and electron microscopical findings. Virchows Archiv A (Pathol. Anat.) 389: 381–395

Schnaidt U, Vykoupil K F, Thiele J, Georgii A 1980b Angioimmunoblastic lymphadenopathy; Histopathology of bone marrow involvement. Virchows Archiv A (Pathol. Anat.) 389: 369–380

Schober R 1982 A case of angioimmunoblastic lymphadenopathy with involvement of the nervous system. Virchows Archiv A (Pathol. Anat.) 395: 109–116

Seigneurin J M, Mingat J, Lenoir G M, Couderc P, Micoud M 1981 Angioimmunoblastic lymphadenopathy after infectious mononucleosis. British Medical Journal 282: 1574–1575

Sharp G C, Irvin W S, Tan E M, Gould R G, Holman H R 1972 Mixed connective tissue disease. An apparently distinct rheumatic disease syndrome associated with a specific antibody to an extractable nuclear antigen (ENA). American Journal of Medicine 52: 148–159

Shearn M A 1971 In: Smith L H (ed) Sjögren's syndrome. (Major problems in Internal Medicine series) Vol. 11. Saunders, Philadelphia, p 124–173

Short C L, Castleman B 1949 Case records of the Massachusetts General Hospital, Case 35391. New England Journal of Medicine 241: 497–500

Short T S 1907 Fatal case of acute lupus erythematosus. British Journal of Dermatology 19: 271–274

Slavin R E, Santos G W 1973 The graft versus host reaction in man after bone marrow transplantation: pathology, pathogenesis, clinical features and implication. Clinical Immunology and Immunopathology 1: 472–498

Stern J O, Dieterich D, Faust M 1982 Disseminated Kaposi's sarcoma: involvement of the GI tract among a group of homosexual men. Gastroenterology 82:1189

Symmers W St C 1956a Primary amyloidosis: a review. Journal of Clinical Pathology 9: 187–211

Symmers W St C 1956b Amyloidosis — Five cases of primary generalised amyloidosis and some other unusual cases. Journal of Clinical Pathology 9: 212–228

Symmers W St C 1978 In: Systemic Pathology 2nd edn, Vol. 2. Churchill Livingstone, Edinburgh, p 693

Taryle D A, Ellis J M 1979 Systemic lupus erythematosus: an unusual case of bilateral hilar lymphadenopathy. Southern Medical Journal 72: 896–897

Teilum G 1945 Miliary epithelioid cell granulomas in lupus erythematosus disseminatus. Acta Pathologica et Microbiologica Scandinavica 22: 73–79

Tribe C R 1966 Amyloidosis in rheumatoid arthritis. In: Hill A G S (ed) Modern Trends in Rheumatology, Butterworths, London, p 121–138

Tschang T P 1976 Nodular malignant lymphoma and amyloidosis. A case report. Cancer 38: 2192–2196

Tung K S, McCormack L J 1967 Angiomatous lymphoid hamartoma: report of five cases with review of the literature. Cancer 20: 525–536

Valdes A J, Blair O M 1976 Angioimmunoblastic lymphadenopathy with dysproteinemia. Immunohistology and ultrastructural studies. American Journal of Clinical Pathology 66: 551–559

Van Vliet G, Vainsel M, Wolter R, Heimann R 1978 Growth failure, refractory anaemia and hyperglobulinaemia: their regression after removal of a mesenteric tumour with the features of giant lymph node hyperplasia, plasma cell type. Acta Paediatrica Belgica 31: 41–44

Virmani R, McAllister H A, Bewtra C, Schulte R D 1982 Intrapericardial giant lymph node hyperplasia. American Journal of Surgical Pathology 6: 475–481

Wallace S L, Feldman D J, Berlin I, Harris C, Glass I A 1950 Amyloidosis in Hodgkin's disease. American Journal of Medicine 8: 552–557

Watanabe S, Shimosato Y, Shimoyama M, Minato K, Suzuki M, Abe M, Nagatani T 1980 Adult T-cell lymphoma with hypergammaglobulinemia. Cancer 46: 2472–2483

Waterson A P 1983 Acquired immune deficiency syndrome. British Medical Journal 286: 743–746

Weisenburger D D 1979 Membranous nephropathy. Its association with multicentric angiofollicular lymph node hyperplasia. Archives of Pathology and Laboratory Medicine 103: 591–594

Westerhausen M, Oehlert W 1972 Chronisches pluripotentielles immunproliferatives syndrom. Deutsche Medicinische Wochenschrift 97: 1407–1413

Wilks S 1856 Cases of lardaceous disease and some allied affections; with remarks. Guy's Hospital Reports 2: 103–132

Woolner L B, McConahey W M, Beahrs O H, Black B M 1966 Primary malignant lymphoma of the thyroid. Review of forty-six cases. American Journal of Surgery 111: 502–523

Worken B, Pearson R D 1953 Hematoxylin bodies associated with allergic angiitis in absence of lupus erythematosus. Archives of Pathology and Laboratory Medicine 56: 293–300

Woodruff J M, Hansen J A, Good R A, Santos G W, Slavin R E 1976 The pathology of the graft versus host reaction (GVHR) in adults receiving bone marrow transplants. Transplantation Proceedings 8: 675–684

WHO Scientific Group 1979 Immunodeficiency. Clinics in Immunology and Immunopathology 13: 296–359

Wright J R, Calkins E, Humphrey R L 1977 Potassium permanganate reaction in amyloidosis. A histologic method to assist in differentiating forms of this disease. Laboratory Investigation 36: 274–281

York J C, Taylor C R, Lukes R L 1981 Monoclonality in giant lymph node hyperplasia. Laboratory Investigation 44:77A (abstract)

Yu G S M, Carson J W 1976 Giant lymph-node hyperplasia, plasma cell type, of the mediastinum with peripheral neuropathy. American Journal of Clinical Pathology 66: 46–53

Zettergren L 1961 Probably neoplastic proliferation of lymphoid tissue (follicular lympho-reticuloma). Reports of 4 cases with a survey of the literature. Acta Pathologica et Microbiologica Scandinavica 51: 113–126

Ziegler J L, Drew W L, Miner R C, Mintz L, Rosenbaum E, Gershow J, Lennette E T, Greenspan J, Shillitoe E, Beckstead J, Casavant C, Yamamoto K 1982 Outbreak of Burkitt's-like lymphoma in homosexual men. Lancet 2: 631–633

9

G.T. Williams

Hodgkin's disease

THE NATURE & ORIGIN OF HODGKIN'S DISEASE

It is now 150 years since Thomas Hodgkin of Guy's Hospital first described the morbid anatomical appearances of the peculiar disease of the lymphoreticular system which bears his name (Hodgkin, 1832). Over the years the remarkably diverse clinical presentation, behaviour and pathology of Hodgkin's disease have perplexed many who have tried to understand the basic nature of the condition, and there remains controversy to this day. Many of the features of the disease suggested to some early investigators that it was a bizarre infection with granulomatous inflammation, while its propensity to invade non-lymphoid tissues, to 'metastasise' and to form solid tumours suggested a truly malignant process to others.

The earliest histopathological description of Hodgkin's disease is attributed to Greenfield (1878) who noted the disruption and destruction of the affected lymph nodes by chronic inflammation and fibrosis, and who recognised the frequent presence of multinucleated cells. In 1898, Sternberg gave a more detailed account of these multinucleated cells, stressing their large size and multilobed nuclei, and in 1902 Dorothy Reed also emphasised their very prominent nucleoli, in a lucid histological description of the disease. The demonstration of Sternberg-Reed cells is now considered to be an essential prerequisite for the diagnosis of Hodgkin's disease, and there is compelling evidence to suggest that these cells, and their mononuclear (and probably precursor) variants, are malignant cells. Sternberg-Reed cells are capable of DNA synthesis and mitosis, and cytogenetic studies have demonstrated aneuploidy and a clonal distribution of marker chromosomes, two of the most fundamental characteristics of neoplasia (Kaplan, 1980, p. 12).

The Sternberg-Reed Cell

There has been much debate over the origin of Sternberg-Reed cells and it is mainly for this reason that the eponymous title, Hodgkin's disease, has survived. Morphological studies suggested to some investigators that Sternberg-Reed cells were derived from transformed B lymphocytes (immunoblasts) (Glick et al, 1976), and the finding of surface and cytoplasmic immunoglobulin was considered at first to support this view (Taylor, 1974). However, more recently it has become apparent that this cytoplasmic immunoglobulin is polyclonal, strongly suggesting that the immunoglobulin is not synthesised by the cells but is taken up by them from the environment (Kadin et al, 1978). This, along with the finding of receptors for immunoglobulin (Fc) and complement (C3) on the surface of Sternberg-Reed cells and the demonstration of phagocytosis of immunoglobulin and immune complexes by these cells, led to the suggestion that they are of macrophage lineage. Further support for this view came from the investigation of Sternberg-Reed-like cells in tissue culture (Kaplan, 1980, p. 70–75) and by electron microscopy (Carr, 1975). Curran & Jones (1978) on the other hand, showed that Sternberg-Reed cells, when stained by a metalophil method, frequently possess delicate dendritic processes similar to those of the normal dendritic reticulum cells of lymph follicles. Since the latter are capable of internalising immunoglobulin and immune complexes these authors suggested that Sternberg-Reed cells might originate from dendritic reticulum cells. Recent evidence from monoclonal antibody studies has suggested that the Sternberg-Reed cell is derived from a hitherto unidentified special type of cell found in small numbers in normal lymph nodes (Stein et al, 1982). Further studies are required to clarify the nature of this elusive cell.

Evidence of disturbed immunity

While there are now good reasons to consider the Sternberg-Reed cell as neoplastic, there is much evidence to suggest that, in Hodgkin's disease, neoplasia occurs in a setting of disordered immunity. Defective T-lymphocyte function has been well demonstrated in many patients with Hodgkin's disease, but it is uncertain whether this precedes the onset of neoplasia or occurs as a consequence of it; the defect is most pronounced in patients with widely disseminated disease, but a proportion of those with localised disease of 'favourable' histological type also show some derangement of cell mediated immunity (Kaplan, 1980, p. 236–279).

The aetiology of Hodgkin's disease is still unknown, but epidemiological studies have suggested the possibility of an underlying infectious agent (Lancet, 1977) although the evidence is not strong. There are almost certainly many factors involved in the pathogenesis. It would appear most likely that in suitably predisposed individuals, perhaps conditioned by age, sex, genetic make up and immune competence, prolonged immunological stimulation with or without an oncogenic agent (such as a virus) leads to the development of the malignant process.

Although Sternberg-Reed cells are a distinctive and consistent cell type in Hodgkin's disease, they are almost certainly not the only neoplastic cells present and they are always accompanied by an admixture of other cell types considered to be non-neoplastic, which include lymphocytes, plasma cells, eosinophils, neutrophils, histiocytes, epithelioid cells and fibroblasts, in varying proportions. A clear relationship exists between the number of Sternberg-Reed cells in the lesions, the density of the accompanying non-neoplastic cells (especially the lymphocytes), and the clinical behaviour of the disease (Rosenthal, 1936; Lukes & Butler, 1966). Generally speaking, there is a steady increase in the number of Sternberg-Reed cells and a corresponding decrease in the number of lymphocytes with advancement of the disease, suggesting a complex interaction between the evolving malignant process and immunological host defence mechanisms.

DEVELOPMENT OF A HISTOLOGICAL CLASSIFICATION OF HODGKIN'S DISEASE (HD)

From the earliest descriptions, it has been clear that the basic histological picture of Hodgkin's disease is one of a disrupted nodal architecture with Sternberg-Reed cells in varying numbers set in a background of reactive inflammatory cells of different types, and with fibrosis of a variable degree. However, there is a wide spectrum of appearances, depending upon the relative proportions of the different constituents, and in view of the great diversity of the clinical presentation and behaviour of Hodgkin's disease, numerous attempts have been made to classify the histological appearances, with the object of relating the histological features at presentation to the behaviour of the disease in an individual patient. This has become of particular importance over the last 30 years, when effective means of treatment with radiotherapy and chemotherapy have been developed.

Rosenthal's classification

The first important contribution was that of Rosenthal (1936), who was the first to recognise the prognostic importance of the density of lymphocytes in Hodgkin's disease. On the microscopical appearances he divided the cases into three groups, 'depending upon the predominance, subordinance and the absence of lymphocytes and lymph nodules'. The average survival time from the onset of the disease in these three groups, treated with radiotherapy, was 4.35, 2.29 and 1.14 years respectively. Rosenthal also noted the inverse relationship between lymphocyte numbers and the frequency of Sternberg-Reed cells.

Jackson & Parker's classification

Jackson & Parker (1944) also divided cases of Hodgkin's disease into three groups, namely paragranuloma, granuloma and sarcoma, with a progressive decrease in the survival time of affected patients. Sternberg-Reed cells were sparse in the paragranuloma group and they were scattered among abundant lymphocytes, with few eosinophils or plasma cells and without necrosis or fibrosis. In the granuloma group Sternberg-Reed cells were numerous, and they were accompanied by all varieties of reactive cells in varying proportions, and often by fibrosis and foci of necrosis. The sarcoma group was characterised by a predominance of proliferating neoplastic 'reticulum cells', many of which had features of Sternberg-Reed cells, but reactive cells were relatively inconspicuous or even absent. Although the prognostic value of this classification was amply confirmed, its practical value in the clinical management of patients was greatly limited by the finding that the vast majority of patients fell into the granuloma group, which had a very variable prognosis.

Smetana & Cohen's classification

Smetana & Cohen (1956) modified Jackson & Parker's classification and improved its practical value by identifying a subgroup of the granuloma type which was distinguished by conspicuous fibrous thickening of the lymph node capsule and marked sclerosis within the node, dividing the tumour tissue into 'pseudofollicles' in which Sternberg-Reed cells were relatively inconspicuous. This subgroup, which was termed 'sclerosing Hodgkin's granuloma', accounted for about 20% of all Hodgkin's granuloma cases and had a significantly better prognosis than the remainder of the granuloma group.

Lukes' classification and the Rye classification

In 1963 Lukes published a classification based on a study of biopsy material from 377 cases of Hodgkin's disease observed in the US Armed Forces in World War 2. He distinguished six histological types and later Lukes et al (1966a) extended the histological descriptions and showed a good correlation between histological type and prognosis. In many ways this classification combines all previous attempts to relate the microscopical features of Hodgkin's disease to prognosis (Hamlin, 1973). Lukes' first two groups (lymphocytic and/or histiocytic (L & H) nodular and diffuse) correspond to the lymphocytic predominance of Rosenthal and include the paragranuloma of Jackson & Parker. The sclerosing Hodgkin's granuloma of Smetana & Cohen forms the basis for the third group, nodular sclerosis. The fourth group, mixed cellularity, represents the classical picture of Hodgkin's disease, while the fifth (diffuse fibrosis) and sixth (reticular) groups derive from the lymphocytic absence of Rosenthal and include the sarcoma of Jackson & Parker.

Lukes' original classification was simplified at the Rye conference in 1965 (Lukes et al, 1966b) to leave four groups, *lymphocytic predominance*, *nodular sclerosis*, *mixed cellularity* and *lymphocytic depletion*. This has become known as the Rye classification and has gained acceptance by both clinicians and pathologists. Table 9.1 gives a comparison between the Rye, Lukes, and Jackson & Parker classifications.

The prognostic value of the Rye classification is indicated in Table 9.2 which shows the percentage of patients in each histological group, their median survival time, and the percentage with clinical stage I disease (limited to one anatomical region) at diagnosis. The figures are obtained from Symmers (1978) and represent mean values from up to ten different series. It is apparent that this classification divides cases of Hodgkin's disease fairly evenly and that the different groups correlate well with clinical staging and prognosis.

Table 9.1 Comparison of the Jackson & Parker, Lukes and Rye classifications of Hodgkin's disease

Jackson & Parker	Lukes	Rye
Paragranuloma	L&H nodular	Lymphocytic predominance
	L&H diffuse	
Granuloma	Nodular sclerosis	Nodular sclerosis
	Mixed cellularity	Mixed cellularity
	Diffuse fibrosis	Lymphocytic depletion
Sarcoma	Reticular	

Table 9.2 Patient distribution, prognosis and clinical stage in relation to histological type of Hodgkin's disease (Rye classification)

Type	Percentage distribution of patients*	Mean survival** (years)	Percentage of patients with clinical stage I**
Lymphocytic predominance	17	7	70
Nodular sclerosis	38	4.5	35
Mixed cellularity	31	1.7	35
Lymphocytic depletion	14	0.8	10

* Mean values from analysis of 10 series
** Mean values from analysis of 4 series
[Figures obtained from Symmers (1978)]

Studies of sequential biopsies from patients with Hodgkin's disease have shown that the nodular sclerosis pattern remains remarkably constant throughout the course of the disease while there is a tendency for lymphocytic predominance to progress to mixed cellularity and for mixed cellularity to progress to lymphocytic depletion, suggesting a gradual failure of the host response to the malignant process (Strum & Rappaport, 1971). This has led to the proposal that nodular sclerosis, which is also distinguished by its high incidence in young females and its propensity for mediastinal involvement, represents a distinctive type of Hodgkin's disease (Franssila et al, 1967).

Cross' classification

Cross (1969), while recognising some of the virtues of the Rye classification, believed that it lacked histological precision, and proposed a new classification in which Hodgkin's disease was divided into three main types, reticular, histiocytic and fibroblastic, with further subdivisions of each type. Although, in Cross' series, there was a good correlation with prognosis, this classification has not gained wide acceptance. Nevertheless, Cross' work does highlight the potential prognostic importance of a pronounced histiocytic and granulomatous reaction, in his opinion of sufficient value to warrant a separate 'histiocytic' type of disease. This histological variant was lost sight of with the merging of Lukes' first two types, into 'lymphocytic predominance' and the dropping of his original term 'lymphocytic and/or histiocytic'.

CLINICAL ASPECTS

Incidence

Hodgkin's disease is the commonest of the malignant lymphomas in most parts of the world, but this is only one of several reasons why it is often considered separately from the non-Hodgkin's lymphomas (see p. 229). In Western Europe, as in the USA, Hodgkin's disease accounts for 40–45% of all malignant lymphomas. The disease is apparently much less common in Japan (Smithers, 1973; Wakasa, 1973).

The *age incidence* shows a remarkably wide range. Very rare under the age of 2, it occurs throughout childhood and adult life with a peak incidence in the third decade and a second, minor peak in the seventh decade. This bimodal curve has been advanced as a reason for regarding Hodgkin's disease as more than one entity (MacMahon, 1957, 1966) — a suggestion which has been refuted by Smithers (1963).

The *sex incidence* shows a preponderance of males in most histological types although nodular sclerosis appears more equally divided between the sexes with a slight bias in favour of females.

Family studies have clearly shown a higher incidence of the disease among first degree relatives than would be expected by chance, but the explanation of this is still unclear.

Presentation

Although Hodgkin's disease may present in many different ways, by far the commonest presentation is with painless enlargement of superficial lymph nodes. Those most frequently involved are the cervical nodes (often in conjunction with mediastinal involvement). Axillary and inguinal nodes are less commonly affected, the latter generally in association with intra-abdominal nodal disease. Presentation with palpable nodes in other sites — pre-parotid, post-auricular, epitrochlear etc., is exceptional.

Attention may be drawn to involved nodes, whether superficial or deep, by the symptom of alcohol-induced pain in sites affected by the disease. Whilst this symptom is not peculiar to Hodgkin's disease, it occurs with greater frequency in HD than in other conditions. Systemic symptoms

— fever, night sweats and loss of weight — are common and these constitute the so-called 'B' symptoms which affect the clinical staging of the patient (qv). Pruritus is another common symptom in Hodgkin's disease, but one which is not necessarily of grave import. Hodgkin's disease is one of the classical causes of 'pyrexia of unknown origin' and the diagnosis may be suspected in a patient presenting with malaise, fever and loss of weight, even in the absence of overt lymphadenopathy. Today, computerised axial tomography (CAT) may help to reveal enlarged, deep-seated nodes (e.g. para-aortic) and laparotomy may be considered justified to obtain a node for biopsy, when there are no enlarged superficial nodes present.

PATHOLOGICAL ASPECTS

Even when there is strong clinical suspicion of Hodgkin's disease, biopsy is necessary, not only to confirm the diagnosis but also to type the disease. In most instances the biopsy tissue will be an excised lymph node: less often, extranodal deposits in bones, lung, liver, skin, retroperitoneum or elsewhere may be taken for biopsy.

Fine needle aspiration cytology has been used increasingly in recent years with a high diagnostic accuracy, especially in centres with a large experience of the technique. In Hodgkin's disease a diagnostic rate of 70% is quoted from some centres (Zajicek, 1974), although such a yield may only be achieved by examining multiple aspiration specimens. The cytological criteria for the diagnosis are the same as in tissue sections, namely the identification of unequivocal Sternberg-Reed cells in an appropriate heterogeneous background of reactive cells and Sternberg-Reed cell variants. Some cytologists have found that Sternberg-Reed cells appear to be more conspicuous in aspirated smears than in histological sections, and that these cells tend to stand out as 'single oaks in open fields' (Söderström, 1966).

Perhaps the biggest disadvantage of the technique is that it seldom allows a confident classification of the type of Hodgkin's disease to be made (Zajicek, 1974). Nodular sclerosis is particularly likely to be misdiagnosed, because the aspirated material is taken selectively from the cellular nodules and consequently the presence of fibrosis fails to be appreciated. For this reason, histological examination of excised tissue is to be preferred.

MACROSCOPIC FEATURES

Lymph nodes involved by Hodgkin's disease are often moderately firm and 'rubbery' in consistency. Even when very large, and individual nodes may measure occasionally up to 10 cm in diameter, they tend to remain discrete, unlike the nodes in some 'non-Hodgkin's' lymphomas. This is not, however, an invariable characteristic and sometimes, even small nodes involved by nodular sclerosing Hodgkin's disease may be matted together and tethered by dense fibrous tissue which may infiltrate surrounding soft tissues and muscle, simulating a chronic inflammatory process. The mimicry of a primarily infective condition may be enhanced by local oedema which at times results in a diffuse swelling, partly or wholly concealing the underlying lymph node disease.

The excised nodes are likewise rather variable. The often rather large nodes of lymphocyte predominant HD naturally tend to be softer in consistency than the nodes in nodular sclerosis, which may be very firm. Fibrosis and nodularity can sometimes be made out with the naked eye on slicing the node. Pale flecks of necrosis may be visible against the homogeneous background of pinkish-white 'fish-flesh' tissue. On occasions, more extensive necrosis or even total infarction of the node may be evident.

HISTOLOGY

Whilst it is sometimes easy to diagnose Hodgkin's disease from a biopsy section, it may on other occasions be extremely difficult, even with good sections. Much depends on the number of Sternberg-Reed cells present in the biopsy. Enough has been said earlier in this chapter to indicate the remarkable diversity of histological appearances in this disease. The differences between the extremes are so great that it might be thought justifiable to question whether one is dealing with more than one type of neoplasm. Despite this, the degree of overlap between one type and another and the observation of how, in a single patient, the histological picture may change, in successive biopsies, from one type to another, have confirmed the belief in the essential unity of Hodgkin's disease.

The one unifying feature which provides the essential common ground in all cases of Hodgkin's disease is the presence of Sternberg-Reed cells. There are, however, several 'variant' forms of Sternberg-Reed cell (see discussion below) which differ from one another sufficiently to make it impossible to give a single accurate description of *the* Sternberg-Reed cell. There is more than a grain of truth in the jocular definition of a Sternberg-Reed cell as 'a cell which two or more competent histopathologists agree to be a Sternberg-Reed cell'. Furthermore, 'typical' Sternberg-Reed cells are sometimes found in non-neoplastic conditions as well as in neoplasms other than Hodgkin's disease (Strum et al, 1970), hence the insistence that

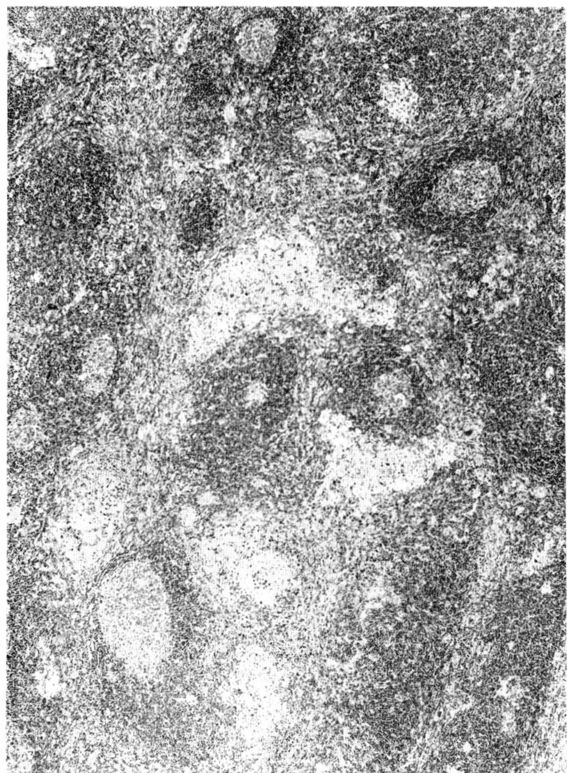

Fig. 9.1 Lymph node in Hodgkin's disease (mixed cellularity type) showing persistent germinal follicles in the presence of widespread infiltration of the interfollicular pulp (H E × 47)

these cells must be present 'in the right setting' to establish a diagnosis of Hodgkin's disease.

There are, indeed, other histological features common to most cases of Hodgkin's disease (HD), regardless of histological type. These are: (1) disturbance in some degree of the normal nodal architecture, commonly, but not invariably, accompanied by some nodularity of the disturbed areas, and (2) a mixed (polymorphic) cellular infiltrate, which at once distinguishes HD from many, but not all, types of non-Hodgkin's lymphoma (NHL). There is a further important histological difference between HD and most NHL which concerns the frequent persistence of reactive germinal follicles in nodes which may be otherwise diffusely infiltrated by Hodgkin's lymphoma (Fig. 9.1). With the single exception of some T cell lymphomas (p. 315), this phenomenon is very rarely seen in NHL. In children and young adults particularly, *the node with Hodgkin's disease may contain many large, active germinal follicles, even within obvious tumour nodules*, and this often overlooked fact is a common source of diagnostic difficulty. Such active follicles are of course seen mainly in lymphocytic predominance and nodular sclerosis. In more advanced disease, although the original follicles may still be recognised, they often show 'burnt-out' germinal centres, containing hyaline eosinophilic deposits.

Sternberg-Reed cells and their variants

Before describing the individual Lukes' types of Hodgkin's disease, it may be helpful to consider in more detail the different forms of Sternberg-Reed (SR) cell met with in Hodgkin's disease (Fig. 9.2). The *classical* SR cell is a large cell 10–40 μm in diameter with abundant cytoplasm, which is weakly eosinophilic or amphophilic and which may appear homogeneous, granular or even vacuolated. The cell differs from a macrophage in having a much larger, polyploid nucleus which is sometimes double, sometimes bilobed or multilobed. The most conspicuous feature of this cell is the very large, inclusion-like, central nucleolus which is acidophil in its staining properties, unlike most nucleoli. The nucleolus may be round, triangular or sausage-shaped and it stands out, not only on account of its size, but because it is often

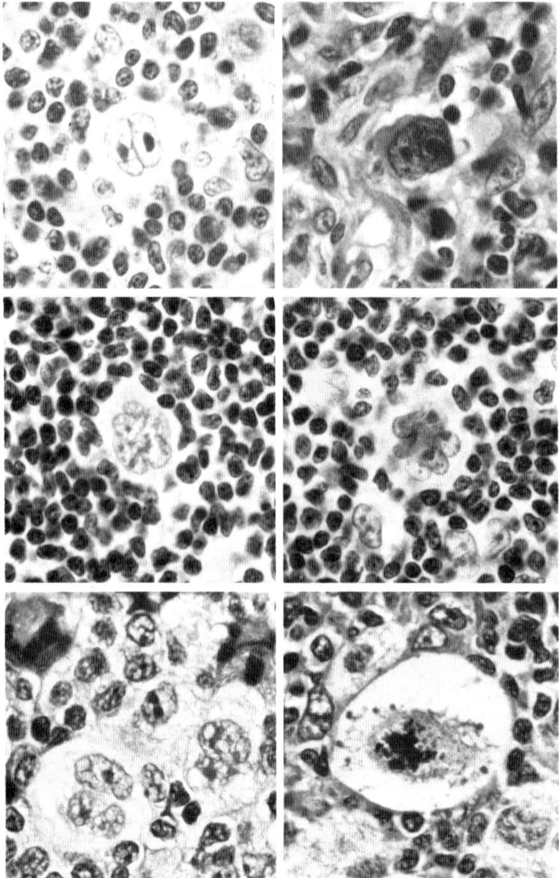

Fig. 9.2 Varieties of Sternberg-Reed cell. (a) classical 'owl's eye' cell with 'mirror-image' nuclei and large acidophilic nucleoli. (b) darkly staining (necrobiotic) variant of classical S-R cell. (c) 'L and H type' — a cell peculiar to lymphocyte predominant Hodgkin's disease with multilobed nucleus and multiple small basophilic nucleoli. (d) a less common variant of the L and H cell with more prominent nucleoli. (e) lacunar cells typical of nodular sclerosing Hodgkin's disease (necrobiotic cell above). Note multilobed nuclei and abundant, pale cytoplasm. (f) another lacunar cell (in mitosis) showing the fully developed lacunar phenomenon. (a)–(f) all H E × 540

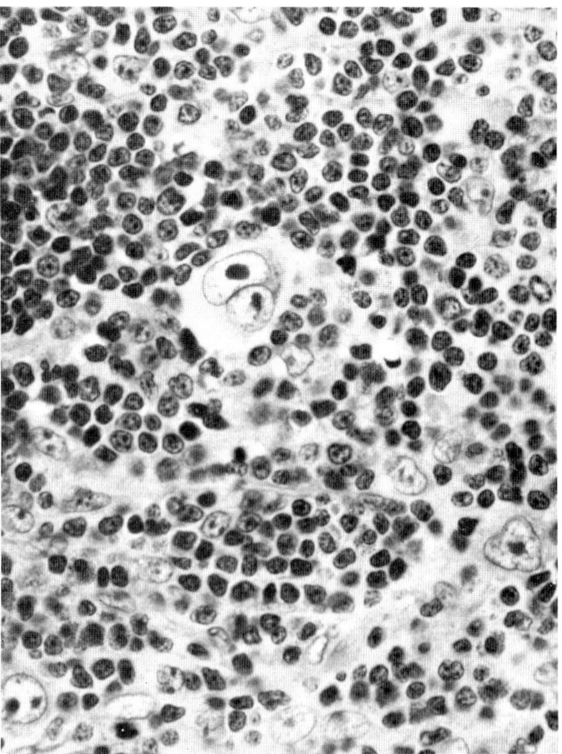

Fig. 9.3 Lymph node in Hodgkin's disease showing a conspicuous Sternberg-Reed cell of classical type. A mononuclear Hodgkin's cell is seen (lower right) and an immunoblast (bottom left). Hodgkin's cells are not diagnostically reliable, but their presence should encourage further search for S-R cells. (H E × 540)

surrounded by a clear halo, separating the nucleolus from the sharply defined nuclear membrane. Binucleate cells with 'mirror-image' nuclei constitute the so-called 'owl's eye' cells (Fig. 9.2a) and even single cells of this type may be readily distinguished with the lower power of the microscope (Fig. 9.3). Many variations of this cell type occur. Mononuclear cells with similar nuclear characteristics (Hodgkin's cells) are frequently met with, but are not diagnostically reliable on their own. Multinucleate forms with bizarre or horseshoe-shaped nuclei are sometimes numerous too, and they may attain a very large size (Fig. 9.4). Exceptionally, all the SR cells are of small size and they then become much more difficult to find. Frequently, a minority of the SR cells have much denser nuclear chromatin, obscuring the nucleoli, and an intensely stained, eosinophilic and pyroninophilic cytoplasm (Fig. 9.2b). All these variants of the 'classical' SR cell, with the exception of the mononuclear type, are, in the right cellular setting, diagnostic of Hodgkin's disease.

Two other variant types of SR cell are characteristic of specific histological types of HD: these are the 'lacunar cell' of nodular sclerosis and the so-called 'L & H' type, which is found in lymphocytic predominance. SR cells of classical type are also found in these forms of HD, but they may

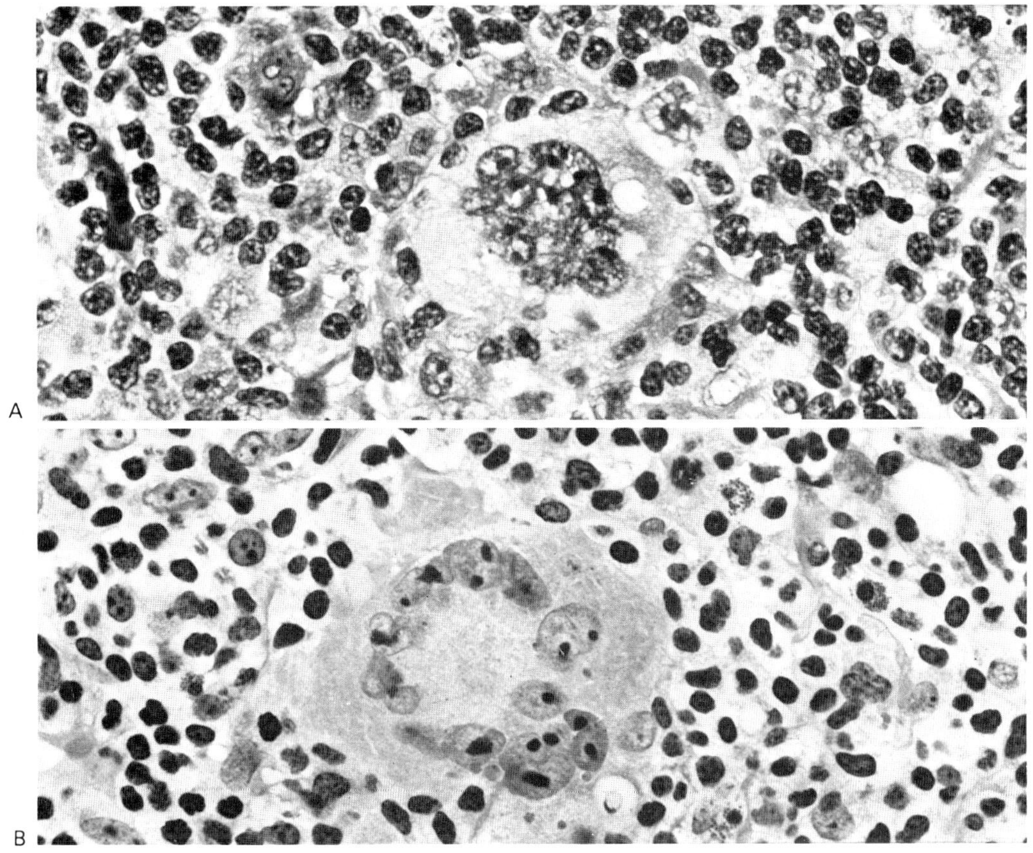

Fig. 9.4 Bizarre giant forms of S-R cell. Such cells are most characteristic of nodular sclerosing Hodgkin's disease. (a) paraffin embedding, (b) resin embedding. (Both H E × 600)

be very scanty. The *lacunar cell* (Fig. 9.2e and f) is so named because imperfect fixation commonly leads to shrinkage of the voluminous, pale staining cytoplasm, leaving a clear halo around the cell which then appears as if suspended in any empty lacuna. The multilobed nucleus often shrinks too and may then appear pyknotic, but when better fixed it is seen to have one or more *basophilic* nucleoli, of smaller size than the nucleoli of the classical SR cell. Imperfect fixation is of course particularly liable to occur in nodular sclerosis, because the thick fibrous capsule of the node and coarse fibrous septa delay penetration of the fixative, unless the node has been sliced before being placed in fixative solution.

The *L & H variant* of the SR cell (Fig. 9.2c and d) is again quite different. These cells vary considerably in size, but are characterised by a large, multilobed nucleus in which the contorted, overlapping lobes have been likened to popcorn by American authors. The nuclear chromatin is finely dispersed and there are one or more *basophilic* nucleoli. The latter are sometimes quite large, but they do not stand out like the nucleoli of the classical SR cell, because they are seldom surrounded by a clear halo. For this reason cells of this type are much less conspicuous than SR cells of classical type and often need the high power of the microscope for their identification.

THE HISTOLOGICAL TYPING OF HODGKIN'S DISEASE

Although the Rye classification distinguishes only four types, there are sufficient histological differences between the two forms of lymphocytic predominance and the two forms of lymphocytic depletion to warrant separate descriptions and thus to adhere to the original Lukes' classification (Lukes, 1963; Lukes & Butler, 1966) in this account. The differential diagnosis will be considered with each type in turn.

Lymphocytic predominance (LP) — nodular type

Synonym:
Lukes' lymphocytic and/or histiocytic (L & H) — nodular

Replacement of the node is often total, but a remnant of uninvolved node may remain as a compressed rim at the periphery (Fig. 9.5). The normal structure is supplanted by a solid mass of lymphocytes with a distinctly nodular arrangement, obliterating the normal follicles and sinuses and often producing considerable enlargement of the node. Closer examination discloses the presence within the nodules of a scattered population of much larger cells with multilobed nuclei and relatively abundant pale staining cytoplasm (Fig. 9.6). These are the 'L & H' type of Sternberg-Reed cell and it may be observed that most of the mitotic activity is in these larger cells. Cells of this type may be scanty or quite numerous, but 'classical' SR cells, when found at all, are always very scarce. Sometimes large reactive macrophages with relatively smaller nuclei and eosinophilic cytoplasm are conspicuous, but their numbers vary from case to case. Such macrophages are occasionally numerous and may be binucleate but they are readily distinguishable from SR cells. At other times, small, localised clusters of epithelioid cells are seen and these tiny granulomas may be seen in a ring formation around the lymphocytic

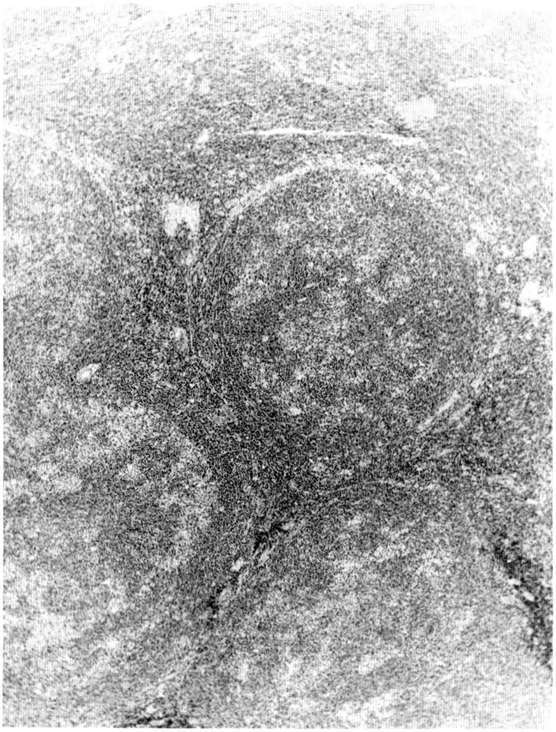

Fig. 9.5 Cervical lymph node biopsy in Hodgkin's disease of nodular lymphocyte predominant type. A rim of compressed uninvolved node is seen above. (H E × 47)

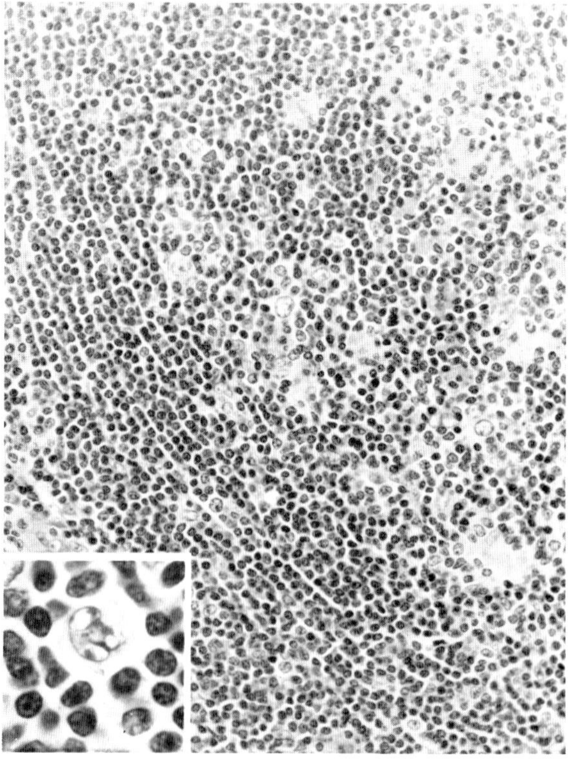

Fig. 9.6 Same node as Fig. 9.5 at a higher magnification to show margin of nodule in nodular L P Hodgkin's disease. Some of the larger, pale cells in the nodule are histiocytes. Inset: L and H type Sternberg-Reed cell from the same node. (H E main figure × 300, inset × 940)

nodules in those cases where the lesion appears to be evolving from 'progressively transformed germinal centres' (see below and Fig. 6.13, p. 94). In the *nodular* form of LP Hodgkin's disease, lymphocytes are always the predominant cell and

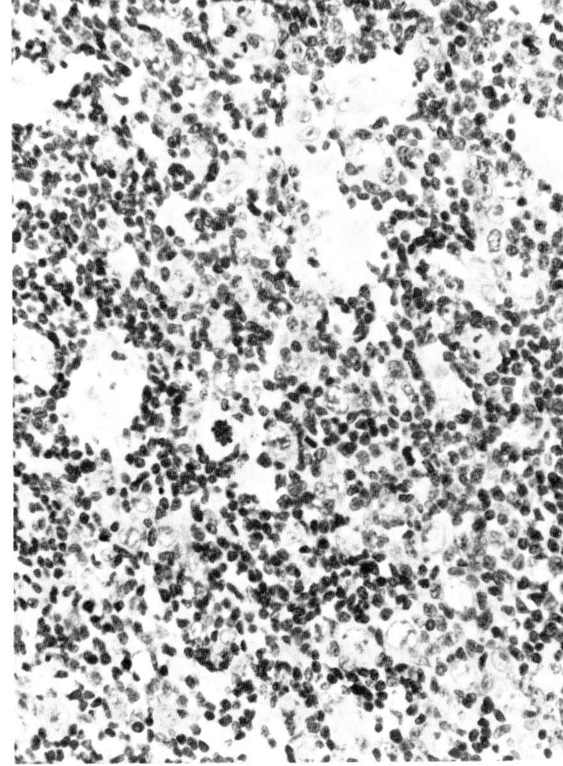

Fig. 9.7 Lymph node from another case of nodular L P Hodgkin's disease showing a larger number of 'blast' type cells and mitoses. There are also large macrophages, but classical S-R cells are not seen. The borderline between lymphocyte predominant and mixed cellularity HD is not sharp. (H E × 300)

one never sees the picture of histiocytic predominance which, at times, characterises the *diffuse* variety. Necrosis and eosinophils are lacking whilst plasma cells are few or absent. Occasionally hyaline deposits containing variable amounts of collagen may be seen, but true fibrosis is absent.

The picture described above may be found in nodes which are known to have been enlarged for months or even years, but as time passes, the number of SR cells tends slowly to increase (Fig. 9.7) and cells of 'classical' type may then appear.

Evolution of LP nodular Hodgkin's disease from progressively transformed germinal centres

Poppema et al (1979) pointed out that this form of Hodgkin's disease which they termed 'Nodular paragranuloma' may appear to evolve from 'progressive transformation' of germinal centres in nodes showing persistent follicular hyperplasia (see p. 91) and we have ourselves observed this sequence on a number of occasions. Since reactive germinal centres may apparently undergo 'progressive transformation' without the subsequent evolution of 'nodular paragranuloma', it is difficult to know precisely what the relationship is between the two lesions, but one conclusion may be drawn — whenever progressively transformed germinal centres are seen in a lymph node biopsy, a careful search for Sternberg-Reed cells of L & H type is mandatory. These cells should be looked for in the lymphoid nodules resulting from the 'transformation' process.

Differential diagnosis. Since reactive germinal follicles are often present in this, as in other types of HD, it is important not to confuse nodular LP HD with a simple reactive node. The problem is only likely to arise in the type of node discussed above, i.e. a node showing progressively transformed germinal centres. In the more fully developed lesion, the nodularity of the process and associated loss of normal architecture will be obvious.

The most frequently encountered difficulty lies in distinguishing nodular LP Hodgkin's disease from follicular lymphoma (ML Cb-Cc follicular). Reticulin staining in both conditions shows a paucity of fibres within the nodules and often condensation of fibres around them, but in HD the nodules tend to be larger and closer together whilst their constituent cells are predominantly lymphocytes, not centrocytes. Typical L & H cells are of course only found in HD. The distinction is further discussed in Chapter 10 (p. 273).

Lymphocytic predominance (LP) — diffuse type

Synonym:
Lukes' lymphocytic and/or histiocytic (L & H) — diffuse

Replacement of the node is more often total in this

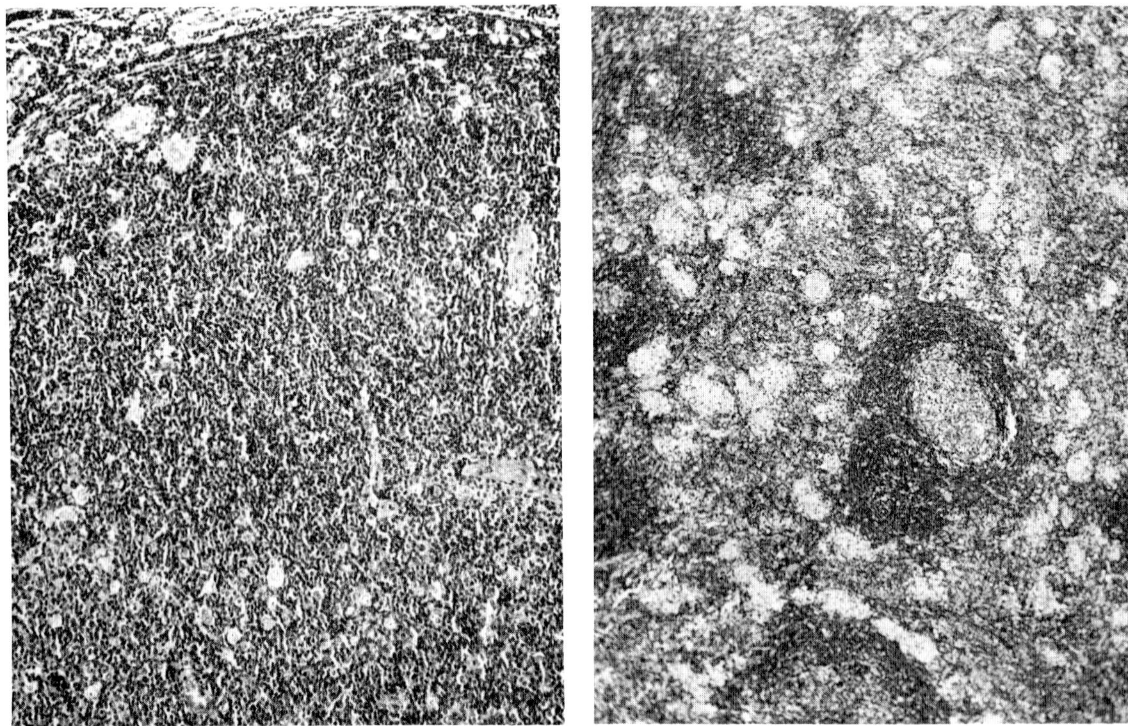

Fig. 9.8 Lymph node in diffuse L P Hodgkin's disease. A patternless sheet of small lymphocytes replaces the normal structure and infiltrates through the capsule (top). Only the presence of scattered, large, pale S-R cells distinguishes this picture from that of a lymphocytic lymphoma. (H E × 120)

Fig. 9.9 Lymphocyte predominant Hodgkin's disease of diffuse type with an abundance of epithelioid cells, forming small clusters like those of toxoplasmosis. Although reactive follicles are present, these do not show the degree of hyperplasia regularly seen in toxoplasmic lymphadenitis, (compare Fig. 6.49, p. 116). (H E × 47)

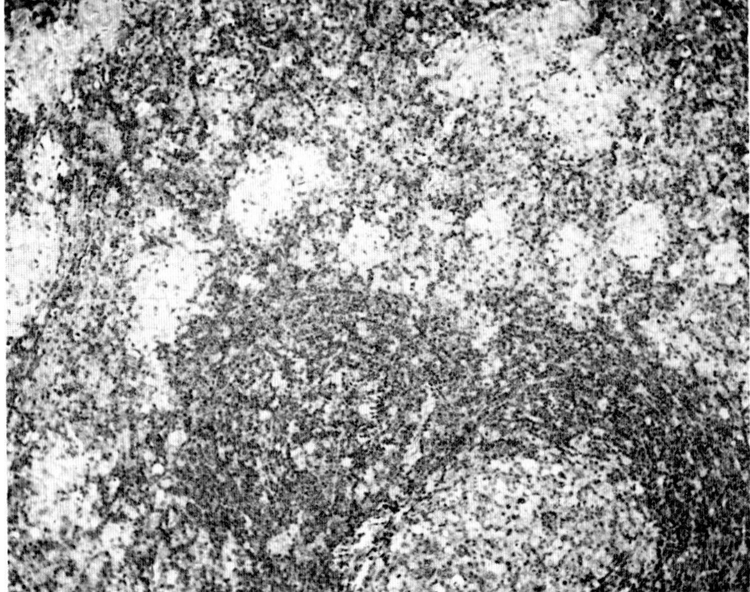

Fig. 9.10 Higher magnification of same node as Fig. 9.9 showing a germinal follicle (top right) (H E × 120)

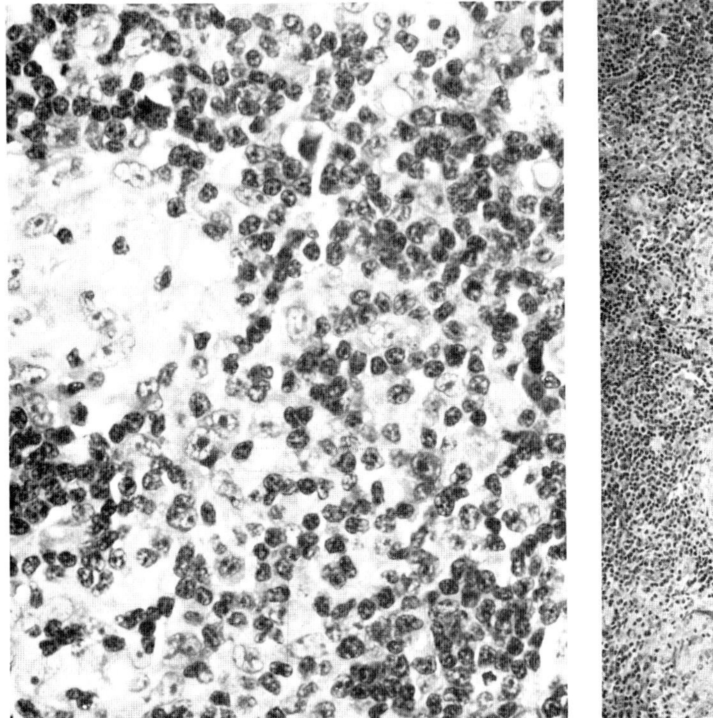

Fig. 9.11 Same node as Figs 9.9 and 9.10 showing a Sternberg-Reed cell of classical type close to a collection of epithelioid cells (left) and a Hodgkin's cell to the right (H E × 470)

Fig. 9.12 Hodgkin's disease of lymphocyte predominant type in which multiple, sharply-defined granulomas are associated with the disease in the node (H E × 120)

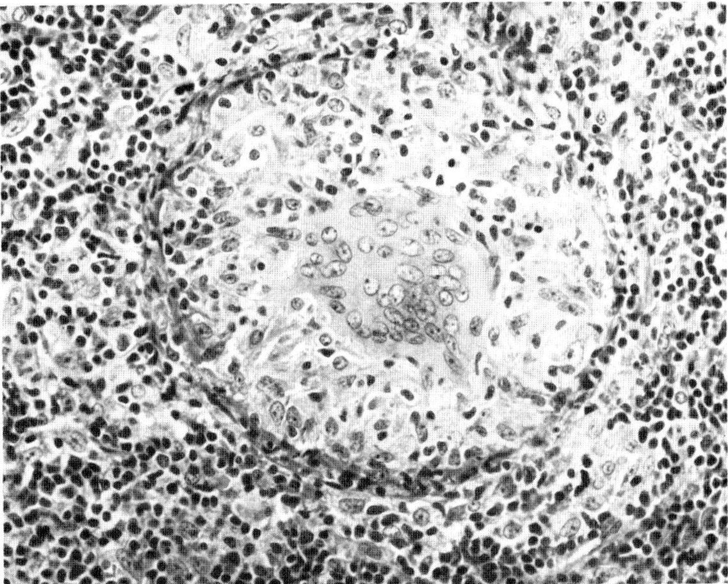

Fig. 9.13 Same node as Fig. 9.12 showing a tuberculoid granuloma at a higher magnification. No evidence of tuberculosis was found in this case. (H E × 300)

variety, although some germinal follicles may remain, as indicated above. The pattern is otherwise diffuse or, at most, only vaguely nodular, and when the nodal architecture is effaced by a diffuse sheet of lymphocytes with infiltration also of the node capsule, the picture may readily be mistaken for that of a 'lymphosarcoma', if the scattered Sternberg-Reed cells are overlooked (Fig. 9.8).

The cellular composition of the infiltrate is more variable than in the nodular type. As a rule, lymphocytes predominate, but histiocytes or epithelioid cells may be very numerous, sometimes forming small clusters resembling those of toxoplasmosis (Figs 9.9, 9.10, 9.11) and sometimes extensive granulomatous areas which may mimic sarcoidosis or tuberculosis very closely (Figs 9.12, 9.13). It is often necessary to search carefully for SR cells which are generally scanty and may lie concealed amongst the epithelioid cells (Fig. 9.11). SR cells of classical type are, however, more often found than in nodular LP HD. At times the epithelioid cells have plump nuclei and conspicuous nucleoli and one may have the impression that they are evolving into SR cells. Small foci of necrosis are occasionally seen in granulomatous areas, heightening the resemblance to tuberculosis. Eosinophils may be present and may even be quite numerous, but neutrophils are generally absent. A few plasma cells may also be seen. As the disease progresses, SR cells and their variants become increasingly numerous and the picture then begins to merge into that of mixed-cellularity HD.

Differential diagnosis. In those examples which are characterised by diffuse lymphocytic proliferation the picture has to be distinguished from that of a lymphocytic lymphoma, but close examination will reveal the presence of SR cells which may be either of the L & H type or the classical type. Positive identification of such cells will clinch the diagnosis of LP HD.

When histiocytes predominate or are a conspicuous feature, it is necessary to distinguish the picture from that of toxoplasmosis, sarcoidosis or tuberculosis, as mentioned above. Once again, the diagnosis of HD rests upon the finding of SR cells, as the mimicry is sometimes quite close. Tuberculosis may of course co-exist with Hodgkin's disease, though the association is less common today than formerly.

Nodular sclerosis (NS)

This is the commonest type of Hodgkin's disease in the Western world, but the relative incidence of the different types seems to vary in different parts of the world (Correa & O'Conor, 1973). As it is understood today, nodular sclerosing Hodgkin's disease differs somewhat from the original concept of nodular sclerosis as envisaged by Smetana & Cohen (1956), the definition today being more broadly based. According to Lukes (1971), the picture is characterised by three features: (1) nodularity, (2) banded sclerosis, and (3) the presence of lacunar cells. Although it is not necessary for all three to be present in order to make this diagnosis, at least two of the features should be seen.

In classical NS the *nodularity* of the process is obvious for the involved node is split up into cellu-

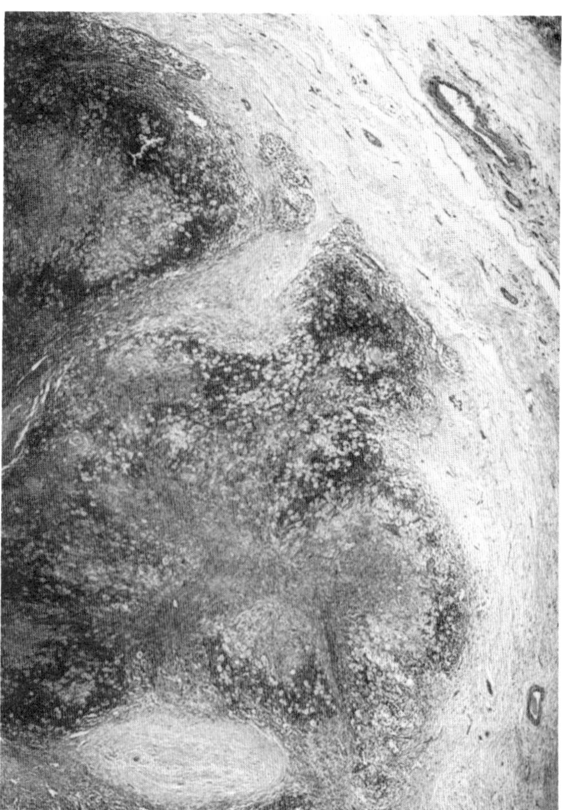

Fig. 9.14 Nodular sclerosing Hodgkin's disease. Segment of node showing gross capsular thickening with collagen bands extending into and subdividing the node. Even at this low magnification individual lacunar cells can be seen around foci of necrosis. (H E × 18)

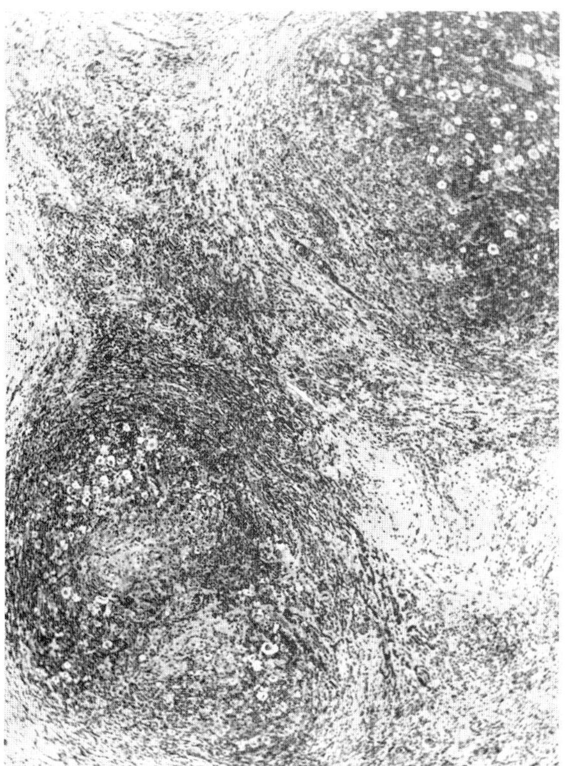

Fig. 9.15 Another case of nodular sclerosis. Lacunar cells can be distinctly seen within the cellular nodules. (H E × 47)

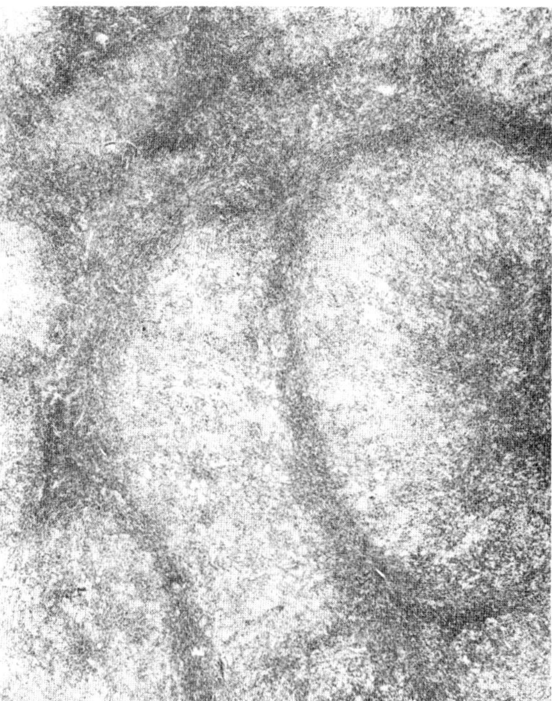

Fig. 9.16 'Cellular phase' of nodular sclerosing Hodgkin's disease showing nodules without sclerosis. An earlier biopsy from this patient showed the typical features of nodular sclerosis. The lacunar cell phenomenon is not seen because of better fixation. (H E × 18)

lar compartments or nodules by broad bands of fibrous tissue (Figs 9.14, 9.15) but the nodularity is also observable in cases where fibrosis is minimal or absent — the so-called 'cellular phase' of NS (Lukes et al, 1966; Kadin et al, 1971) (Fig. 9.16).

The degree of *sclerosis* varies widely, not only from case to case, but within the nodes of a single patient. At one extreme, dense collagenous fibrosis may replace the greater part of the node, leaving only small isolated nodules of cellular tissue. At the opposite extreme, fibrosis may be confined to collagenous thickening of the node capsule and perhaps one or two slender bands of fibrous tissue passing for a short distance into the node from the capsule. Concentric 'onion-peel' rings of collagen round small arteries are a commonly observed and useful sign in cases where fibrosis is otherwise slight (Fig. 9.17). The essential feature of the sclerosis in NS is that the collagen is laid down in parallel bundles, so that it appears birefringent when viewed with polarised light. This property distinguishes this type of fibrosis from the irregular fibre deposition seen in the diffuse fibrosis type of HD.

Lacunar cells (Fig. 9.18) have already been described on pages 202–3. Whilst SR cells of this type are particularly characteristic of nodular sclerosis, they are not entirely confined to NS and may be seen, generally in smaller numbers, in mixed cellularity HD (Marshall et al, 1976). In classical cases of NS with septate fibrosis of the node, lacunar cells are often plentiful and may be picked out readily under the low power of the microscope. They often tend to congregate together in the centres of the tumour nodules, which helps to define the individual nodules in the 'cellular phase' of NS.

Not only is there great variability in the degree of sclerosis in NS, but the cell picture is equally variable. Despite this, the process is generally eas-

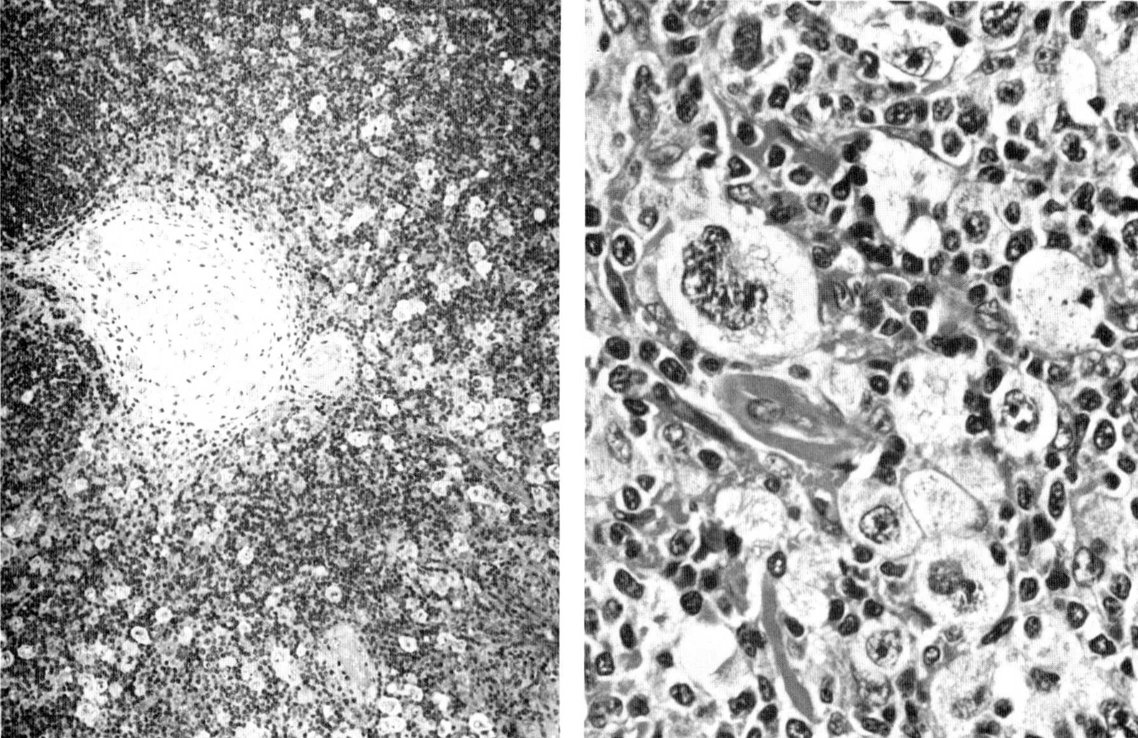

Fig. 9.17 Concentric periarterial fibrosis in nodular sclerosing Hodgkin's disease. The node capsule was also thickened and the consequent delayed fixation accounts for the clear definition of the lacunar cells. (H E × 120)

Fig. 9.18 Lacunar cells in nodular sclerosing Hodgkin's disease. Note strands of hyaline collagen within the cellular nodule and outlining a capillary. (H E × 600)

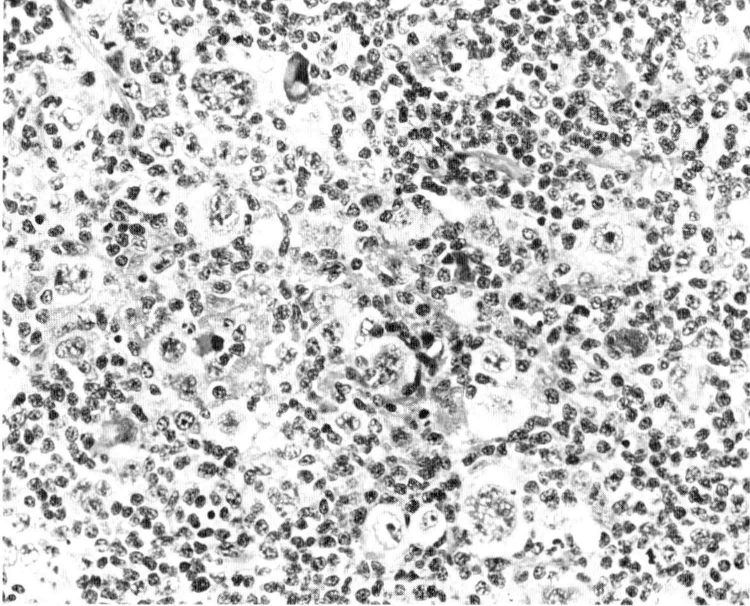

Fig. 9.19 Nodular sclerosing Hodgkin's disease. Many variants of the Sternberg-Reed cell may be seen in this field and most have copious cytoplasm. (H E × 300)

ily recognised as Hodgkin's disease. The large, lacunar cells stand out conspicuously and classical SR cells are commonly found too, whilst sometimes there are bizarre multinucleate variants of giant size (Fig. 9.19). Although cellular pleomorphism of the SR cells is the rule, one is occasionally struck by the monomorphism of these cells and when they are predominantly of mononuclear type, and arranged in solid clusters, confusion with secondary carcinoma or melanoma may occur (Fig. 9.20).

Necrosis is very common (Fig. 9.21) and varies from necrosis of individual SR cells to massive necrosis of almost the entire node. Solid clusters of lacunar cells are particularly liable to undergo necrosis and when this is accompanied, as it often is, by heavy polymorph infiltration, the lesions may be mistaken for abscesses and the true nature of the process may be overlooked (Fig. 9.22). It is worthy of note that nodular sclerosing HD may provoke an inflammatory response in the affected tissues, which is independent of the extent or even the presence of necrosis. There may sometimes be significant periadenitis around affected nodes, accompanied by fibrinous exudation (Fig. 9.23, p. 212).

The background population of cells in NS shows as much variation as the SR cells themselves. At one end of this spectrum, there is a preponderance of lymphocytes, amongst which scattered lacunar cells may be seen. At the other end, solid masses of lacunar cells may have all but supplanted the lymphocyte population. Plasma cells are frequently numerous, especially at the margin of the nodules and often in adjacent, uninvolved nodes. Eosinophils are generally found too, sometimes in huge numbers. Heavy tissue eosinophilia may be found, both with (Fig. 9.24) and without extensive necrosis in the nodes. Although considerable numbers of histiocytes and 'indeterminate' cells may

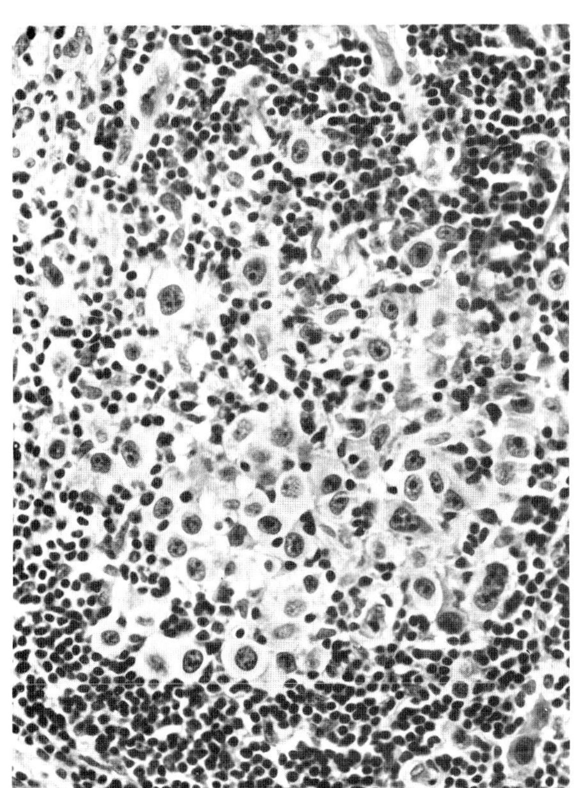

Fig. 9.20 A cluster of rather uniform lacunar cells in another case of nodular sclerosing HD. Solid clusters like this may be mistaken for secondary carcinoma. (H E × 300)

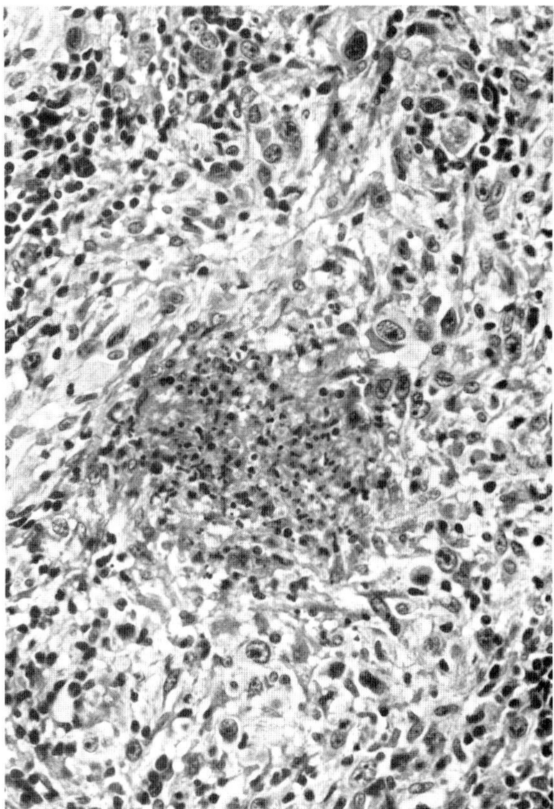

Fig. 9.21 A small focus of necrosis in the centre of a cluster of lacunar cells and spindle cells in nodular sclerosing HD (H E × 300)

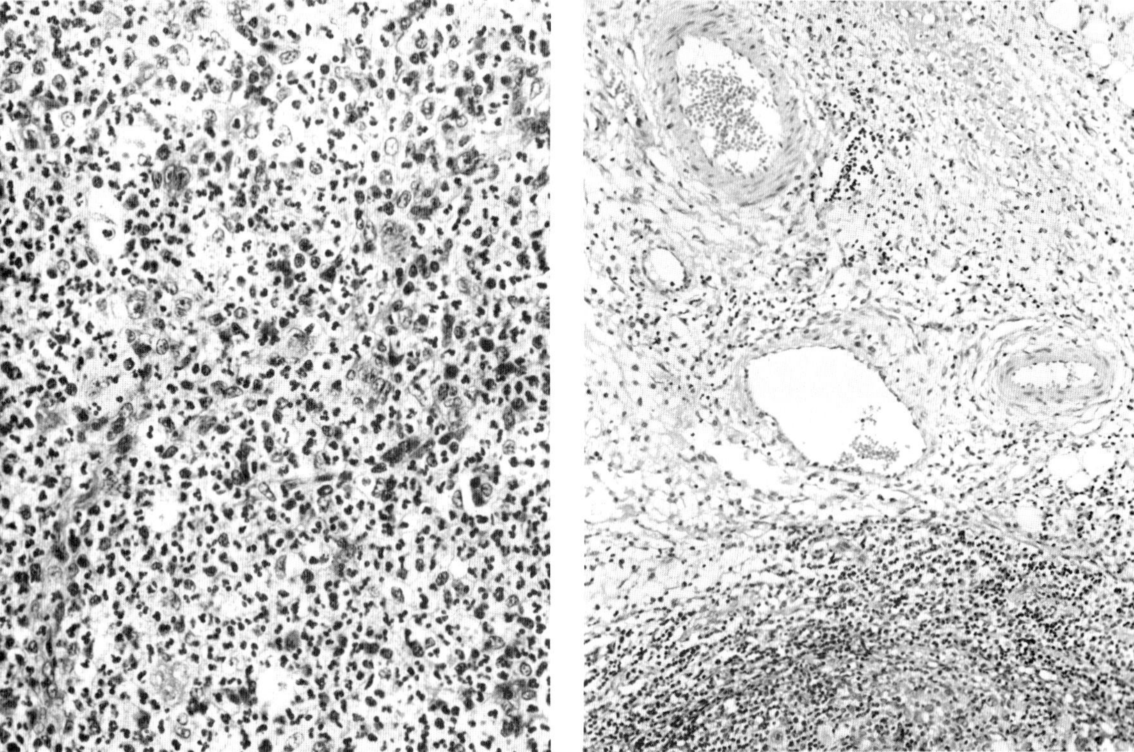

Fig. 9.22 Extensive necrosis with heavy polymorph infiltration in nodular sclerosing HD. Such lesions may be mistaken for abscesses if the occasional Sternberg-Reed cells (upper left) are overlooked. (H E × 300)

Fig. 9.23 Periadenitis with fibrinous exudation around a lymph node containing Hodgkin's disease of nodular sclerosing type. This may result in fixation and matting of nodes. (H E × 120)

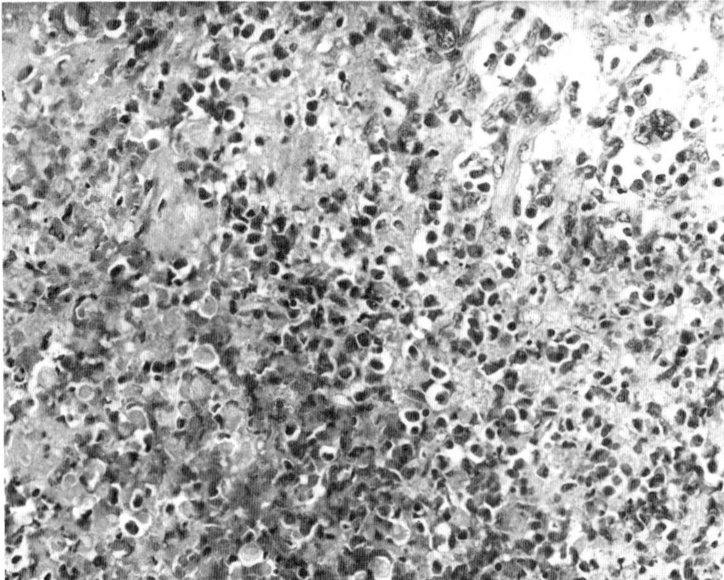

Fig. 9.24 Massive eosinophil infiltration with eosinophilic necrosis (below) in nodular sclerosing HD. With the exception of a solitary Sternberg-Reed cell (top right) practically all the cells in this field are eosinophils. (H E × 300)

sometimes be found within the affected nodes, these cells tend to mingle with the SR cells and seldom form discrete granulomatous foci as they do in diffuse LP HD.

Progression of lesion in NS and relation to stage of disease

Unlike the other types of HD, in nodular sclerosis there is very little relationship between the histological changes and the stage of the disease. In other words, prediction of the stage of advancement of the disease from the histological picture is quite unreliable and once a diagnosis of nodular sclerosing HD is established by biopsy, more reliance must be placed on the clinical and pathological stage of the disease than upon the relative proportions of lymphocytes and Sternberg-Reed cells in the biopsy in assessing prognosis. Only when the histological picture approaches one or other extreme of the wide range of appearances in nodular sclerosis do the changes give a fair indication of prognosis.

It was at one time assumed that the sclerosing process was progressive and that the 'cellular phase', as it has since come to be called, represented 'early' Hodgkin's disease, while advanced sclerosis represented 'late' HD. This, too, is now known to be untrue and an 'early' biopsy is just as likely to show sclerosis as a 'late' biopsy is to show the cellular phase.

Differential diagnosis. The possibilities of confusion of NS with suppurative lymphadenitis or with metastatic carcinoma and melanoma have already been mentioned. In those cases characterised by heavy eosinophilia, it is important not to mistake HD for benign lesions such as eosinophilic lymphadenitis and eosinophilic granuloma (see discussion of differential diagnosis of HD MC on p. 214).

Nodular sclerosis in the cellular phase is sometimes mistaken for HD LP nodular. Both show a nodular pattern, but typically the SR cells in NS are of lacunar type — larger and with more voluminous cytoplasm than L & H type cells. Furthermore, they tend to congregate at the centres of the neoplastic nodules, in a way which is seldom seen in nodular LP HD.

Mixed cellularity (MC) Hodgkin's disease

The histological picture here is often described as 'classical Hodgkin's disease'. The process is diffuse rather than nodular and typically the whole or the greater part of the node is involved, although remnants of reactive follicles may still be seen, especially in younger patients (Figs 9.1, 9.25). The cellular infiltrate is characterised by its

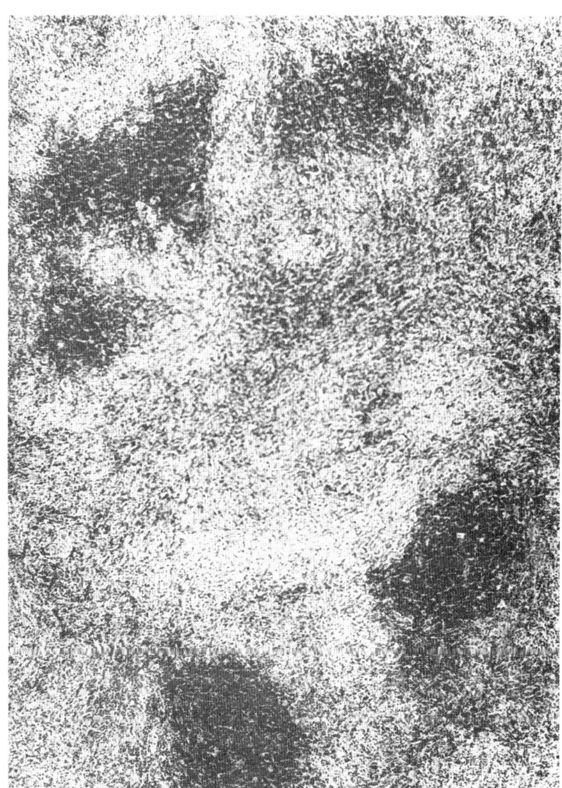

Fig. 9.25 Mixed cellularity Hodgkin's disease in an adult showing some residual collections of lymphocytes (without germinal centres) despite advanced infiltration of the node. H E × 47)

polymorphism. The lymphocyte population is noticeably diminished and there is a corresponding increase of Sternberg-Reed cells and their mononuclear variants, amongst which mitoses, sometimes of atypical form, are readily found. Histiocytes may be conspicuous, especially in those cases which have evolved from a previous granulomatous stage (Fig. 9.26) and the distinction

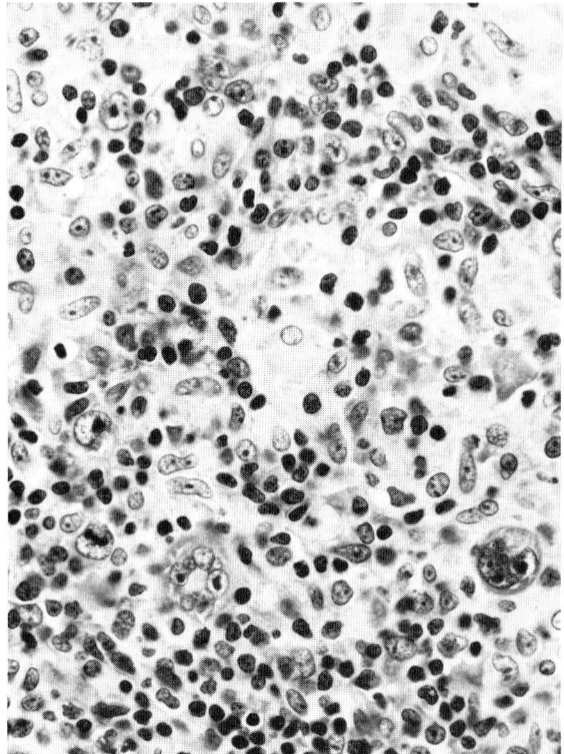

Fig. 9.26 Mixed cellularity HD showing a diversity of cell types with two S-R cells (lower field) and several Hodgkin's cells. The abundant histiocytes suggest that this may have evolved from a previous L and H stage. (H E × 470)

from LP HD of diffuse type is not sharp, being based chiefly on the number of SR cells present. In addition, there are often numerous histiocyte-like cells of indeterminate type (Fig. 9.27). The SR and Hodgkin's cells are scattered indiscriminately amongst the other cellular elements and do not form solid clusters as they often do in nodular sclerosis. They are seen against a background of eosinophils and plasma cells, either of which may be very numerous or relatively scarce. The latter tend to congregate towards the periphery of the lesions whilst eosinophils mingle with the neoplastic cells. Neutrophils are seen chiefly in relation to foci of necrosis, which are often present although frequently small.

Differential diagnosis. The diagnosis in MC HD is generally easy, as the conspicuous SR cells and polymorphic cell picture catch the eye. Where eosinophils are very numerous, the picture must be distinguished from that of eosinophilic lymphadenitis (p. 88) and eosinophil granuloma (Histiocytosis X) (p. 363). Occasional examples of NHL — especially ML lymphoplasmacytoid and ML immunoblastic may show a comparable degree of cellular polymorphism and rare examples of the latter (especially in the gastrointestinal tract) may be associated with a striking eosinophilia, but the demonstration of *typical* SR cells will usually make the diagnosis clear. Sternberg-Reed-like cells may also be seen sometimes in metastatic renal carcinoma or other neoplasms, but confusion is only likely to arise if there is an associated eosinophilia. Perhaps the greatest difficulty is encountered in distinguishing MC HD from immunoblastic (angioimmunoblastic) lymphadenopathy, in which a comparable degree of cellular polymorphism may be found with occasional SR-like cells and bizarre plasma cells which may be confused with SR cells (see p. 183).

Pathologists often find difficulty in deciding between mixed cellularity and nodular sclerosis in

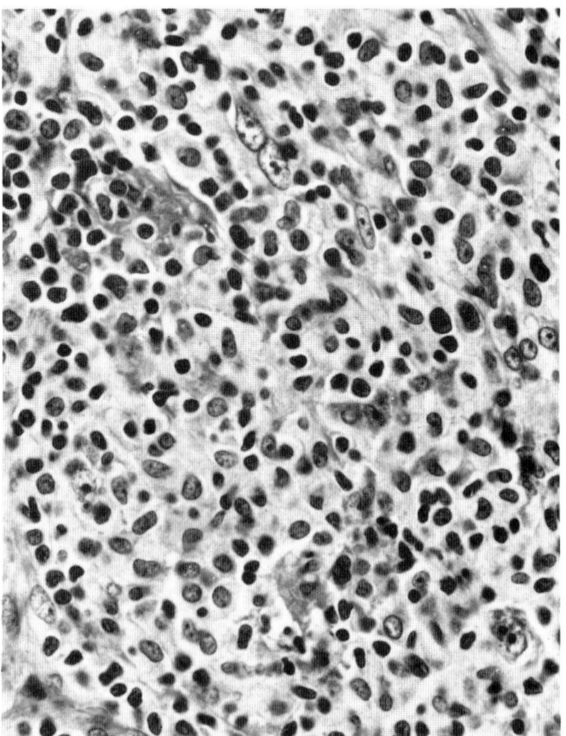

Fig. 9.27 Another case of M C Hodgkin's disease showing a Sternberg-Reed cell (bottom right) and many 'indeterminate' cells. Lymphocytes are markedly reduced in number. (H E × 470)

those cases of Hodgkin's disease where neither nodularity nor sclerosis is an outspoken feature and where the cell picture is 'mixed'. With increasing experience, it will be found that more cases will be put into the nodular sclerosis category and fewer into mixed cellularity, but there will remain some instances which are a matter of personal judgement (see Neiman, 1978).

Lymphocytic depletion (LD) — Lukes' diffuse fibrosis type (DF)

Just as the histological picture of lymphocyte predominance corresponds very largely to early, Stage I, Hodgkin's disease, so, conversely, lymphocyte depletion is generally found in advanced, Stage III or IV disease. Patients presenting this picture almost invariably have 'B' symptoms and often show evidence of immune paresis. The lymphocyte count in the peripheral blood is reduced.

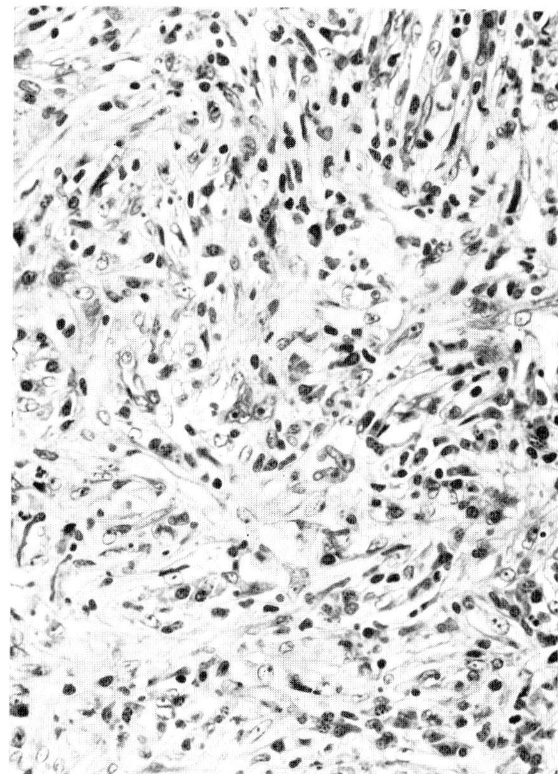

Fig. 9.28 Lymphocytic depletion Hodgkin's disease of diffuse fibrosis type. The normal structure is replaced by a sheet of haphazardly arranged spindle-cells and capillaries, with some plasma cells, eosinophils and scattered Sternberg-Reed cells. (H E × 300)

In the biopsy section, no trace of the original node structure remains; follicles have by now disappeared and sinuses are obliterated, indeed it may be difficult to recognise from the histological appearances that this has ever been a lymph node (Fig. 9.28). A diffuse or vaguely nodular mass of haphazardly arranged, pale-staining, spindle cells makes up the bulk of the tissue and against this background, scattered, often bizarre, giant-cells are seen, which may be recognisable as SR cells although they commonly show nuclear hyperchromatism. Atypical mitoses are frequently present. Lymphocytes are thinly scattered amongst the spindle cells, along with eosinophils and a few plasma cells. Areas of necrosis are often present, but these generally evoke no reaction.

The palely stained appearance of such a node is due not only to the dearth of lymphocytes, but to a general cellular depletion accompanied by a diffuse increase of fine, argyrophilic, intercellular fibres and amorphous proteinaceous material. As Lukes recognised (Lukes, 1963), the picture of a disorderly, fine fibrosis, revealed by silver staining, is quite different from the septate fibrosis seen in nodular sclerosis (Fig. 9.29). Very little of the fibre stains pink with Van Gieson's stain and there is no birefringence when the section is viewed by polarised light.

Differential diagnosis. The diagnosis of HD may already be known or at least suspected by the time the patient presents with advanced disease of this type. However, even when there is no prior knowledge, the picture is so distinctive that the pathologist will seldom have any difficulty in making the correct diagnosis. The bizarre giant cells and mitotic activity immediately suggest a neoplasm and the only other neoplasm for which this is likely to be mistaken is a malignant fibrous histiocytoma.

Treatment of Hodgkin's disease by radiotherapy or chemotherapy results in a histological picture of cell depletion, but this differs from the picture of DF. In treated HD, areas formerly occupied by neoplastic tissue are replaced by almost acellular, eosinophilic, hyaline material, whilst any parts of the node which had not been infiltrated still show a more or less normal structure (Fig. 9.30).

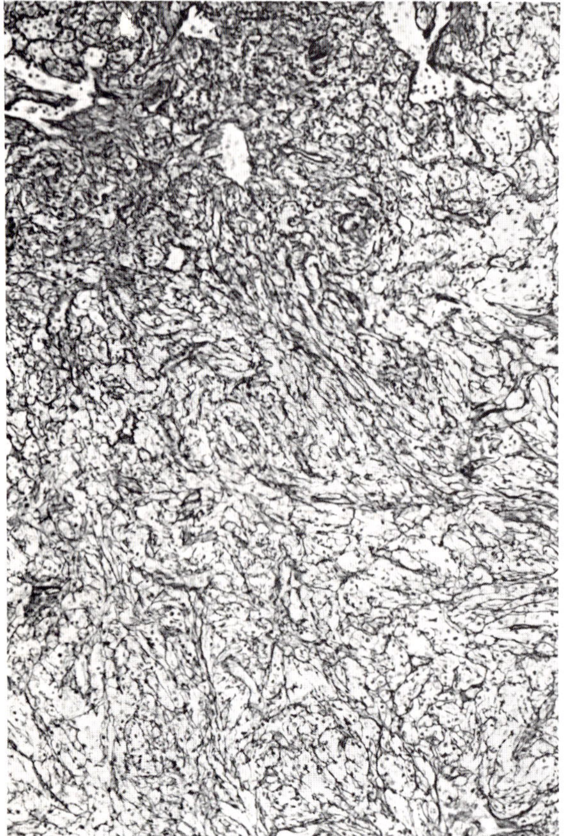

Fig. 9.29 L D Hodgkin's disease of diffuse fibrosis type. Node from another case showing the disorderly fine fibrosis which characterises this form of the disease. (Gordon and Sweets reticulin × 120)

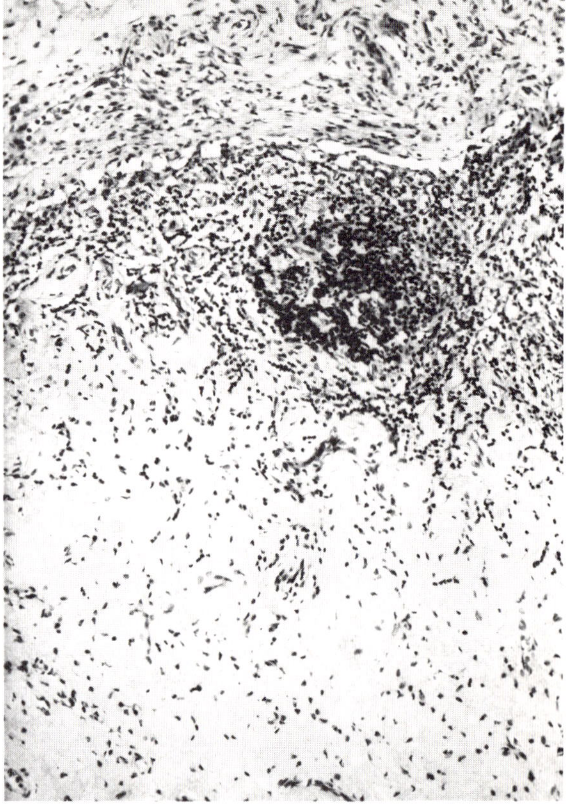

Fig. 9.30 Lymph node previously occupied by Hodgkin's disease after effective therapy. Involved areas of the node show cellular depletion and replacement by hyaline material whilst an uninvolved follicle remains. The picture is quite distinct from that of untreated L D Hodgkin's disease (compare with Fig. 9.28). (H E × 120)

Lymphocytic depletion (LD) — Lukes' reticular type (RT)

As with HD DF, this type generally corresponds to advanced disease with 'B' symptoms. It occurs chiefly in older subjects. In the affected lymph nodes, there is again total loss of normal architectural features, with severe lymphocyte depletion, but instead of overall cell depletion and fibrosis there is massive infiltration by pleomorphic Sternberg-Reed cells and mononuclear 'blast' cells, showing a high mitotic rate (Fig. 9.31). Many of the tumour giant-cells are very atypical and classical Sternberg-Reed cells may be hard to find. This uncommon picture corresponds to the 'Hodgkin's Sarcoma' of Jackson & Parker (1944). Necrosis is commonly seen and there may be infiltration of the tumour by eosinophils and neutrophils, as well as large macrophages. Other parts of the node may still show traces of unmistakeable Hodgkin's disease with areas of fibrosis which help to confirm the diagnosis (see below). Indeed, although the picture described above may be seen in 'pure' form, on other occasions one sees examples of lymphocyte depletion which are intermediate between the diffuse fibrosis and the reticular types.

Differential diagnosis. The differential diagnosis between HD of reticular type and ML immunoblastic of pleomorphic type is often difficult, and it may be impossible to reach a firm decision based on morphology alone. As mentioned above, Sternberg-Reed cells in this stage of HD are often

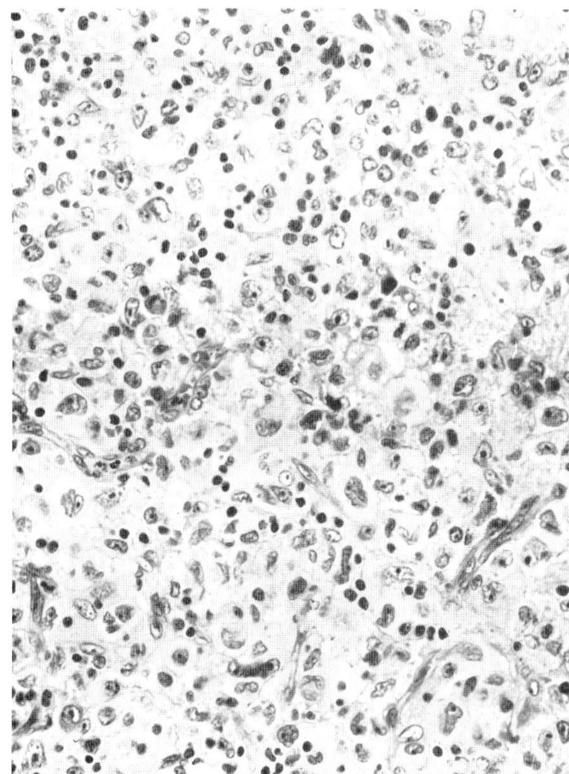

Fig. 9.31 Lymphocytic depletion Hodgkin's disease of reticular type. The picture corresponds to that of 'Hodgkin's sarcoma', showing a pleomorphic cellular neoplasm with many Hodgkin's and Sternberg-Reed type cells. (H E × 300)

highly atypical and besides this, neoplastic giant-cells of this type are not peculiar to HD. One may be tempted to make a diagnosis of 'Hodgkin's sarcoma' in a lymphoreticular neoplasm showing extreme pleomorphism. But it should be remembered that some peripheral T cell lymphomas may be equally pleomorphic (see p. 323) and it is probably only justifiable to diagnose of LD Hodgkin's disease of reticular type in cases where clear evidence of Hodgkin's disease is seen alongside the pleomorphic neoplasm or where an earlier biopsy has shown unequivocal Hodgkin's disease (but see discussion below).

Progression of histological changes

As already indicated, nodular sclerosis does not usually show the same evolutionary sequence as is observed in other types of Hodgkin's disease. In the latter, the direction of change is always the same, viz: lymphocytic predominance → mixed cellularity → lymphocytic depletion — never the reverse, although of course the initial lymph node biopsy in any given patient may show MC or even LD disease. Thus not every patient shows evidence of having passed through a stage of lymphocytic predominance and, likewise, the rate of progression of the disease is very variable, being very slow, as a rule, in those whose initial biopsy shows the changes of LP nodular disease (Figs 9.32, 9.33). As Lukes (1963) pointed out, there is good correlation between histological picture and clinical stage in all types of HD, except nodular sclerosis. LP, especially the nodular variety, corresponds often to Stage I HD, whilst MC and especially LD are usually found in Stages III and IV.

In contrast to the gradual evolutionary process outlined above, there is occasionally evidence of a

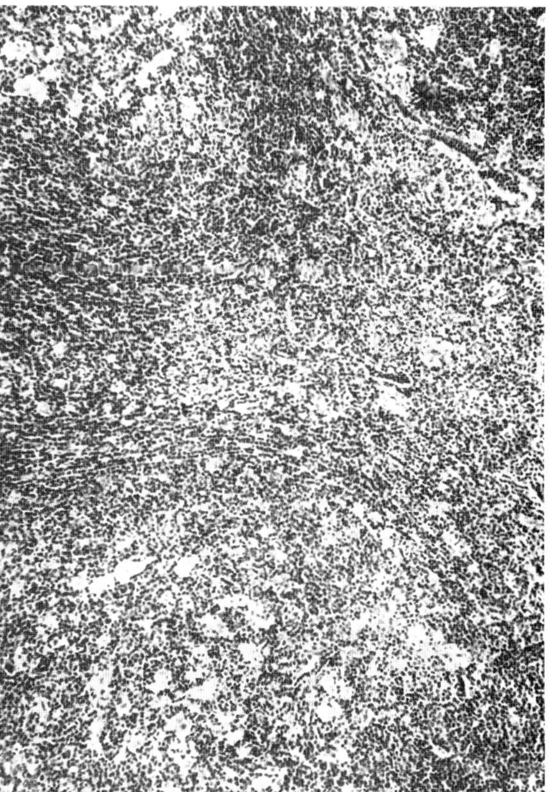

Fig. 9.32 Cervical lymph node biopsy from a young man showing L P Hodgkin's disease of nodular type. He was treated by radiotherapy on a 250 Kv machine and the disease remitted (see Fig. 9.33). (H E × 120)

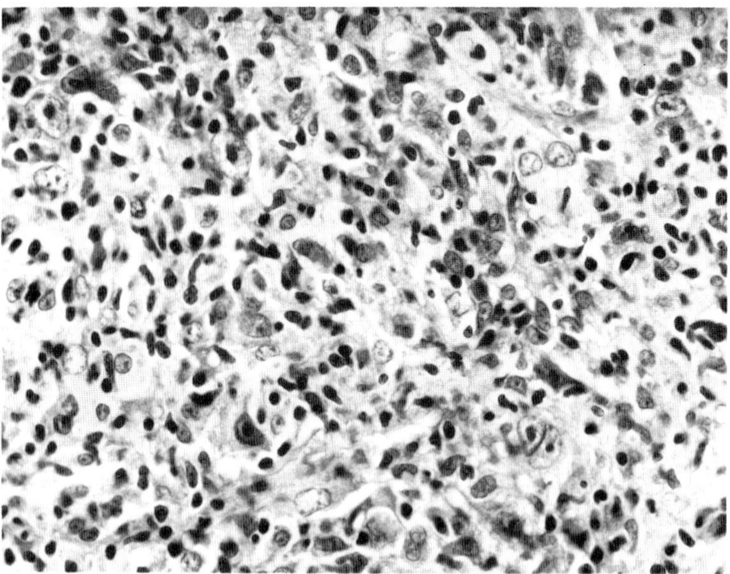

Fig. 9.33 Inguinal node biopsy from the same man as in Fig. 9.32 but 23 years later, showing lymphocytic depletion Hodgkin's disease of reticular type. Although the length of this disease-free interval is remarkable, the sequence is not unusual. (H E × 470)

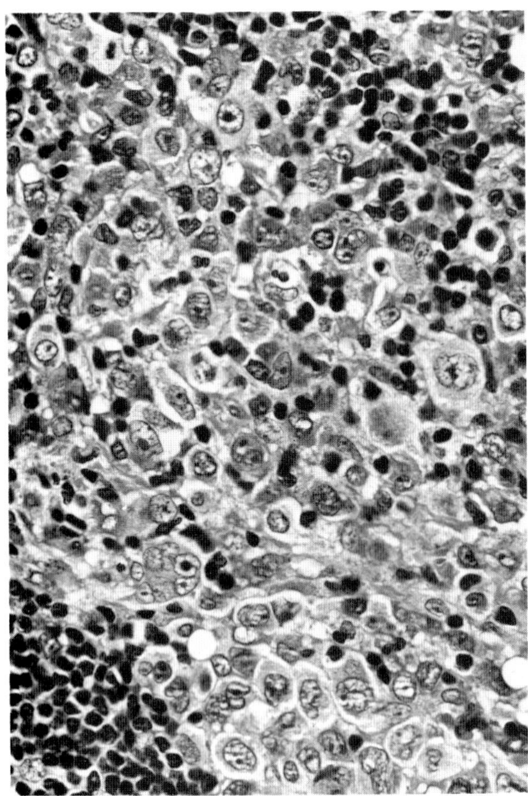

Fig. 9.34 Lymph node biopsy showing nodular sclerosing HD with solid sheets of lacunar cells. Note large S-R cell (lower left). (H E × 470)

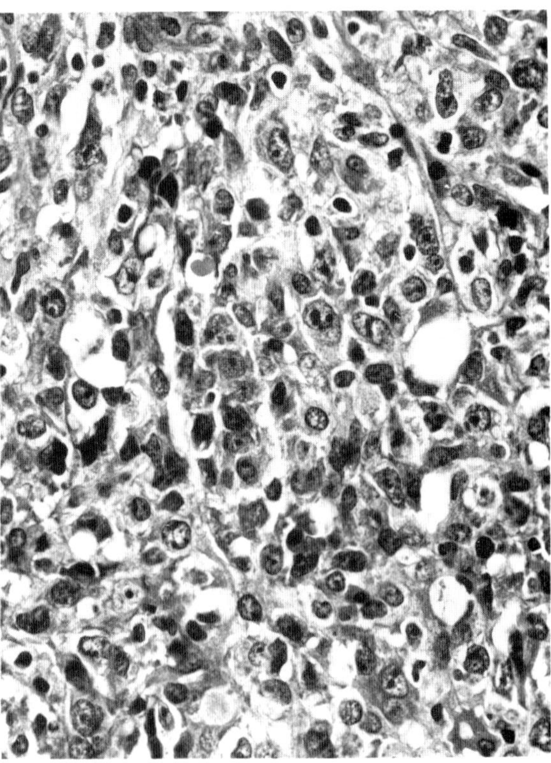

Fig. 9.35 Further lymph node biopsy from the same patient as Fig. 9.34 and taken soon afterwards, following poor response to therapy. The node was extensively necrotic, but viable areas such as this showed the picture of an immunoblastic sarcoma (ML immunoblastic). (H E × 470)

rapid transformation of the neoplasm into a high grade malignant lymphoma, usually of immunoblastic type (Figs 9.34, 9.35). The process generally begins focally, in a single node or group of nodes, or in the spleen. It is recognised histologically by the appearance of solid sheets of immunoblast-type cells, the monomorphism of which often contrasts strikingly with the pleomorphic infiltrate of HD. Transformation of this type may occur at any stage in the evolution of Hodgkin's disease and seems to be independent of the lymphocyte population at the time. It is thus clearly distinguishable, both temporally and morphologically, from LD Hodgkin's disease. The process may well be analogous to the transformation of low grade lymphomas of other types into high grade malignant lymphomas (see Ch. 10, p. 269). It is not known whether this is due to the emergence of a new clone of neoplastic cells or to what extent the occurrence of the phenomenon in HD may be attributable to impaired cell-mediated immunity.

Significance of the different cell types in HD

The reciprocal relationship between lymphocytes and Sternberg-Reed cells, first commented on by Rosenthal, supports the suggestion that the lymphocytes in LP disease are in some way acting in a defensive capacity — perhaps controlling the proliferation of the neoplastic cells. The control is imperfect, of course, as is evidenced by the slow multiplication of Sternberg-Reed cells and the loss of cell-mediated immunity which accompanies this. In LP Hodgkin's disease there is often an absolute lymphocytosis in the peripheral blood although in general the lymphocyte count is depressed in HD (Aisenberg, 1965). Also the amount of lymphoid tissue throughout the body may be increased in LP HD, even when the disease itself appears to be of very limited extent. In one personally observed instance, a readily palpable spleen was removed in the course of staging laparotomy. The organ, which weighed over 400 g, showed a diffuse increase of lymphocytes in the white pulp when sectioned. There was no evidence of its involvement by Hodgkin's disease.*

Plasma cells are in a different category. Absent from the nodes in the early stages, plasma cells tend to increase with progression of the disease and the decline of lymphocytes. They are often very numerous in advanced and progressing disease, congregating especially at the periphery of the lesions. There is additional evidence of antibody synthesis in HD, in the occurrence of immune-complex disorders (glomerulonephritis and possibly demyelinating disease).

Eosinophils are a common, but variable ingredient of the cell picture in HD. As with plasma cells, their presence in very large numbers seems to be a bad prognostic sign and is associated with progressive disease. They are often numerous when pruritus is a troublesome symptom. Neutrophils are found chiefly in relation to necrosis in the nodes.

Epithelioid histiocytes and the occurrence of granulomas

In common with a great many malignant neoplasms, HD often attracts a large population of macrophages. These are of course particularly numerous around areas of necrosis. In addition to phagocytic histiocytes, epithelioid cells are a major feature of the histological picture in many cases of HD, especially in the LP diffuse and MC types and in the 'Lennert type' (qv). The significance of this high concentration of epithelioid cells is unknown, but it has been suggested that it is due to the production of a macrophage 'migration inhibition factor' by the lymphoid cells (Lennert, 1978). When splenectomy became a common procedure in the staging of Hodgkin's disease, it was discovered that excised spleens quite often showed multiple, small, epithelioid cell granulomas in the white pulp, in the absence of other evidence of involvement by HD (Kadin et al, 1970, 1971). Focal granulomas of this type may be scanty or very numerous and occasionally they are large enough to be visible to the naked eye. They may be found also in other sites — liver, abdominal nodes (Fig. 9.36) and bone marrow. Although these granulomas are usually found in patients whose

* Sometimes biopsy of an enlarged superficial node, in a patient who is in remission after treatment for Hodgkin's disease, will show only reactive lymphoid hyperplasia with prominent follicles. This provides a cogent argument for rebiopsy, before it is assumed that the disease has relapsed.

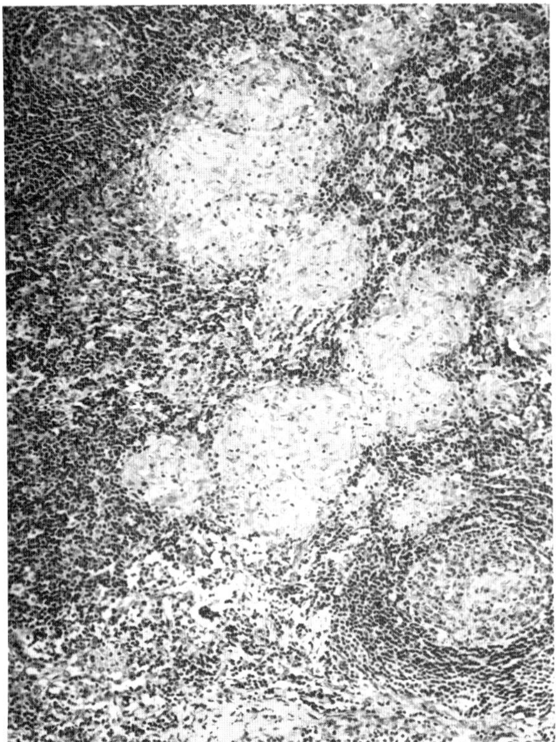

Fig. 9.36 Multiple small granulomas in the coeliac lymph node, taken at splenectomy and staging laparotomy from a man of 21 who had Hodgkin's disease of nodular sclerosing type. The spleen was enlarged and contained many such granulomas, together with one small focus of HD. No evidence of HD was found either in the coeliac node or in the liver, biopsy of which showed multiple granulomas of the same type. (H E × 120)

diagnostic lymph node biopsy has shown an abundance of epithelioid cells, this is not invariably so. There is no evidence that such granulomas precede the appearance of Hodgkin's disease in the same sites, or that their occurrence adversely affects the prognosis, indeed it has been suggested that the reverse may be true (O'Connell et al, 1975).

Lennert's lymphoma and Hodgkin's disease

In 1968 Lennert & Mestdagh described under the title of 'epithelioid cellular lymphogranulomatosis' the lesion which has since become known as Lennert's lymphoma. The lesion was characterised by loss of normal architecture in the affected nodes and by uniformly distributed small clusters of epithelioid cells. Sternberg-Reed cells were either absent or present in very small numbers, nevertheless the authors proposed that this represented a special variety of Hodgkin's disease.

The evidence today suggests that 'epithelioid cellular lymphogranulomatosis' represents certainly more than one and, most probably, several different diseases (see p. 322). Whilst many such cases are almost certainly not examples of HD, a few do appear to be of this nature and the presence (or absence) of undoubted Sternberg-Reed cells is the only reliable distinguishing characteristic, when the histological features may otherwise look remarkably alike. The exact status of this variant of Hodgkin's disease in relation to other types has yet to be defined, but it differs from Lukes' diffuse L & H type (LP — diffuse) both clinically and pathologically. Clinically, it is commoner in older

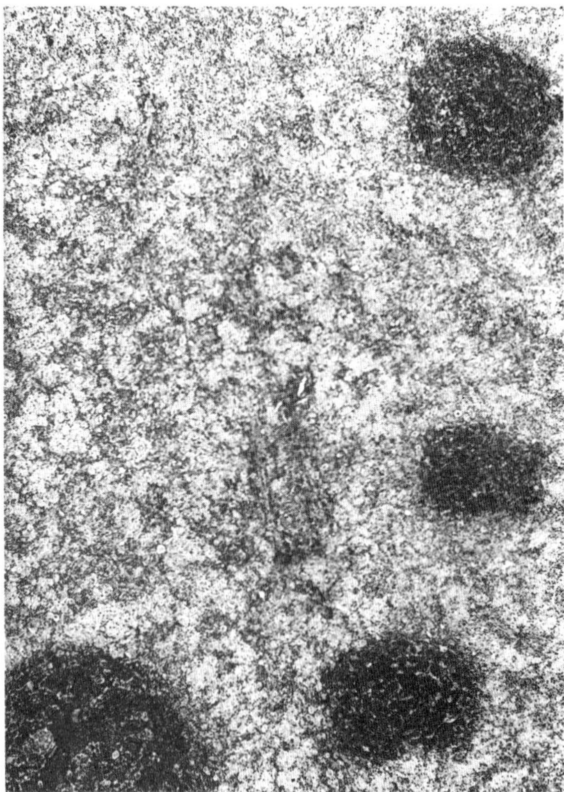

Fig. 9.37 Hodgkin's disease simulating 'Lennert's lymphoma' (lymphoepithelioid lymphoma). Some follicles persist and the interfollicular pulp is filled with uniformly distributed, small, epithelioid cell clusters — more closely packed than those typically seen in HD of diffuse L P type and yet appearing discrete. (Compare with Figs 8.28, p. 180; 10.26, p. 246; 12.33, p. 321) (H E × 47)

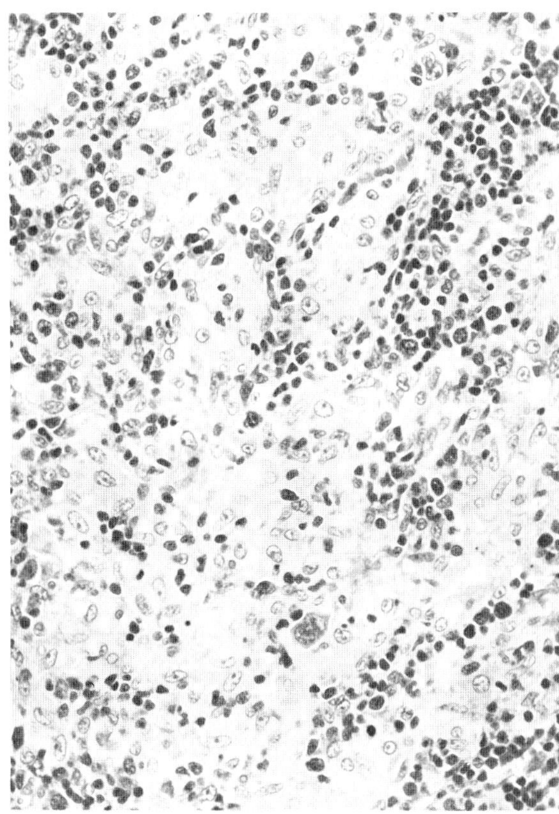

Fig. 9.38 Lymph node biopsy from another case of Hodgkin's disease with a close mimicry of 'Lennert's lymphoma'. The patient was a man of 61. In this instance Sternberg-Reed cells (top right and lower centre) were not difficult to find amidst the coalescent epithelioid cell clusters. (H E × 300)

subjects and usually presents as advanced disease with 'B' symptoms, having a much graver prognosis than L & H disease. Pathologically, it is characterised, as stated above, by a remarkably uniform and diffuse distribution of small epithelioid cell clusters amongst which small numbers of typical Sternberg-Reed cells are seen (Figs 9.37, 9.38). Lymphocytes are reduced in number, but plasma cells are often present (for differential diagnosis see pp. 322–3). The numbers of epithelioid cells may fluctuate and the picture may switch to that of LD Hodgkin's disease with the disappearance of the epithelioid cell clusters.

Amyloid and 'Para-amyloid' in HD

Different patterns of collagenous fibrosis in nodes affected by HD have already been discussed, as well as the deposition of amorphous protein in the diffuse fibrosis type of lymphocytic depletion disease. In addition, it is not uncommon to find, usually in HD of long standing, nodes which are partially or extensively replaced by a meshwork of amorphous, hyaline material, the meshes of which are sparsely populated by lymphocytes. The change, often referred to as 'hyalinosis' (para-amyloid), occurs spontaneously and is independent of treatment. This condition, and the much rarer occurrence of amyloidosis in HD, are discussed in chapter 8 (pp. 170–173).

SPREAD OF HODGKIN'S DISEASE

The weight of evidence suggests that HD begins in a single focus, nearly always a lymph node. and spreads centrifugally from that source by lymphatic channels. One does not often see direct evidence of such spread in the form of lymphatic permeation or sinus infiltration in newly involved nodes, although both may be observed from time to time. However, the observation of Peters (Peters. 1950; Peters et al, 1966), that the recurrence rate could be markedly reduced by extending radiotherapy fields to cover adjacent lymph node groups as well as those affected, confirmed that this is the main route of spread of the disease. In fact, the system of 'staging', on which treatment programmes are planned, is based on the assumption that Hodgkin's disease, at least in its early stages, spreads in a predictable manner by lymphatic pathways. Thus, primary mediastinal disease, commonly found in nodular sclerosis, spreads first to cervical nodes*. Primary abdominal disease spreads to supraclavicular nodes, bypassing the thoracic nodes, and so on. It is equally apparent that haematogenous spread is common and it is generally presumed that this is the route by which the spleen and bone marrow become affected. Invasion of vein walls by Hodgkin's tissue

* A special instance of local lymphatic spread of nodular sclerosis deserves mention here. Sometimes disease in the thymus or anterior mediastinal nodes spreads directly into adjacent ribs, or through intercostal muscles, to present as a tumour of the thoracic wall. Spread into adjacent muscles in this type of HD has been alluded to already on p. 200.

was found in 6 to 14% of involved lymph nodes by Rappaport et al (1971b) and occurred in all types except lymphocytic predominance. The finding was associated with an increased incidence of extranodal involvement. Commonly HD remains confined to lymph nodes, spleen, liver and bone marrow — at least for a long period of time, but ultimately it may spread to lungs, gastrointestinal tract, adrenals, kidneys, meninges — and indeed almost anywhere, although very rarely to the CNS.

Although there are occasional reports of Hodgkin's disease arising primarily in extranodal sites, it is clear from studying such reports that there have been many cases of mistaken identity and genuine instances of primary extranodal Hodgkin's disease appear to be very rare indeed.

STAGING OF HODGKIN'S DISEASE

The treatment for HD adopted in many centres today is so dependent upon an accurate knowledge of the stage of the disease, that staging procedures are regularly undertaken at or soon after the time of diagnosis. The Ann Arbor system of staging (Carbone et al, 1971) is now widely used. In this there are four stages, each divided into A and B categories, depending upon the absence (A) or presence (B) of constitutional symptoms (fever, night sweats and loss of weight). The reader is referred to the original report for the niceties of this classification, but essentially Stage I represents disease confined to a single lymph node region, Stage II is disease involving two or more lymph node regions on the same side of the diaphragm, in Stage III there is lymph node involvement on both sides of the diaphragm (for this purpose the spleen is counted as a lymph node region) and in Stage IV there is spread to extra-lymphatic tissues, often on a wide scale.

Clinical staging in Hodgkin's disease is notoriously inaccurate and when staging laparotomy was introduced, this procedure was found in one series to change the stage in 25 to 50% of patients (Sutcliffe et al, 1976). Details of staging procedures are out of place here, but suffice it to say, that lymphangiography, CAT scanning, ultrasonic scanning, laparotomy with biopsy and sometimes thoracotomy with biopsy may each have a part to play in determining the extent of the disease, so that treatment may be planned accordingly. If some simpler investigation, such as a marrow aspiration or liver biopsy show that either of these sites is involved, then, by definition, the patient has Stage IV disease and further tests are unnecessary since chemotherapy is the only possible treatment for such advanced disease.

The detection of splenic involvement is in most instances dependent upon histological examination of the excised organ, for size alone is a very inaccurate index of involvement (Rosenberg, 1971) and even the most sophisticated scanning techniques are little better. Because of the importance of deciding whether or not the spleen is involved and because it is difficult to irradiate the spleen satisfactorily without injuring the left kidney, splenectomy has become a routine part of the staging laparotomy procedure in adults. In children, however, there appears to be a significant risk of fatal bacterial septicaemia and meningitis when splenectomy has been performed (Chilcote et al, 1976) and it is now generally felt that in childhood this risk outweighs the advantages of knowing whether the organ is involved and of removing a potential site of HD.

At a staging laparotomy operation, the paraortic, iliac and other groups of lymph nodes are inspected and biopsies are taken of any suspicious nodes, the sites of excised nodes being marked by tantalum clips to aid subsequent radiological detection. Particular attention needs to be paid to upper abdominal nodes, such as the coeliac group, as these are generally not detectable by lymphangiography. (They are better visualised by CAT scanning). A wedge biopsy is also taken from the liver and some advocate a needle biopsy as well. These may be taken from any suspicious-looking areas or, if none is seen, at random.

Examination of staging laparotomy specimens

Some brief comments on this topic may be helpful to any pathologists not already versed in the procedure.

Spleen. Preferably the organ should be received in the laboratory fresh so that it may be inspected and weighed by the pathologist. It should then be sliced cleanly with a large sharp knife into slices not more than 1 cm thick and these should be laid flat on formalin-soaked cotton wool in a large dish, deep enough for the slices to be subsequently covered with formalin to allow proper fixation. If, at the first cut, it is obvious that the spleen contains tumour deposits, then serial slicing of the whole organ is obviously unnecessary. If, on the other hand, tumour involvement is not immediately apparent, it is important to ensure that the discovery of tiny deposits is not jeopardised by poor fixation or bad technique. After allowing the spleen slices to fix overnight, each slice may then be further sliced into 2 mm slices. It is impossible to cut even slices of the required thinness without prior fixation and it is necessary to cut them as thin as this, since the smallest deposits that may be picked up with the naked-eye are about 2 mm in diameter. The individual spleen slices should be minutely inspected for pale nodules of larger size than the Malpighian bodies and suspicious areas should be taken for histological examination. Whilst single nodules may be found in very early infiltration, more often, small clusters of nodules occur, due to spread of the disease in the white pulp. Occasionally, tiny pale foci may turn out on section to be granulomas of the type described on page 219 or to consist merely of hyperplastic lymphoid tissue.

Lymph nodes. Any large nodes that are not obviously infiltrated by HD on macroscopic examination, should be sliced so that the whole node is embedded and sectioned, for sometimes involvement is focal and may even require interval sections for its detection. Even when all the excised nodes are obviously involved, all should be examined histologically and the type of disease present compared with that in the diagnostic lymph node biopsy. Often the lower abdominal and pelvic nodes will show an oleogranulomatous reaction resulting from lymphangiography. The presence of the oily contrast medium and associated macrophage reaction does not interfere with the detection of Hodgkin's deposits, for the premise upon which lymphangiography is based is that the contrast medium fails to enter areas of the node where the sinuses are compressed or obliterated. In LP Hodgkin's disease, abdominal nodes may be large and fleshy, but histological examination may show only an increased content of lymphocytes and no evidence of disease. On other occasions, enlargement of nodes may be due to granulomas of the type described on page 219, but it is obvious that meticulous search must be made for SR cells. Again, eosinophils are often encountered without other evidence of HD. In MC or LD Hodgkin's disease, uninvolved nodes are often small with a reduction of lymphocytes, but sometimes an increase of plasma cells.

Liver. Hodgkin's deposits of microscopic size may sometimes be found in expanded portal tracts, when macroscopic evidence of disease is lacking, but a word of warning is necessary about misinterpreting small portal infiltrates as indicating HD, when these infiltrates consist only of lymphocytes and/or eosinophils and macrophages. Such infiltrates are commonly seen in HD and the same remarks apply to liver biopsies as have been made in relation to abdominal nodes. It cannot be stressed too strongly that a diagnosis of Hodgkin's disease must be based, here as elsewhere, upon the discovery of Sternberg-Reed cells in an appropriate cellular setting. If the appearances are thought to be suspicious of HD, interval sections should be examined (Rappaport et al, 1971a). Liver involvement by Hodgkin's disease probably never occurs in the absence of splenic deposits (Rosenberg, 1971).

Bone marrow. Although marrow examination is not strictly related to staging laparotomy, it is an important part of the staging procedure, and a bone biopsy is often performed at the same time as laparotomy. The same remarks apply to the interpretation of marrow biopsies as to soft tissue biopsies, but it is often more difficult to recognise Sternberg-Reed cells in a marrow trephine. This is mainly for technical reasons, the cells being poorly preserved after many decalcification procedures. Focal deposits in the marrow may be recognised by the absence of fat cells within them and the increased content of fibre, confirmed by reticulin staining. High power examination of such foci reveals the pleomorphic character of the infiltrate and mitoses may be evident. In a good quality preparation there should seldom be difficulty in identifying SR and Hodgkin's cells. In advanced disease, there is sometimes total replacement of the normal marrow in the biopsy by Hodgkin's tissue and areas of necrosis may be seen. There may or may not be an excess of eosinophils.

Post-treatment staging laparotomy

In some centres and in selected patients, staging laparotomy may be carried out *after* Hodgkin's disease has been treated, instead of before treatment (Sutcliffe et al, 1978). The object of this is to determine whether there is still evidence of active disease which requires further treatment. In resected spleens or lymph node biopsies, taken in such circumstances, areas of successfully treated HD may be seen as foci or massive areas of structureless hyaline material sparsely populated by lymphocytes, with macrophages, sometimes containing haemosiderin pigment (see Fig. 9.30). The picture is readily distinguishable from that of lymphocytic depletion HD (diffuse fibrosis type). Sometimes, alongside such areas, evidence of still active HD may be seen, with SR cells and mitoses indicating that the original disease has not been eradicated. The presence of granulomas, in the absence of SR cells, is not sufficient to indicate that the disease is still active.

Opportunist infections in HD

It has long been appreciated that patients with Hodgkin's disease are specially subject to certain infections and in recent years the defect in cell-mediated immunity which accompanies the disease, has been demonstrated. In former times, when tuberculosis was rife in Britain, many patients with HD developed tuberculosis and the lesions of both diseases could be seen side by side. This combination is much rarer today, but certain fungal infections, notably cryptococcosis, still occur from time to time in patients with uncontrolled HD — not necessarily in sites affected by the disease. Pneumocystis carinii pneumonia is also prone to occur and may be the terminal event. As might be expected, there is also increased susceptibility to some viral infections, such as Herpes zoster.

Association of Hodgkin's disease with other neoplasms

The increased incidence of second neoplasms in patients who have, or who have had, Hodgkin's disease is not readily explicable by any single, straightforward mechanism. The longer survival of patients treated by modern regimes has undoubtedly increased the incidence of such forms of neoplasia, and two reasons have been advanced for this increase: (1) an oncogenic effect of radiotherapy and chemotherapy, (2) an impairment of host immune surveillance, resulting both from therapy and from the disease itself. In some instances a second neoplasm has appeared relatively early in the disease and does not appear therefore to have been provoked by treatment given for HD. In many other instances, however, the second neoplasm has followed after the Hodgkin's disease has been successfully ablated by treatment. Second neoplasms in HD may be considered under two headings:

1. Other malignant lymphomas and leukaemias

The association of Hodgkin's disease with other types of malignant lymphoma, although rare, is nevertheless well documented in the case of two low grade B cell neoplasms, namely chronic lymphocytic leukaemia (B-CLL) and follicular, centroblastic-centrocytic lymphoma (Kim et al, 1977). The former combination (HD and CLL) has sometimes been confused with blastic transformation in CLL (Richter's syndrome), from which, however, it is clearly distinguishable, despite the occasional presence of 'Sternberg-Reed-like' cells in the latter (Foucar & Rydell, 1980), (Figs 9.39, 9.40). When Hodgkin's disease is combined with centroblastic-centrocytic follicular lymphoma, the two lymphomas may appear concurrently or sequentially and in the former case they may involve the same or separate sites.

In the two instances cited above the development of a second lymphoreticular neoplasm may occur whether or not treatment has been given and is thus independent of any possible oncogenic effect of treatment. On the other hand, the occasional development of a high-grade immunoblastic lymphoma in the course of Hodgkin's disease (see p. 219) generally follows treatment of the latter by radiotherapy or chemotherapy or both. Krikorian et al (1979) described the occurrence of high grade malignant

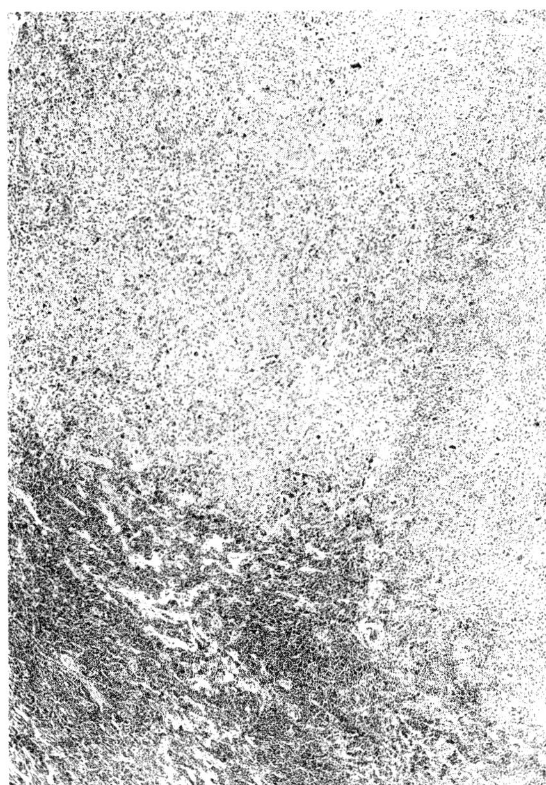

Fig. 9.39 Hodgkin's disease (above in chronic lymphocytic leukaemia of B-cell type (below). This cervical node biopsy was performed because of recent enlargement of the node in a patient who had been known for some years to have B-CLL. (H E × 47)

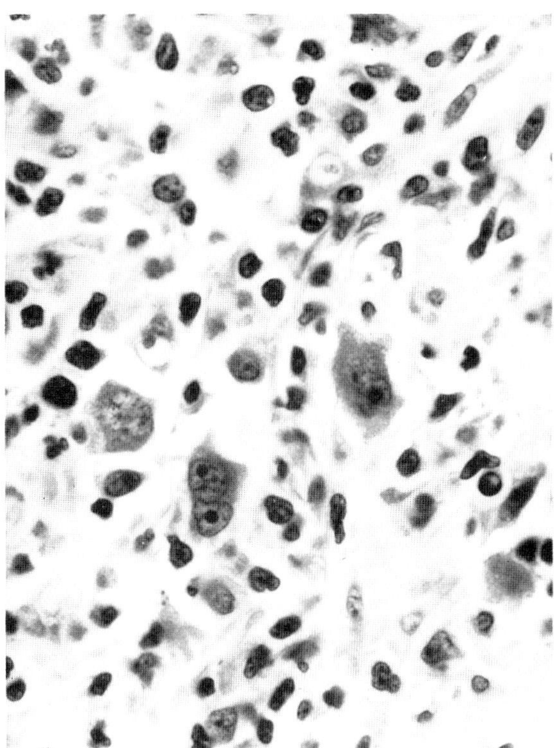

Fig. 9.40 Higher power view of the focus of Hodgkin's disease seen in Fig. 9.39. Two typical Sternberg-Reed cells are shown. (H E × 750)

lymphomas in six patients, all of whom had previously been treated for Hodgkin's disease by radiotherapy and chemotherapy and in none of whom evidence of HD existed at the time the second lymphoma developed.

The most frequently recorded second neoplasm in treated Hodgkin's disease is acute leukaemia, generally of myeloblastic, myelomonocytic or monocytic types (Rosner & Grunwald, 1975). The role of radiation damage in inducing these forms of neoplasia is well recognised. Conversely, the rare development of Hodgkin's disease following successful treatment of acute lymphoblastic leukaemia has also been reported (Woodruff et al, 1977).

2. Non-lymphomatous neoplasms

A variety of second neoplasms of other types has been recorded in patients with Hodgkin's disease. Some of these are very unusual, particularly having regard to the age of the subject. We have seen a rapidly fatal fibrosarcoma which originated in the uterine cervix of a young woman, 8 years after treatment for Hodgkin's disease. At necropsy there was disseminated fibrosarcoma, but no evidence of residual Hodgkin's disease.

An association of HD with Kaposi's sarcoma is well recognised (see p. 153) and may be related to the patient's immunodeficient state. Eosinophilic granuloma (Histiocytosis X) has also been found in lymph nodes containing HD, more commonly than would be expected if this were a chance association.

PROGNOSIS

Hodgkin's disease is an outstanding example of a neoplasm which was formerly almost uniformly fatal, but in which the outlook has been transformed by a much more aggressive approach to treatment, in which pathological staging of the disease plays a vital part. Radiotherapy is the cornerstone of treatment for localised disease and combination chemotherapy is generally given for disseminated disease. With rationally planned treatment, the mortality has been drastically reduced, even in advanced disease. A substantial proportion of the residual mortality is due to inadequate or badly planned treatment in the early stages, patients dying of uncontrolled Hodgkin's disease, opportunist infections or both. Few die of other neoplasms.

REFERENCES

Aisenberg A C 1965 Lymphocytopenia in Hodgkin's disease. Blood 25: 1037–1042

Carbone P P, Kaplan H S, Musshoff K, Smithers D W, Tubiana M 1971 Report of the committee on Hodgkin's disease staging classification. Cancer Research 31: 1860–1861

Carr I 1975 The ultrastructure of the abnormal reticulum cells in Hodgkin's disease. Journal of Pathology 115: 45–50

Chilcote R R, Baehner R L, Hammond D et al 1976 Septicemia and meningitis in children splenectomized for Hodgkin's disease. New England Journal of Medicine 295: 798–800

Correa P, O'Conor G T 1973 Geographic pathology of lymphoreticular tumours: summary of survey from the geographic pathology committee of the international union against cancer. Journal of the National Cancer Institute 50: 1609–1617

Cross R M 1969 Hodgkin's disease: histological classification and diagnosis. Journal of Clinical Pathology 22: 165–182

Curran R C, Jones E L 1978 Hodgkin's disease: an immunohistochemical and histological study. Journal of Pathology 125: 39–51

Foucar K, Rydell R E 1980 Richter's syndrome in chronic lymphocytic leukaemia. Cancer 46: 118–134

Fransilla K O, Kalima T V, Voutilainen A 1967 Histologic classification of Hodgkin's disease. Cancer 20: 1594–1601

Glick A D, Leech J H, Flexner J M, Collins R D 1976 Ultrastructural study of Reed-Sternberg cells. American Journal of Pathology 85: 195–208

Greenfield W S 1878 Specimens illustrative of the pathology of lymphadenoma and leucocythaemia. Transactions of the Pathological Society of London 29: 272–304

Hamlin I M E 1973 Histological type and grade. In: Smithers D W (ed) Hodgkin's disease, Churchill Livingstone, Edinburgh, ch 6, p 40–52

Hodgkin T 1832 On some morbid appearances of the absorbent glands and spleen. Medico-Chirurgical Transactions 17: 68–114

Jackson H, Parker F 1944 Hodgkin's disease. 1. General considerations. New England Journal of Medicine 230: 1–8

Kadin M E, Donaldson S S, Dorfman R F 1970 Isolated granulomas in Hodgkin's disease. New England Journal of Medicine 283: 859–861

Kadin M E, Glatstein E, Dorfman R F 1971 Clinicopathological studies of 117 untreated patients subjected to laparotomy for the staging of Hodgkin's disease. Cancer 27: 1277–1294

Kadin M E, Stites D P, Levy R, Warnke R 1978 Exogenous immunoglobulin and the macrophage origin of Reed-Sternberg cells in Hodgkin's disease. New England Journal of Medicine 299: 1208–1214

Kaplan H S 1980 Hodgkin's Disease, 2nd edn. Harvard University Press, Cambridge, Massachusetts

Kim H, Hendrickson M R, Dorfman R F 1977 Composite lymphoma. Cancer 40: 959–976

Krikorian J G, Burke J S, Rosenberg S A, Kaplan H S 1979 Occurrence of non-Hodgkin's lymphoma after therapy for Hodgkin's disease. New England Journal of Medicine 300: 452–458

Lancet (Editorial) 1977 Risk factors in Hodgkin's disease. Lancet 1: 888–889

Lennert K 1978 Classification of non-Hodgkin's lymphomas. In: Malignant lymphomas other than Hodgkin's disease. Springer-Verlag, Berlin, Part 3, p 95

Lennert K, Mestdagh J 1968 Lymphogranulomatosen mit konstant hohem Epithelioidzellgehalt. Virchows Archiv A (Pathol Anat) 344: 1–20

Lukes R J 1963 Relationship of histologic features to clinical stages in Hodgkin's disease. American Journal of Roentgenology 90: 944–955

Lukes R J 1971 Criteria for involvement of lymph node, bone marrow, spleen and liver in Hodgkin's disease. Cancer Research 31: 1755–1767

Lukes R J. Butler J J 1966 The pathology and nomenclature of Hodgkin's disease. Cancer Research 26: 1063–1083

Lukes R J, Butler J J, Hicks E B 1966a Natural history of Hodgkin's disease as related to its pathologic picture. Cancer 19: 317–344

Lukes R J, Craver L F, Hall T C, Rappaport H, Ruben P 1966b Report of the Nomenclature Committee. Cancer Research 26:1311

MacMahon B 1957 Epidemiological evidence on the nature of Hodgkin's disease. Cancer 10: 1045–1054

MacMahon B 1966 Epidemiology of Hodgkin's disease. Cancer Research 26: 1189–1200

Marshall A H E, Matilla A. Pollock D J 1976 A critique and case study of nodular sclerosing Hodgkin's disease. Journal of Clinical Pathology 29: 923–930

Neiman R S 1978 Current problems in the histopathologic diagnosis and classification of Hodgkin's disease. Pathobiology Annual 13(2): 289–328

O'Connell M J, Schimpff S C, Kirschner R H, Abt A B, Wiernik P H 1975 Epithelioid granulomas in Hodgkin's disease, a favourable prognostic sign? Journal of the American Medical Association 233: 886–889

Peters M V 1950 A study of survivals in Hodgkin's disease treated radiologically. American Journal of Roentgenology 63: 299–311

Peters M V, Alison R E, Bush R S 1966 Natural history of Hodgkin's disease as related to staging. Cancer 19: 308–316
Poppema S, Kaiserling E, Lennert K 1979 Hodgkin's disease with lymphocytic predominance nodular type (nodular paragranuloma) and progressively transformed germinal centres — a cytohistological study. Histopathology 3: 295–308
Rappaport H, Berard C W, Butler J J, Dorfman R F, Lukes R J, Thomas L B 1971a Report to the committee on histopathological criteria contributing to staging of Hodgkin's disease. Cancer Research 31: 1864–1865
Rappaport H, Strum S B, Hutchison G, Allen L W 1971b Clinical and biological significance of vascular invasion in Hodgkin's disease. Cancer Research 31: 1794–1798
Reed D M 1902 On the pathological changes in Hodgkin's disease, with especial reference to its relation to tuberculosis. Johns Hopkins Hospital Reports 10: 133–196
Rosenberg S A 1971 A critique of the value of laparotomy and splenectomy in the evaluation of patients with Hodgkin's disease. Cancer Research 31: 1737–1740
Rosenthal S R 1936 Significance of tissue lymphocytes in the prognosis of lymphogranulomatosis. Archives of Pathology 21: 628–646
Rosner F, Grunwald H 1975 Hodgkin's disease and acute leukaemia. American Journal of Medicine 58: 339–353
Smetana H F, Cohen B M 1956 Mortality in relation to histologic type in Hodgkin's disease. Blood 11: 211–224
Smithers D W 1963 Some inferences about the origin of tumours derived from their age distribution. Clinical Radiology 14: 418–423
Smithers D W 1973 Prevalence and age distribution. In: Hodgkin's disease. Churchill Livingstone, Edinburgh, ch 2, p 11, Fig. 2.1
Söderström N 1966 Fine-Needle Aspiration Biopsy. Almqvist & Wiksell, Stockholm
Stein H et al 1982 Identification of Hodgkin and Sternberg-Reed cells as an unique cell type derived from a newly-detected small-cell population. International Journal of Cancer 30: 445–459
Sternberg C 1898 Uber eine eigenartige unter dem Bilde der Pseudoleukaemie verlaufende Tuberculose des lymphatischen Apparates. Zeitschrift für Heilkunde 19: 21–90
Strum S B, Park J K, Rappaport H 1970 Observation of cells resembling Sternberg-Reed cells in conditions other than Hodgkin's disease. Cancer 26: 176–190
Strum S B, Rappaport H 1971 Interrelations of the histologic types of Hodgkin's disease. Archives of Pathology 91: 127–134
Sutcliffe S B J, Katz D R, Stansfeld A G, Shand W S, Wrigley P F M, Malpas J S 1978 Post-treatment laparotomy in the management of Hodgkin's disease. Lancet 2: 57–60
Sutcliffe S B J et al 1976 Intensive investigation in management of Hodgkin's disease. British Medical Journal 2: 1343–1347
Symmers W St C 1978 The Lymphoreticular System. In: Symmers W St C (ed) Systemic Pathology, vol 2, 2nd edn. Churchill Livingstone, Edinburgh. Ch 9, p 788, Table 9.11
Taylor C R 1974 The nature of Reed-Sternberg cells and other malignant 'reticulum' cells. Lancet 2: 802–807
Wakasa H 1973 Hodgkin's disease in Asia, particularly in Japan. National Cancer Institute Monograph 36: 15–22
Woodruff R K et al 1977 Hodgkin's disease occurring during acute leukaemia in remission. Lancet 2: 900–903
Zajicek J 1974 Aspiration biopsy cytology, part 1: cytology of supradiaphragmatic organs. In: Wied G L (ed) Monographs in Clinical Cytology, 4th vol, Karger, Basel, ch 4, p 90

A.G. Stansfeld

Non-Hodgkin's lymphomas: low grade B-cell lymphomas

INTRODUCTION

The malignant lymphomas other than Hodgkin's disease — commonly but not euphoniously referred to as the 'non-Hodgkin's lymphomas' (NHL) — are a diverse group of neoplasms which present in a variety of different ways. Whilst lymphadenopathy is the commonest mode of presentation in this group of neoplasms, an extra-nodal presentation is by no means rare, indeed in certain categories of malignant lymphoma it is the rule rather than the exception. For example, Burkitt's lymphoma classically presents with a tumour in the jaw, or gonads, or other extra-nodal site and nodal involvement may be insignificant or lacking throughout. Likewise, the presenting feature in hairy cell leukaemia (leukaemic reticuloendotheliosis) is commonly splenomegaly and nodal involvement is often minimal in this disease. Moreover, whilst it is customary to think of a malignant lymphoma as a solid tumour, whether arising in lymph nodes, or tonsil, or gut, or elsewhere, lymphoid neoplasms may present as a diffuse infiltration of bone marrow, or blood (leukaemia), with or without infiltration of other organs, such as spleen, or liver. It is quite illogical to exclude neoplasms presenting in this way from consideration, just because the patient is referred to the haematologist, rather than to the surgeon for lymph node biopsy. It would be just as irrational to exclude those forms of lymphoid neoplasia where the presenting features are those of a hyperviscosity syndrome, resulting from the production of excessive quantities of an abnormal immunoglobulin by the neoplastic cells (e.g. Waldenström's macroglobulinaemia). Pursuing this line of argument, myeloma is properly regarded as a malignant lymphoma, although, for practical reasons, it is generally excluded from classifications of the malignant lymphomas, being strictly a tumour of the bone marrow in the great majority of instances.

Geographical and racial differences in incidence of NHL

Malignant lymphomas probably occur in all races, but the relative incidence of different types of malignant lymphoma varies in different parts of the world and in different races. Burkitt's lymphoma may be cited as an example of a neoplasm with a distinctive geographical distribution (Burkitt, 1958). Similarly there is a high incidence of B-cell lymphomas of the gut in parts of the Middle East, related to the occurrence of α-chain disease in these areas (Seligmann et al, 1968). Recent studies have indicated that there is a relatively high incidence of certain T-cell lymphomas in the Japanese (e.g. Suchi et al, 1979) and in blacks from the Caribbean (Catovsky et al, 1982). In the Western world, a large majority of NHL appear to arise from B-lymphocytes or their precursors, but in parts of Japan, T-cell lymphomas are more frequent than B-cell lymphomas (Mitsui et al, 1983).

Age and sex differences in incidence of NHL

One very important fact to note is that practically all malignant lymphomas occurring in childhood, with the exception of Hodgkin's disease, are high grade, blast-cell neoplasms. All the common low-grade B-cell NHL are essentially neoplasms of adult life, being rare under the age of 25 and practically unknown under the age of 18. Most types of malignant lymphoma show a higher incidence in males, but the sex difference is not particularly striking, except in the case of the T-lymphoblastic (convoluted cell) lymphoma (see p. 287), which has been variously estimated as two to six times commoner in males. On the other hand, the virus associated pleomorphic T-cell lymphomas are, in some series, commoner in females (see Ch. 12).

Comparative incidence of NHL and Hodgkin's disease

Remarks concerning the relative incidence of different types of malignant lymphoma in different parts of the world apply also to the relative frequency of NHL and Hodgkin's disease. In Europe and North America, Hodgkin's disease is undoubtedly the commonest type of malignant lymphoma. The ratio of Hodgkin's disease to NHL is approximately 44:56 in Western Europe (Lennert, 1978) and the figures appear to be similar in the North American continent, whilst in Japan Hodgkin's disease is comparatively rare (Smithers, 1973).

Clinical differences between NHL and Hodgkin's disease

Generally speaking, it is impossible for the clinician to make a confident diagnosis of Hodgkin's disease, as opposed to a malignant lymphoma of another kind, when confronted with a patient who presents with lymph node enlargement, and the diagnosis must obviously be based upon the histopathological (or cytological) findings. Nevertheless, there may be strong grounds for suspecting that the disease is in fact Hodgkin's disease, especially when the patient is a child or young adult. Pruritus and alcohol induced pain are both much more frequently encountered in Hodgkin's disease than in other types of lymphoma and the same applies to a lesser extent with the occurrence of fever, night sweats and weight loss. The distinction is far from absolute and 'B' symptoms occur in other varieties of malignant lymphoma from time to time. The reverse of course also applies. The clinical situation may strongly point to some other type of lymphoma rather than Hodgkin's disease. Generalised lymphadenopathy at presentation is more characteristic of the non-Hodgkin's lymphomas in general and involvement of certain extra-nodal sites, such as Waldeyer's ring, gastrointestinal tract and skin, is much less frequent in Hodgkin's disease than in some NHL.

CLASSIFICATION AND TERMINOLOGY OF NHL

Since a diagnosis of malignant lymphoma rests ultimately upon the pathological findings in a biopsy of affected tissue, it is natural that these diseases should be classified in pathological terms.

Various attempts at classification have been made over the years from the early studies of Robb-Smith (1938) and Gall & Mallory (1942) to the 1966 classification of Rappaport. In the past decade a spate of classifications has appeared — some based solely on descriptive features, some taking account of the functional characteristics of the cells as well (Dorfman, 1974; Bennett et al, 1974; Gérard-Marchant et al, 1974; Lukes & Collins, 1974, 1975). Knowledge of the immune system has now advanced to a point where functional aspects of the neoplastic cells may be usefully incorporated into a classification of malignant lymphomas, although there are several reasons why a classification based primarily on cell function, such as that proposed by Hansen & Good (1974) is still unsatisfactory. We do not yet know enough about the functional characteristics of the various types of lymphoid cell in relation to their morphology to be able to describe these neoplasms in purely functional terms and a significant proportion of malignant lymphomas are composed of cells which lack functional markers ('null cells') and thus cannot be assigned to either a B-cell or a T-cell category. For the present, cell morphology must remain the essential basis for classifying malignant lymphomas.

An ideal system of classification must be: (1) readily understandable to clinicians as well as to pathologists; (2) clinically relevant in its ability to predict behaviour and prognosis; (3) reproducible in the hands of those applying it, and (4) scientifically accurate in terms of the concepts upon which it is based. We believe that, of the various systems of classification in current use today, that based on the ideas of Lennert — the *Kiel classification*

Table 10.1 Malignant lymphomas (ML) Kiel classification (revised)

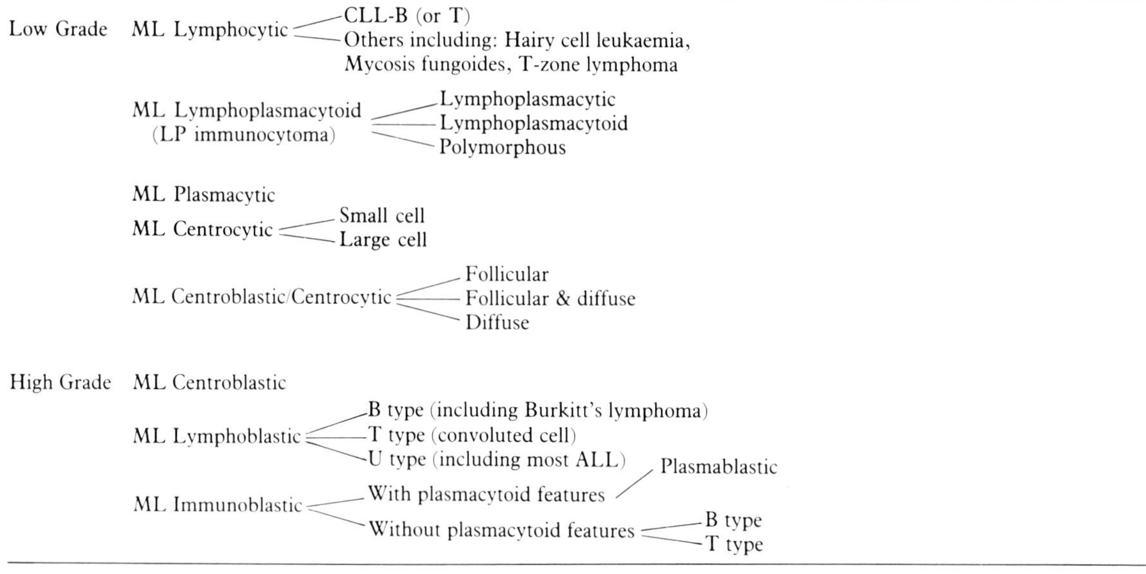

Grade	Type	Subtype	
Low Grade	ML Lymphocytic	CLL-B (or T)	
		Others including: Hairy cell leukaemia, Mycosis fungoides, T-zone lymphoma	
	ML Lymphoplasmacytoid (LP immunocytoma)	Lymphoplasmacytic	
		Lymphoplasmacytoid	
		Polymorphous	
	ML Plasmacytic		
	ML Centrocytic	Small cell	
		Large cell	
	ML Centroblastic/Centrocytic	Follicular	
		Follicular & diffuse	
		Diffuse	
High Grade	ML Centroblastic		
	ML Lymphoblastic	B type (including Burkitt's lymphoma)	
		T type (convoluted cell)	
		U type (including most ALL)	
	ML Immunoblastic	With plasmacytoid features	Plasmablastic
		Without plasmacytoid features	B type
			T type

NB Both Low Grade and High Grade include a category of ML Unclassified (LG or HG)
(Malignant Histiocytoma and Malignant Histiocytosis are classified as reticulosarcomas
See Chapter 14)

(Gérard-Marchant et al, 1974; Lennert, 1978, 1981) — comes closest to fulfilling these ideals, and this system will be used here (Table 10.1).

In the description of the different types which follows, synonyms will be given and an attempt will be made to indicate how closely the various terms applied do in fact correspond with one another. It would be quite misleading to pretend that there is now a very wide measure of agreement over the various categories of NHL and that only terminological differences remain to be settled between the proponents of the six or so current classifications (see Appendix on the Working Formulation for Clinical Usage, p. 398). In some areas there is indeed a considerable measure of agreement and the terms used by different authors are strictly synonymous with one another, but in other areas there are still wide, and even fundamental, divergences concerning the very existence of certain categories of malignant lymphoma, as well as the boundaries between one type and another. The difficulties of translation from one classification to another are compounded by the use of similar terms in different senses by different authors. Thus 'poorly differentiated lymphocytic lymphoma' in the British National Lymphoma Investigation classification (Bennett et al, 1974) implies a high grade blast cell tumour (Kiel — lymphoblastic), whilst the same term is used in the Rappaport classification for a much less aggressive tumour of centrocytes, whether nodular or diffuse in pattern. It is thus necessary to mention which classification is being used when such terms are applied.

The whole concept of differentiation, as applied to lymphoid cells, may be called into question, since the stem cell, whence all other lymphoid and perhaps myeloid cells also are derived, is morphologically indistinguishable from the so-called 'well differentiated' lymphocyte. Moreover, transformation of a small lymphocyte into a blast cell may be regarded as a step in the direction of differentiation of that particular cell line. For these reasons it is better to avoid a terminology which makes assumptions about the degree of differentiation of the neoplastic cells. Equally inappropriate is the use of the term 'atypical' (Dorfman, 1974) when applied to the lymphoid cells of germinal centres which have irregularly shaped nuclei. Naming these same cells 'prolymphocytes'

(WHO Classification, 1976) is to be deplored, since this term has long been used in a totally different sense by haematologists. 'Cleaved follicle-centre cell' as employed by Lukes & Collins (1975), is clumsy and it is the nucleus that is 'cleaved', not the whole cell. Furthermore the clefts in the nucleus are not always visible. The author prefers the term centrocyte for this cell. It has the merits of brevity and clarity, drawing attention to the normal situation of these distinctive lymphoid cells within the germinal centres, whilst not carrying any undesirable connotation. The blast cell of the germinal centres is, in the author's view, best termed a centroblast.

It is certainly true that the rate of turn-over of blast cells is much more rapid than that of lymphoid cells in the resting phase, and this is reflected in the varying rates of growth of malignant lymphomas. Those tumours which consist largely or entirely of blast cells are much faster growing as a rule than those composed mainly of cells in the resting phase. Recognition is taken of this fact in the Kiel subdivision of the non-Hodgkin's malignant lymphomas into two broad groups of 'low grade' and 'high grade'. Within each group, the terminology reflects the main cell composition. Thus the low grade lymphomas end in the suffix '-cytic' or '-cytoid', whilst the high grade lymphomas end in the suffix '-blastic'.

The various categories of malignant lymphoma differ from one another not only in their age and sex incidence, their rate of growth and the nature of their constituent cells, but also in their manner of presentation, the frequency with which they involve different tissues (lymph nodes, spleen, marrow, blood, skin etc.), the presence or absence of overt immunological abnormalities and the response of the neoplasm to treatment. It is therefore desirable to achieve as accurate a designation of each neoplasm as possible and here the use of additional staining methods, immunocytochemistry, electron microscopy and other ancillary tests may be valuable adjuncts to routine light microscopy. Even where all these facilities are employed and impeccable sections are available for study, it is not always possible to make a definitive diagnosis of the type of malignant lymphoma. To some extent this is a reflection on the imperfections of our present system of classification, but it is also important to recognise the remarkable diversity in the tumours derived from lymphoid cells and, whilst it would be untrue to say that no two tumours are alike, it is undoubtedly true that not a few lymphomas do not fit neatly into any one morphological category, but appear to be intermediate between one class and another. Borderline tumours are encountered between certain of the low grade B-cell lymphomas, for example, between ML centroblastic-centrocytic and ML centrocytic, and between each of these and ML lymphoplasmacytoid. Equally there are borderline tumours in the high grade group, e.g. between ML centroblastic and ML immunoblastic.

It is not only necessary to recognise the occurrence of such borderline tumours, it is also important to be aware of the possibility that the appearances presented by a single lymph node biopsy may represent a transitional phase in the evolution of a malignant lymphoma. In certain tumours, some lymphoplasmacytoid lymphomas for example, it is not uncommon for the initial biopsy to show a background of inflammatory cell infiltration and this may at times be of such intensity as to obscure the presence of the underlying neoplasm. The inflammatory cell infiltration is often a passing phase and in subsequent biopsies it tends to diminish or disappear. Perhaps a parallel instance is the progressive emergence of the picture of malignant lymphoma in successive lymph node biopsies from a patient presenting initially with the picture of (angio) immunoblastic lymphadenopathy (p. 181–2).

A different phenomenon is the transformation of an initially low grade malignant lymphoma into a high grade tumour. This is a well recognised occurrence in those low grade malignant lymphomas which have a blast-cell component, and it is particularly frequently encountered in ML centroblastic-centrocytic. Such 'blastic transformation' is much less common with ML lymphocytic — B-CLL, and ML lymphoplasmacytoid. The phenomenon only occurs with the greatest rarity in ML centrocytic in which blast cells are absent or extremely scarce.

It follows, from what has been said above, that at the present time it is essential to retain a category of 'unclassified' in any system of classification of the malignant lymphomas and, for practical reasons it is useful to subdivide, where possible, the unclassified tumours too into low grade and high grade. There may, of course, be differing reasons why a malignant lymphoma is designated as unclassified (or unclassifiable). Not only are there instances, as cited above, when the tumour cannot be accurately designated, despite adequate sections, but there are the far more numerous occasions where, for a variety of reasons, the biopsy section is not adequate to allow an accurate diagnosis. The importance of making an accurate diagnosis dictates that, in such circumstances, either better sections should be prepared from the original biopsy material or a fresh biopsy taken, as appropriate. So long as these unclassified malignant lymphomas are recorded as such by the pathologist, it is always possible to pick them out for review at a later date, at which time some of the cases may be classifiable. If, however, a tumour which is properly unclassifiable is forced into a pigeon hole where it does not really fit, it may be lost for ever and its inclusion in an inappropriate category may distort the figures when cases in that category are analysed.

LOW-GRADE B-CELL LYMPHOMAS

ML LYMPHOCYTIC

In this variety of malignant lymphoma the cells are predominantly lymphocytes, whether of B- or T-type, and blast cells constitute at most a minor component of the neoplasm. Exactly how many sub-types should be included under this heading is still a matter for debate, but two points are agreed by the proponents of the Kiel classification: (1) most lymphocytic lymphomas are B-cell neoplasms, and (2) in these B-lymphocytic lymphomas, the predominant cells are morphologically lymphocytes, with round nuclei and a dense nuclear chromatin. The cells display surface immunoglobulin (SIg) but do not contain cytoplasmic immunoglobulin (CIg). If CIg is demonstrable in more than a very occasional cell, the neoplasm should be classified under the next heading — lymphoplasmacytoid lymphoma, whether or not a monoclonal immunoglobulin is demonstrable in the serum. In this regard, the concept of the Kiel classification differs from that of some other authors (e.g. Pangalis et al, 1977). Plasma cells may occasionally be found in B-lymphocytic lymphomas, but are of mature type and are polyclonal, both types of light chain being represented on immunoperoxidase staining. It should also be stressed that these neoplasms do not contain lymphoid cells of germinal centre type (centrocytes and centroblasts), except where remnants of the original node structure persist.

Much the commonest variety of B-lymphocytic lymphoma is B-type chronic lymphocytic leukaemia (B-CLL) and it is still uncertain whether there is a clearly separable entity of B-lymphocytic lymphoma which does not progress to B-CLL, as maintained by Pangalis et al (1977). It is widely believed that hairy cell leukaemia (leukaemic reticuloendotheliosis) is a B-lymphocytic neoplasm and it has been accorded this status in the Kiel classification (Table 10.1). We feel, however, that there is still some uncertainty about the nature of the neoplastic cells in this condition which justifies caution. In view of its primarily haematological presentation this entity will be considered in Chapter 13 (p. 340).

The T-cell lymphocytic lymphomas are undoubtedly rarer. They will be considered along with other peripheral T-cell lymphomas in Chapter 12.

ML LYMPHOCYTIC — B-TYPE (B-type Chronic Lymphocytic Leukaemia) (B-CLL)

Synonyms:
ML lymphocytic, well differentiated, diffuse.
ML Small lymphocytic type.
Chronic lymphatic leukaemia.

This is one of the commonest forms of malignant lymphoma, the presentation of which is generally with chronic lymphocytic leukaemia. Essentially a disease of adults past middle life, the symptoms are sometimes those of anaemia — fatigue and breathlessness. Significant lymphadenopathy may or may not be present. Thus the diagnosis is usually made by the haematologist and, in the UK, lymph node biopsy is seldom undertaken if the diagnosis appears straightforward. In West Germany the practice is different and lymph node biopsy is performed much more commonly, even when a diagnosis of CLL has already been made on the haematological findings (Lennert, 1978 p. 106). This may seem an unnecessary infliction upon the patient, but it does ensure that a correct diagnosis is made in every case. Where lymph node biopsy is not performed, a proportion of the patients who are diagnosed as having CLL, in fact have some other type of malignant lymphoma with circulating neoplastic cells (Galton, 1974).

On rare occasions, lymph node enlargement precedes the development of leukaemia and, when this happens, the diagnosis will probably depend upon lymph node biopsy. The morphological appearances in the lymph nodes are similar, whether or not there is an absolute lymphocytosis (defined as > 4000 lymphocytes/mm^3) in the peripheral blood. In non-leukaemic cases, the interval between the appearance of lymphadenopathy and the development of leukaemia varies from months to several years and some patients may never develop CLL as defined above. A higher proportion of non-leukaemic than leukaemic cases present with *localised* lymphadenopathy, but there do not appear to be any other significant differences between the two groups (Pangalis et al, 1977). One can only speculate at the present time as to whether the rare non-leukaemic form of B-lymphocytic lymphoma is a distinct entity or not. A definite answer to this question must await further detailed studies of the cells in such cases.

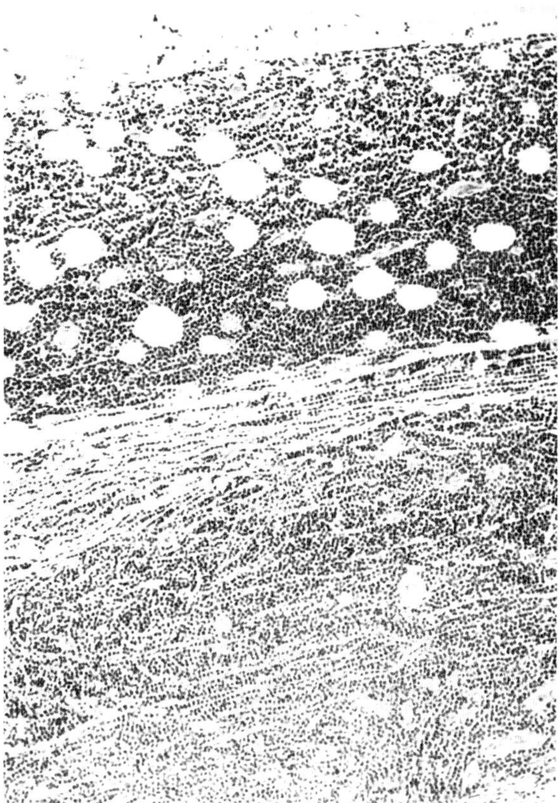

Fig. 10.1 Lymph node in B-lymphocytic lymphoma (B-CLL) showing typically diffuse pattern of infiltration of node (below) and of capsule and surrounding adipose tissue (above) by uniform small lymphocytes. (H E × 120)

Lymph node changes

Macroscopic. As stated above, the degree of lymphadenopathy is very variable but, when present, it is generally widespread and at times appears to involve every node in the body. The nodes are soft as a rule and discrete, even when massively enlarged. The cut surface is soft, pale pink in colour and bulges above the cut edge of the capsule (see Fig. 5.1, p. 68).

Histology. Typically the normal architectural features of the node are effaced by a featureless and closely packed mass of rather uniform-appearing small round cells. These cells fill every crevice of the node, obliterating the follicles and sinuses and often infiltrating the capsule and spreading into the hilar or surrounding adipose tissue (Fig. 10.1). The infiltration is characteristically non-destructive—a displacement of the pre-existing cell population, although the reticulin pattern is altered, the reticulin framework of the node being expanded, often uniformly, so that the sites of former sinuses and follicles are no longer discernible (Fig. 10.2). Only occasionally, in the 'tumour-forming' type of CLL (qv), is there significant distortion or compression of the reticulin framework.

On closer examination of the cells, these may be less uniform than appears at first sight. The great majority are small lymphocytes, generally slightly larger than the average size of lymphocytes in a normal node, with round or ovoid nuclei, a dense nuclear chromatin and rarely visible nucleolus. The cytoplasm is very scanty and hardly visible, staining feebly with Giemsa and being non-

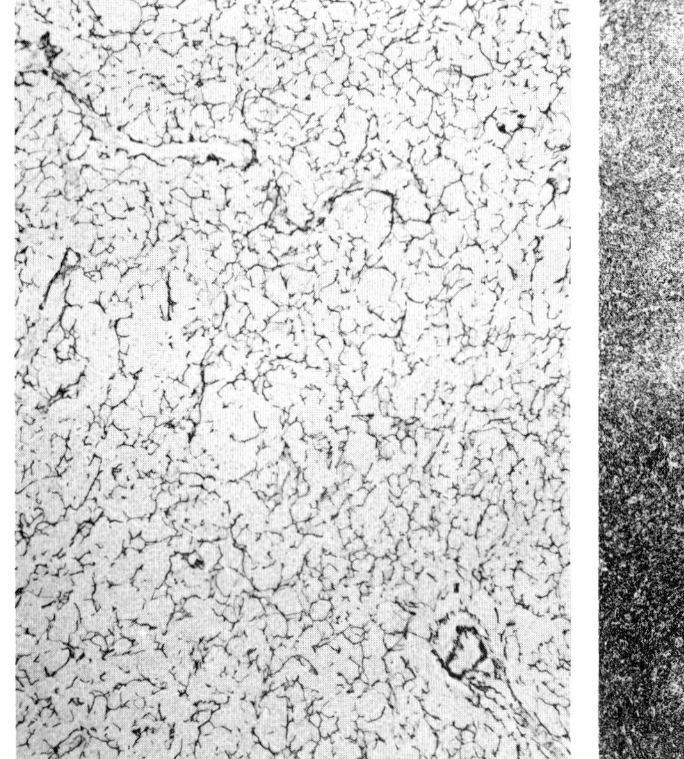

Fig. 10.2 Lymph node in B-lymphocytic lymphoma (B-CLL) showing reticulin pattern. (Compare with Fig. 12.11, p. 308) (Gordon and Sweets reticulin × 120)

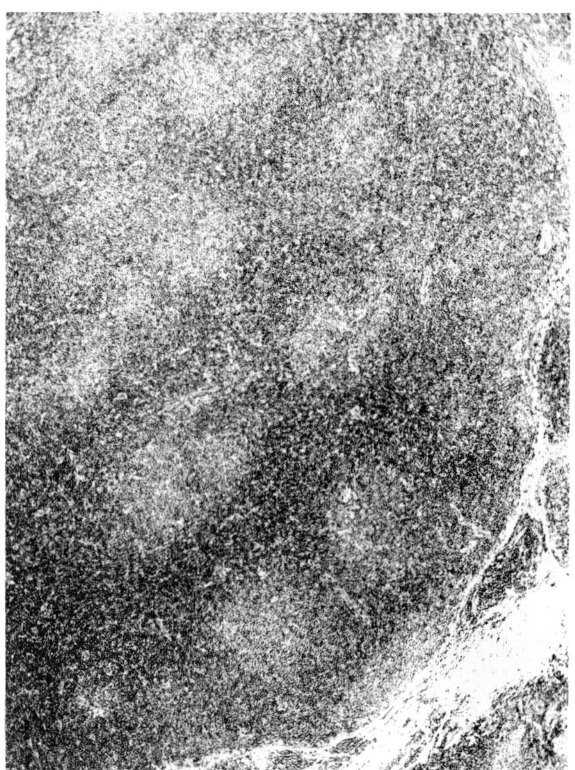

Fig. 10.3 Lymph node in B-lymphocytic lymphoma (B-CLL) showing poorly defined, pale pseudo-follicles (proliferation centres). (Compare with Fig. 10.53, p. 263.) (H E × 47)

Fig. 10.4 Same node as Fig. 10.3 at a higher magnification (H E × 120)

pyroninophilic with methyl-green pyronin (MGP). In many instances, however, there is a minority population of blast cells amongst the prevailing lymphocytes. The blast cells may be scattered singly or may be found in small, evenly distributed foci known as pseudo-follicles or proliferation centres (Fig. 10.3). These growth centres are generally smaller than true follicles and are much less well defined, but in a well fixed preparation they stand out as paler staining areas against the darker background of lymphocytes (Fig. 10.4). In each proliferation centre the blast cells lie singly amongst cells intermediate in size and appearance between the lymphocytes and the blast cells. Mitoses are generally scanty in B-CLL but tend to be concentrated in the proliferation centres. The blast cells are typically rather small with a 'vesicular' nucleus containing a prominent central nucleolus (Figs 10.5, 10.6). The scanty cytoplasm stains rather weakly in comparison with that of an immunoblast and Lennert (1978, p. 121) has termed these cells 'para-immunoblasts'. The intermediate cells, in which a small nucleolus is often visible, have been called 'prolymphocytes' (Lennert, 1978, p. 122)*, since morphologically they resemble the cells of prolymphocytic leukaemia (Galton et al, 1974).

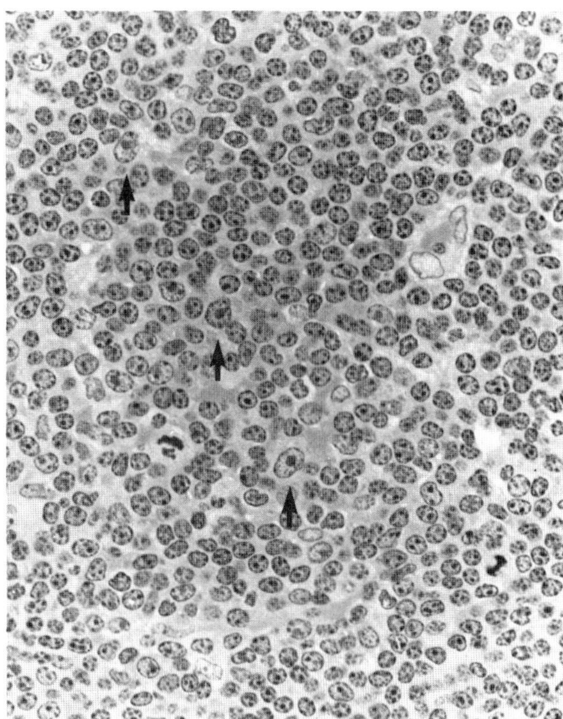

Fig. 10.6 Semi-thin section (resin embedded) from another case of B-lymphocytic lymphoma (B-CLL) showing a small proliferation centre and scattered paraimmunoblasts (arrows) in the midst of a uniform population of small lymphocytes. Note two mitotic figures and a small vessel (upper right). (H E × 600)

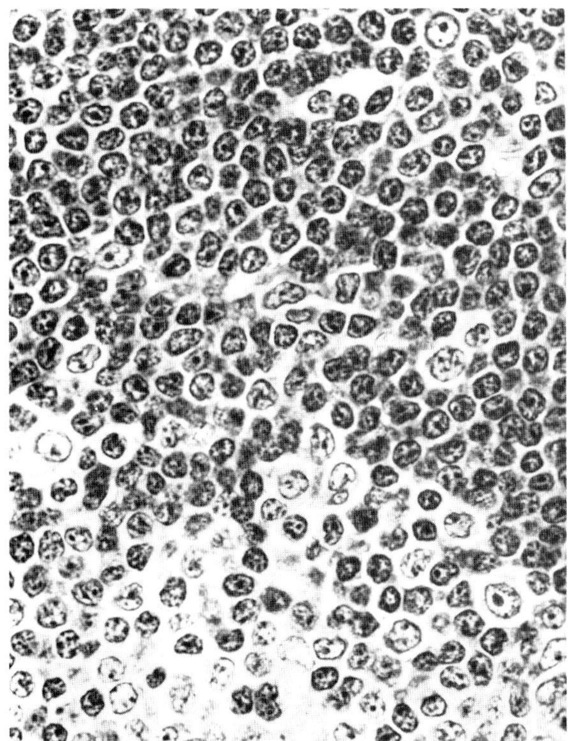

Fig. 10.5 Margin of a proliferation centre in B-lymphocytic lymphoma (B-CLL) showing the contrast between lymphocytes (above), prolymphocytes and paraimmunoblasts (Giemsa × 750)

In a minority of cases, the proliferation centres may be larger, even partially confluent, with an increased number of blast cells, sometimes of more variable type, and an increased number of mitoses. Lukes & Collins (1975) refer to the 'accelerated phase' of B-CLL in such cases and there is evidence that the progress of the disease is more rapid when this picture is found (Figs 10.7, 10.8). Occasionally, bizarre giant blast cells, resembling

* It should be emphasised that the term prolymphocyte is used here in the sense generally understood by haematologists and not in the same sense as that of the WHO classification (1976). The latter cell is a centrocyte.

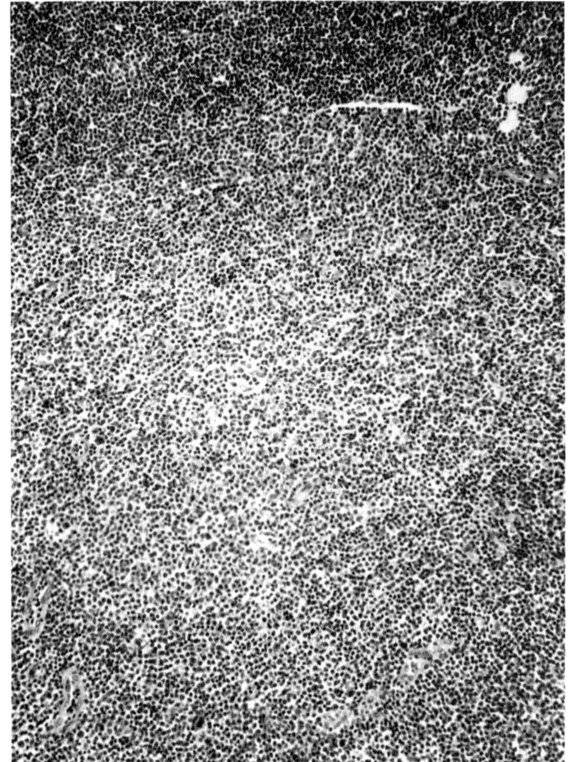

Fig. 10.7 Lymph node in B-lymphocytic lymphoma (B-CLL), 'accelerated phase', showing part of a large proliferation centre with typical small lymphocytes (above) (H E × 120)

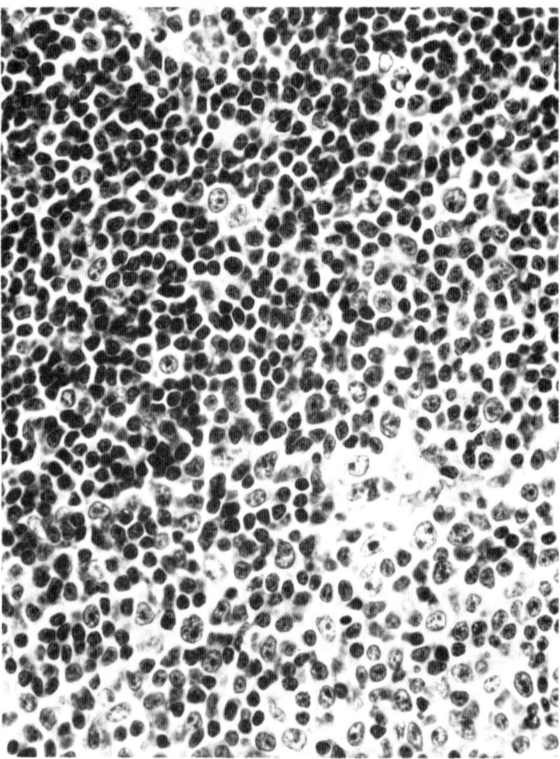

Fig. 10.8 Same lymph node as Fig. 10.7 showing an increased number of 'blast' cells in comparison with typical B-CLL (H E × 470)

Sternberg-Reed cells, may be found scattered amongst the small lymphocytes (Fig. 10.9). The finding is of interest in view of the well documented, though rare, association of Hodgkin's disease with B-CLL (see p. 244). The presence of confluent masses of atypical blast cells may signal the transformation of B-CLL into a high grade malignant lymphoma, generally of immunoblastic type (Richter's syndrome) (Fig. 10.10). The incidence of this transformation has been estimated at somewhere over 3% (Armitage et al, 1978).

Variant forms of B-CLL

'Tumour-forming' B-CLL (Lennert, 1978). As already indicated, in most instances of B-CLL the neoplastic cells mingle intimately with the cells of the infiltrated tissue whether this be a lymph node, bone marrow, spleen, liver or other organ. There

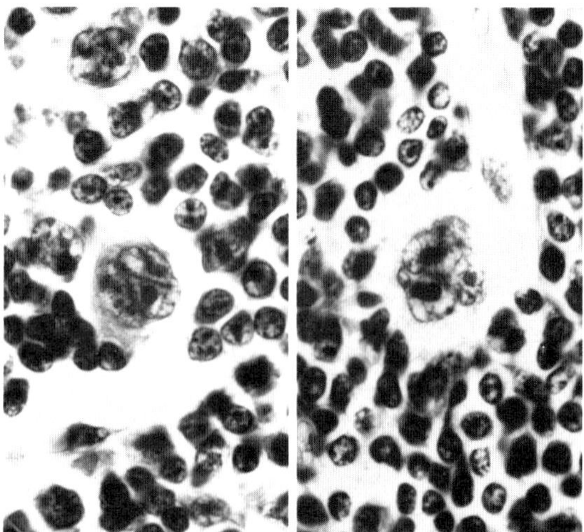

Fig. 10.9 Two fields from the spleen of an otherwise typical case of B-CLL showing large Sternberg-Reed-like blast cells amongst the lymphocytes of the white pulp infiltrate (H E × 940)

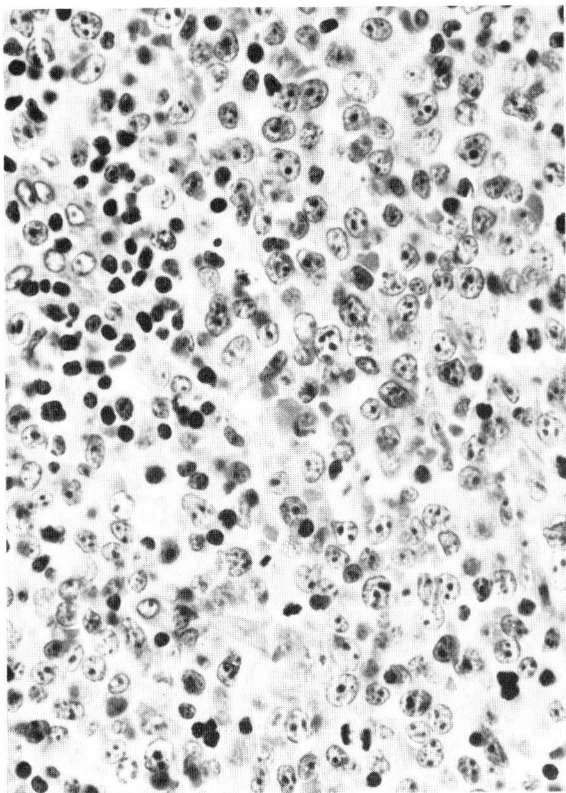

Fig. 10.10 Lymph node showing transformation of B-lymphocytic lymphoma (B-CLL) into a high grade immunoblastic lymphoma (so-called Richter's syndrome). Scattered lymphocytes persist amongst the blast cells. The bone marrow in this case showed diffuse infiltration by small lymphocytes at the time this biopsy was taken. (H E × 480)

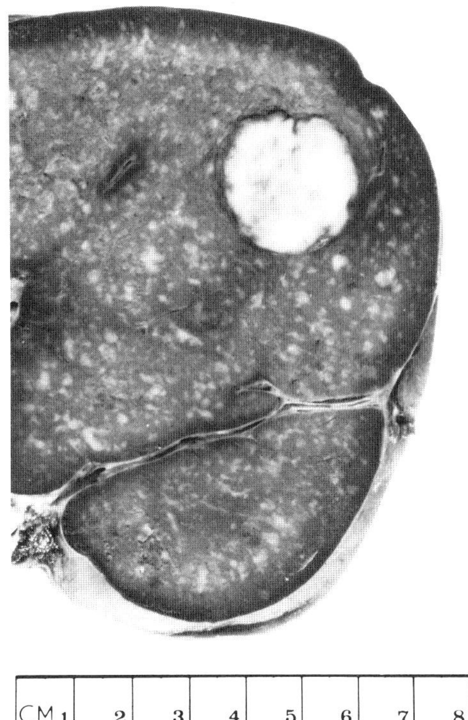

Fig. 10.11 Slice of spleen from a case of 'tumour-forming' B-CLL showing a discrete tumour mass as well as diffuse expansion of the white pulp characteristic of leukaemic infiltration

may be local aggregation of lymphocytes, for example, in the portal tracts of the liver, but the infiltration is essentially diffuse and non-destructive in type. The term 'leukaemic infiltration' is commonly used to describe this form of infiltration. Infrequently, the cells tend to adhere together to form expanding tumourous masses in addition to the diffuse type of infiltration (Fig. 10.11). The cells of these tumours are morphologically similar to those of the diffuse infiltrate but the prognosis in such cases is worse than that of classical B-CLL (Lennert, 1978, p. 115). The explanation of this cell cohesiveness in B-CLL is not known.

*Prolymphocytic leukaemia**. In typical B-CLL a large majority of the cells in the lymph nodes are small lymphocytes and larger sized lymphoid cells (prolymphocytes and para-immunoblasts) constitute a minor component. Rarely, prolymphocytes are the dominant cell type not only in the nodes and spleen, but also in the bone marrow and peripheral blood (Fig. 10.12). This disease is characterised by marked hepato-splenomegaly, very high prolymphocyte counts in the peripheral blood and a uniformly poor prognosis and lack of response to treatment (Galton et al, 1974). It is not certain whether there is a corresponding aleukaemic form of this rare variant of B-CLL. A prolymphocytic type of T-CLL has also been described (see p. 308).

Prognosis in B-CLL

In many instances B-CLL is a relatively indolent disease and in the elderly patient death frequently occurs from intercurrent disease rather than directly from the lymphomatous process. On the other hand, death may be indirectly hastened by

* See footnote on p. 235

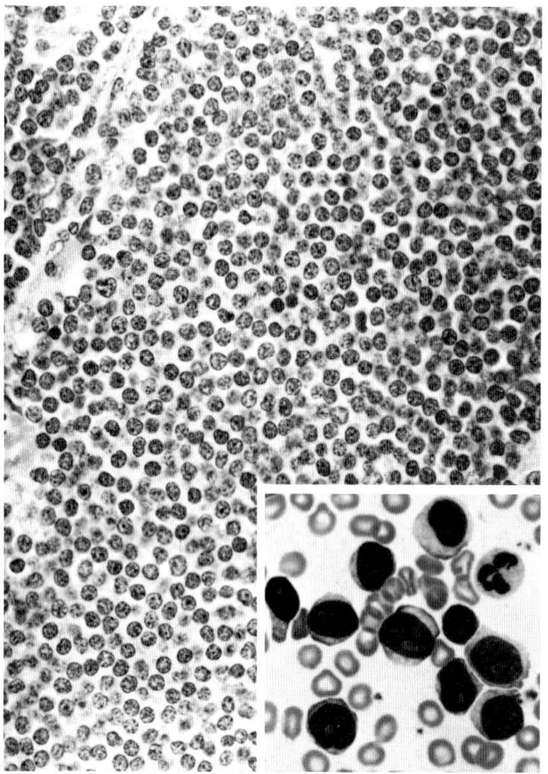

Fig. 10.12 Prolymphocytic leukaemia. Dilated lymph sinus filled with prolymphocytes in a lymph node biopsy from a patient with this condition. (H E × 470) Inset: prolymphocytes in the peripheral blood of this patient. (May-Grünwald Giemsa × 800)

B-CLL, owing to increased susceptibility to infection. Viral infections, such as herpes zoster, commonly occur and there is evidence too of an increased susceptibility to cancer (Gunz & Angus, 1965). On other occasions, death may be more immediately attributable to the condition itself and/or the attendant anaemia. Bad prognostic features are: (1) a variable cell picture in the lymph node biopsy with increased numbers of blast cells and/or large proliferation centres; (2) a tendency to form localised tumours; (3) a high peripheral blood lymphocyte count; (4) the cytological/histological picture of the prolymphocytic variant.

Differential diagnosis of B-CLL

It is pertinent to consider first the haematological aspects of the differential diagnosis. The finding of an excess of small lymphoid cells in the blood and/or marrow all too often has led to an uncritical diagnosis of chronic lymphocytic leukaemia, when a more careful examination of the cells might have shown them to have notched (cleaved) nuclei. Lymph node biopsy in such cases will reveal the histological picture of ML centroblastic-centrocytic type or sometimes ML centrocytic type. Occasionally, hairy cell leukaemia may be mistaken for CLL, but again a careful examination of the blood or marrow smears, if necessary with acid phosphatase staining after tartrate treatment, should make the distinction clear.

The histological diagnosis of B-CLL in a lymph node biopsy is not generally difficult with a good section, unless the picture is atypical. If fixation is poor, there may be difficulty in distinguishing other types of small cell lymphoma — ML centrocytic (p. 253) or lymphoplasmacytoid (p. 240) in particular, either of which may be accompanied by 'leukaemia'. The small celled T-lymphoblastic (convoluted cell) lymphoma should seldom be a problem since this is usually found in the young while B-CLL is a disease of late adult life. Unless fixation is very poor, the high mitotic rate in the lymphoblastic tumour is an obvious distinguishing feature. The differential diagnosis of B-CLL and T-CLL is considered in Chapter 12 (p. 308).

ML LYMPHOPLASMACYTOID
(Lymphoplasmacytoid Immunocytoma)

Synonyms:
ML plasmacytoid lymphocytic.
Diffuse lymphoma lymphocytic, well differentiated, with plasmacytoid features.
Diffuse lymphosarcoma, lymphoplasmacytic.
Waldenström's macroglobulinaemia (= one variety).

This is a group of neoplasms all of which are, by definition, of B-cell origin. They have features in common with ML lymphocytic of B-cell type, but are distinguished by the fact that many of the cells show evidence of plasma cell differentiation in varying degree, and *cytoplasmic* immunoglobulin (CIg) synthesis, not merely SIg as in B lymphocytic lymphoma.

Presentation. The neoplasms of this group differ from one another not only in the details of their cell composition (qv), but also in their mode of presentation and the latter is only partly determined by the histological and cytological sub-type. In some instances the patient may experience episodes of bacterial infection due to impaired immunity before the neoplasm becomes apparent, but the neoplasm itself often presents in one of three ways:

(1) With a *tumour* — this may be primarily within a lymph node or nodes but it is not uncommonly extranodal. On occasions, gross splenomegaly, in the absence of lymphadenopathy, is the presenting feature. Or there may be a solitary, extranodal tumour in orbit, salivary gland, lung, Waldeyer's ring, gastrointestinal tract, thyroid or skin — in each case with or without regional node involvement. In contrast to plasmacytoma, localised tumours of this type seldom seem to arise primarily in the bone marrow. One of the most interesting sites of extranodal involvement is the brain, which may be the primary seat of the disease, no other organ being involved. Certainly some, and probably many of the tumours of the brain which have been reported as microgliomas, are in fact lymphoplasmacytoid lymphomas (Jellinger et al, 1975).

(2) With a *chronic lymphoid leukaemia* resembling B-CLL. The clinical presentation here may closely resemble that of B-CLL, although the cell count in the peripheral blood is generally lower than that found in the average case of B-CLL. Leukaemia is much less common in lymphoplasmacytoid lymphoma than in B-lymphocytic lymphoma.

(3) With a *hyperviscosity syndrome*. This of course relates to those patients who have severe paraproteinaemia and in whom lymphadenopathy or splenomegaly are generally insignificant (Waldenström's syndrome). The physician may first be alerted by the discovery of a very high erythrocyte sedimentation rate or rouleaux formation in the blood, in the course of investigating a patient for non-specific symptoms of ill-health — fatigue, loss of weight, repeated respiratory infections, for example. Sometimes the hyperviscosity of the blood may lead to visual disturbances due to blockage of retinal vessels by 'shunting' of agglutinated red cells — a phenomenon which can be observed with an ophthalmoscope. At other times the increased blood viscosity may promote venous thrombosis in various parts of the body. It should be noted that paraproteinaemia is by no means an invariable accompaniment of lymphoplasmacytoid lymphoma, being found in one-quarter to one-third of all cases (Lennert, 1978, p. 220). When it occurs, the immunoglobulin class of the protein responsible for the 'M' band in the serum is of course the same as that found in the neoplastic cells. This immunoglobulin is generally an IgM, with either kappa or lambda light chains (but not both), in contradistinction to the paraprotein of myeloma which is generally IgG. Rarely a lymphoplasmacytoid lymphoma is found which is secreting IgG or IgA (Papadimitriou et al, 1979).

Development of ML lymphoplasmacytoid in immunodefective states

The remarks above concerning the presentation of this group of lymphomas apply to a majority of tumours of this class, which seem to arise *de novo*, without any antecedent contributory factors. It is, however, a significant fact that the great majority of the malignant lymphomas reported as occurring against a background of autoimmunity, immunodeficiency, or immunosuppression, are either of this type or belong to the closely related category of ML B-immunoblastic (Lukes & Collins, 1975). There is sometimes suggestive evidence of a viral 'trigger' being concerned in the process, as in the association of EBV infection with the X-linked lymphoproliferative syndrome of Purtilo (1980) (see p. 129). It has been speculated that different viruses might start off a train of B-lymphocytic proliferation, in the absence of effective T-lymphocyte control, which could culminate in the development of a B-cell lymphoma (Purtilo, 1980).

Whatever the mechanism underlying the development of malignant lymphomas in some organ-specific autoimmune diseases, the site of the tumour is clearly determined in most instances of this kind by the location of the preceding lymphoproliferative reaction. Thus autoimmune thyroiditis (Hashimoto's disease) may be complicated by a lymphoplasmacytoid lymphoma arising in the thyroid and Sjögren's syndrome may lead to the development of a similar tumour in a salivary gland. In other immunodefective states, whether inborn or acquired, malignant lymphomas may arise almost anywhere in the body, not necessarily in lymphoid organs.

Lymph node changes

Macroscopic. As already noted, lymphadenopathy is not invariably a feature of this type of lymphoma, the presentation of which may be extranodal (see above). When lymphadenopathy is present it is very variable in degree, being sometimes widespread, sometimes localised. There are no macroscopic features which distinguish the nodes from those of any other type of malignant lymphoma.

Histology. The normal architectural features of the node are generally obscured, but not always to the same degree as is usual in B-CLL. Sinuses may still be discernible and are sometimes dilated. Isolated germinal follicles may still remain in some areas, even when the bulk of the node is infiltrated by the tumour (Fig. 10.13). In some cases, blood vessels are very conspicuous, either on account of vascular proliferation, or because they are outlined by hyaline deposits, or both.

As a rule, the pattern of the tumour is diffuse throughout (Fig. 10.13), but sometimes it is distinctly nodular in parts, though seldom to a degree which is likely to cause confusion with centroblastic-centrocytic, follicular lymphoma (Fig. 10.14). The nodularity may be accentuated by strands of hyaline fibrosis, radiating from the centres of the nodular foci. Pseudo-follicles (proliferation centres) are much less conspicuous than in B-CLL, but may be found in over 50% of cases (Papadimitriou et al, 1979).

The impression gained from low power examination of the node varies from case to case. At times, the picture is strikingly uniform — a diffuse infiltration by small cells which appear to be all of similar size. In other instances, there is a great

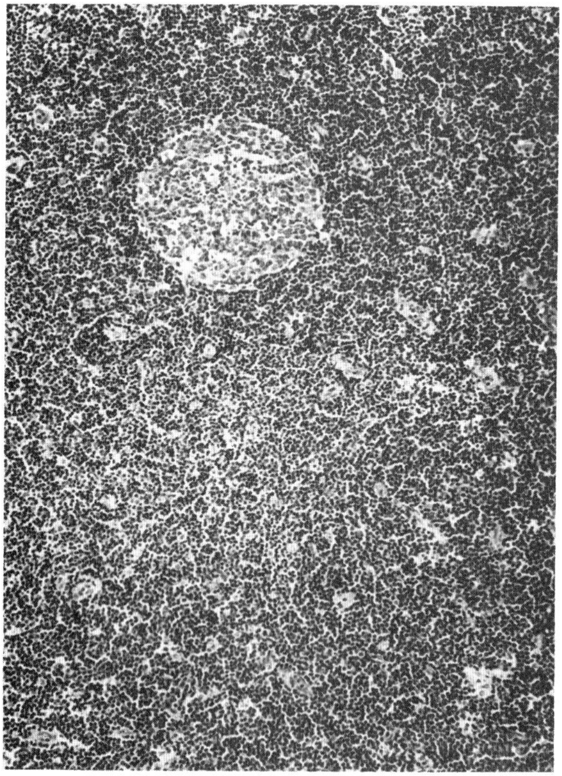

Fig. 10.13 Residual germinal follicle in a lymph node infiltrated by lymphoplasmacytoid lymphoma (H E × 120)

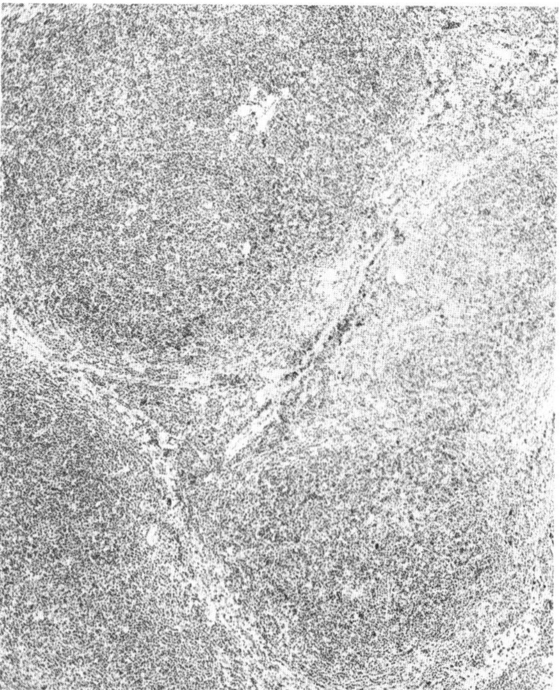

Fig. 10.14 Lymph node infiltrated by lymphoplasmacytoid lymphoma showing a distinctly nodular pattern. The nodules do not correspond to pre-existing follicles and the picture is unlikely to be confused with that of centroblastic-centrocytic follicular lymphoma. (H E × 47)

diversity in cell size and appearance. Indeed, there is probably a wider range of appearances in this group of malignant lymphomas than in any other, with the exception of Hodgkin's disease and certain T-cell lymphomas.

Essentially all the lymphoplasmacytoid lymphomas are composed of a mixture of lymphocytes, plasma cells and cells with intermediate characteristics between the two — lymphoplasmacytoid cells. These may be intermingled, but quite frequently some degree of segregation is seen, with groups of plasma cells or lymphoplasmacytoid cells alternating with groups of lymphocytes (Fig. 10.15). Blast cells, sometimes resembling the 'para-immunoblasts' of B-CLL, sometimes larger immunoblasts, are an almost constant feature, although in varying numbers. Mast cells are frequently increased, sometimes conspicuously so, and the picture may be further modified by a population of reactive macrophages, or epithelioid cells, the latter often in considerable numbers. Add to these variations in the cell picture the occasional occurrence of proteinaceous deposits, amyloid or para-amyloid, perhaps with secondary collagenisation, and some idea of the range of appearances may be gained.

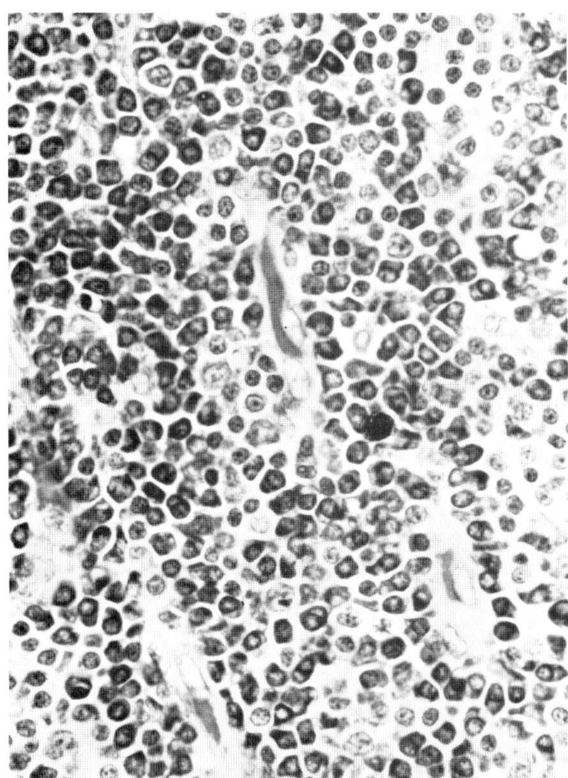

Fig. 10.15 *Lymphoplasmacytic* sub-type of immunocytoma with a predominant population of plasma cells (darker cells) and lymphoid cells. The black cell to the right of centre is a mast cell. Pleural tumour. (Giemsa × 500)

Three main histological sub-types of lymphoplasmacytoid lymphoma may be distinguished, namely, a *lymphoplasmacytic type*, a *lymphoplasmacytoid type* and a *polymorphic* (*or mixed*) *type*. These differ from one another not only in their histological characteristics, but also, to some extent, in their presentation and behaviour. Any one of the three sub-types may be associated with a paraproteinaemia (generally IgM) but this is most often seen in the lymphoplasmacytic sub-type. A chronic lymphoid leukaemia, on the other hand, is more often associated with the lymphoplasmacytoid sub-type. The rarely observed tendency of immunocytomas to undergo blast cell transformation is, not unnaturally, most frequent with the polymorphic sub-type.

1. Lymphoplasmacytic sub-type.

In this, a high proportion of the neoplastic cells show obvious plasmacytoid characteristics, indeed they may be typical plasma cells with round, excentric nuclei, a perinuclear 'hof' and abundant strongly staining cytoplasm (Figs 10.15, 10.16). Variable numbers of the plasma cells may contain in their cytoplasm brightly eosinophilic, usually PAS-positive, homogeneous globules (Russell bodies) which are composed largely of immunoglobulin within distended cisternae (Fig. 10.17). Exceptional tumours show a predominance of Russell body cells.

In addition to plasma cells, there is, however, always a certain proportion of lymphocytes in these tumours and generally a small number of immunoblasts (Fig. 10.17) which may contain the same light chain class as the plasma cells on immunoperoxidase staining. Mast cells are frequently increased (Fig. 10.18).

In cases of 'Waldenström's macroglobulinaemia' the histological picture is usually that of this type, less often that of the lymphoplasmacytoid sub-type.

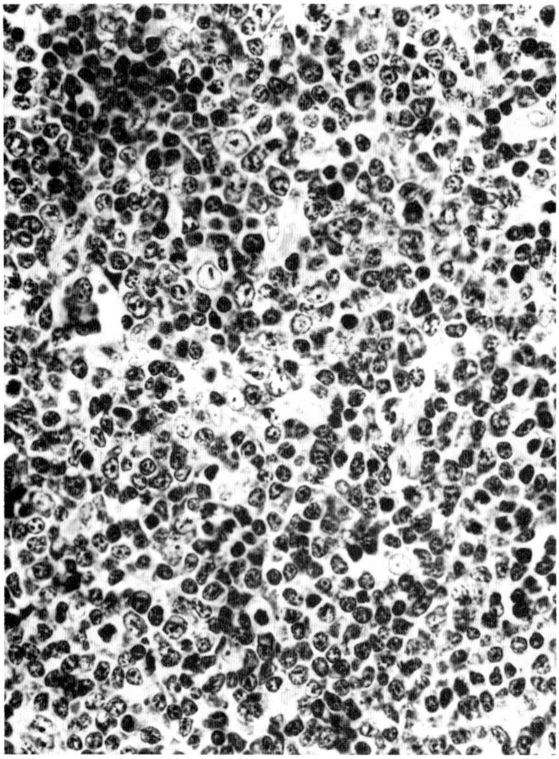

Fig. 10.16 Inguinal lymph node biopsy from a woman of 74 showing a lymphoplasmacytoid lymphoma of *lymphoplasmacytic* sub-type. The margin of a residual follicle is seen (top left). Most of the neoplastic cells show obvious plasmacytoid differentiation. Some blast cells are present. (Giemsa × 470)

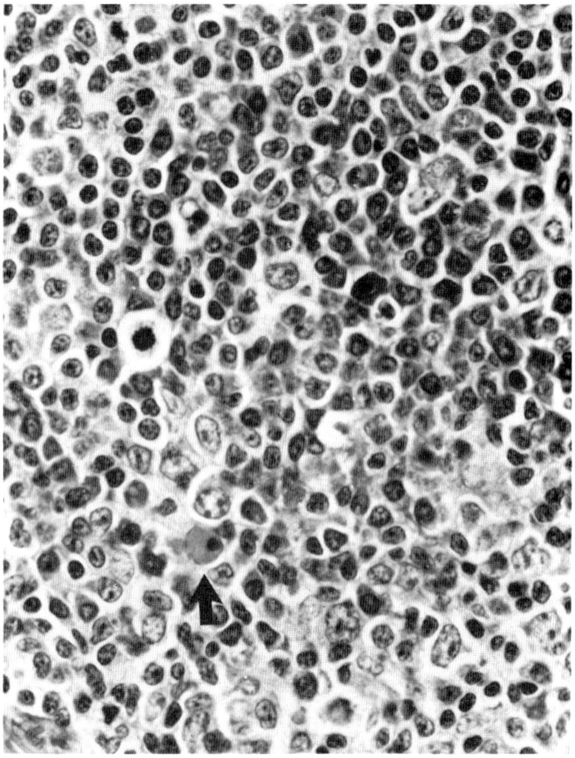

Fig. 10.17 Lymphoplasmacytoid lymphoma showing a characteristically heterogeneous cell population of lymphocytes, plasma cells, lymphoplasmacytoid cells and 'blast' cells. One cell contains a Russell body (arrowed). (PAS × 600)

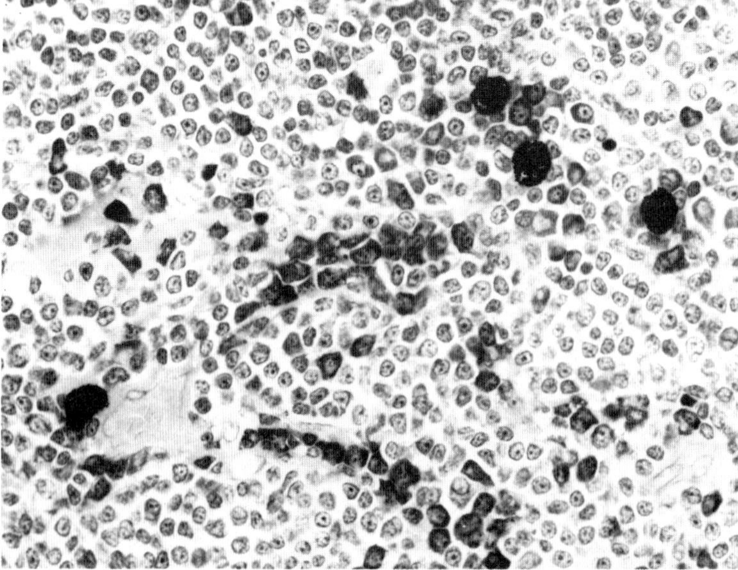

Fig. 10.18 Another lymphoplasmactyoid lymphoma (paraspinal mass) showing several heavily granulated mast cells in the tumour. These appear black in the illustration. Plasma cells are a shade lighter. (Giemsa × 470)

2. Lymphoplasmacytoid sub-type.

In this sub-type a small number of plasma cells may be seen, but typically the cells are of smaller size — only marginally larger than the lymphocytes, which are also present, so that close inspection may be necessary to pick out the plasmacytoid features of the lymphoplasmacytoid cells and thus to distinguish the picture from that of ML lymphocytic (Figs 10.19, 10.20). In those cases presenting with a leukaemic blood picture, the cells in the peripheral blood smears may be indistinguishable from the lymphocytes of B-CLL by light microscopy. On the other hand, the nucleus of lymphoplasmacytoid cells may show the coarsely clumped, 'clock-face' chromatin pattern of a plasma cell, even when the cell has very little cytoplasm. A proportion of the cells, however, show

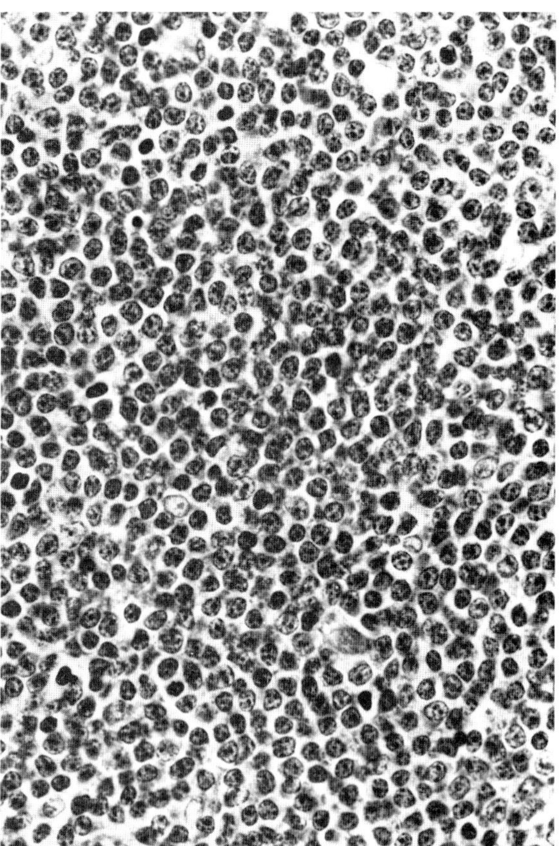

Fig. 10.20 Another case of lymphoplasmacytoid lymphoma of *lymphoplasmacytoid* sub-type showing relative monomorphism of the tumour cells. Close inspection at a high magnification is needed to detect plasmacytoid characteristics in many of the nuclei. (Giemsa × 470)

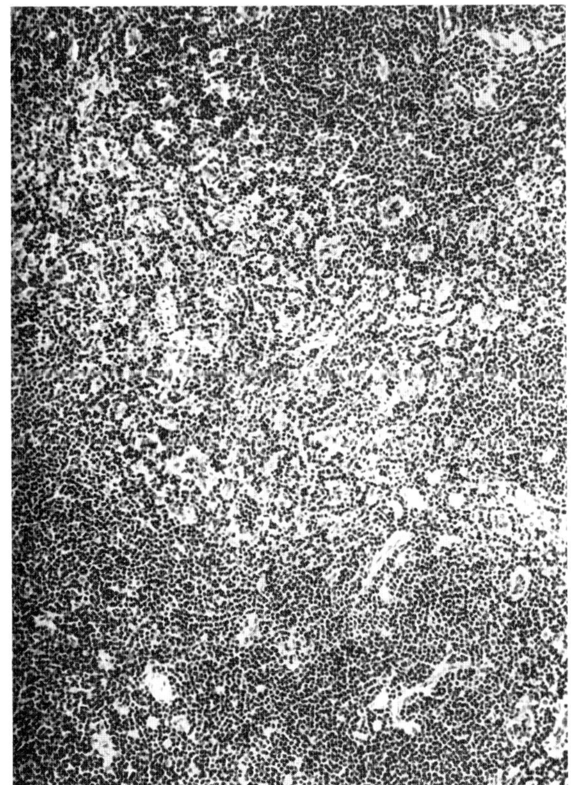

Fig. 10.19 Lymph node biopsy showing a lymphoplasmacytoid lymphoma composed of small, rather uniform lymphoplasmacytoid cells. The picture of this magnification is not unlike that of B-CLL except for outlining of small vessels (centre of field) due to hyaline thickening of their walls. (H E × 120)

rather more cytoplasm which stains strongly even with haematoxylin and eosin, but shows up even better with methyl-green pyronin or Giemsa staining. On electron microscopy, these cells, like those of the lymphoplasmacytic sub-type, can be seen to contain cytoplasmic strands of rough endoplasmic reticulum (Fig. 10.21), sometimes with cisternae distended by moderately electron dense material.

Sometimes the presence of Russell bodies may immediately distinguish a small-celled malignant lymphoma as belonging to this category, but Russell bodies are often scanty and may be absent in this sub-type. The recognition of Russell bodies and of the similar, apparently intranuclear inclusions known as Dutcher bodies, is greatly facili-

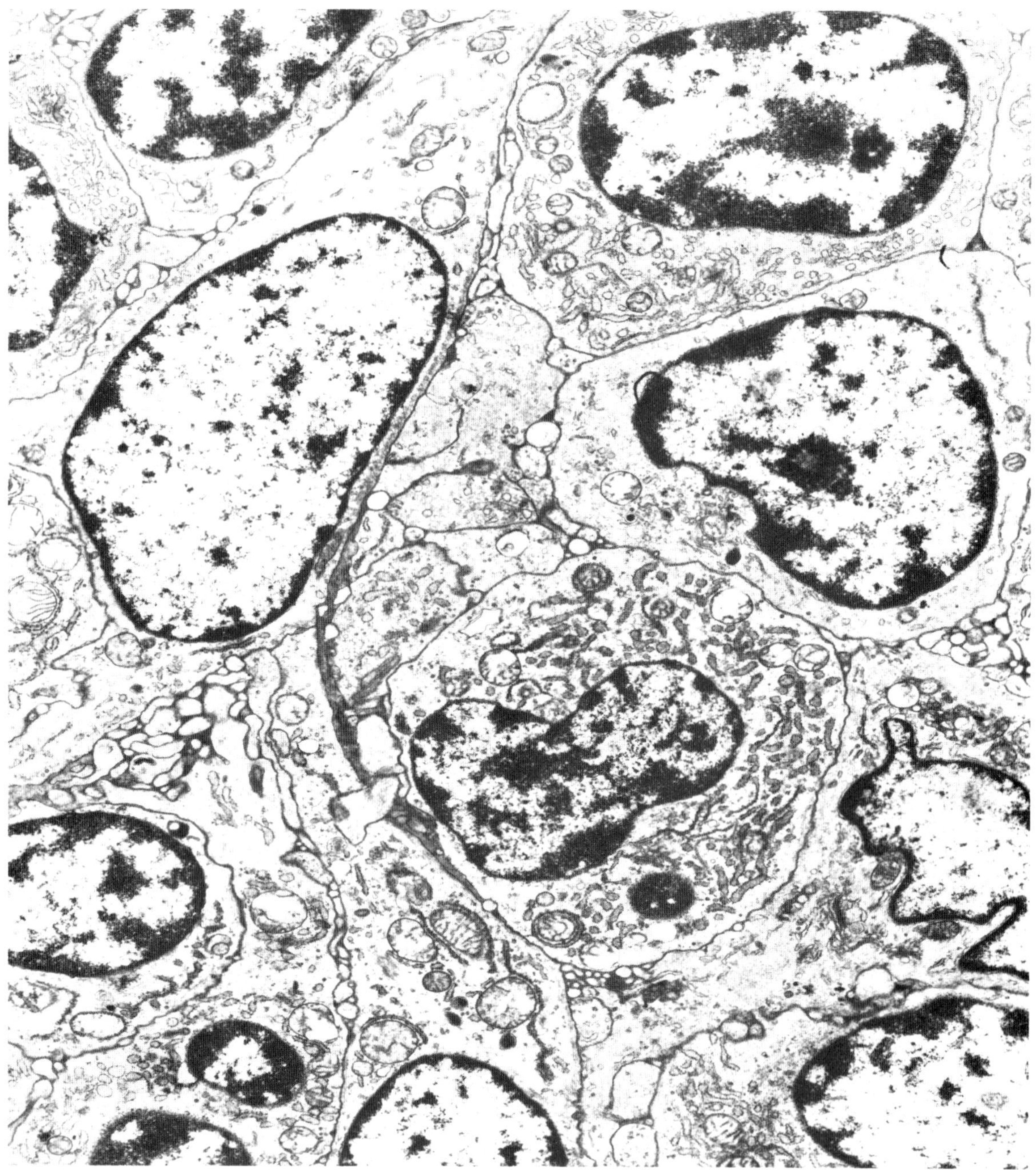

Fig. 10.21 Electron micrograph of a lymphoplasmacytoid lymphoma (same case as Fig. 10.16) showing short lengths of rough endoplasmic reticulum in the cytoplasm of many cells. Note the plasmacytoid character of the nucleus at top right.

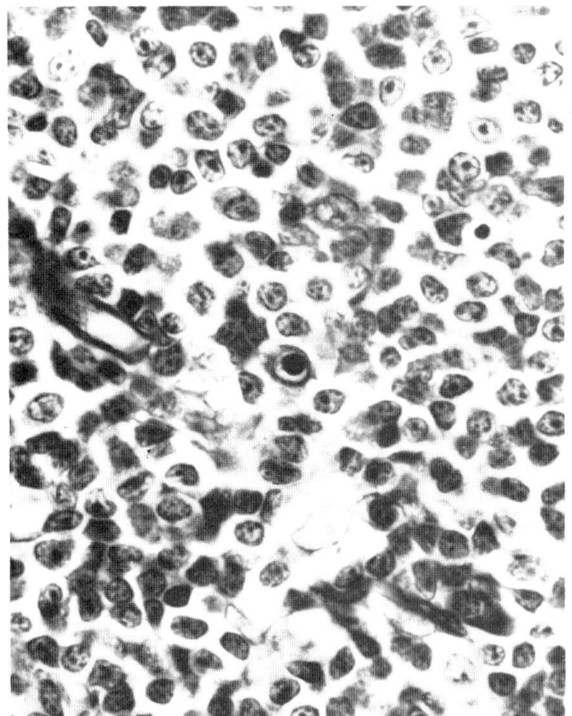

Fig. 10.22 Lymphoplasmacytoid lymphoma showing a prominent, PAS-positive, intranuclear Dutcher body in the centre of the field (PAS × 940)

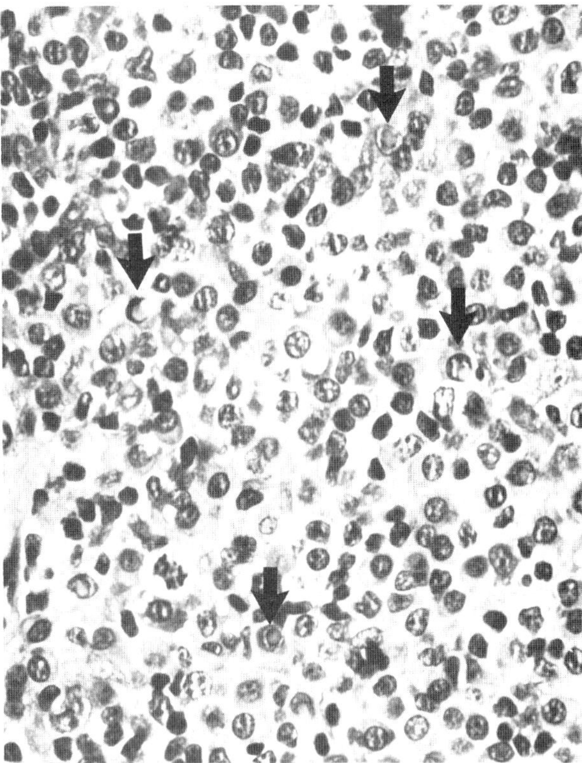

Fig. 10.23 Lymphoplasmacytoid lymphoma showing obvious plasmacytoid features in many cells and also numerous Dutcher bodies (arrows). Nasal tumour. (H E × 600)

tated by the use of the PAS stain, since both these bodies are generally strongly PAS positive and thus stand out clearly against the contrasting background (Fig. 10.22). Dutcher bodies, like Russell bodies, consist mainly of intracellular immunoglobulin, although they are often negative with the immunoperoxidase technique. Although they appear to be intranuclear and may be recognised in an HE stained section as clear, non-staining intranuclear vacuoles, they are in fact situated in 'nuclear pockets' — cytoplasmic invaginations of the nucleus, as can be shown by electron microscopy. The cells containing Dutcher bodies often resemble centrocytes rather than plasma cells, which can be linked to the fact that nuclear pockets are typical of the former, and are not ordinarily found in plasma cells. In some instances, however, a considerable number of Dutcher bodies may be found, regardless of the other morphological features of the cells (Fig. 10.23). The demonstration of Dutcher bodies is virtually diagnostic of an immunoglobulin-secreting B cell lymphoma, generally but not always of this class (see pp. 260, 271). The Russell body is less specific, especially when present in small numbers.

A variable but generally small population of immunoblasts is present in this as in the first sub-type.

3. Polymorphic (mixed) sub-type.

As the name implies, this sub-type is characterised by a more polymorphic cell picture than either of the other two. The plasma cells and lymphoplasmacytoid cells often show great variation and giant forms with two or more nuclei are common. There is also a substantially increased number of blast cells and these too may show marked pleomorphism, with giant binucleate forms which may be mistaken for Sternberg-Reed cells (Fig. 10.24). Mitotic activity is more evident in the polymorphic sub-type and mitoses are at times quite frequent

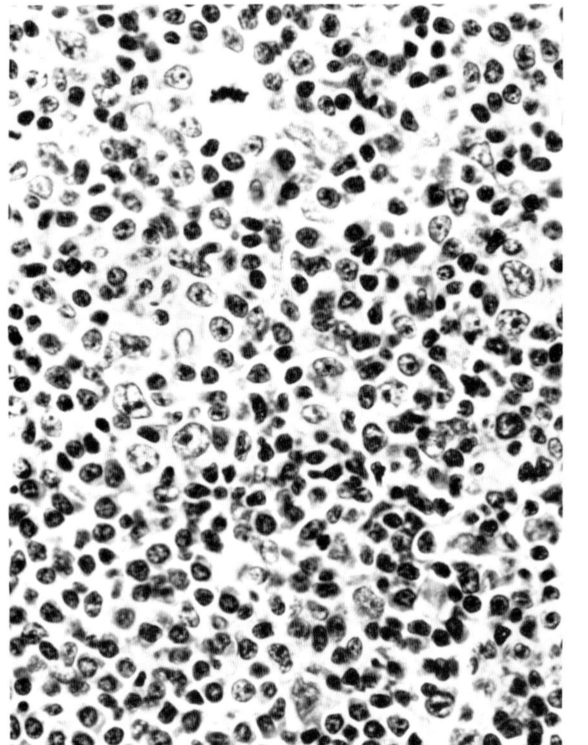

Fig. 10.24 Lymphoplasmacytoid lymphoma of *polymorphic* sub-type showing a relatively high proportion of blast-type cells and some mitoses, as well as plasmacytoid cells (H E × 470)

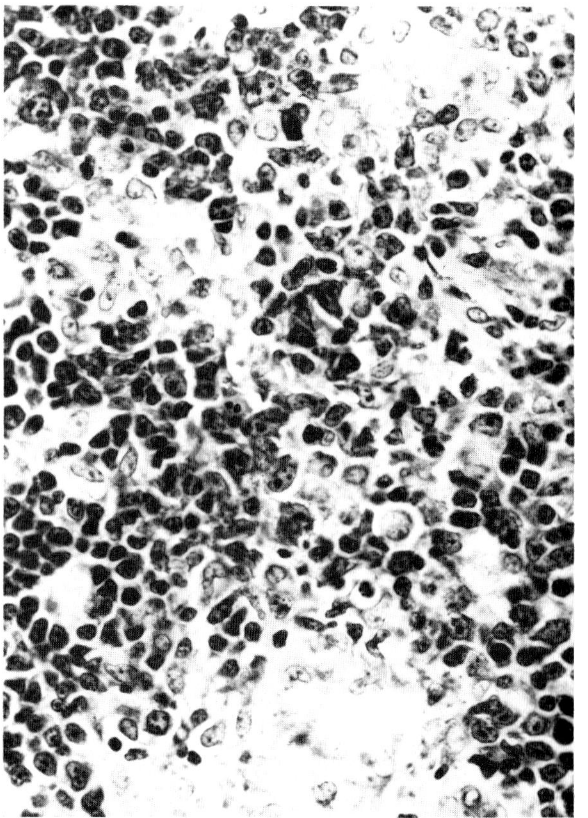

Fig. 10.25 Lymphoplasmacytoid lymphoma showing aggregates of epithelioid cells in the tumour (Giemsa × 470)

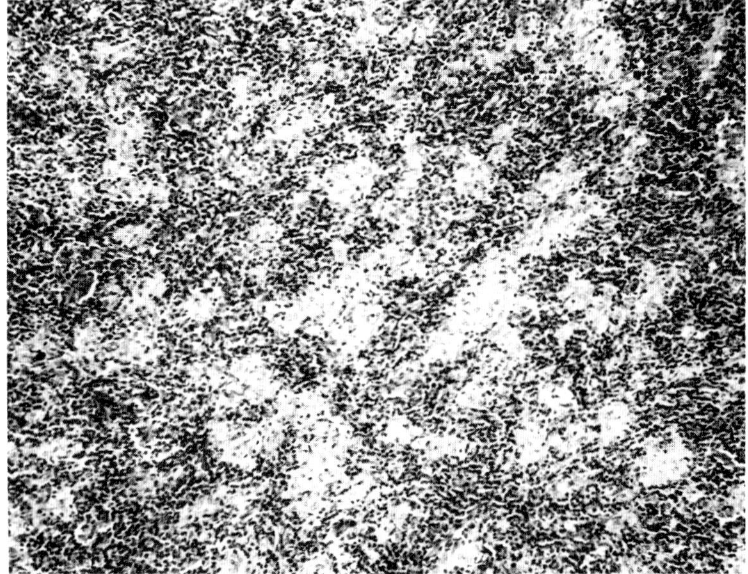

Fig. 10.26 Lymph node biopsy showing a lymphoplasmacytoid lymphoma in which small clusters of epithelioid cells were a dominant feature, producing a mimicry of Hodgkin's disease and lymphoepithelioid lymphoma (H E × 170)

and may be atypical. Lymphocytes are again present in variable numbers, but some of the smaller lymphoid cells have the morphological features of centrocytes, thus further increasing the cell diversity. Reactive macrophages and sometimes clusters of epithelioid cells may be an additional feature (Fig. 10.25).

The occurrence of epithelioid cell clusters in lymphoplasmacytoid lymphoma has been alluded to above. Exceptionally these may be very numerous and distributed throughout the greater part of the tumour (Figs 10.26, 10.27), resulting in a picture which closely resembles that of 'Lennert's lymphoma' (see p. 322 for discussion on differential diagnosis). Immunocytomas of this type are distinguishable from the true lymphoepithelioid lymphoma, and from rare cases of Hodgkin's disease showing a similar pattern, by the background population of plasma cells and lymphoplasmacytoid cells. Some cases of angioimmunoblastic lymphadenopathy (lymphogranulomatosis X) may be very difficult to distinguish on morphological criteria, but here the plasma cells are polytypic on immunostaining, not monotypic as in immunocytomas.

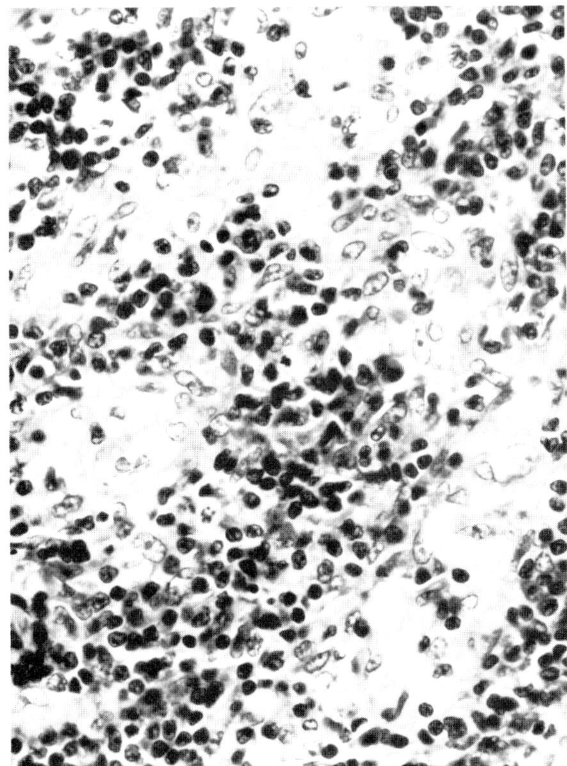

Fig. 10.27 Same node as Fig. 10.26 at a higher magnification to show plasmacytoid cells between the epithelioid cell clusters (H E × 470)

The picture is not invariably as mixed as the above description might suggest. Cellular pleomorphism may be less marked, but the diagnosis may be justified by the relatively high proportion of blast cells in the tumour. When this is so, there may be difficulty in distinguishing between a polymorphic immunocytoma and a high grade malignant lymphoma of immunoblastic type. The presence of obviously neoplastic (monoclonal) plasma cells, intermixed with the blast cells, serves to place the tumour in this category. On the other hand, the presence of solid sheets of immunoblasts may denote transformation into an immunoblastic lymphoma (see Fig. 11.26, p. 295).

Proteinaceous deposits.
As already observed, immunoglobulin secretion by the neoplastic cells may be evidenced not only by the presence of CIg in the cells (Russell bodies and Dutcher bodies), but also by the presence of extracellular deposits of proteinaceous material. This may be seen in its simplest form as a brightly eosinophilic, PAS positive, homogeneous coagulum in still patent lymph sinuses. Sometimes, however, there are more solid appearing deposits of homogeneous protein in sinuses or more widely dispersed throughout the tumour (Figs 10.28. 10.29). Deposits of this type are most frequently encountered in the lymphoplasmacytic sub type. The deposits may give some or all of the staining reactions of amyloid and in these cases they may evoke a foreign body giant-cell reaction (see Fig. 8.15, p. 172). The more widely dispersed eosinophilic material generally fails to stain or stains only feebly with amyloid stains and is often referred to as para-amyloid. Deposits of this kind may outline the blood vessels and the reticulin framework of the node (Fig. 10.30) and may show secondary collagenisation in varying degree, as indicated by fuchsinophilia with Van Gieson's stain. Deposits of the same kind may of course be seen in extranodal lymphoplasmacytoid lymphomas.

Prognosis. As might be expected, lymphoplasmacytoid lymphomas show a wide range of behav-

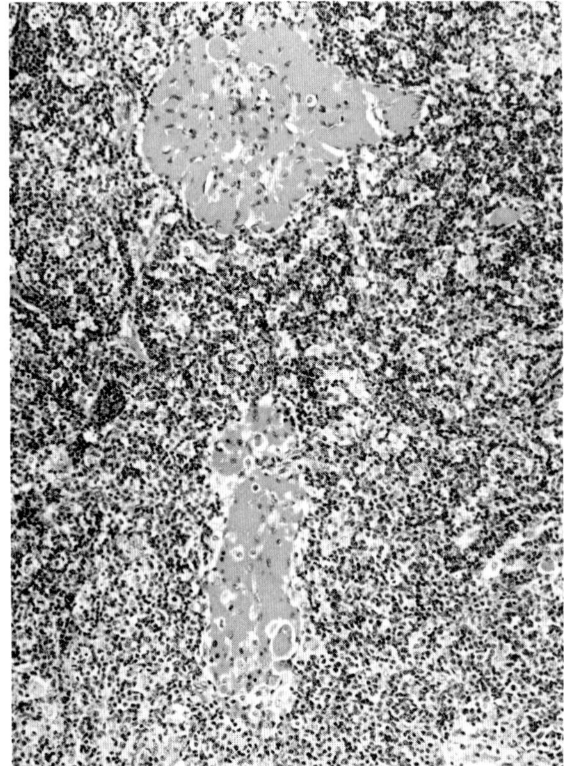

Fig. 10.28 Lymph node biopsy from another case of lymphoplasmacytoid lymphoma with paraproteinaemia, showing solid eosinophilic coagulum in dilated lymph sinuses (H E × 120)

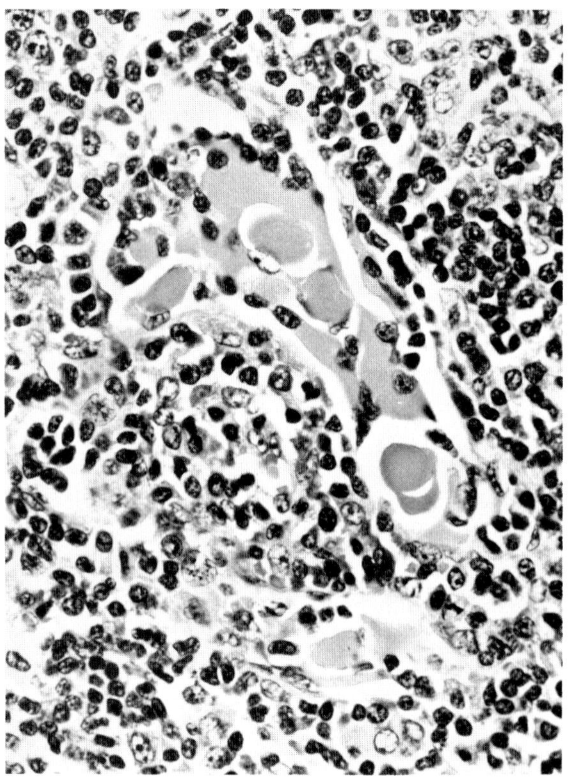

Fig. 10.29 Same node as Fig. 10.28 showing solid blocks of homogeneous proteinaceous material in a lymph sinus (H E × 470)

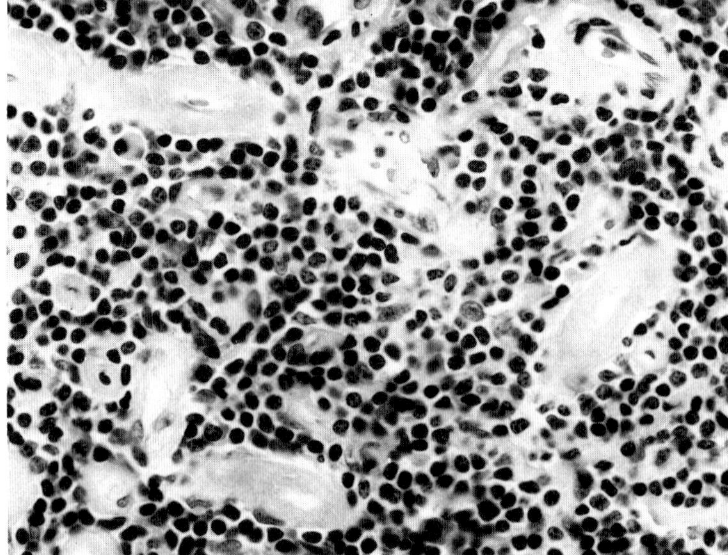

Fig. 10.30 Another case of lymphoplasmacytoid lymphoma in which all the small blood vessels of the node showed deposits of amyloid-like material in their walls. Note Russell-body cell (upper left). (H E × 470)

iour, but in general the prognosis is worse than it is for the B-lymphocytic lymphomas (Brittinger et al, 1977). Some of the extranodal tumours of this type, e.g. those arising in the orbit or the lung, may behave in a very indolent fashion, but those presenting primarily with lymphadenopathy, especially when the tumour is of the polymorphic sub-type, tend to have a much shorter survival. Death may be due to pneumonia or other intercurrent infection. Transformation into a high grade B-immunoblastic lymphoma is a relatively rare occurrence.

Differential diagnosis. The histological picture of the *lymphoplasmacytoid sub-type* in a lymph node biopsy has to be distinguished from those of ML lymphocytic and ML centrocytic of small cell type, both of which show a diffuse infiltration of the node by small lymphoid cells. A detailed study of the cells, however, with the use of Giemsa or methyl-green pyronin stains will reveal the plasmacytoid features, so characteristic of an immunocytoma. PAS staining is also useful in the demonstration of Dutcher bodies, while immunostaining with the PAP method may be useful in determining the monoclonal nature of the cells. On occasions a lymphoplasmacytoid lymphoma may contain very conspicuous blood vessels which may give an impression of a T-lymphocytic lymphoma/leukaemia, although the cell morphology is different.

The *lymphoplasmacytic sub-type* has to be distinguished on the one hand from a reactive plasmacytosis and on the other hand from a plasmacytoma (qv). If obviously reactive germinal follicles are a conspicuous feature this clearly favours a diagnosis of reactive plasmacytosis. However, small reactive centres may sometimes persist in lymphoplasmacytic lymphoma and, where doubt exists, the demonstration of monoclonality by PAP immunostaining may be required to resolve the doubt. Absence of follicles is equally unhelpful, for this again fails to discriminate between a reactive plasmacytosis of extreme degree and a low grade lymphoma of this type. The presence in the infiltrate of a complete range of maturing plasma cells, from plasmablasts and even immunoblasts, through to fully mature Marschalkó plasmacytes, favours a reactive plasmacytosis, for in a lymphoplasmacytic lymphoma, the plasma cells tend to be mainly of one type, that is, at a single stage of maturation. Once again, PAP immunostaining is the final arbiter in difficult cases for, in reactive states, the plasma cells are always polyclonal.

A plasmacytoma, whether arising primarily in the bone marrow (myeloma) or outside it, consists only of plasma cells and contains neither plasmablasts, nor lymphocytes.

The *polymorphic sub-type* of immunocytoma, depending on its cell composition, has to be distinguished from Hodgkin's disease, a high grade malignant lymphoma of immunoblastic type and especially when large numbers of epithelioid cells are present, from 'Lennert's lymphoma' (see p. 322) and from immunoblastic lymphadenopathy. The first two of these differential diagnoses have already been mentioned in the description of this sub-type. The high proportion of plasmacytoid cells in an immunocytoma distinguishes this from Lennert's lymphoma, but the distinction from immunoblastic lymphadenopathy (lymphogranulomatosis X) may at times be difficult. The characteristic vascular arborisation of the latter is not, however, seen in an immunocytoma, although blood vessels may be a prominent feature of the latter.

Finally, those cases of lymphoplasmacytoid lymphoma showing amyloid deposits in the node biopsy have to be distinguished from primary amyloidosis of lymph nodes (see p. 170), whilst diffuse para-amyloid infiltration should not be mistaken for simple scarring on the one hand or lymphocyte depleted Hodgkin's disease on the other. Careful examination of the cells should prevent these mistakes.

ML PLASMACYTIC

Synonyms:
Plasmacytoma.
Extramedullary plasmacytoma.

This type of lymphoma was not included in the original Kiel classification but later discussion among the authors of the classification made clear that it should be included as a separate category. The plasmacytic lymphomas are composed exclusively of plasma cells and *contain neither lympho-*

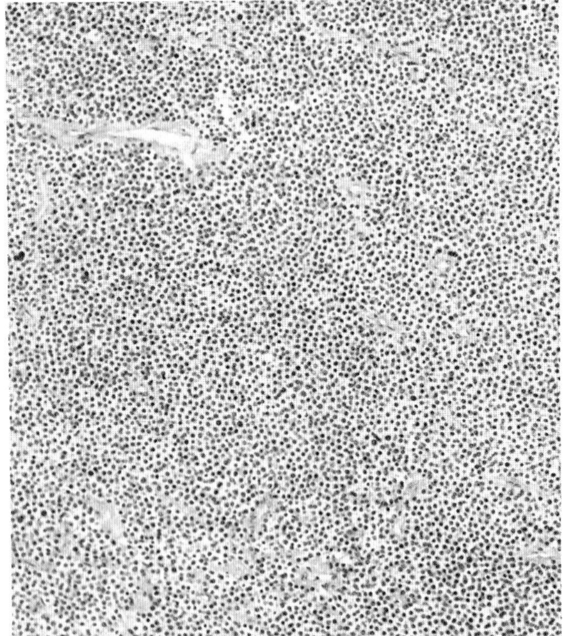

Fig. 10.31 Lymph node biopsy showing a plasmacytic lymphoma (extramedullary plasmacytoma). Note the striking uniformity of the cells. (H E × 120)

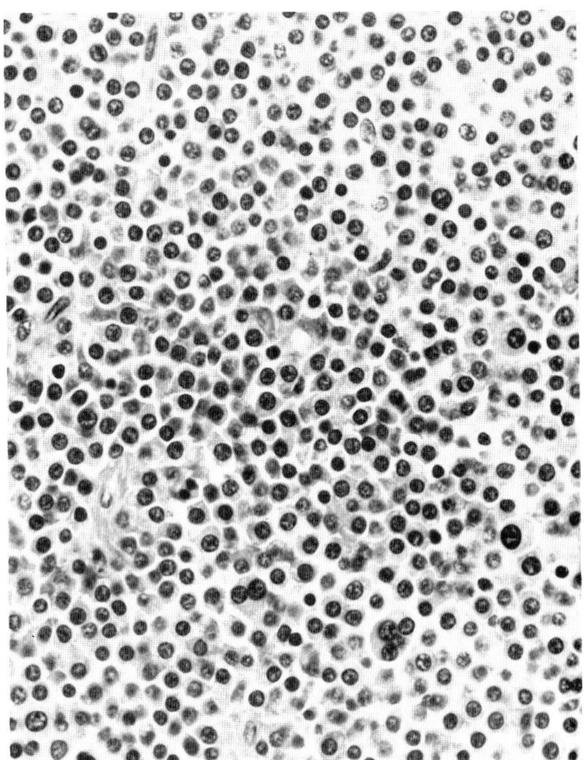

Fig. 10.32 Same node as Fig. 10.31 at a higher magnification. The cells are all plasma cells — there are no lymphocytes or lymphoplasmacytoid cells and no plasmablasts. (H E × 470)

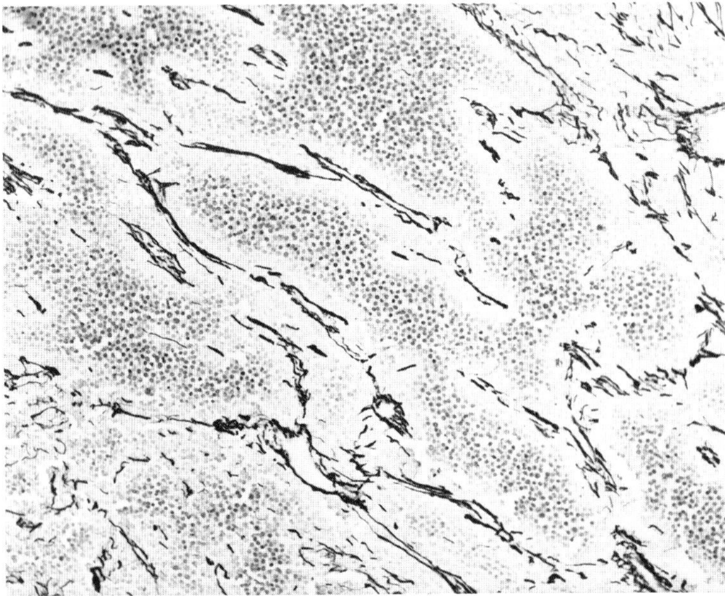

Fig. 10.33 Same node as Figs 10.31 and 10.32. Silver impregnation shows a coarse network of argyrophil fibres (compare with Fig. 11.34, p. 298). (Gordon and Sweets reticulin × 120)

cytes nor blast cells, i.e. all the neoplastic cells are of the same stage of maturity and are often strikingly uniform. Excluding those tumours which arise in the bone marrow (myeloma), ML plasmacytic occurs most frequently as a primary tumour of the gastrointestinal tract. Tumours of this class occasionally arise in the respiratory tract, the nasal passages, Waldeyer's ring or elsewhere, but are very rare as primary tumours of lymph nodes. Care must be exercised in excluding the possibility that an apparently primary lymph node plasmacytoma is not in fact a metastasis from a latent bone marrow tumour.

Histology. The node biopsy shows diffuse infiltration by plasma cells, generally of very uniform type (Fig. 10.31). Whilst the cells are readily identified as plasma cells (Fig. 10.32), they are often immature and atypical forms may be seen. Mitoses are infrequent in nodal plasmacytomas. The reticulin pattern is distinctive and the tumour cells are enclosed in a coarse network of fibres (Fig. 10.33).

Prognosis. The primary plasmacytomas of lymph nodes seem generally to behave in a rather indolent manner. A single lymph node is often involved and simple excision of the node may be curative. On the other hand, the disease may subsequently make its appearance in the bone marrow, so the distinction from primary myeloma is not always easy.

Differential diagnosis. (See under ML lymphoplasmacytoid — lymphoplasmacytic sub-type, p. 249.)

ML CENTROCYTIC

Centrocytic lymphoma was first recognised as a distinct variety of diffuse malignant lymphoma by Lennert under the title of germinocytoma (Lennert et al, 1975). Centrocytes in a reactive germinal centre vary appreciably in size, although there is as yet no indication that there are functional differences between the larger and smaller cells of this class. However, in many malignant lymphomas of centrocytic type we find that the tumour is composed, either of small centrocytes, or of large centrocytes, the cells in a single tumour often exhibiting quite a narrow range of cell size. There are of course exceptions to this rule and in certain centrocytic lymphomas the cells do vary quite markedly in size, nevertheless the separation of two different sub-types of centrocytic lymphoma is justified on more grounds than just the matter of cell size, for there are other morphological and behavioural differences which will emerge in the account which follows. The differential diagnosis is also peculiar to each sub-type, so the two sub-types will be considered separately.

Small-celled Centrocytic Lymphoma

Synonyms:
Small cleaved follicle centre cell lymphoma.*
ML poorly differentiated lymphocytic, diffuse.
Diffuse lymphoma, lymphocytic, intermediate differentiation.
Diffuse lymphosarcoma, prolymphocytic.

The cells composing this neoplasm resemble the small centrocytes of germinal centres in their morphology but their surface markers are sometimes intermediate between those of germinal centre centrocytes and the B-lymphocytes of the mantle zone (see p. 55). They show larger amounts of SIg (of single light chain type as a rule) than the cells of B-CLL, but CIg is absent or present in trace quantities only.

Incidence and presentation

Although less common than either B-lymphocytic or centroblastic-centrocytic lymphomas, these neoplasms are not rare and in our experience occur with approximately the same frequency as lymphoplasmacytoid lymphomas.

As with other low grade malignant lymphomas of B-cell type, the small-celled centrocytic lymphomas may present in several different ways:

(1) With lymph node swellings, which may be localised to a single group, but are often more widespread.

(2) With extranodal tumours, most commonly occurring in the gastrointestinal tract, which may show remarkably extensive involvement.

* This term is employed by Lukes & Collins (1975) for both ML centrocytic and ML centroblastic-centrocytic of the Kiel classification and these authors do not distinguish ML centrocytic as a separate type.

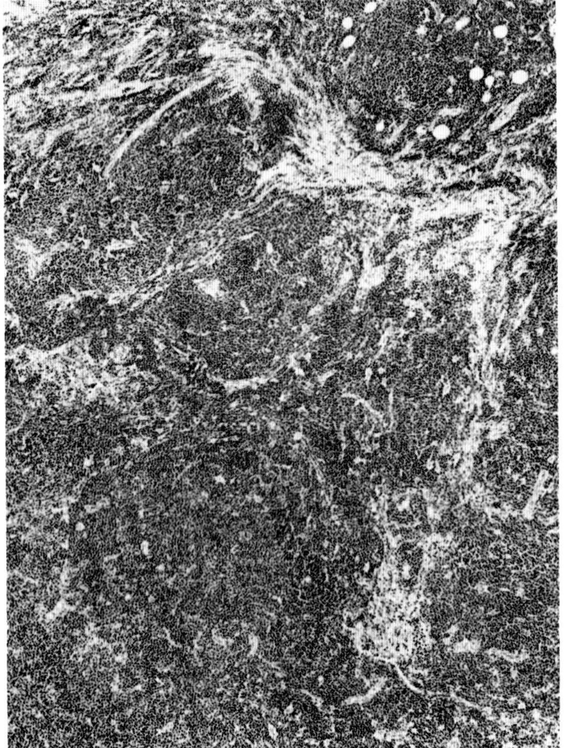

Fig. 10.34 Lymph node replaced by small-celled centrocytic lymphoma. There is a vaguely nodular pattern in parts of the tumour, but this is not borne out by reticulin staining. The cells appear very uniform. Note areas of hyaline fibrosis. (H E × 60)

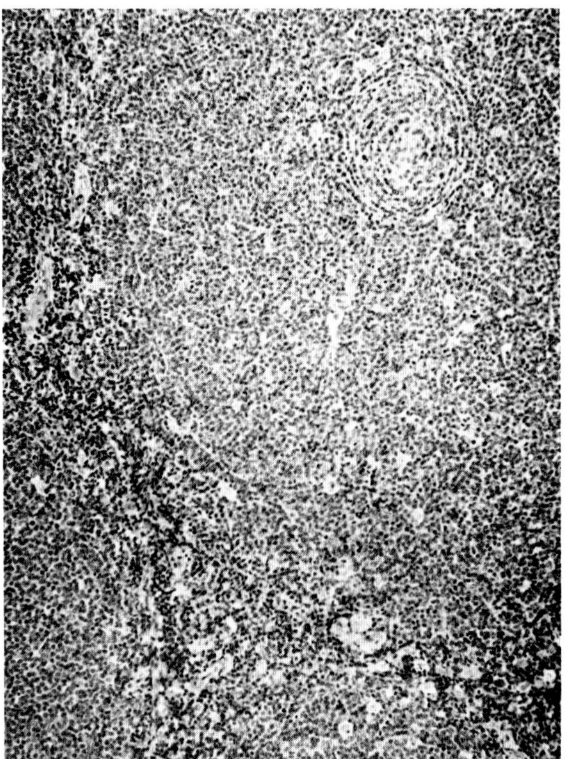

Fig. 10.35 ML centrocytic showing a nodular pattern with a mantle of neoplastic centrocytes surrounding the remains of a small germinal follicle in which the cells were polytypic on immunostaining. This pattern was found in a part of the tumour only and in a subsequent biopsy the pattern of the tumour was diffuse throughout. (H E × 120)

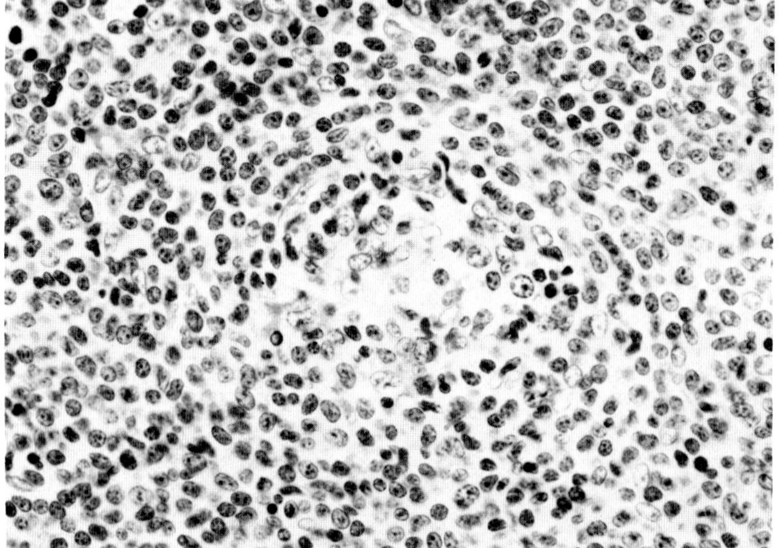

Fig. 10.36 Higher power view of the top right hand corner of field in Fig. 10.35. Note the contrast between the uniformity of the neoplastic centrocytes and the non-neoplastic germinal centre cells in the middle. (H E × 470)

(3) With a chronic lymphoid leukaemia, which may be mistaken for B-CLL.

(4) With massive splenomegaly, generally accompanied by a leukaemic blood picture.

Lymph node changes

Macroscopic. There are no distinctive features in the involved lymph nodes. In gastrointestinal tract lesions, the disease tends to present as lymphomatous polyposis with diffuse infiltration of the mucosa.

Histology. The normal architectural features of the node are usually effaced by a diffuse infiltrate of very uniform appearing small lymphoid cells (Fig. 10.34). Although it is usual to see replacement of the whole node by the neoplastic cells, there may sometimes be remnants of reactive follicles and, in some instances, one may have the impression that the neoplastic process has originated in the mantle zone of the follicle and extended outwards, leaving the original germinal centre or part of it intact (Figs 10.35, 10.36) (see under differential diagnosis p. 257). The pattern of the tumour is diffuse, but in focal areas there may be a tendency to nodular aggregation of the cells, resulting in poorly defined rounded masses, with a certain resemblance to primary follicles (Fig. 10.34). Rarely a more marked follicular pattern is seen, but this is seldom present throughout and in most instances there is no difficulty in distinguishing the picture from that of centroblastic-centrocytic lymphoma. Reticulin staining is sometimes helpful in making this distinction, for whilst the silver stain nearly always accentuates the follicular pattern in a centroblastic-centrocytic lymphoma, outlining the separate follicles, the reverse is often the case with those centrocytic lymphomas which show a nodular pattern, that is to say, silver staining makes the pattern less rather than more apparent.

At first sight, the picture may be mistaken for that of B-CLL, especially if there is leukaemia, but in a well fixed, well stained preparation, with reasonably thin sections, three distinguishing features may be noted:

(1) The cell picture is remarkably uniform and there are neither proliferation centres nor blast cells. Despite this, mitoses may be quite numerous.

(2) The cells are perceptibly larger than the cells of B-CLL, having more cytoplasm and an irregular, often angular and elongate nucleus, as opposed to the round nucleus of the lymphocyte (Fig. 10.37). Furthermore, the nuclear chromatin is less dense and a small central nucleolus is sometimes visible (Fig. 10.38). In lymph node imprints or blood smears, the 'cleaved' nucleus is very apparent in a proportion of the cells. Nuclear clefts are more difficult to make out in sections examined by light microscopy, and may appear as darker streaks or lines. Nuclear irregularities are readily seen on electron microscopy.

(3) A very commonly observed feature, and one which is characteristic of this tumour, is hyaline collagenous thickening of the capillary walls in in-

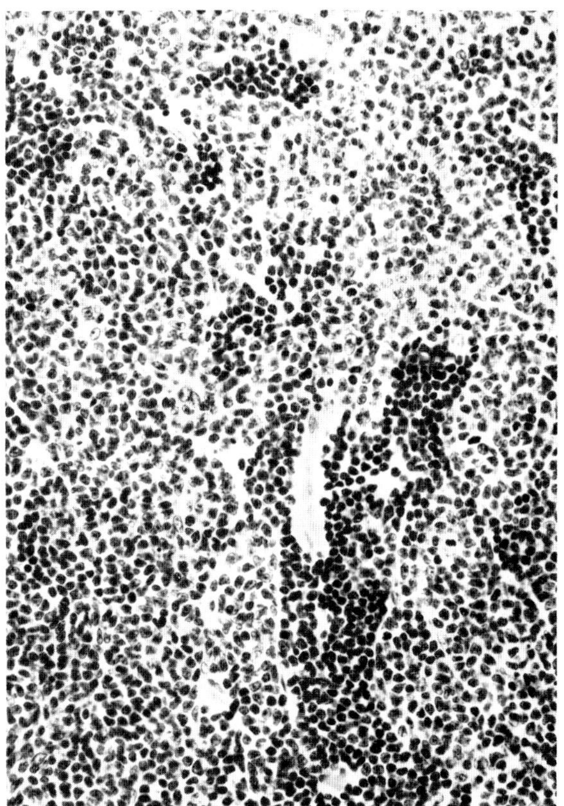

Fig. 10.37 Small-celled centrocytic lymphoma showing the contrast between the larger, paler neoplastic centrocytes and the smaller, darker residual lymphocytes in the node (H E × 300)

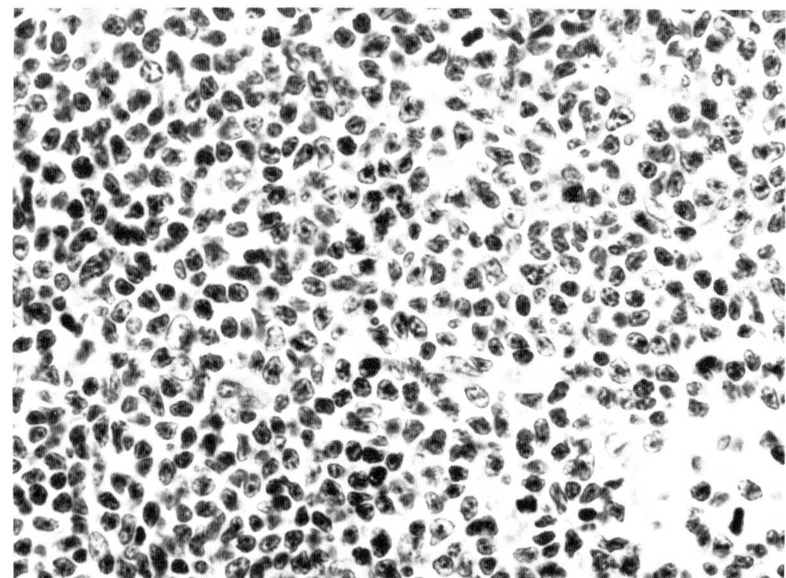

Fig. 10.38 ML centrocytic. The irregular shape of the nuclei can be clearly seen. A small nucleolus is often visible. (H E × 600)

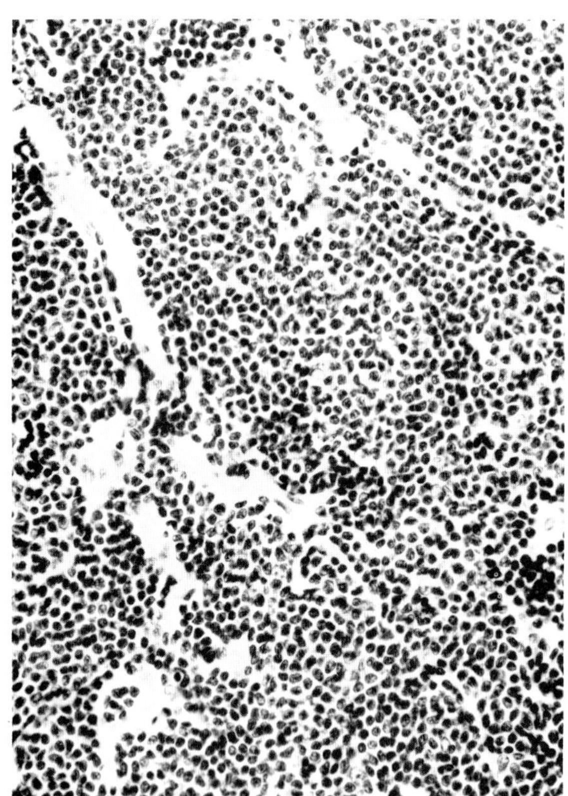

Fig. 10.39 ML centrocytic of small-celled type showing hyaline thickening of vessel walls — a distinctive feature of this tumour (H E × 300)

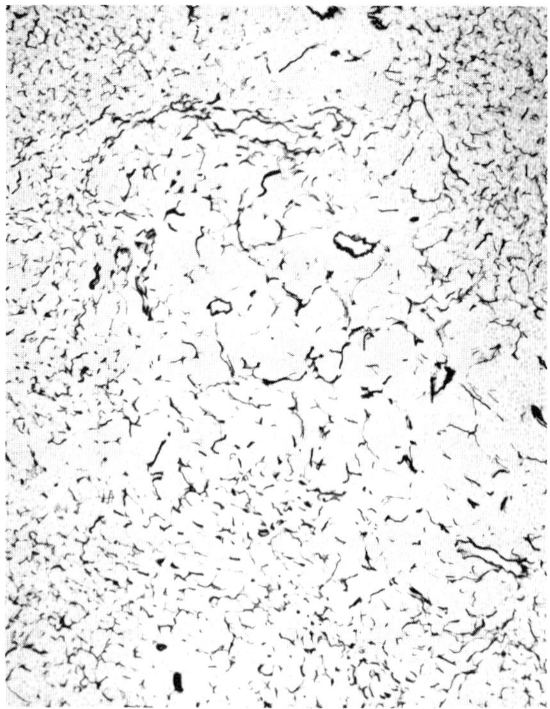

Fig. 10.40 Reticulin pattern of small-celled centrocytic lymphoma showing focal expansion of the reticulin framework around the blood vessels the walls of which are heavily outlined (Gordon and Sweets reticulin × 120)

filtrated regions of the node. This can easily be picked up with H & E staining (Fig. 10.39). Reticulin staining shows a general paucity of fibres in the tumourous areas with coarse, black strands representing thickened capillary walls (Fig. 10.40).

The progressive replacement of the lymph node by the centrocytic tumour results in diminution or disappearance of lymphocytes and most other cell types. As with other germinal centre-cell lymphomas, dendritic reticulum cells are found in association with the neoplastic centrocytes, but they are hard to distinguish by light microscopy. Centroblasts are absent or present in such small numbers that they are difficult to detect except where remnants of reactive follicles are present. Plasma cells are sometimes seen in small numbers, but these are generally reactive, i.e. polyclonal with immunostaining. From time to time, the monotony of the cell picture is relieved by the presence of isolated large macrophages, scattered through the tumour (Figs 10.41, 10.42).

The same cytological features distinguish the small-celled centrocytic lymphomas arising in the gut or elsewhere. With splenic involvement, whilst the neoplastic infiltrate appears to be centred on the white pulp in a diffuse manner, it commonly spreads outside, with progressive loss of distinction between white and red pulp, both macroscopically and microscopically. Localised tumour deposits are rarely, if ever, seen.

Related types of lymphoma — 'intermediate' and 'mantle-zone' lymphomas

Largely on the basis of marker studies, Jaffe et al (1977) distinguished a group of malignant lym-

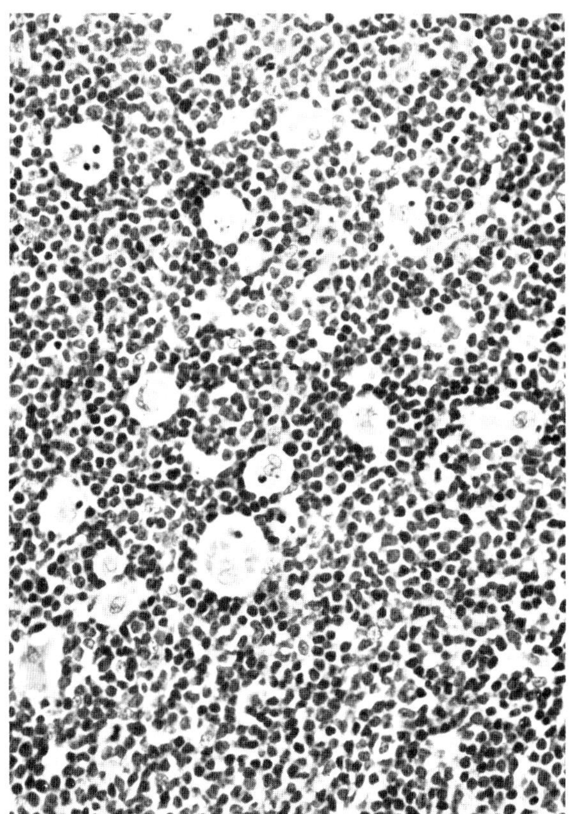

Fig. 10.41 Centrocytic lymphoma with a high content of large macrophages, many containing ingested nuclear fragments. This was a consistent finding in repeat biopsies from this patient. (H E × 300)

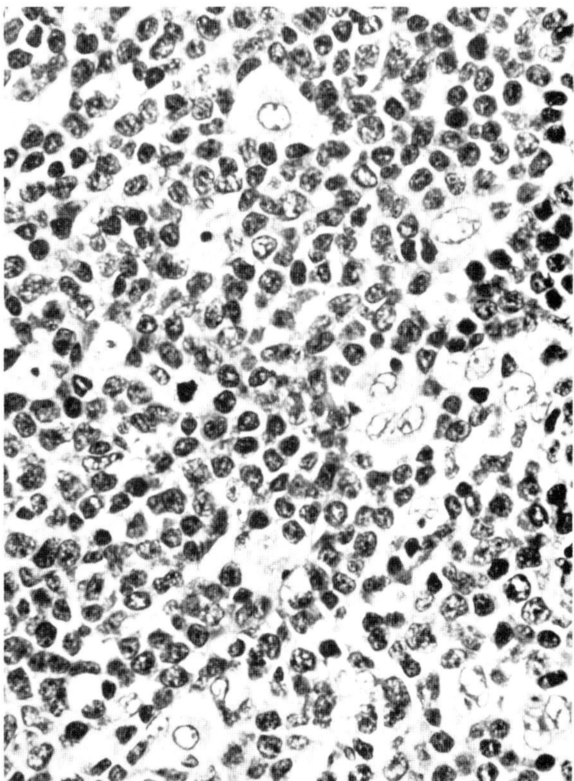

Fig. 10.42 Another case of centrocytic lymphoma in which active histiocytes are a prominent feature. Care should be taken not to mistake this type of picture for Hodgkin's disease. (H E × 470)

phomas of 'intermediate differentiation' which, in the authors' opinion, showed pathological and immunological features intermediate between those of follicular (nodular poorly differentiated lymphocytic) and lymphocytic (well differentiated lymphocytic) lymphomas. The authors deduced that lymphomas of this type were derived from cells of the mantle zone.

A large series of cases of 'intermediate lymphoma' diagnosed on morphological criteria, was published by Weisenburger et al (1981) and the same group in a later study (Weisenburger et al, 1982) described 12 cases in which a similar neoplasm 'appeared to arise from the mantle zone of secondary follicles'. As noted above (p. 253), we have seen the same pattern in the early stages of centrocytic lymphoma, whereas subsequent biopsies from the same patients have shown the typical histological features of diffuse centrocytic lymphoma (Swerdlow et al, 1983). Lennert (1978) had earlier drawn attention to the same phenomenon.

Very rarely, malignant lymphomas of mantle-zone type can initially be associated with large reactive (polyclonal) germinal centres (Palutke et al, 1982) (Fig. 10.43).

Prognosis. As with other low grade, B-cell lymphomas, the prognosis of the small-celled centrocytic lymphoma varies within fairly wide limits, but in general it is appreciably worse than ML lymphocytic, ML lymphoplasmacytoid and ML centroblastic-centrocytic. Although remissions occur with treatment, relapse is almost invariable with currently available therapy, and sooner or later death results from dissemination of the neoplasm. If fresh biopsies are taken at each relapse, it may be observed that the neoplastic cells gradually increase in size and become more pleomorphic (Fig. 10.44), but the phenomenon of blast-cell

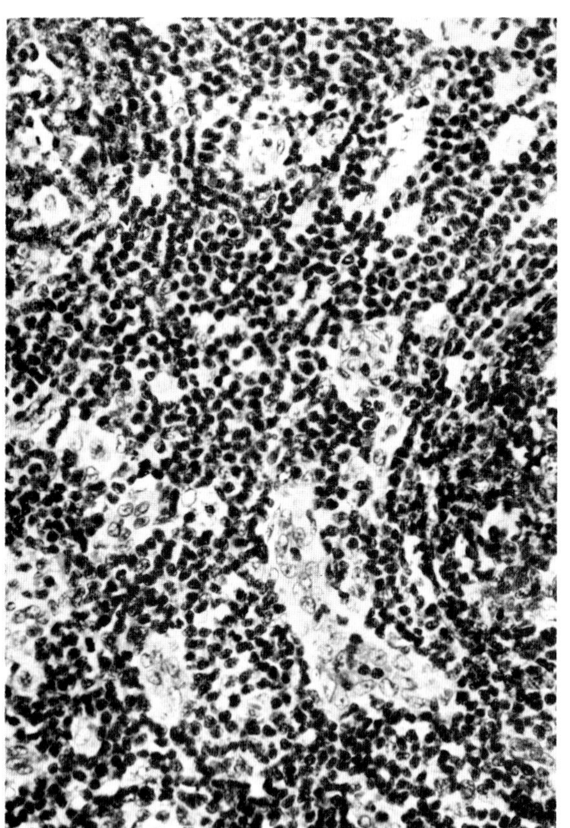

Fig. 10.43 'Mantle-zone lymphoma' — a variant of ML centrocytic. The margins of two reactive germinal follicles are shown (top left and middle right) and the neoplastic infiltrate lies between. (H E × 300)

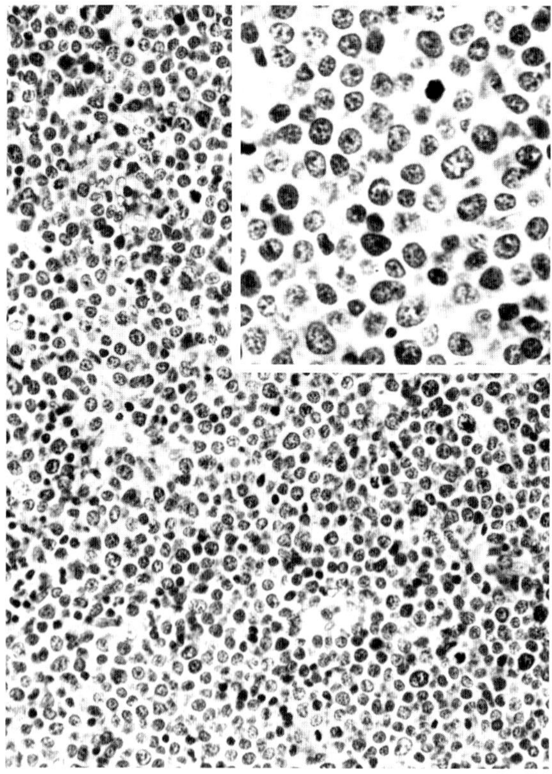

Fig. 10.44 Anaplastic centrocytic lymphoma. Repeat biopsy of relapsed disease 2 years after treatment for an initially typical small-celled centrocytic lymphoma. The cells are now larger and more variable with a higher mitotic rate. (H E main figure × 300, inset × 600)

transformation does not seem to occur (c.f. ML centroblastic-centrocytic). A high mitotic rate appears to influence the prognosis adversely (Swerdlow et al, 1983).

Differential diagnosis. Small-celled centrocytic lymphoma needs to be distinguished first from other low-grade malignant lymphomas of B-cell type — ML lymphocytic, ML lymphoplasmacytoid and ML centroblastic-centrocytic and secondly, from T-lymphoblastic lymphoma (convoluted cell tumour), and from a rare, monomorphic type of peripheral T-cell lymphoma.

Attention has already been drawn to the monotony of the cell picture in this sub-type of centrocytic lymphoma. The total absence or very small number of blast cells distinguishes this from the other low grade lymphomas, even when the tumour presents a suggestively follicular growth pattern. It has to be acknowledged, however, that rare borderline cases between small-celled centrocytic lymphoma and centroblastic-centrocytic lymphoma do occur and exceptionally a single lymph node biopsy may show the distinctive features of ML centrocytic in one part and ML centroblastic-centrocytic in another.

In ML centrocytic, detailed study of the cells reveals the irregular outline of the nuclei, but the 'cleaved' nuclei of this tumour should not be mistaken for the 'convoluted' nuclei of a T-lymphoblastic lymphoma (see p. 289). With poor quality sections this error can be made more easily than might be imagined, particularly with a centrocytic lymphoma showing marked mitotic activity. In this context, the age of the patient is an important consideration. The other type of T-cell lymphoma which may be confused with a centrocytic lymphoma is the rare, monomorphic, peripheral T-cell lymphoma composed of 'centrocyte-like' cells (see pp 60, 309). This tumour occurs in adults, but the nuclei are more irregular than those of centrocytes and hyalinisation of blood vessels is lacking.

Large-celled Centrocytic Lymphoma

Synonyms:
Large cleaved follicle centre cell lymphoma.
Diffuse histiocytic lymphoma (some cases).

Alone among the large-celled malignant lymphomas, this tumour is exclusively composed of large centro*cytes* and as with the small-celled sub-type, centroblasts are absent or, at most, exceedingly scanty. Not surprisingly, perhaps, the prognosis is better than it is in any of the high-grade, blast-cell lymphomas (Strauchen et al, 1975), yet it is certainly a more aggressive tumour than other lymphomas of low-grade type, including the small-celled centrocytic lymphoma. Although the average size of the cells of a small-celled centrocytic lymphoma may increase in the course of a patient's disease, there is relatively little overlap between the large-celled and small-celled sub-types and there is generally little difficulty in assigning a tumour to one or other category. As mentioned above, there are other significant differences between the two sub-types of centrocytic lymphoma, which raises the question of whether there are more fundamental differences between these two tumours than the mere question of cell size.

Incidence and presentation

The large-celled centrocytic lymphoma is a less common type of malignant lymphoma than the small-cell sub-type and its presentation is different. It presents more often as a localised tumour, whether in a lymph node or in an extranodal site, such as gastrointestinal tract, thyroid or Waldeyer's ring. With the exception of Burkitt's lymphoma (and plasmacytoma), this tumour appears to present more frequently as a solitary bone lesion than any other type of B-cell malignant lymphoma and probably most of the reported examples of 'reticulum cell sarcoma' of bone are lymphomas of this type. Large-celled centrocytic lymphomas may also arise in unusual extranodal sites and we have encountered three instances in women where the tumour presented with diffuse infiltration of the vaginal wall. A leukaemic presentation is rarely observed and if the spleen is involved, this generally takes the form of localised tumour deposits. Similarly, localised tumours may be found in the gastrointestinal tract, rather than the diffuse infiltration which is characteristic of the small-celled centrocytic lymphoma. Although the large-celled centrocytic lymphoma generally arises *de novo*, tumours of this type may rarely develop from a pre-existing centroblastic-centrocytic lymphoma (see p. 270) (Figs 10.45, 10.46).

Histology. The pattern of the tumour is always diffuse without any hint of a follicular arrangement and the neoplastic cells resemble large centrocytes in their morphology (Fig. 10.46). The nuclei are relatively large and are often highly irregular in outline. They may appear more or less rounded or ovoid in the absence of sclerosis, but in sclerosing tumours (qv) they are often angular and elongate in shape (Fig. 10.47). The nuclear chromatin is moderately dispersed and there are one or more small, centrally placed, inconspicuous nucleoli. Mitoses may be relatively numerous. The cytoplasm is fairly abundant, but stains weakly with Giemsa or MGP. As in the small-celled sub-type, blast cells are absent or extremely scanty.

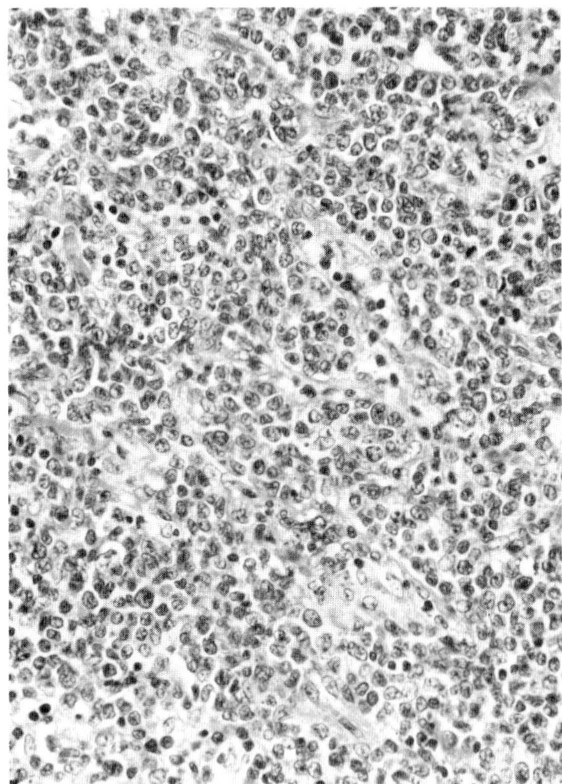

Fig. 10.45 Large-celled centrocytic lymphoma which was found in a lymph node biopsy at clinical relapse in a man of 74. An earlier lymph node biopsy taken 14 years previously had shown a typical centroblastic-centrocytic follicular lymphoma but with a preponderance of large centrocytes in the neoplastic follicles. The tumour shown is diffuse and the cells are almost exclusively large centrocytes. (H E × 300)

A frequently observed feature of these tumours is a fine 'compartmentalising' sclerosis readily apparent in HE stained sections (Fig. 10.48), but emphasised on reticulin staining (Bennett, 1975). This type of fibrosis is particularly characteristic of the large-celled centrocytic lymphoma and is quite different from the 'banded' fibrosis sometimes seen in centroblastic-centrocytic lymphomas (see p. 272).

As indicated above, the cytological picture is relatively 'pure'. Reactive macrophages and a few plasma cells of polyclonal type may sometimes be a feature. The presence of scattered dendritic reticulum cells provides further support for the suggested histogenesis of the tumour.

Prognosis. Although, in the untreated case, the large-celled centrocytic lymphoma behaves in an aggressive manner, this tumour is generally responsive to therapy and perhaps because it is so often a localised tumour, the prospects of 'cure' are probably better than they are with almost any

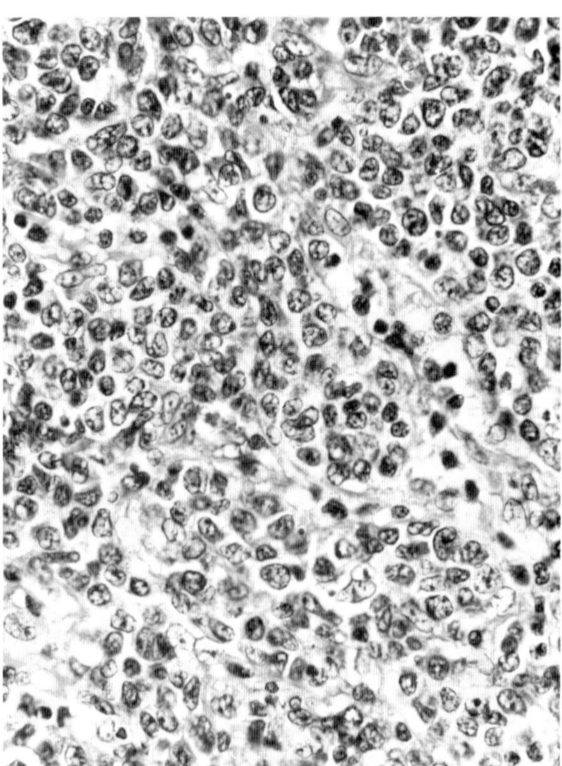

Fig. 10.46 Higher magnification of centre of field shown in Fig. 10.45 to show detailed morphology of cells and delicate 'compartmentalising' sclerosis (H E × 470)

other type of B-cell lymphoma. Rosas-Uribe & Rappaport (1972) drew attention to the relatively slow progression and better prognosis of the sclerosing 'diffuse histiocytic' lymphomas, in comparison with other 'diffuse histiocytic' lymphomas. The relatively good prognosis of localised 'reticulum cell sarcoma' of the long bones is attested by many reports (e.g. Boston et al, 1974). As with the small-celled centrocytic lymphoma, blastic transformation does not seem to occur.

Differential diagnosis. In poorly fixed preparations and in certain sites, the possibility of confusion with undifferentiated carcinoma may arise, but in an adequate biopsy the distinction should seldom be a problem. The distinction between this and other types of large-celled malignant lymphoma is more likely to present difficulties, especially with poor fixation which may result in 'vesicular' nuclei. High grade malignant lymphomas of immunoblastic or polymorphic centroblastic types consist predominantly of obviously blastic

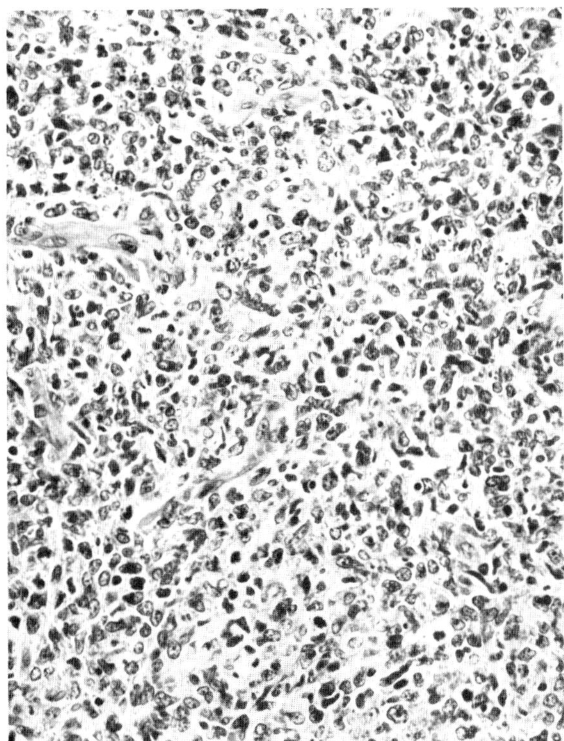

Fig. 10.47 Another large-celled centrocytic lymphoma showing irregular and often elongate nuclei with small nucleoli (subcutaneous tumour) (H E × 300)

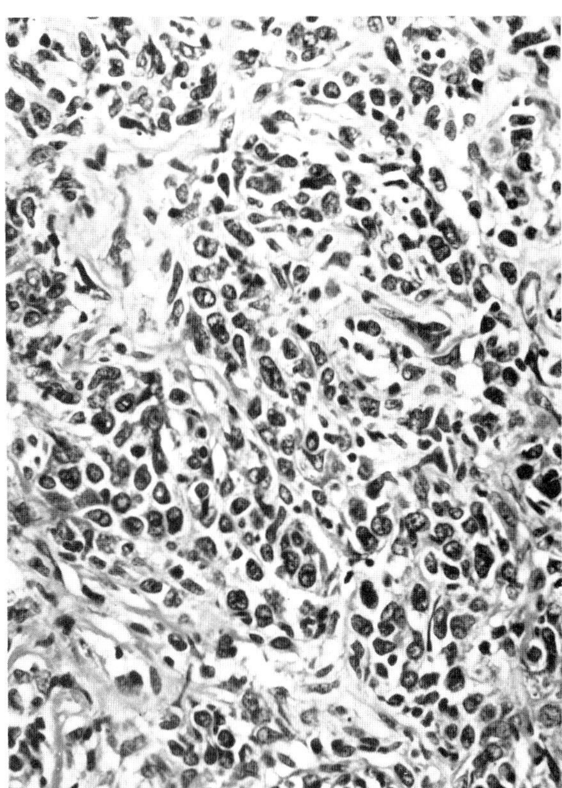

Fig. 10.48 Inguinal lymph node biopsy from a woman of 20 showing 'compartmentalising' sclerosis in a large-celled centrocytic lymphoma. A simultaneous biopsy of a lytic lesion in the homolateral femur showed tumour of the same type. (H E × 300)

cells with much more prominent nucleoli and strongly basophilic (Giemsa) or pyroninophilic (MGP) cytoplasm, in contrast with the weakly staining cytoplasm of large centrocytes. A proportion of centrocytes are of course found in the polymorphic centroblastic lymphomas, but always in these circumstances, associated with centroblasts and immunoblasts, so the picture is not monomorphic.

True histiocytic neoplasms (malignant histiocytoma/malignant histiocytosis) may sometimes be mistaken for large-celled centrocytic lymphomas and *vice versa*, but the distinction can be made by immunostaining for muramidase (p. 37) or, if fresh biopsy material is available, by staining frozen sections for non-specific esterase or acid phosphatase. Each will give negative results with centrocytic lymphomas, but positive results with histiocytic neoplasms.

ML CENTROBLASTIC-CENTROCYTIC (ML Cb-Cc)

This common type of B-cell malignant lymphoma is characterised by two important features: (1) the neoplasm almost always shows, in whole or in part, a follicular pattern, (2) the neoplastic follicles are composed essentially of a mixture of centrocytes and centroblasts, usually with the former predominating. There is abundant evidence that the neoplastic follicles of the tumour are the counterpart of normal secondary follicles as originally proposed by Lennert (1973). Not only are the neoplastic cells morphologically similar by light and electron microscopy to the centrocytes and centroblasts of reactive germinal centres (Levine & Dorfman, 1975), but they also show the same surface marker characteristics as their normal counterparts. Occasionally a proportion of the cells show CIg as well as SIg, and this trait is seen in extreme form in the rare variant known as a signet-cell or signet-ring cell lymphoma (Kim et al, 1978; van den Tweel et al, 1978).

A significant feature of centroblastic-centrocytic lymphoma is the consistent finding that a relatively high proportion of the cells in a cell suspension mark as T-cells (up to 40% or more). This is so even when a section of the same node shows apparently total replacement by what is clearly a B-cell neoplasm, and the finding is in sharp contrast to that in ML centrocytic, in which T-cells are present in much smaller numbers. This observation adds a further cogent argument for making a clear distinction between the two types of lymphoma (Tolksdorf et al, 1980). It has been found that the presence of T (helper) cells is necessary for the development of normal reactive follicles (Davies et al, 1969), and it may perhaps be inferred that the follicular organisation of this tumour is likewise dependent upon T-cells. Certainly in many instances the node biopsy section shows the preservation of well developed T-zones, with prominent venules, lying between the neoplastic follicles.

The degree of 'follicularity' of these tumours varies greatly, as do the size, definition and other features of the neoplastic follicles. Nevertheless, present evidence seems to support the idea that, contrary to the thesis put forward by Rappaport et al (1956), all malignant lymphomas which display a clear cut follicular pattern (as distinct from a non-specific nodularity), belong to a single category, regardless of variations in the cell composition. Furthermore, although it is customary to distinguish cases in which the whole of the biopsy section shows a follicular pattern, from those in which the pattern is partly follicular and partly diffuse, and to record the relative proportions of each, there is, at present, no good evidence that variations in *the pattern alone* influence the behaviour of the tumour or the prognosis. Variations in the *cell picture* in different parts of the biopsy are of much greater significance and in reporting on centroblastic-centrocytic lymphomas, it is important not merely to record the approximate proportions of centroblasts to centrocytes but to note a relative increase in blast cells when comparing one area of the biopsy with another, or a fresh biopsy with previous biopsies from the same patient. A loss of follicular pattern which is accompanied by a marked increase of centroblasts, especially if the latter are present in solid clusters, may signal transformation of the tumour into a high grade, centroblastic lymphoma. A gradual blurring of the follicular pattern may be found in successive biopsies from an individual patient, with increasing pleomorphism of the neoplasm, but without evidence of actual blast-cell transformation. Thus loss of an originally follicular pattern is a common development, which may or may not signify blastic transformation of the tumour, and which may be found in one node whilst adjacent nodes may still show the follicular pattern and cytological features of the original tumour.

Although there appear to be rare tumours composed of centrocytes and centroblasts in which the pattern is *entirely* diffuse *from the outset*, it is uncertain whether these tumours are really the same entity, differing only in their incapacity to form follicular structures, or are a different class of neoplasm. For this reason, these diffuse tumours will be described separately.

ML Centroblastic-Centrocytic — follicular; follicular and diffuse

Synonyms:
Follicular lymphoma

(Older terms: Brill-Symmers disease; Giant follicle lymphoma; Follicular lymphoblastoma)
Nodular lymphomas (lymphocytic; mixed — lymphocytic and histiocytic; histiocytic)
Follicle centre cell lymphomas (FCC) (see footnote on p. 251).

Incidence and presentation

This is one of the commonest types of malignant lymphoma, excluding Hodgkin's disease, with which it is very rarely associated. As with all the other low-grade B-cell lymphomas, centroblastic-centrocytic lymphomas are essentially tumours of adults, being uncommon under the age of 25 and virtually unknown under the age of 18. The incidence in the two sexes is almost equal.

The usual mode of presentation is with lymphadenopathy, which may initially affect one group of nodes, or even one node, but which is more frequently found to be widespread at the time of presentation. The spleen is quite often palpable too, and massive splenomegaly is occasionally a presenting feature. An extranodal presentation is relatively less frequent than it is in ML centrocytic or ML lymphoplasmacytoid, but, from time to time, patients present with a mass in the gastrointestinal tract, retroperitoneal connective tissue, skin, Waldeyer's ring, thyroid or some other site. Occasionally too, the disease may come to light through the discovery of a chronic lymphoid leukaemia on blood examination, although physical examination in these circumstances will almost always reveal the presence of a significant lymphadenopathy. Close scrutiny of the leukaemic cells in a peripheral blood film will show them to have the typical notched nuclei of centrocytes. Even in the absence of a leukaemic blood picture, marrow involvement is very commonly found at the time of initial presentation, the lymphomatous foci showing a characteristically paratrabecular distribution in a trephine biopsy.

Macroscopic features. The individual lymph nodes in centroblastic-centrocytic lymphoma may be quite large (up to 5 cm or more in diameter), but generally appear discrete rather than matted. Usually the cut surface of the node presents a uniform, solid, whitish appearance, typical of lymphomas in general, and only occasionally can a follicular pattern be seen with the naked eye. Exceptionally, lymphatic obstruction by the growth may result in gross dilatation of still patent lymph sinuses within the node, imparting a sponge-like appearance to the cut surface (Fig. 10.49). Lymphatic obstruction in abdominal nodes, with resultant chylous ascites, probably occurs more frequently with centroblastic-centrocytic lymphoma than with other types of NHL.

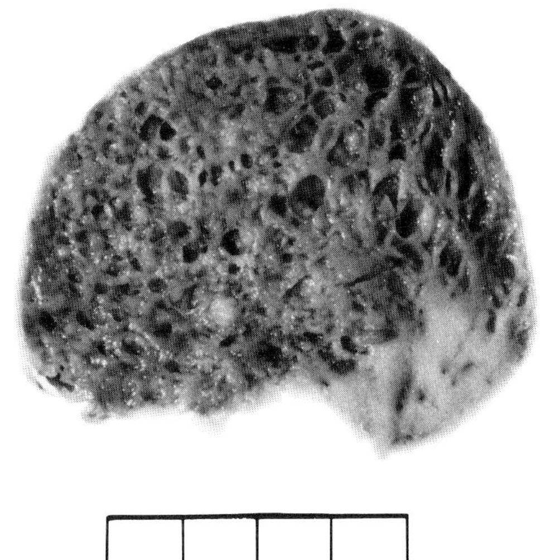

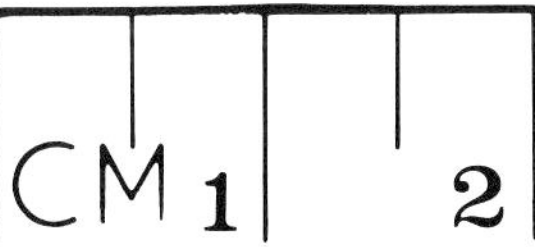

Fig. 10.49 An inguinal lymph node biopsy replaced by centroblastic-centrocytic lymphoma which shows a sponge-like texture of the cut surface due to dilatation of the lymph sinuses (a rare finding) (see Fig. 10.51).

Histology. As a rule, the neoplasm occupies practically the whole of the node biopsy section and it is not unusual to see extension through the capsule into the surrounding fat (Fig. 10.50). Sometimes lymph sinuses can still be made out and, rarely, these are dilated (Fig. 10.51). When the node is only partially involved by the growth and residual non-neoplastic follicles are seen, these generally appear inactive and sometimes atrophic (Fig. 10.52). There is no evidence that follicular hyperplasia precedes the development of follicular lymphoma (Rappaport et al, 1956) and transition of one into the other probably never occurs. This is important, since it implies that, if the section shows large and obviously hyperplastic germinal

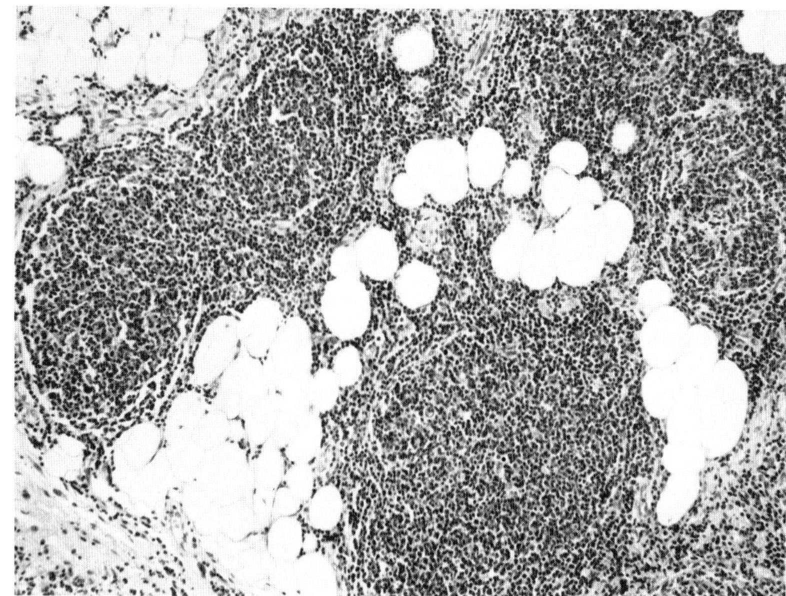

Fig. 10.50 Extracapsular extension of neoplastic follicles in a centroblastic-centrocytic follicular lymphoma (H E × 120)

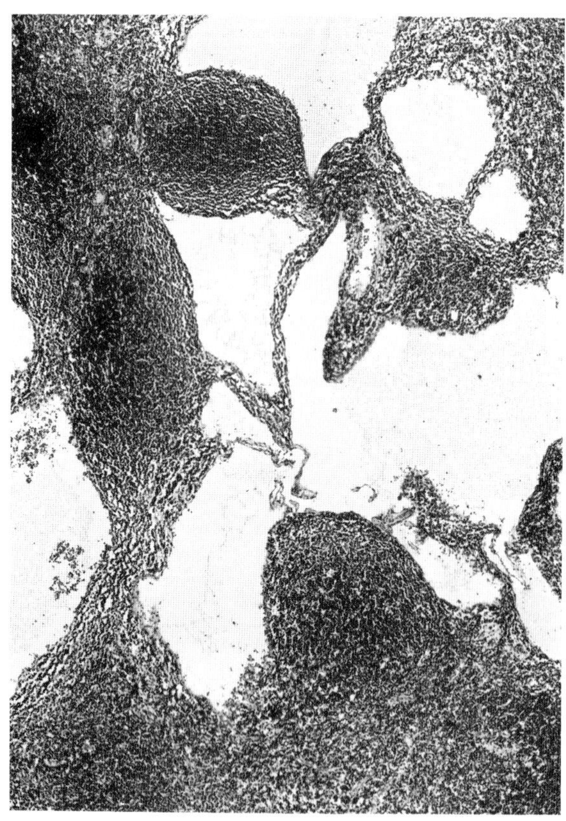

Fig. 10.51 Dilatation of lymph sinuses in a centroblastic centrocytic follicular lymphoma (same case as Fig. 10.49). The neoplastic follicles are poorly defined. (H E × 47)

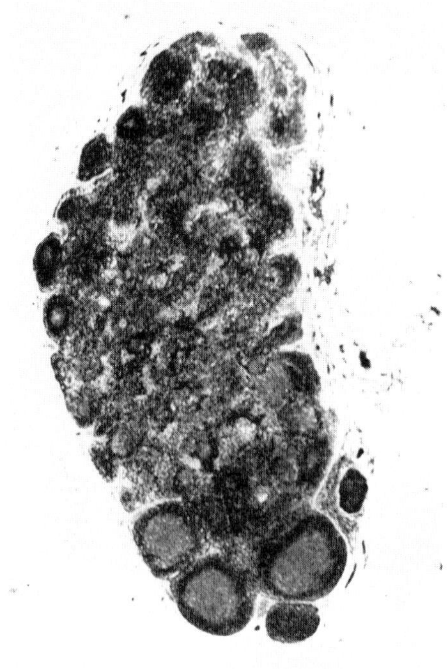

Fig. 10.52 A small lymph node showing partial involvement by follicular lymphoma (lower pole). Residual normal follicles are small and inactive. (H E × 6)

centres in one area, then more dubious follicular structures in another part of the same node are very unlikely to be neoplastic follicles. Differences in fixation can create marked differences in the appearance of hyperplastic, as of neoplastic follicles, even in a single section. Between the neoplastic follicles of a centroblastic-centrocytic lymphoma, T-cell areas, characterised by prominent venules, can often be made out, although these areas can easily be obscured by overlying small centrocytes (see below).

Follicular pattern. The follicular pattern of the neoplasm is often better seen with a hand lens than under the microscope and, in doubtful cases, reticulin staining is useful in revealing the pattern with greater clarity (Figs 10.53, 10.54). It is, of course, essential to distinguish neoplastic from reactive follicles and further to distinguish the follicular pattern of ML Cb-Cc from the nodular pattern which is a feature of some types of Hodgkin's disease and of some other NHL (see under differential diagnosis). The diagnosis is very easy to make at times and difficult at other times.

The main difficulty lies in the variability of neoplastic follicles on the one hand and of reactive germinal follicles on the other. The range of appearances which may be found in each is such that there is a degree of overlap between them and none of the distinguishing characteristics commonly cited is, by itself, absolutely reliable (see Table 10.2). In classical examples of reactive follicular hyperplasia or of centroblastic-centrocytic follicular lymphoma, the diagnosis should present no problem, but in difficult cases it is necessary to take into account *all* the features and weigh up the evidence accordingly. (There may, of course, be ancillary evidence in favour of a malignant lymphoma or of a reactive process.)

Although extracellular acidophilic precipitates are more often seen in reactive germinal centres

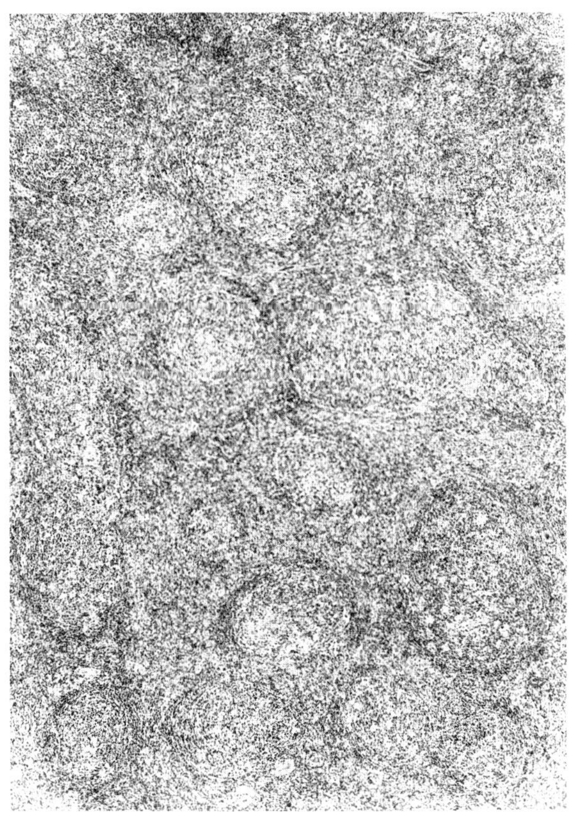

Fig. 10.53 Follicular centroblastic-centrocytic lymphoma with characteristically poorly-defined follicles (H E × 47)

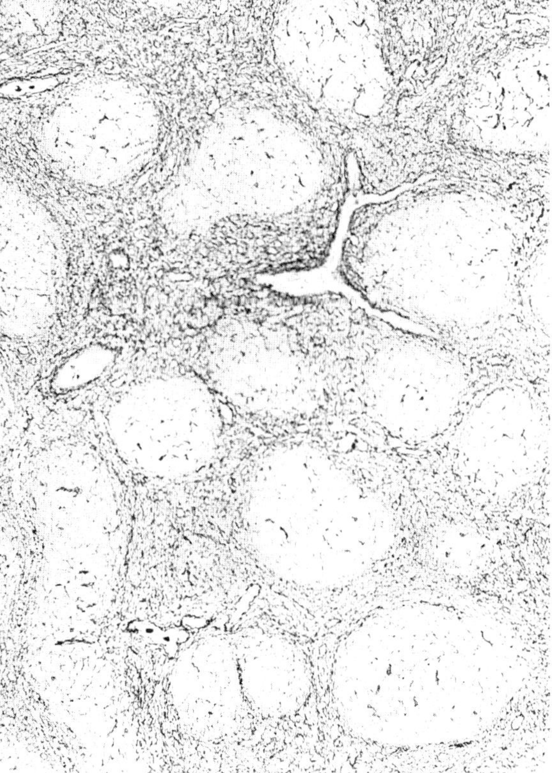

Fig. 10.54 Same lymph node as Fig. 10.53 showing how reticulin staining improves the definition of the follicles (Gordon and Sweets reticulin × 47)

Table 10.2 Distinguishing features between follicular hyperplasia and follicular lymphoma (centroblastic-centrocytic) (modified after Rappaport, 1966)

Character	Follicular hyperplasia	Follicular lymphoma
Nodal architecture	Essentially preserved	May be obliterated
Distribution of follicles	Predominantly cortical	Evenly distributed throughout
Extracapsular spread of follicles	Absent or very limited	Often present
Size of follicles	Variable often large	Tends to be fairly uniform in any given case
Shape of follicles	Frequently irregular	Usually regular and rounded
Definition of follicles	Usually sharp	Often poorly defined
Lymphocyte mantle	Present unless follicles very large	Frequently absent, narrow if present
Reticulin	Not compressed around follicles	Compressed around follicles
Polarity of cells within follicles	Present	Absent
Acidophil extracellular deposits in follicles	Often present	Occasionally present
'Starry sky' pattern in follicles	Frequent	Occasionally seen, usually absent
Mitoses in follicles	Often numerous, typical	Generally fewer, may be abnormal
Cellular atypia	Absent	May be present
Distribution of centrocytes	Confined to follicles	Often present in interfollicular pulp
Plasma cells	Often numerous in interfollicular pulp	Absent or scanty

than in neoplastic follicles, they are by no means rare in the latter. Neoplastic follicles rarely if ever exhibit any polarity (p. 75), but this feature is not invariably seen in reactive germinal centres. Whilst the cytological features may be helpful in differentiating neoplastic and reactive follicles, even these cannot always be relied upon in a really difficult case. If the biopsy section shows clear evidence of extension of follicles beyond the capsule and out into the surrounding fat, then it can generally be assumed that the process is neoplastic (Fig. 10.50).

The neoplastic follicles of ML Cb-Cc in any given case may be large or small (Figs 10.55, 10.56), uniform or variable in size, regular or irregular in shape, entirely discrete or partially confluent (Fig. 10.57), sharply defined or poorly defined, closely packed or widely spaced. The diagnosis of lymphoma is easy when the node is filled with closely-packed, uniform, small, regular, but poorly defined follicles, and fortunately this is a common pattern (Fig. 10.53). The distinction from reactive follicular hyperplasia is much more difficult in the minority of cases where the follicles are more widely spaced, variable in size, irregular in outline and thrown into relief by a surrounding mantle of small lymphocytes (Fig. 10.55). Occasionally the follicles may be so bizarre and ir-

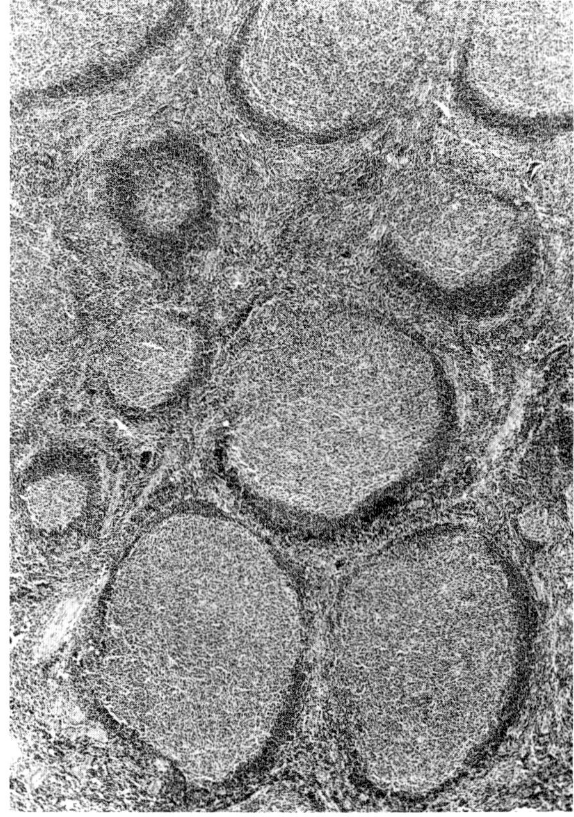

Fig. 10.55 Follicular centroblastic-centrocytic lymphoma with large follicles, each outlined by a mantle of lymphocytes. Note the absence of a 'starry-sky' pattern. (H E × 47)

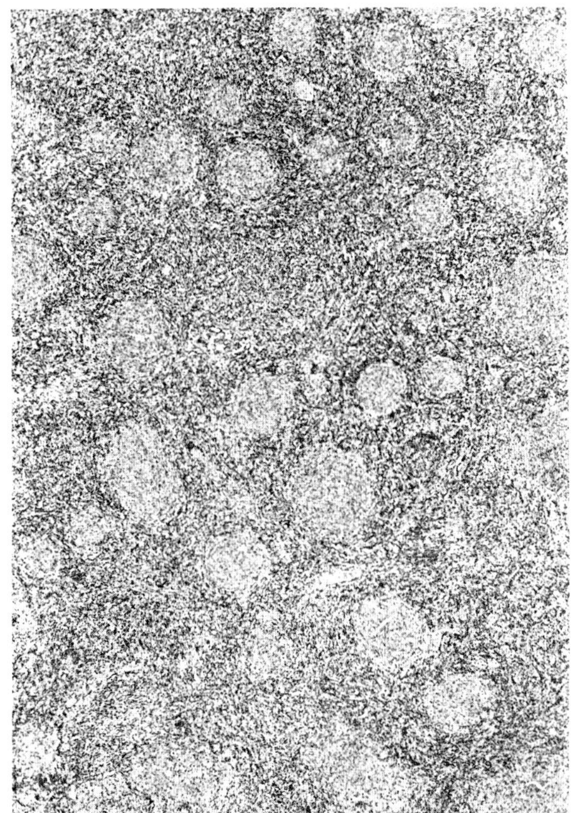

Fig. 10.56 Follicular centroblastic-centrocytic lymphoma with small, less well defined follicles (H E × 47)

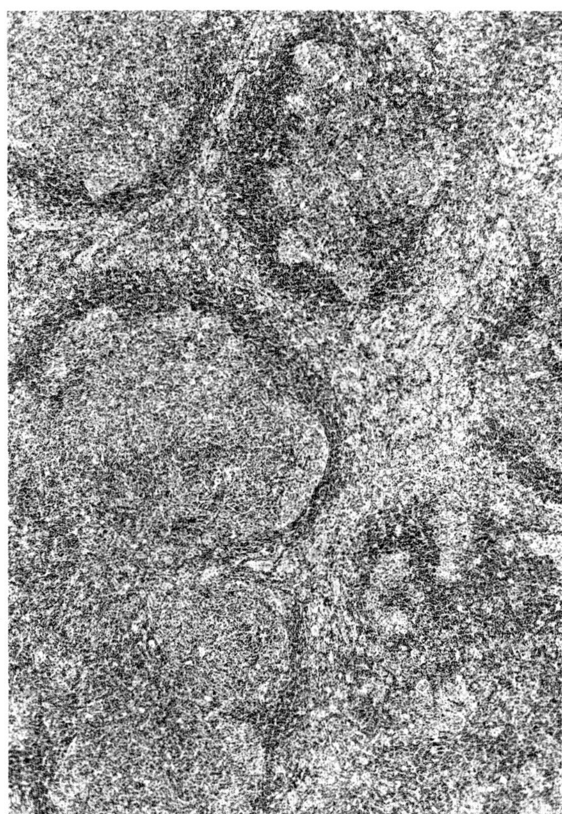

Fig. 10.57 Follicular centroblastic-centrocytic lymphoma with irregular, partially confluent follicles (H E × 47)

regular in shape that they may not be recognised as follicles at all (Fig. 10.58). The sparse reticulin within these follicles, revealed by silver impregnation, and the cell composition will assist in the recognition of such atypical neoplastic follicles.

Occasionally a lymph node biopsy may show an abrupt change in the follicular pattern of a follicular centroblastic-centrocytic lymphoma (Fig. 10.59). Such cases have been sometimes wrongly categorised as examples of composite lymphoma (Kim et al, 1977).

As already indicated, a follicular pattern may be evident throughout the tumour or may be limited to a part of the biopsy section only. When the tumour is partly follicular and partly diffuse in pattern, it is important to decide whether the cells in the diffuse areas are essentially the same as those in the follicular areas or whether the neoplasm is showing signs of transformation.

Cell picture. In contrast to ML centrocytic, the cell picture in ML centroblastic-centrocytic tends to be much more variable. Not only is there always a certain proportion of centroblasts in the neoplastic follicles, but in an individual case there is often more variation in the size of the centrocytes too.

In most cases, small centrocytes predominate and make up the greater proportion of the cells composing the follicles. When this is so, the edges of the follicles are generally indistinct, for there is often no surrounding mantle of lymphocytes, and small centrocytes 'overflow' in considerable numbers into the interfollicular pulp (Fig. 10.60). In tumours which are partly follicular and partly diffuse, the diffuse areas are usually composed largely of small centrocytes which may be indistinguishable morphologically from those in the follicles, although sometimes the extrafollicular cells are

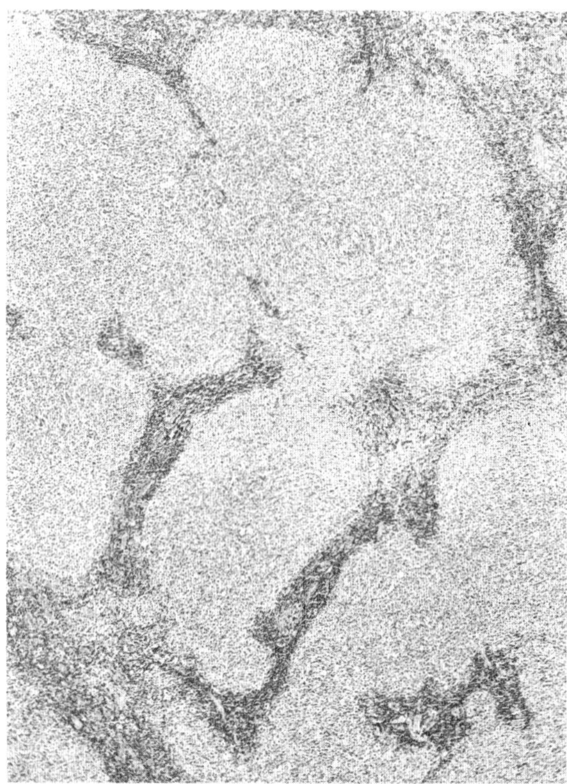

Fig. 10.58 Follicular centroblastic-centrocytic lymphoma with large, irregular follicles. Their pale staining and sharp definition is due to a preponderance of large centrocytes (see Fig. 10.64). (H E × 47)

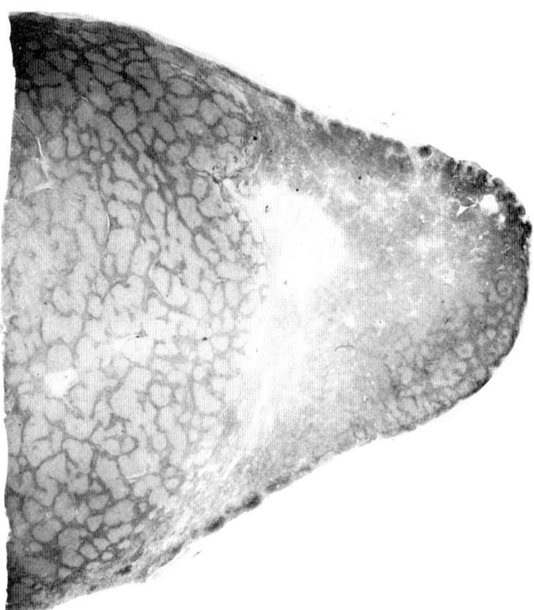

Fig. 10.59 Abrupt change in the follicular pattern and follicular size in a centroblastic-centrocytic follicular lymphoma. Both halves of the section are involved by lymphoma and this change does not imply the emergence of a different type of lymphoma. (H E × 4)

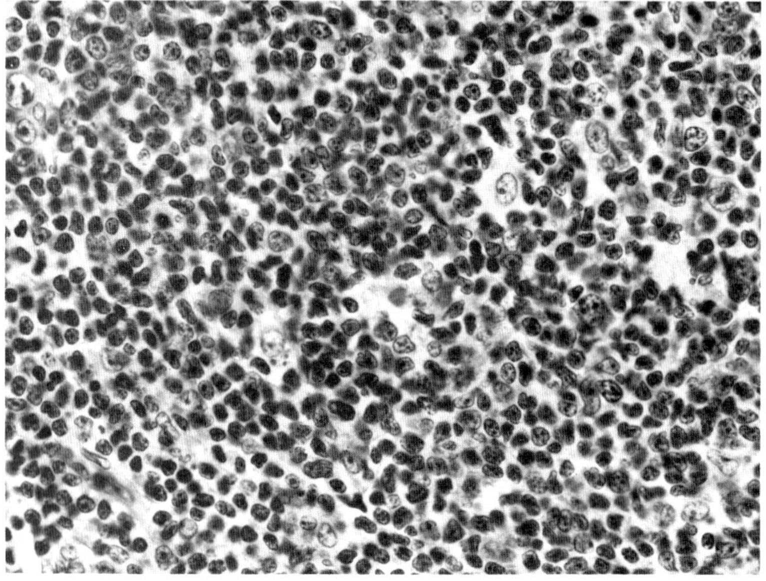

Fig. 10.60 Part of a neoplastic follicle composed predominantly of small centrocytes and containing few centroblasts. The ill-defined margin of the follicle is seen in the lower left hand corner and there are many centrocytes outside the follicle. A single immunoblast is seen in the follicle (right). Few histiocytes are seen. (H E × 470)

smaller. It is this small centrocyte form of ML Cb-Cc which is most often associated with Stage 4 disease (marrow, spleen and liver involvement and/or a leukaemic blood picture) at the time of diagnosis. The small centrocytes of the follicles resemble the cells of the small-cell type of centrocytic lymphoma in their elongate and irregular ('cleaved') nuclei, but there is amongst them a proportion of T-cells which may have even more irregularly shaped nuclei and more cytoplasm.

Centroblasts are the other essential ingredient of the neoplastic follicles. They may be few in number and are sometimes quite difficult to spot, especially when the sections are thick, but there is no difficulty in picking them out in semi-thin sections of resin embedded tissue (Fig. 10.61). Generally these centroblasts resemble the centroblasts of reactive germinal centres, having large, round, 'vesicular' nuclei with peripherally placed nucleoli and scanty basophilic cytoplasm. Occasionally there are some blast cells with very prominent central nucleoli more like those of immunoblasts. Moreover, even when the proportion of blast cells is quite small, there may occasionally be highly atypical, giant or binucleate forms, which can be easily mistaken for Sternberg-Reed cells (Fig. 10.62).

Besides these main constituents of the neoplastic follicles, the latter also contain, like their normal counterparts, some dendritic reticulum cells (Fig. 10.63), as can be shown by electron microscopy. The two other cell types which are sometimes present in small numbers are reactive (polyclonal) plasma cells and macrophages. The

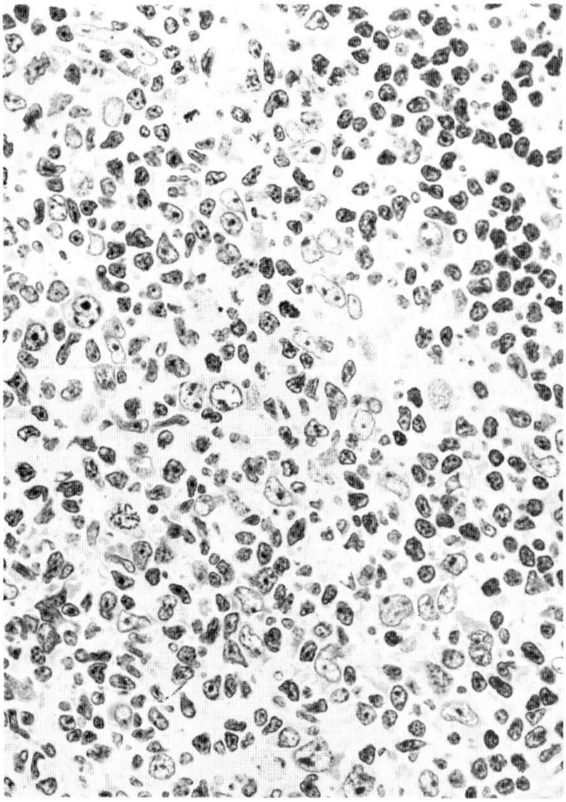

Fig. 10.61 Part of a neoplastic follicle from another case of follicular centroblastic-centrocytic lymphoma showing a much higher proportion of centroblasts than Fig. 10.60. Centrocytes and centroblasts are much more readily identified in this semi-thin section of resin-embedded tissue. Note lymphocytes in surrounding mantle (top right). (Compare with Fig. 5.13, p. 77) (H E × 470)

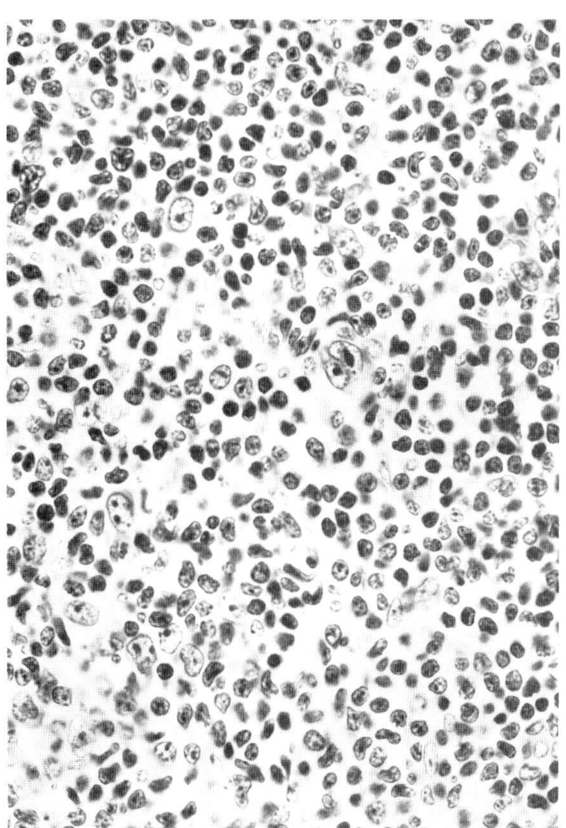

Fig. 10.62 A single binucleate blast cell resembling a Sternberg-Reed cell is seen in this neoplastic follicle from another case of follicular centroblastic-centrocytic lymphoma. (H E × 470)

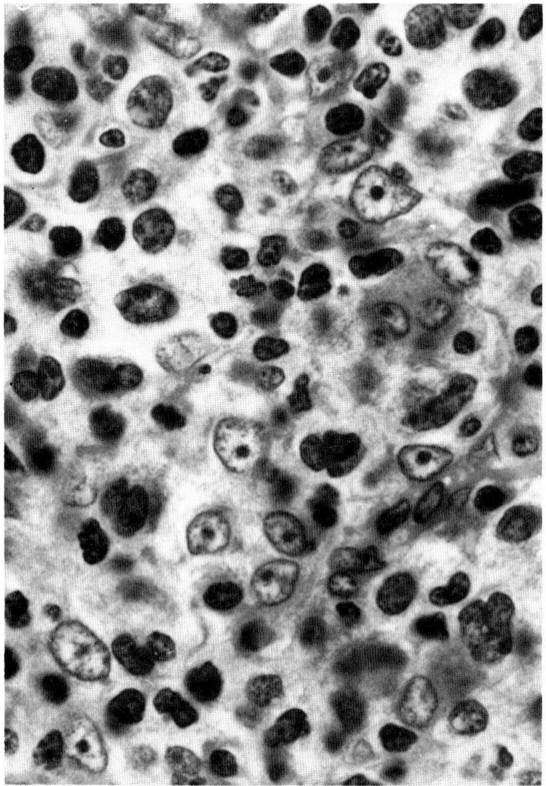

Fig. 10.63 Dendritic reticulum cells are regularly found in the neoplastic follicles of ML Cb-Cc. In this instance they are unusually numerous and are readily identified by their thick nuclear membranes, clear nuclear sap and prominent central nucleoli. (H E × 940)

latter are seldom a conspicuous feature, but nevertheless they may contain nuclear fragments and may be sufficiently numerous on occasions to impart a 'starry sky' pattern to the neoplastic follicles. Occasionally, small epithelioid cell clusters may be found in centroblastic-centrocytic lymphoma, as in most types of malignant lymphoma, but when present they are focally distributed and are not found throughout the tumour.

Variations in centrocytes

Whilst, in any single case, the size and appearances of the centrocytes (and hence of the follicles) tends to be fairly consistent throughout, there is marked variation from case to case in this regard. Sometimes, medium-sized, and occasionally, large, centrocytes predominate, instead of the more usual predominance of small centrocytes (Figs 10.58, 10.64). In the large-centrocytic variant, the follicles appear paler and more sharply demarcated than those of the smaller cell variety, for the large centrocytes have more cytoplasm and show less tendency to spread outside the follicles. By the same token, the large centrocytic variety presents less often with marrow involvement or Stage 4 disease. This large centrocytic variety is included in Rappaport's 'histiocytic nodular' category (Rappaport, 1966), along with some instances of centroblastic lymphoma.

The size of the individual centrocytes, *per se*, does not seem to be related to the proportion of centroblasts in the neoplastic follicles, nor does it appear to relate to the tendency to transform into a high-grade, blastic lymphoma, or the speed with which such transformation occurs. There is, how-

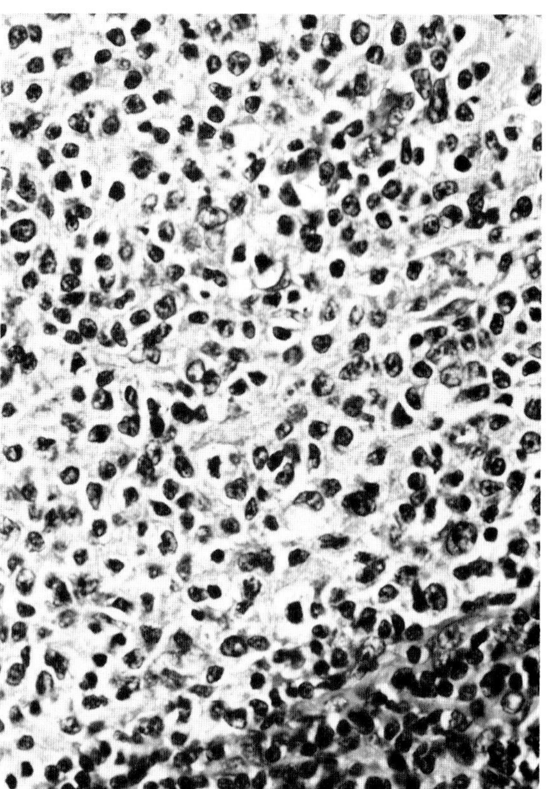

Fig. 10.64 Same case as Fig. 10.58. The neoplastic follicles in this case of centroblastic-centrocytic follicular lymphoma are composed mainly of large centrocytes and centroblasts are scanty. In the Rappaport classification this would be classed as a nodular histiocytic lymphoma. (H E × 470)

ever, one cellular variant which may possibly be distinguishable and which broadly corresponds with Rappaport's 'mixed lymphocytic and histiocytic nodular' category. In this, there is not only a somewhat higher proportion of centroblasts than in the average case, but there seems to be a wider range than usual in the size of the centrocytes which accentuates the impression of a 'mixed' cell population (Fig. 10.61). There is insufficient evidence at the present time to decide whether this picture represents a distinct variety of centroblastic-centrocytic lymphoma, or whether it may be a stage in the transformation process, but there is some evidence that patients whose biopsies present this picture may have a better response to therapy (Lister et al, 1978).

Variations in centroblasts

Contrary to what might be expected, centroblasts generally form a much smaller proportion of the cell population in neoplastic follicles than they do in the germinal centres of reactive follicles. They are sometimes very scanty indeed (1–2%) and are then difficult to find. It is, however, usual to see 3–10% of centroblasts, intermingled with the predominating centrocytes from which they are readily distinguished, especially with Giemsa staining or in a semi-thin section (Fig. 10.61). Sometimes a higher proportion of centroblasts is seen — up to 30% or more of the cells in the neoplastic follicles, but if these are intermingled with centrocytes and do not present atypical features, the finding does not invariably imply impending blast-cell transformation of the neoplasm. Only when solid clumps of centroblasts are found, or when many of the blast cells are highly atypical (Fig. 10.65), does a high centroblast count signify probable blast-cell transformation (Lennert, 1978, p 353). The presence of isolated, atypical centroblasts, which may be mistaken for Sternberg-Reed cells, has already been mentioned (p. 267). The mitotic rate within the neoplastic follicles roughly parallels the number of centroblasts, although this does not necessarily imply that all the dividing cells are centroblasts. Mitoses are often, but by no means always, fewer in number than in a briskly reactive germinal centre.

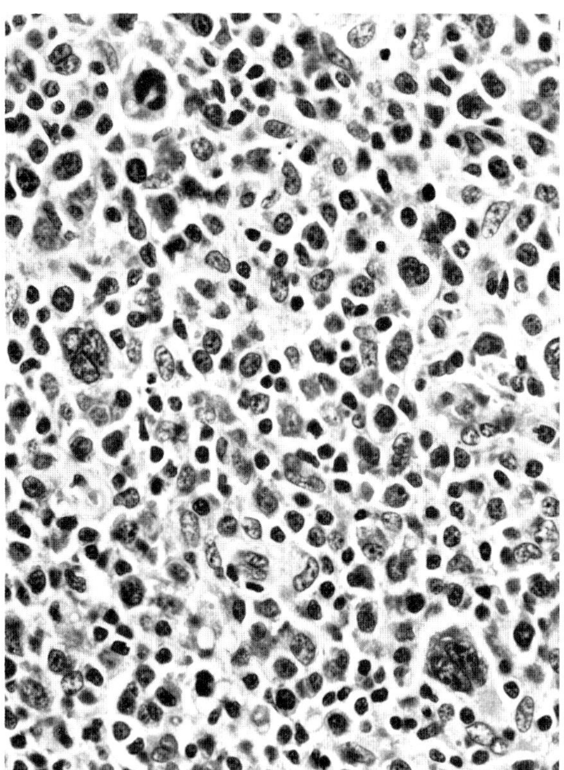

Fig. 10.65 Follicular centroblastic-centrocytic lymphoma showing a large proportion of atypical blast-type cells. Transformation into a high grade, pleomorphic, immunoblastic lymphoma was found in a subsequent biopsy. (H E × 470)

Blast cell transformation

This phenomenon occurs with greater frequency in centroblastic-centrocytic lymphoma than in any other variety of low-grade B-cell malignant lymphoma. Lennert (1981) found blastic transformation in 40% of cases examined at post mortem. The frequent occurrence of such transformation has been known for many years. The interval between the time of the initial diagnosis of centroblastic-centrocytic lymphoma and its transformation into a high grade blast-cell (usually centroblastic) malignant lymphoma is extremely variable and may be anything from a few months up to 12–15 years or even more. At times, the initial lymph node biopsy, from a patient who has had no prior evidence of lymphoma, may show a high-grade centroblastic or immunoblastic lymphoma in one part and clear evidence of a centroblastic-centrocytic follicular lymphoma in another, suggesting that blast-cell transformation occurred almost simultaneously with the development of the malignant lymphoma.

Not only is there a variable time interval between the appearance of the initial lymphoma and its transformation, but the actual rate of transformation may vary greatly also, as can be demonstrated sometimes in patients who have had serial lymph node biopsies (Cullen et al, 1979). Transformation may appear abruptly in a single group of nodes which may be observed to enlarge rapidly. Alternatively, successive biopsies, taken over a period of a year or more, in a patient with relapsing disease, may demonstrate a progressive loss of follicular pattern, accompanying a progressive increase of blast cells with increasing cellular atypia (Figs 10.66, 10.67).

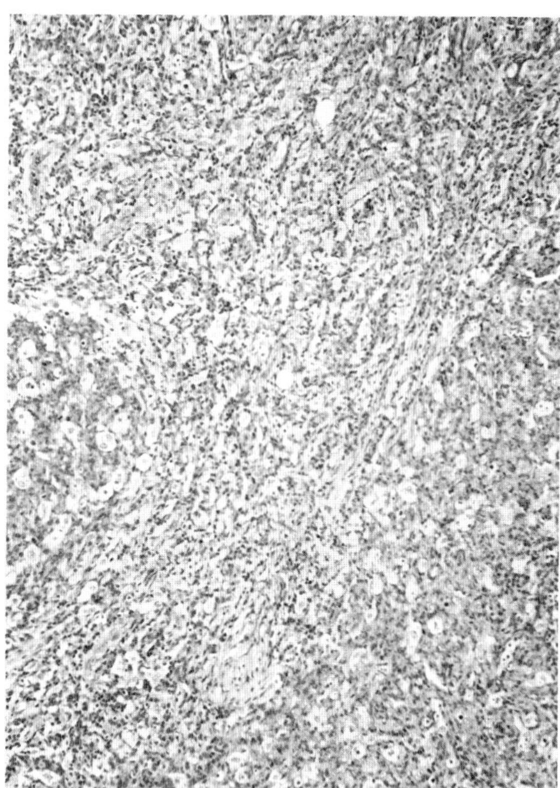

Fig. 10.66 Repeat lymph node biopsy in a woman of 64 in whom successive biopsies had shown a gradual change from a typical follicular centroblastic-centrocytic lymphoma with well defined follicles and scanty blast cells into the type of picture seen here. Remnants of a follicular structure remain but much of the tumour showed loss of follicular pattern. (H E × 120)

Uncommonly, a centroblastic-centrocytic follicular lymphoma may 'transform' into a diffuse large-cell centrocytic lymphoma, instead of into a blast-cell lymphoma (see p. 257 and Figs 10.45, 10.46). Blast-cell transformation is the usual sequel, but the morphology of the resultant high grade lymphoma varies greatly. The tumour may be composed entirely of small or medium sized centroblasts (ML centroblastic), or there may be a mixture of centroblasts and immunoblasts (ML centroblastic-polymorphic), or the cells may be exclusively immunoblasts of medium or large size (ML immunoblastic) (see Figs 11.24, 11.25, p. 294).

The recognition that blast cell transformation has occurred, or is occurring, in a patient, previously known to have centroblastic-centrocytic follicular lymphoma, is not difficult as a rule and

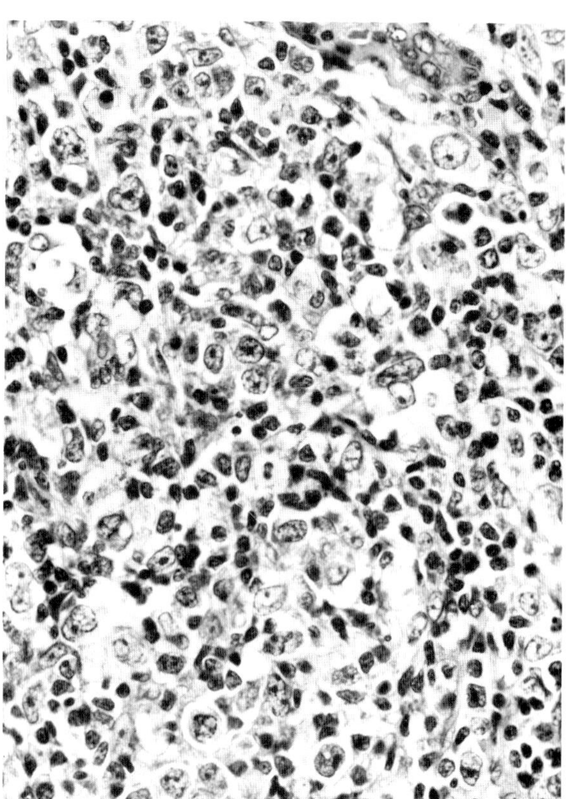

Fig. 10.67 Another field from the same biopsy as Fig. 10.66 at a higher magnification. Blast cells are numerous, but they are still interspersed with centrocytes. (H E × 470)

the phenomenon may be suspected by the clinician before biopsy, although not invariably so (Cullen et al, 1979). The appearance of compact clusters or sheets of blast cells within a still follicular tumour may herald the event, and occasionally a proportion of the original neoplastic follicles may show 'in situ' transformation, that is, they may be filled with centroblasts which have not yet infiltrated the interfollicular tissue (see Fig. 11.2, p. 279). More often, the biopsy section will show complete effacement of the original follicular pattern by a diffuse sheet of blast cells with numerous mitoses and frequently the tumour will have already spread through the capsule into the surrounding tissue.

Immunoglobulin secretion

Surface marker studies in cases of centroblastic-centrocytic lymphoma regularly show SIg of monoclonal type on the neoplastic centrocytes and occasionally there may be evidence of CIg in such tumours as well. This may be seen in the form of vacuoles or globules, either within the cytoplasm or in nuclear pockets of the neoplastic centrocytes. Rarely this phenomenon is present in such striking degree as to have achieved separate recognition under the title of 'signet-ring cell lymphoma'. As to whether such separation is warranted remains to be seen when more cases have been reported.

It would seem that there are at least two distinct varieties of *signet-ring cell lymphoma*. In one of these, the cells have obvious plasma cell characteristics and the cytoplasmic globules consist of IgM. In the other, the cells are equally clearly centrocytes and the vacuoles contain IgG (Kim et al, 1978). The first type is obviously a variant form of lymphoplasmacytoid lymphoma and should be classified as such. We have observed a remarkable instance of the second variety in a woman aged 35

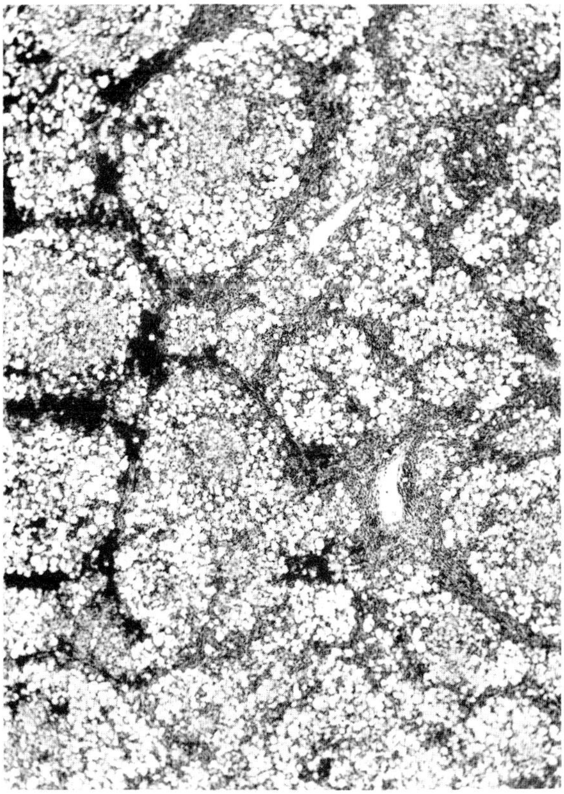

Fig. 10.68 Follicular centroblastic-centrocytic lymphoma of signet-ring cell type. A large proportion of the neoplastic cells show clear vacuoles in which traces of monotypic IgG could be demonstrated by immunostaining. (H E × 47)

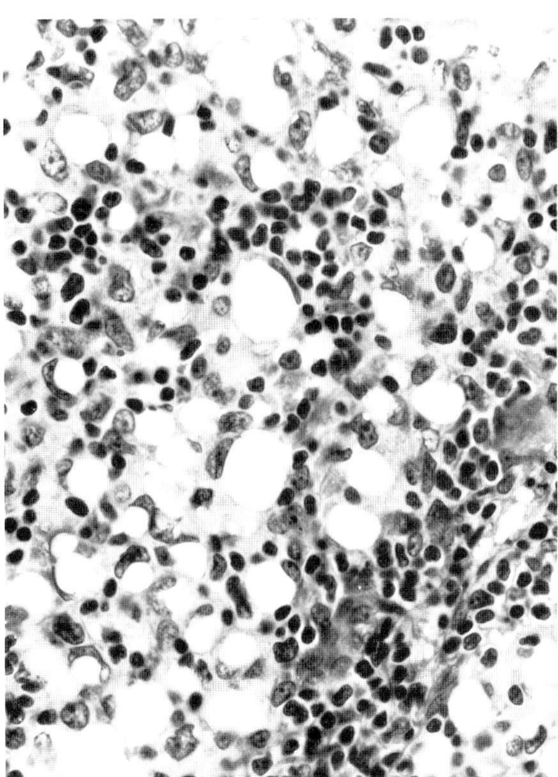

Fig. 10.69 Higher power view of same node as Fig. 10.68 showing margins of two follicles. The intracellular location of the vacuoles can be seen. (H E × 470)

in whom successive biopsies of malignant nodes over a period of more than 6 years have shown a centroblastic-centrocytic follicular lymphoma, with large, apparently empty, vacuoles in a high proportion of the neoplastic centrocytes (Figs 10.68, 10.69).

Sclerosis

Some degree of sclerosis is not uncommon in centroblastic-centrocytic follicular lymphoma, more particularly in inguinal and abdominal nodes (Bennett & Millett, 1969) (Fig. 10.70). The sclerosis may be striking and band-like, simulating the pattern of nodular sclerosing Hodgkin's disease, but this degree of sclerosis is much less common within lymph nodes than outside them. Not infrequently an involved node at the centre is free of fibrosis, whereas the surrounding extranodal infiltrate has provoked marked sclerosis. When much fibrosis is present, the follicular pattern of the tumour is often broken up and irregular within the fibrotic areas, although it may still be obvious in the non-fibrotic parts of the same tumour (Fig. 10.70). It is important to bear this in mind when interpreting biopsies of sclerotic lymphomas from sites such as the retroperitoneum. The significance of fibrosis in centroblastic-centrocytic lymphoma is still uncertain. Bennett (1975) found a slower progression of the disease in patients whose initial biopsy section showed fibrosis, than in those patients whose biopsy section did not show fibrosis, and this finding has been confirmed by others (Lennert, 1978, p. 337 et seq.).

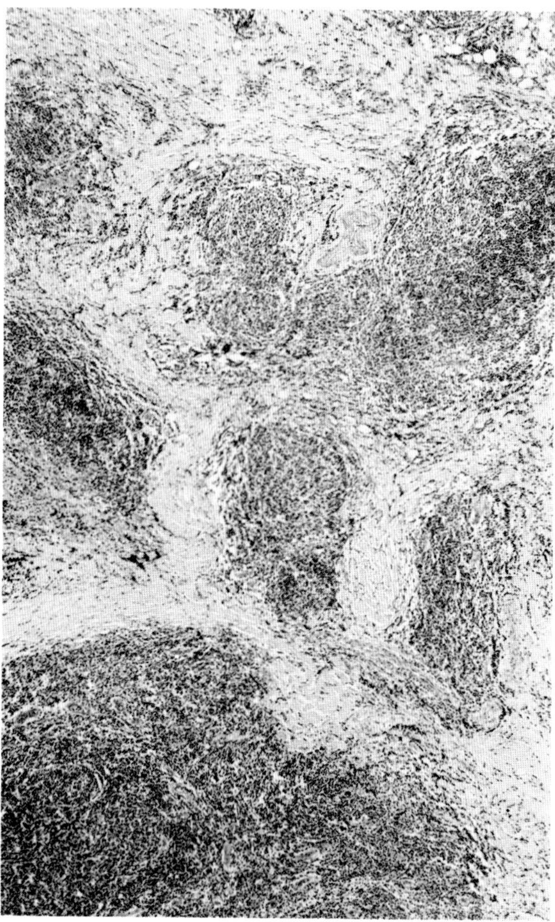

Fig. 10.70 Follicular centroblastic-centrocytic lymphoma with banded sclerosis. The follicular pattern of the tumour is less obvious in the sclerotic areas. (H E × 47)

A much less common pattern of spontaneous fibrosis is sometimes seen, in which hyalinised fibrous scars occupy the centres of neoplastic follicles (Fig. 10.71). In one such case observed by the author, collagenisation appeared to follow the deposition of extracellular immunoglobulin in the follicles (Fig. 10.72). Total replacement of the neoplastic follicles by hyaline material may be seen in biopsies of patients with centroblastic-centrocytic follicular lymphoma, following treatment of the disease with cytotoxic drugs.

Prognosis. Although varying within wide limits, the prognosis in terms of length of survival is generally better in centroblastic-centrocytic follicular lymphoma than in any other class of low grade NHL except for ML lymphocytic. Ultimately most patients with widespread disease die from its effects. The disease may be controlled by therapy, often over many years, but very few patients are cured. It is difficult to judge the effects of therapy, for the progress of the disease may sometimes be very slow in the untreated patient. On the other hand, progress may occasionally be unexpectedly rapid. Rapid deterioration may be due, as already indicated, to transformation of the initially low-grade lymphoma into a high-grade tumour of centroblastic, immunoblastic or large-cell centrocytic type. When transformation occurs, as it does ultimately in many cases, survival is usually measurable in months. Other adverse prognostic features include bulky tumour masses, whether in

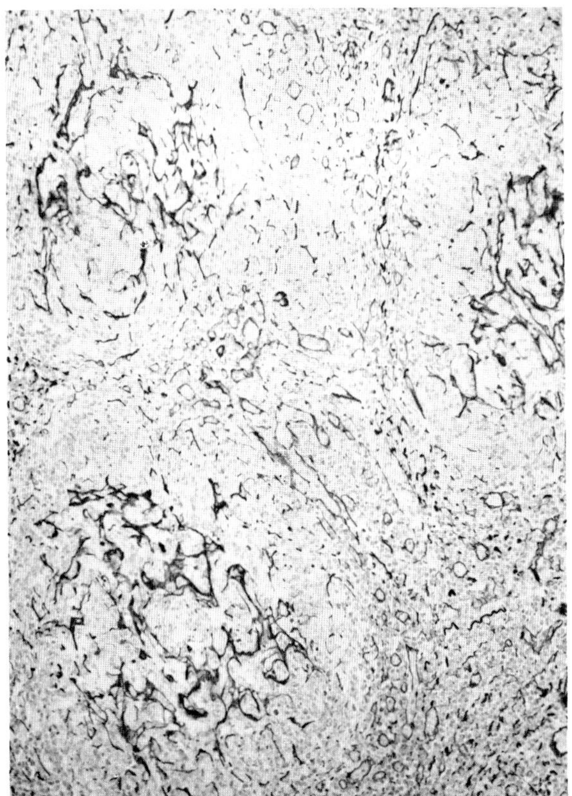

Fig. 10.71 Sclerosis within the follicles of a follicular centroblastic-centrocytic lymphoma — probably a sequel of immunoglobulin production by the tumour (Gordon and Sweets reticulin × 120)

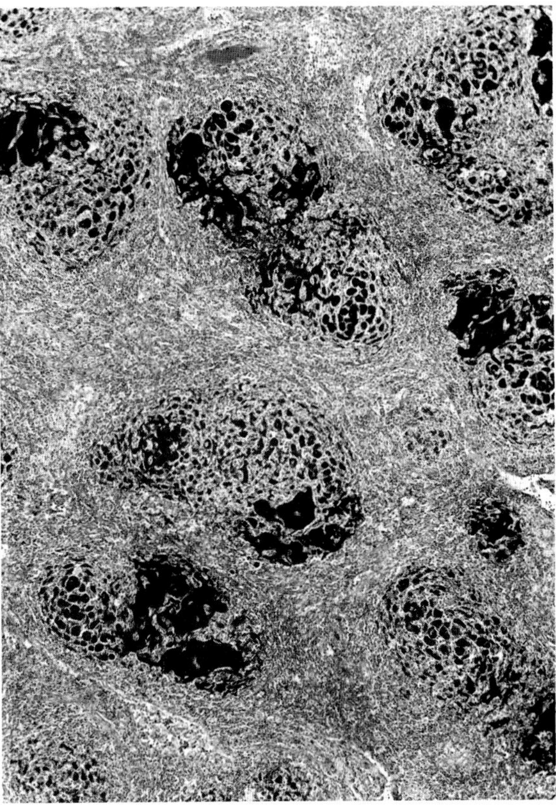

Fig. 10.72 Strongly PAS-positive amorphous deposits within the neoplastic follicles of a centroblastic-centrocytic follicular lymphoma. A weak reaction for monotypic IgG was obtained on immunostaining. (PAS × 47)

lymph nodes or elsewhere, and high peripheral blood lymphoid cell counts.

Differential diagnosis. The chief problem in differential diagnosis relates to the distinction of neoplastic follicles from reactive follicles and this has already been discussed (see p. 264). Of less importance, as regards the consequences of a mistaken diagnosis, is the problem of distinguishing centroblastic-centrocytic follicular lymphoma from other types of malignant lymphoma. Three lymphomas in particular are liable to be confused with centroblastic-centrocytic follicular lymphoma. These are the nodular form of lymphocyte predominant Hodgkin's disease, ML centrocytic and occasionally ML lymphoplasmacytoid. Provided the follicular pattern of the tumour is recognised, it is unlikely that other types of malignant lymphoma will cause difficulty*. The proliferation centres of B-CLL are less well defined structures than neoplastic follicles and the cells here are lymphocytes, not centrocytes (see p. 235).

In *nodular lymphocyte predominant Hodgkin's disease*, the background cells are always lymphocytes, except where remnants of reactive follicles persist. The nodules here are often larger than the follicles of ML Cb-Cc and, more importantly, one nodule adjoins the next with a narrower intervening T-zone area than that usually found in ML Cb-Cc. The characteristic L & H type of Sternberg-Reed cell is generally quite different from a centroblast, but the problem of Sternberg-Reed-like cells in ML Cb-Cc has already been mentioned (p. 267). Usually, however, the correct diagnosis can be

* Except for a rare variant of 'mantle-zone' lymphoma which appears to be a form of ML centrocytic (see p. 255).

reached without difficulty by the pathologist who is mindful of the possibilities.

The differentiation of ML Cb-Cc from ML Cc has already been discussed on page 257. It is very unusual for lymphoplasmacytoid lymphomas to show a sufficiently nodular pattern for confusion to arise on this account (p. 240). The problem of the rare 'signet-cell lymphomas' has already been discussed (p. 271). In the exceptional case of ML Cb-Cc in which the biopsy shows a high proportion of blast cells, there may be difficulty in deciding whether transformation is occurring or not. This point is discussed on page 270.

ML Centroblastic-Centrocytic — diffuse

As mentioned in the introduction to this section (p. 260) the great majority of centroblastic-centrocytic lymphomas display a follicular pattern, at least in part or at some stage in the course of their development. Occasional malignant lymphomas are found which show no trace of a follicular pattern, but which appear to consist of a mixture of centrocytes and centroblasts, with the former predominating (Figs 10.73, 10.74). These may be classified as ML Cb-Cc diffuse. In a recent critical re-appraisal of tumours which we had classified in this way, we found that several were clearly examples of ML centrocytic containing occasional blast-type cells, some of which might have been the residue of reactive follicles, caught up in the tumour. Others were found to be from patients in whom a previous biopsy had shown an obvious follicular lymphoma. Most of the remainder appeared to have been misdiagnosed (unpublished data). Thus, in the author's experience, this is a very rare type of malignant lymphoma and, indeed, its existence as a clearly recognisable entity is, we believe, open to question. One such tumour,

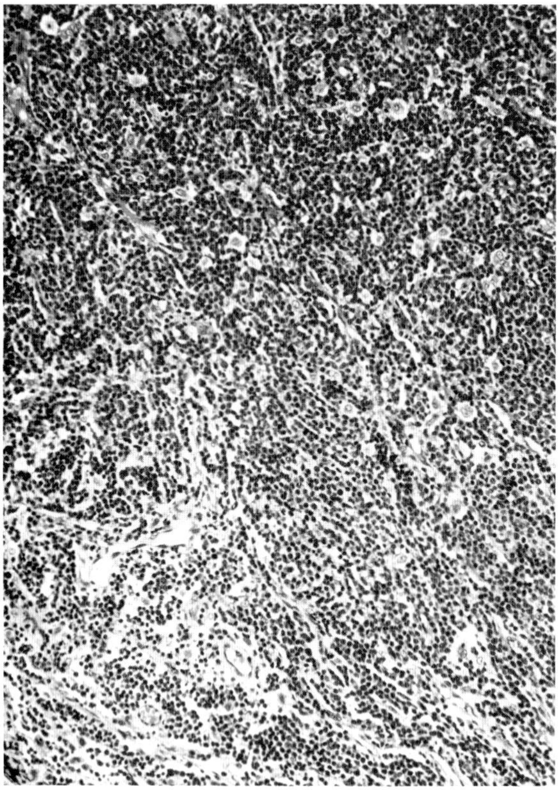

Fig. 10.73 Lymph node biopsy showing a diffuse centroblastic-centrocytic lymphoma. The cells here are predominantly of centrocytic type, but scattered centroblasts can be seen. (H E × 120)

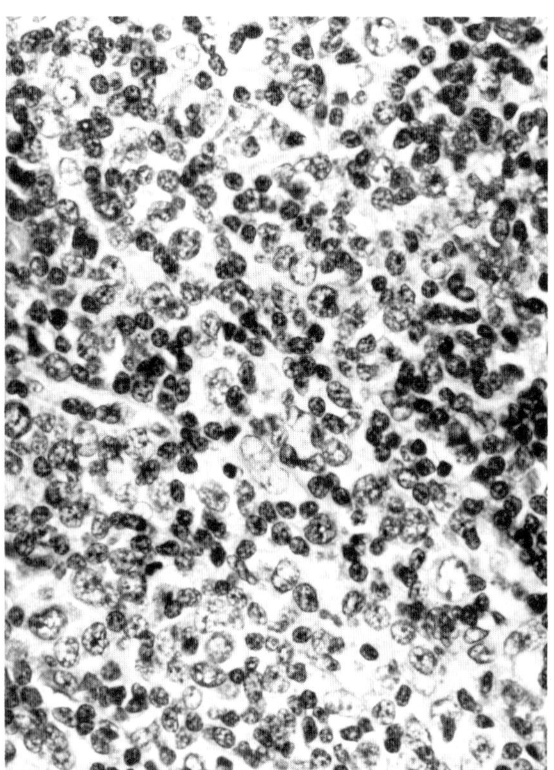

Fig. 10.74 Another case of diffuse centroblastic-centrocytic lymphoma at a higher magnification showing a mixture of centrocytes and centroblasts (H E × 470)

in a middle-aged man, displayed a relatively high proportion of centroblasts in the initial biopsy. This transformed rapidly and, a few months later, a second biopsy showed an overwhelming preponderance of centroblasts. The patient died shortly afterwards.

REFERENCES

Armitage J O, Dick F R, Corder M P 1978 Diffuse histiocytic lymphoma complicating chronic lymphocytic leukemia. Cancer 41: 422–427

Bennett M H 1975 Sclerosis in non-Hodgkin's lymphomata. British Journal of Cancer 31: Supplement II: 44–52

Bennett M H, Millett Y L 1969 Nodular sclerotic lymphosarcoma — a possible new clinico-pathological entity. Clinical Radiology 20: 339–343

Bennett M H, Farrer-Brown G, Henry K, Jelliffe A M 1974 Classification of non-Hodgkin's lymphomas. Lancet 2: 405–406 (Letter to the Editor)

Boston H C, Dahlin D C, Ivins J C, Cupps R E 1974 Malignant lymphoma (so-called reticulum cell sarcoma) of bone. Cancer 34: 1131 — 1137

Brittinger G, Bartels H, Bremer K et al 1977 Retrospektive untersuchungen zur klinischen bedeutung der Kiel-klassifikation der malignen non-Hodgkin-lymphome. Strahlentherapie 153: 222–228

Burkitt D 1958 A sarcoma involving the jaws in African children. British Journal of Surgery 46: 218–233

Catovsky D, Greaves M F, Rose M et al 1982 Adult T-cell lymphoma-leukaemia in blacks from the West Indies. Lancet 1: 639–643

Cullen M H, Lister T A, Brearley R L, Shand W S, Stansfeld A G 1979 Histological transformation of non-Hodgkin's lymphoma. Cancer 44: 645–651

Davies A J S, Carter R L, Leuchars E, Wallis V 1969 The morphology of immune reactions in normal, thymectomised and reconstituted mice. Immunology 17: 111–126

Dorfman R F 1974 Classification of non-Hodgkin's lymphomas. Lancet 1: 1295–1296 (Letter to the Editor)

Gall E A, Mallory T B 1942 Malignant lymphoma. A clinico-pathologic survey of 618 cases. American Journal of Pathology 18: 381–429

Galton D A G 1974 The chronic leukaemias. In: Hardisty R M and Weatherall D J (eds) Blood and its disorders. Blackwell Scientific, Oxford. Ch 21, p 974

Galton D A G, Goldman J M, Wiltshaw E 1974 Prolymphocytic leukaemia. British Journal of Haematology 27: 7–23

Gérard-Marchant R, Hamlin I, Lennert K, Rilke F, Stansfeld A G, van Unnik J A M 1974 Classification of non-Hodgkin's lymphomas. Lancet 2: 406–408 (Letter to the Editor)

Gunz F W, Angus H B 1965 Leukemia and cancer in the same patient. Cancer 18: 145–152

Hansen J A, Good R A 1974 Malignant disease of the lymphoid system in immunological perspective. Human Pathology 5: 567–599

Jaffe E S, Braylan R C, Nanba K, Frank M M, Berard C W 1977 Functional markers: a new perspective on malignant lymphomas. Cancer Treatment Reports 61: 953–962

Jellinger K, Radaszkiewicz T, Slowik F 1975 Primary malignant lymphomas of the central nervous system in man. Acta Neuropathologica (Berlin), Supplement 6: 95–102

Kim H, Hendrickson M R, Dorfman R F 1977 Composite lymphoma. Cancer 40: 959–976

Kim H, Dorfman R F, Rappaport H 1978 Signet ring cell lymphoma — a rare morphologic and functional expression of nodular (follicular) lymphoma. American Journal of Surgical Pathology 2: 119–132

Lennert K 1973 Follicular lymphoma — a tumour of the germinal centers. GANN monograph on Cancer Research 15: 217-231

Lennert K, in collaboration with Mohri N; Stein H, Kaiserling E, Müller-Hermelink H K 1978 Malignant Lymphomas other than Hodgkin's Disease. Springer-Verlag, Berlin

Lennert K 1981 Histopathology of non-Hodgkin's lymphomas. Springer-Verlag, Berlin

Lennert K, Stein H, Kaiserling E 1975 Cytological and functional criteria for the classification of malignant lymphomata. British Journal of Cancer 31: Supplement II 29–43

Levine G D, Dorfman R F, 1975 Nodular lymphoma: an ultrastructural study of its relationship to germinal centers and a correlation of light and electron microscopic findings. Cancer 35: 148–164

Lister T A, Cullen M H, Beard M E J et al 1978 Comparison of combined and single-agent chemotherapy in non-Hodgkin's lymphoma of favourable histological type. British Medical Journal 1: 533–537

Lukes R J, Collins R D 1974 Immunologic characterization of human malignant lymphomas. Cancer 34: 1488–1503

Lukes R J, Collins R D 1975 New approaches to the classification of the lymphomata. British Journal of Cancer 31. Supplement II 1–28

Mitsui T, Kikuchi M, Eimoto T, Nishiuchi M, Toyooka R 1983 Non-Hodgkin's lymphoma in North Western Kyushu island of Japan. Acta Pathologica of Japan 33: 71–88

Palutke M, Eisenberg L, Mirchandari I, Tabacza P, Husain M 1982 Malignant lymphoma of small cleaved lymphocytes of the follicular mantle zone. Blood 59: 317–322

Pangalis G A, Nathwani B N, Rappaport H 1977 Malignant lymphoma, well differentiated lymphocytic — its relationship with chronic lymphocytic leukemia and macroglobulinemia of Waldenström. Cancer 39: 999–1010

Papadimitriou C S, Müller-Hermelink U, Lennert K 1979 Histologic and immunohistochemical findings in the differential diagnosis of chronic lymphocytic leukemia of B-cell type and lymphoplasmacytic/lymphoplasmacytoid lymphoma. Virchow's Archiv A (Path Anat and Histol) 384: 149–158

Purtilo D T 1980 Epstein-Barr-Virus-induced oncogenesis in immune-deficient individuals. Lancet 1: 300–303

Rappaport H 1966 Tumors of the hematopoietic system. In: Atlas of Tumor Pathology, Section III, Fascicle 8, Armed Forces Institute of Pathology, Washington DC

Rappaport H, Winter W J, Hicks E B 1956 Follicular lymphoma — a re-evaluation of its position in the scheme of malignant lymphoma based on a survey of 253 cases. Cancer 9: 792–821

Robb-Smith A H T 1938 Reticulosis and reticulosarcoma: a histological classification. Journal of Pathology and Bactériology 47: 457–480
Rosas-Uribe A, Rappaport H 1972 Malignant lymphoma, histiocytic type with sclerosis (sclerosing reticulum cell sarcoma). Cancer 29: 946–953
Seligmann M, Danon F, Hurez D et al 1968 Alpha chain disease: a new immunoglobulin abnormality. Science 162: 1396–1397
Smithers D W 1973 Prevalence and age distribution. In: Hodgkin's disease, Churchill Livingstone, Edinburgh, ch 2, p 11, Fig. 2.1
Strauchen J A, Young R C, De Vita V T et al 1978 Clinical relevance of the histopathologic subclassification of diffuse 'histiocytic' lymphoma. New England Journal of Medicine 299: 1382–1387
Suchi T, Tajima K, Nanba K et al 1979 Some problems on the histiopathological diagnosis of non-Hodgkin's malignant lymphoma — a proposal of a new type. Acta Pathologica of Japan 29: 755–776
Swerdlow S H, Habeshaw J A, Murray L J, Dhaliwal H S, Lister T A, Stansfeld A G 1983 Centrocytic lymphoma: a distinct clinicopathologic and immunologic entity. American Journal of Pathology 113: 181–197
Tolksdorf G, Stein H, Lennert K 1980 Morphological and immunological definition of a malignant lymphoma derived from germinal-centre cells with cleaved nuclei (centrocytes). British Journal of Cancer 41: 168–182
van den Tweel J G, Taylor C R, Parker J W, Lukes R J 1978 Immunoglobulin inclusions in non-Hodgkin's lymphomas. American Journal of Clinical Pathology 69: 306–313
Weisenburger D D, Nathwani B N, Diamond L W, Winberg C D, Rappaport H 1981 Malignant lymphoma, intermediate lymphocytic type — a clinicopathological study of 42 cases. Cancer 48: 1415–1425
Weisenburger D D, Kim H, Rappaport H 1982 Mantle-zone lymphoma — a follicular variant of intermediate lymphocytic lymphoma. Cancer 49: 1429–1438
World Health Organization 1976 Histological and cytological typing of neoplastic diseases of haematopoletic and lymphoid tissues. Mathé G, Rappaport H, in collaboration with O'Conor G T, Torloni H. In: International Histological Classification of Tumours No 14, World Health Organization, Geneva

11

A.G. Stansfeld

High grade malignant lymphomas

INTRODUCTION

The subdivision of the non-Hodgkin's lymphomas into low grade and high grade categories was described in the last chapter as a central feature of the Kiel classification (p. 230). The neoplastic cells in the high grade malignant lymphomas are either transformed lymphoid cells or primitive precursor cells of the lymphoid system. Both may be termed 'blasts' and in both instances a high mitotic index reflects the rapid rate of cell turnover and generally rapid growth of the tumours arising therefrom. Despite some similarities, there are, however, important differences between these two classes of cell. Transformed lymphoid cells are generally larger and have more cytoplasm than primitive precursor lymphoid cells. Malignant lymphomas arising from transformed cells correspond in the main to Rappaport's 'histiocytic' lymphoma category (which also includes ML centrocytic of large cell type) (Rappaport, 1966). The use of the term 'histiocytic' to describe large cell lymphomas in general is still widespread, despite universal recognition of the fact that the vast majority of such neoplasms are composed of transformed lymphoid cells, usually of B-cell type. The malignant lymphomas of primitive, precursor lymphoid cells have been classed in the Rappaport classification as 'undifferentiated', in the case of Burkitt's lymphoma and the morphologically similar 'non-Burkitt's' type. The precursor T-cell tumours have more recently been labelled 'lymphoblastic' in the amended Rappaport classification (Nathwani et al, 1976) although they were originally included in the 'poorly differentiated lymphocytic' category (Rappaport, 1966).

In the Kiel classification three main classes of high-grade malignant lymphoma are recognised, namely, centroblastic, immunoblastic and lymphoblastic, and each of these is subdivided into two or more categories. Whilst the subdivisions of the lymphoblastic lymphomas distinguish primitive tumours arising from fundamentally different cell types B, T or U (= unclassified), the subdivisions of the centroblastic and immunoblastic lymphomas (transformed cells) are much less clearly defined and, in the light of further knowledge, the boundaries may need to be redrawn. At the present time, when the diagnosis rests mainly on morphological criteria, it seems wise to distinguish more rather than fewer categories, where genuine morphological and/or behavioural differences seem to exist. It may well be that further experience will, in due course, reduce the number of categories, if it is proved that two tumours with relatively minor differences in morphology are fundamentally similar in cell composition and behaviour.

The 'peripheral' (or 'adult') T-cell lymphomas are, as a group, less well defined than the B-cell lymphomas. It is clear however that some classes of peripheral T-cell lymphoma are just as aggressive in behaviour as many of the 'high-grade' B cell lymphomas, although initially at least, they may contain only a minority of 'blast' cells. Some of these categories have yet to be accommodated in the Kiel classification. The peripheral T-cell lymphomas are discussed in Chapter 12. Lymph node neoplasms of histiocytic origin are dealt with in Chapter 14.

ML CENTROBLASTIC (ML Cb)

Synonyms:

'Histiocytic' lymphoma, nodular and diffuse (some examples).

Follicle centre cell lymphoma, large, non-cleaved. Large cell lymphoma, diffuse (some examples).

This type of B-cell malignant lymphoma is composed exclusively or predominantly of blast-type cells which resemble the centroblasts of reactive germinal centres. Currently the centroblastic lymphomas are split into two morphological variants — (1) a **Monomorphic** (or pure) **sub-type**, where the cells are all blasts of similar morphology, and (2) a **Polymorphic sub-type** in which the prevailing centroblasts are intermingled with centrocytes, a small proportion of immunoblasts and sometimes cells showing plasmacytoid characteristics. In our experience tumours of this sub-type are more prone to arise in extranodal sites than the monomorphic sub-type. The Kiel classification (Lennert, 1978, p 346–360) further subdivides centroblastic lymphomas into: (a) *Primary* centroblastic lymphomas — high grade lymphomas arising *de novo*, that is, not preceded by a low grade tumour of centroblastic-centrocytic type, and (b) *Secondary* centroblastic lymphomas, which result from blastic transformation in a centroblastic-centrocytic lymphoma (see p. 269). These two types may be morphologically indistinguishable, but it remains to be seen whether there are any differences between them, other than the manner in which they appear to arise.

Incidence and presentation

In the Kiel lymph node registry data (Lennert, 1981) centroblastic lymphomas account for about 5% of malignant lymphomas other than Hodgkin's disease. By far the largest proportion occur in adult life. We have not noted a marked difference in incidence in the two sexes.

ML centroblastic may present within lymph nodes or in extranodal sites. *Secondary* centroblastic lymphomas (i.e. arising by transformation of a pre-existing centroblastic-centrocytic lymphoma) generally present with nodal swellings and are sometimes characterised clinically by the sudden, accelerated growth of a single node or group of nodes in a patient already known to have a follicular lymphoma. On the other hand, *primary* centroblastic lymphoma may present with lymphadenopathy or with extranodal tumours, e.g. in gastrointestinal tract, Waldeyer's ring, thyroid or elsewhere. As already mentioned, these extranodal tumours are often of the polymorphic sub-type.

Macroscopic features. There are no macroscopic features which distinguish centroblastic from other malignant lymphomas and the diagnosis rests upon the histological picture.

Histology. 1. Primary centroblastic lymphomas. These tumours generally appear primarily in lymph nodes, often in a single node or group of nodes. Less frequently the growth may present in a tonsil or other extranodal site. Although, in the initial stages, the malignant centroblasts may be mixed with the residual lymphoid cells of the node (Fig. 11.1), they tend to form solid sheets of blast-type cells, generally of fairly uniform size and appearance. The pattern of the tumour is usually diffuse, but sometimes a part of

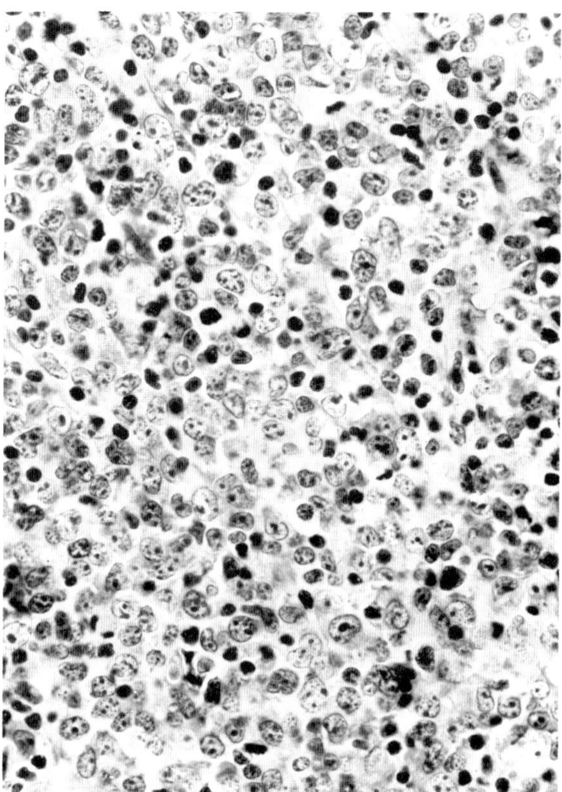

Fig. 11.1 Lymph node from a woman of 70 showing ML centroblastic with a diffuse pattern. There is a scattering of lymphocytes amongst the blast cells. (H E × 470)

the tumour in the node exhibits a clear cut follicular pattern (Fig. 11.2).

In the *monomorphic* sub-type, practically all the neoplastic cells resemble centroblasts (Fig. 11.3), having a relatively large, round or oval, 'vesicular' nucleus with several nucleoli at the periphery of the nucleus and a small amount of basophilic and pyroninophilic cytoplasm. Mitoses are numerous and sometimes atypical in form. As with all high-grade malignant lymphomas, the tumours generally have a large content of macrophages, which often contain nuclear debris, as in reactive germinal centres (Fig. 11.4).

In the *polymorphic* sub-type of ML centroblastic, whilst most of the neoplastic cells have the morphology of centroblasts, these are intermixed with large centrocytes and there are intermediate forms between the two. In addition, a small proportion of immunoblasts is present and occasionally cells showing distinct plasmacytoid differentiation

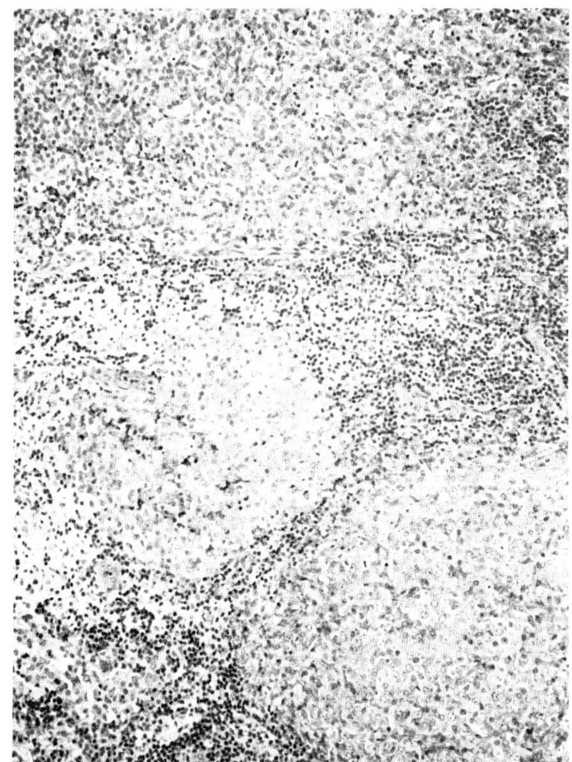

Fig. 11.2 Lymph node from a man of 50 showing ML centroblastic with a partly follicular pattern (H E × 120)

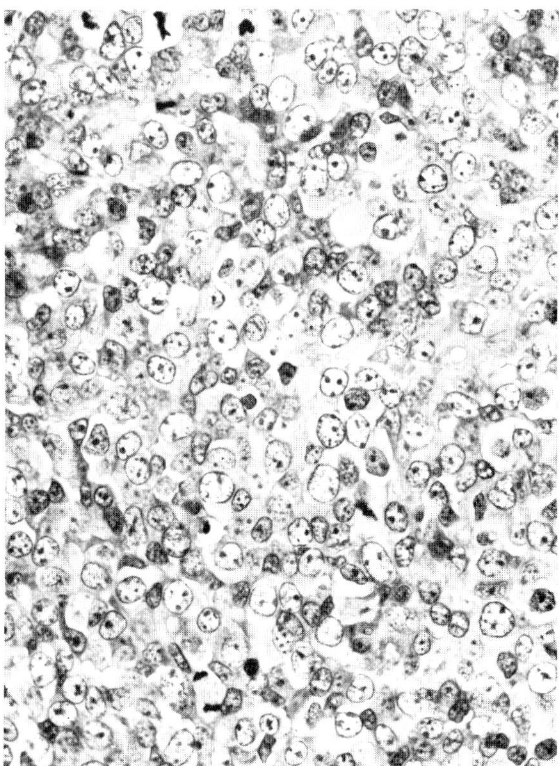

Fig. 11.3 Part of the same node as Fig. 11.2 showing cellular detail in ML centroblastic of monomorphic sub-type. The cells resemble the centroblasts of reactive germinal centres, having large round nuclei and several medium-sized, often peripheral nucleoli. Note mitoses. (H E × 470)

(Fig. 11.5). In either sub-type, occasional, bizarre, giant blast cells may be seen (Fig. 11.6).

2. *Secondary centroblastic lymphomas.* This term is applied to those centroblastic lymphomas which arise as a result of blastic transformation in a centroblastic-centrocytic lymphoma. Secondary centroblastic lymphomas probably occur with greater frequency than primary centroblastic lymphomas, whether of monomorphic or polymorphic sub-type. In a patient previously known to have had a low-grade centroblastic-centrocytic lymphoma a fresh biopsy may show evidence of blast cell transformation in a part or the whole of the section (see p. 270). Even in the absence of a previous history of lymphoma, the biopsy section may sometimes show distinct traces of a follicular pattern in part of the section, whilst other parts are overrun by a diffuse sheet of centroblasts. It is of course

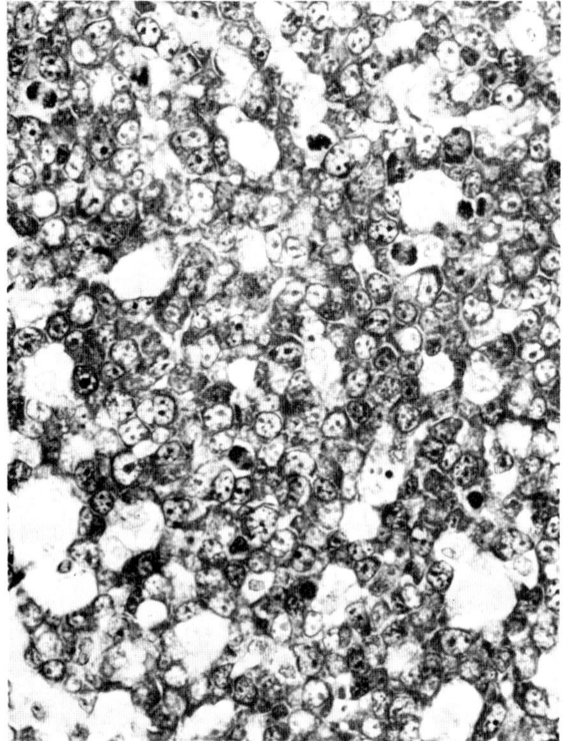

Fig. 11.4 Supraclavicular lymph node from a woman of 52 showing ML centroblastic of diffuse pattern. The resemblance to a germinal centre is heightened by the presence of many large macrophages which are very lightly stained in contrast with the strongly basophilic neoplastic centroblasts. (Giemsa × 470)

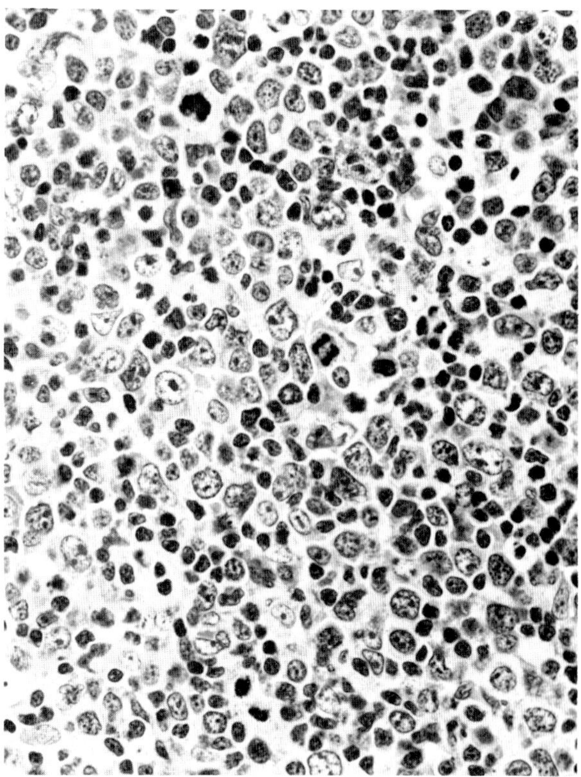

Fig. 11.5 Lymph node from a case of ML centroblastic of polymorphic sub-type. The cells are much more variable than in the monomorphic sub-type and include an occasional immunoblast, centrocytes and some plasmacytoid cells, as well as centroblasts. (H E × 470)

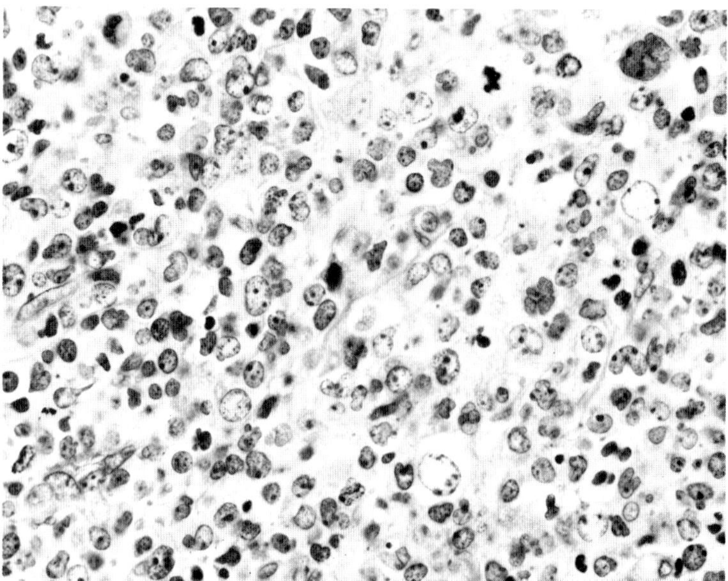

Fig. 11.6 ML centroblastic of polymorphic sub-type showing marked variation in cell size and a large, bizarre blast cell (top right) (Male aged 63). (H E × 470)

necessary to establish that such follicles are part of the neoplasm and not residual normal follicles, but, as pointed out earlier (see p. 261), it is very unusual to see prominent reactive follicles alongside a malignant lymphoma of germinal centre-cell origin. Whilst occasionally these neoplastic follicles are filled entirely with blast cells (Fig. 11.7), more often an admixture of centrocytes with centroblasts in the follicles confirms that one is dealing with a secondary centroblastic lymphoma. On other occasions, of course, the whole node may be diffusely infiltrated by neoplastic centroblasts.

The morphology of the blast cell tumour which results from the transformation of a centroblastic-centrocytic lymphoma is variable (see p. 270), (Lennert, 1978, p 345–359; Cullen et al, 1979). All the cells may show the features of centroblasts or they may resemble immunoblasts, having large, central nucleoli, or they may be a mixture of the two (Fig. 11.8). In any event, mitoses are generally numerous and often atypical.

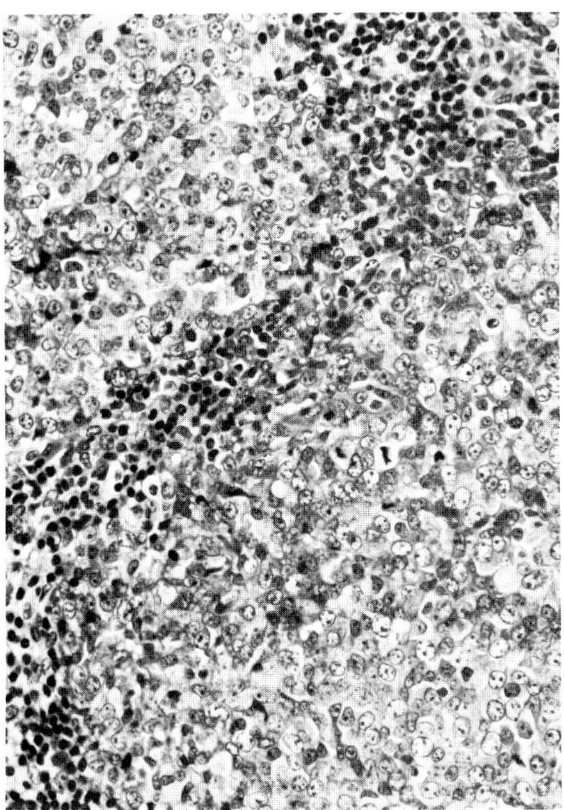

Fig. 11.7 Secondary centroblastic lymphoma showing 'follicular' aggregates of centroblasts (same case as Figs 11.2 and 11.3) (H E × 300)

We have found in several instances that the transformation of a centroblastic-centrocytic lymphoma into a centroblastic lymphoma has been accompanied by a change in the phenotype of the cells with at least a temporary phase of gross T-cell preponderance, even when morphologically the cells appear to be nearly all centroblasts (Habeshaw et al, 1979). The precise significance of this observation is uncertain.

Prognosis. The prognosis of ML centroblastic was formerly very bad, survival being measurable often in months rather than years. However, with the introduction of more effective forms of combination chemotherapy, the prognosis is now comparable with that of the large-cell type of centrocytic lymphoma and a proportion of patients appear to be cured by such treatment.

Differential diagnosis. The identification of a malignant lymphoma as ML centroblastic generally depends upon the availability of good sections of well fixed tissue. If such are not available it may be impossible to distinguish ML centroblastic from other high-grade malignant lymphomas (ML lymphoblastic and ML immunoblastic), from large-cell centrocytic lymphomas (when poor fixation has resulted in nuclear 'ballooning') or even from some reactive conditions. Given reasonable sections, the main problem is in distinguishing ML centroblastic from ML immunoblastic and, occasionally, from ML lymphoblastic of 'B' type. Neoplastic centroblasts are often smaller than neoplastic immunoblasts and are more comparable in size with the relatively large lymphoblasts of the B-lymphoblastic lymphomas. Size alone is not, however, an absolute criterion. The nuclear size is often much the same in centroblasts and immunoblasts, but the latter usually have more cytoplasm than centroblasts while B-lymphoblasts have the same amount or less. The density of the nuclear chromatin in the centroblast is much less than that in the B-lymphoblast, as a result of which the small, generally multiple, and often peripheral nucleoli of the centroblast stand out quite clearly. Nucleoli may be difficult to distinguish in B lymphoblasts because of the denser chromatin. In the neoplastic immunoblast, the nucleolus is usually solitary and very large, often appearing

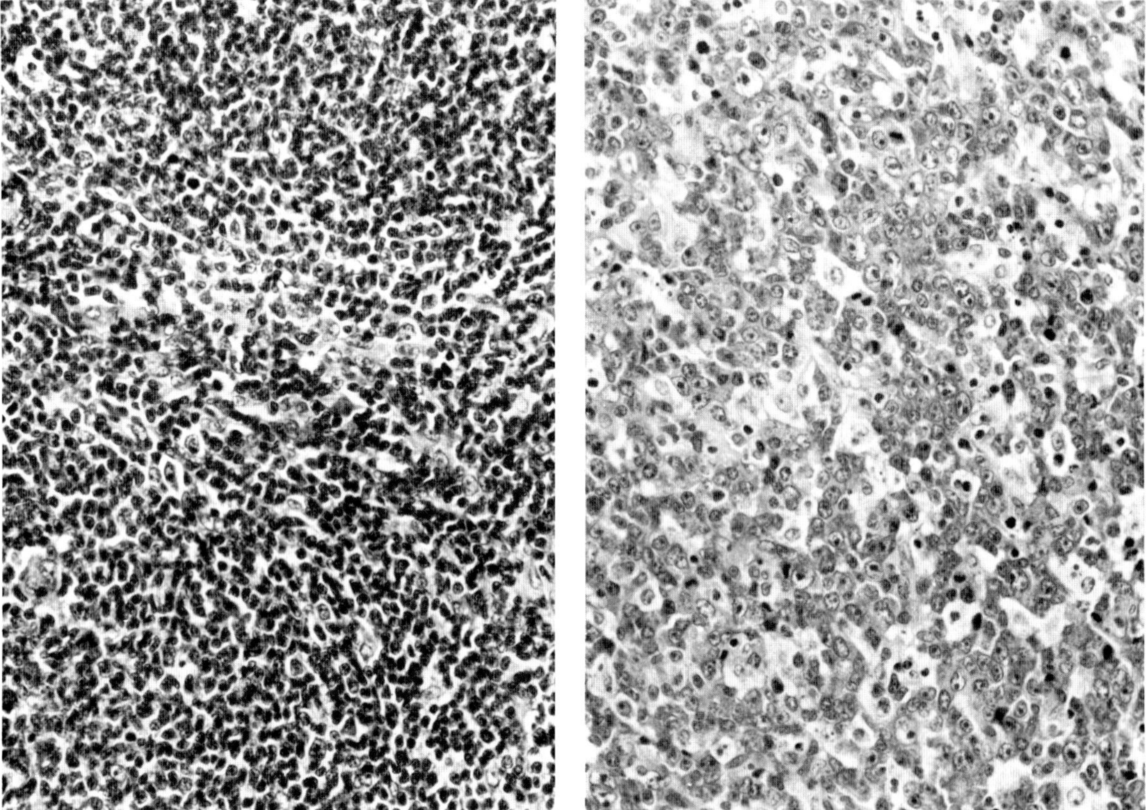

Fig. 11.8 (a) and (b) Transformation of centroblastic-centrocytic, follicular malignant lymphoma (a) into polymorphic centroblastic malignant lymphoma of diffuse pattern (b). The two lymph node biopsies were one year apart. ((a) and (b) both H E × 300)

central in position. It stands out very clearly by reason of its size and the contrast between nucleolus and pale nuclear sap.

ML LYMPHOBLASTIC (ML LB)

In the Kiel classification, three different types of lymphoblastic lymphoma are distinguished, namely, a B-type, a T-type and a U-(unclassified) type, in which the cells are devoid of both B and T surface markers. Following the introduction of monoclonal antibodies specific for T cells, some of the previously unclassified lymphoblastic lymphomas which fail to form E rosettes have been shown to be of T cell origin.

The lymphoblastic lymphomas have in common the fact that in each case the neoplastic cells are of primitive type, having no recognisable counterpart in the lymphoid cells of post-natal life. Whilst this may not be true of all B-lymphoblastic lymphomas, it is certainly true in the case of T-lymphoblastic lymphomas (convoluted cell lymphomas) in which the neoplastic cells share common surface characteristics and enzyme activity with a particular stage in the development of thymic lymphocytes (Stein et al, 1976). These primitive blast cells are of medium or small size, with very scanty cytoplasm and a relatively large, deeply staining nucleus, which at once distinguishes the cells from those of other high grade malignant lymphomas (ML centroblastic and ML immunoblastic) derived from transformed lymphoid cells. In view of the embryonic origins of the cells in the lymphoblastic lymphomas, it is understandable that this group of lymphomas have their highest incidence in infancy and childhood.

Because the three classes of lymphoblastic lymphoma differ from one another in both morphology and behaviour, each will be described separately.

ML Lymphoblastic — B-type (including Burkitt's lymphoma)

Synonyms:
ML undifferentiated — Burkitt type.
ML undifferentiated — non-Burkitt (some examples).
ML poorly differentiated lymphocytic (BNLI classification).
Burkitt's lymphoma.
Follicle centre cell lymphoma, small non-cleaved (Lukes & Collins).

The type of high-grade malignant lymphoma which was first recognised by Burkitt as occurring endemically in tropical Africa (Burkitt, 1958), is now known to occur sporadically in Europe and North America and is probably of worldwide distribution, although comparatively rare outside the endemic areas (across tropical Africa and parts of New Guinea). The romantic story of the discovery of the Epstein-Barr virus (EBV) and its association with Burkitt's lymphoma and infectious mononucleosis has been well documented (Epstein et al, 1964; Henle et al, 1968) and will not be repeated here. Some authors maintain that the term Burkitt's lymphoma should only be used for those cases occurring within endemic areas or in which there is proof of EBV infection. Such proof is nearly always lacking in non-endemic cases and it has been suggested that these might be called 'Burkitt's lymphoma-like' or 'of Burkitt type'. Others are prepared to use the term Burkitt's lymphoma for all tumours with the characteristic morphology, regardless of whether or not EBV is shown to be associated.

At a conference of pathologists in Bethesda, USA, in 1967, it was agreed by the participants that Burkitt's lymphoma should be designated 'undifferentiated (Berard et al, 1969), but it later became clear that the neoplastic cells synthesise immunoglobulin — a property of B-cells (Minowada et al, 1967). Lukes & Collins (1973) have argued that Burkitt's lymphoma is derived from the small non-cleaved cells of germinal centres but Lennert denies identity of these lymphoma cells with centroblasts although admitting that Burkitt's lymphoma with its 'starry sky' appearance is reminiscent of an active germinal centre. The problem of the histogenesis of this tumour is discussed at length by Lennert (Lennert, 1978, p 364–367) who concludes that it may be derived from a precursor-type cell found in germinal centres. Interestingly, Magrath (1974) claimed to have found both B and T surface characteristics on neoplastic lymphoblasts from African cases of Burkitt's lymphoma, and this observation has been confirmed by Stein (Stein & Tolksdorf, 1977). It seems that the term 'undifferentiated' as applied to this tumour, may be appropriate after all.

Aside from the question of histogenesis of Burkitt's lymphoma, is the problem of whether the European and American cases of B-type lymphoblastic lymphoma, which do not contain the EBV genome, are really the same tumour. There are certainly clinical differences in regard to the age of onset and type of presentation which will be discussed in the next section.

Incidence and presentation

In the endemic areas of tropical Africa, Burkitt's lymphoma is the commonest malignant tumour of childhood, whilst acute lymphoblastic leukaemia is rare. The frequency of these two diseases relative to one another is reversed in Europe and North America. Whilst B-lymphoblastic lymphoma is everywhere much commoner in children than in adults, the peak incidence occurs earlier in African subjects than in North Americans — mean age 9.1 years and 12.2 years (Levine et al, 1975). The sex ratio is approximately 2 ♂:1 ♀.

The classical mode of presentation of African Burkitt's lymphoma, especially in young boys, is with a rapidly growing tumour in the jaw. The fact that this presentation is so seldom seen in white races may be a reflection of the later age of onset of the tumour in the latter. In African subjects the tumour commonly presents in the ovaries in girls, and less frequent sites are retroperitoneum, bones other than the jaws, thyroid, salivary glands and breast (Wright, 1970). A noticeable feature is the

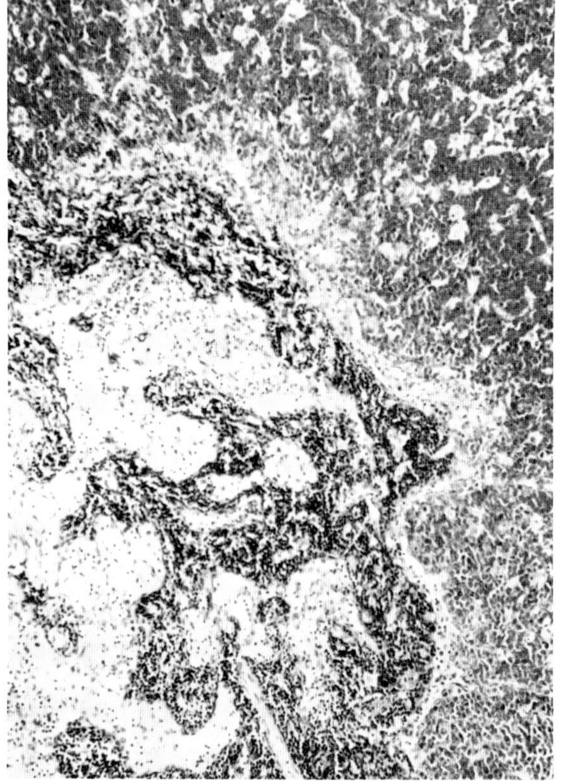

Fig. 11.9 B-lymphoblastic lymphoma, Burkitt type, from a Chinese male of 20. The neoplasm (top and right of field) completely envelops a mesenteric lymph node (bottom left) but does not invade it. Such behaviour is characteristic of Burkitt's lymphoma. (H E × 120)

comparative rarity of lymph node involvement (Fig. 11.9).

In B-lymphoblastic lymphomas occurring outside endemic areas, not only is the peak incidence in somewhat older children, but the age spread is much wider and occasional cases may be met with throughout adult life, particularly under the age of 50. The presentation tends to be different too. In children especially, the commonest presentation is with an intestinal tumour, generally in the lower ileum (Levine et al, 1982). Whilst other extranodal sites, such as those listed above, may also be involved, it is noteworthy that lymph nodes are more frequently involved than in African cases and the disease may occasionally present with cervical lymphadenopathy (Levine et al, 1982).

Tumours of long bones may present with spontaneous fractures and tumours of the spine with paraplegia. Involvement of the CNS is well recognised when the neoplasm relapses after treatment but leukaemia is exceptional and is then generally preterminal.

Macroscopic features. The tumour tissue, whether in an extranodal site or in lymph nodes, presents a featureless, pale pink or white appearance on section and the cut surface may show areas of necrosis. Tumours of the gut may have produced intussusception, in which case the tumour will be found to involve all coats of the intestinal wall and perforation may have occurred. The mucosal surface is nearly always ulcerated in these intestinal tumours, and sometimes necrosis is so extensive that it is possible to miss the fact that the perforation is due to a neoplasm. Even when the ileocaecal lymph nodes are grossly enlarged, they are not necessarily involved by lymphoma.

Histology. In a well fixed preparation, the neoplastic cells of the B-lymphoblastic lymphoma ap-

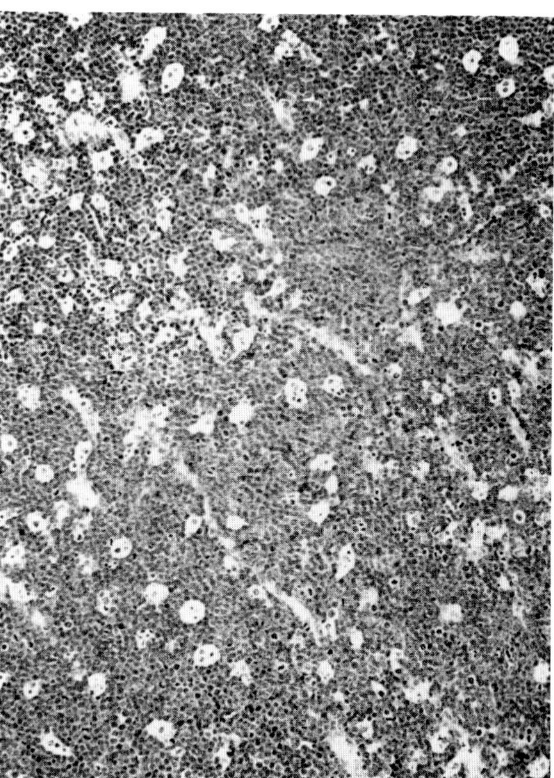

Fig. 11.10 B-lymphoblastic lymphoma (Burkitt's tumour) from the jaw of a four and a half year old Indian girl living in Nigeria. Abundant macrophages impart a 'starry sky' pattern to the tumour. (H E × 120)

pear cohesive, forming a solid sheet which is broken only by clear holes, occupied by large pale-staining macrophages, which often contain ingested nuclear debris, or even whole pyknotic nuclei (Figs. 11.10, 11.11). The 'starry sky' appearance, thus imparted, is one of the best known characteristics of Burkitt's lymphoma, but it should be noted that a similar appearance may be seen in other high grade malignant lymphomas from time to time. Furthermore, even in Burkitt's lymphoma, the number of 'stars' in the 'sky' is very variable and they may be absent or inconspicuous in some parts. The neoplastic cells are medium-sized blast-type cells which are distinguishable by their relatively large nuclei and scanty cytoplasm. The latter stains intensely with pyronin and is strongly basophilic with Giemsa, due to the rich content of polyribosomes (Fig. 11.12). The cytoplasm also frequently contains fat vacuoles, stainable with Oil Red O in imprint preparations. These are rarely visible in conventional sections, but can often be seen in semi-thin sections after resin embedding. Whilst the nuclei may appear round or oval at a low magnification, they are often highly irregular in outline when studied more closely. The cells are, nonetheless, easily distinguished from those of the T-lymphoblastic lymphoma (convoluted cell tumour). The nuclear chromatin is relatively dense and coarse, often partially obscuring the rather small nucleoli which may be single or multiple. Mitoses are very numerous, reflecting the rapid rate of cell turnover and generally rapid growth of the tumour (Fig. 11.11).

The high macrophage content of the tumour also mirrors the rate of cell turnover and tendency to spontaneous necrosis of the neoplastic cells. Whilst necrosis is often piecemeal, affecting iso-

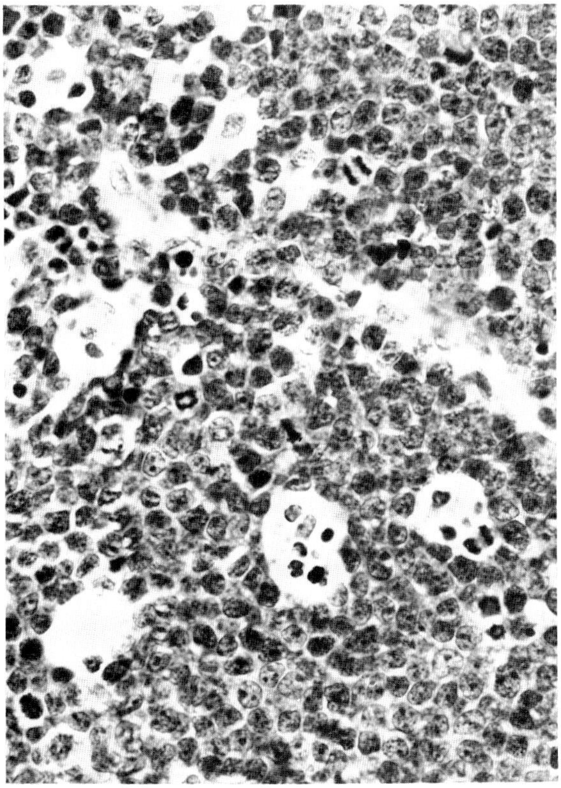

Fig. 11.11 Same tumour as Fig. 11.10 at higher magnification. The neoplastic cells form a cohesive sheet, interrupted by large macrophages containing nuclear debris. Note frequent mitoses. (H E × 470)

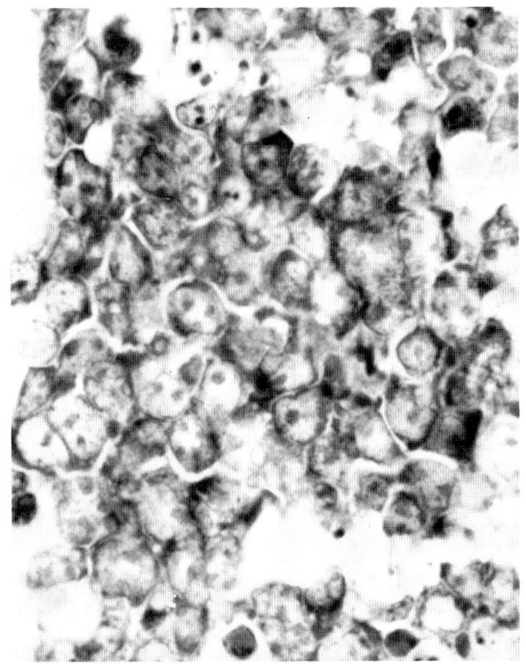

Fig. 11.12 B-lymphoblastic lymphoma, Burkitt type. Part of a large abdominal tumour probably arising in the ileocaecal region, but here infiltrating muscle, from a European male of 36. Note large nuclei, relatively prominent nucleoli and intensely basophilic cytoplasm of cells. (Giemsa × 940)

lated cells throughout the tumour, it may be on a more extensive scale, affecting large areas, which then may appear littered with nuclear fragments. In extreme cases where little viable tumour remains the true nature of the lesion may not be appreciated (Fig. 11.13).

Prognosis. A dramatic response to treatment with cyclophosphamide or methotrexate has often been observed in African Burkitt's lymphoma in children but the tumours have frequently relapsed. Prior to the introduction of chemotherapy the tumours were almost uniformly rapidly fatal. However, rare cases of spontaneous remission have been reported (Burkitt & Kyalwazi, 1967). The response to therapy of Burkitt type lymphoblastic lymphoma in non-endemic areas has generally been very disappointing, particularly in adult patients. Remissions have most often been obtained in children with primary tumours of the intestine, but much depends on the stage of the disease at the time of diagnosis. Spread of the tumour to lymph nodes materially worsens the prognosis.

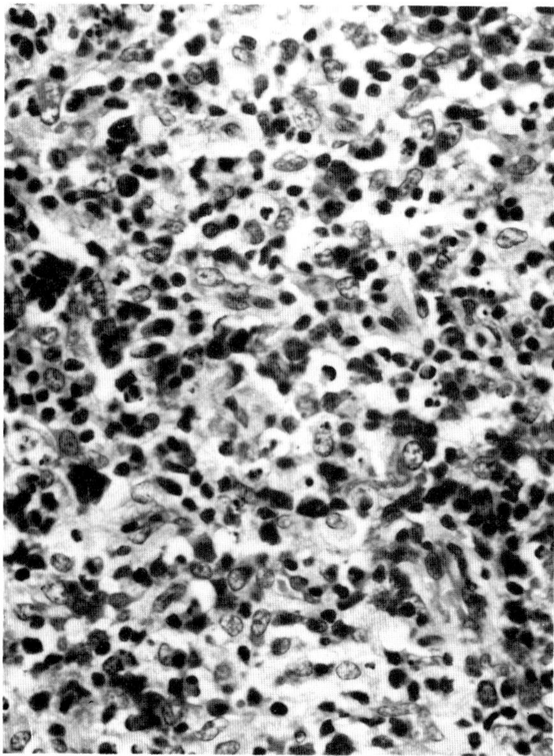

Fig. 11.13 B-lymphoblastic lymphoma with spontaneous necrosis. Section of a nasal tumour from a boy of 7. Extensive necrosis and macrophage infiltration obscure the true nature of the tumour, which is represented only by isolated groups of darkly staining cells. (The diagnosis had been missed in an earlier lymph node biopsy because of extensive necrosis.) Soon after the nasal biopsy was taken, perforation of a similar tumour in the ileocaecal region occurred and the bowel tumour also showed widespread necrosis which was no doubt responsible for the perforation. (H E × 470)

Differential diagnosis. B-lymphoblastic lymphomas are most likely to be confused with other types of high-grade lymphoma — not only other types of lymphoblastic lymphoma (T-lymphoblastic and unclassified lymphoblastic), but also with centroblastic and small cell variants of B-immunoblastic lymphoma. The much more prominent nucleoli should serve to distinguish the latter. In occasional cases of infectious mononucleosis in childhood, the cellular infiltrate in a node biopsy may be sufficiently monomorphic to cause confusion with a lymphoblastic lymphoma, but this mistake is less likely to be made if the node is removed intact and the whole picture observed.

ML Lymphoblastic — T type

Synonyms:
ML Lymphoblastic.
Malignant lymphoma of convoluted lymphocytes (Lukes).
Thymic lymphoma (Collins et al, 1979).
Convoluted cell lymphoma.
Sternberg's leukosarcoma.

Recognised as a distinct entity by Barcos & Lukes in 1973 (published 1975), this highly aggressive neoplasm is composed of primitive T-lymphocytes, identified as prothymocytes in some instances and thymocytes in others, by their surface marker and enzyme histochemical characteristics (Stein et al, 1980). The thymic origin of the cells is reflected in the frequency of an anterior mediastinal tumour. It is closely allied to T-type acute lymphoblastic leukaemia which may occur both with and without associated solid tumour formation. In most instances a large proportion of the neoplastic cells form spontaneous 'E-rosettes' with sheep erythrocytes.

Incidence and presentation

The T-lymphoblastic lymphomas are fairly uncommon tumours, comparable in frequency with the B-lymphoblastic lymphomas in non-endemic areas. There is no published evidence of a specific racial or geographical predisposition. Although occasional cases are met with in adults, the main incidence is in children and adolescents, and it is more than twice as common in boys as in girls. The classical mode of presentation is with a large anterior mediastinal mass, with or without pleural effusions. There are commonly enlarged lymph nodes also, in the supraclavicular fossae, axilla or elsewhere, biopsy of which will confirm the diagnosis. Not infrequently lymphadenopathy may occur without a thymic tumour. The marrow and peripheral blood are often normal at the time of presentation, but within a short space of time, the marrow may be flooded with T-lymphoblasts and overt acute lymphoblastic leukaemia quickly follows. Extranodal presentations other than with a thymic tumour are uncommon, but the disease frequently becomes generalised, to involve many organs when the leukaemic phase sets in. CNS involvement is common at this stage.

On occasions, the acute leukaemia presents first or concurrently with the discovery of a mediastinal mass. At other times the process is strictly leukaemic throughout, without a solid tumour phase.

Macroscopic features. There are no distinctive macroscopic appearances in lymph nodes, but even when involved by tumour these may be quite small and may appear normal to the naked eye. Later, large, soft greyish-white nodes are the rule.

Histology. In the early stages, infiltration of affected nodes is frequently patchy, the infiltrating cells mingling with normal elements, so that architectural disturbance is not immediately apparent and close scrutiny may then be required to detect the presence of the neoplasm (Fig. 11.14). When the node is only partially infiltrated, it may be observed that the periphery of the cortex and especially the follicles (B-zones) are spared. Soon, however, the normal architecture becomes progressively effaced by a diffuse cellular infiltrate which spreads into the capsule and trabeculae and out into the surrounding fat (Fig. 11.15). Diffuse infiltration of trabeculae is particularly characteristic, with parallel columns of cells lying between the spread out collagen bundles of the expanded trabecula (Fig. 11.16). This same pattern may be seen in acute lymphoblastic leukaemia of 'common type' and in acute myeloblastic leukaemia.

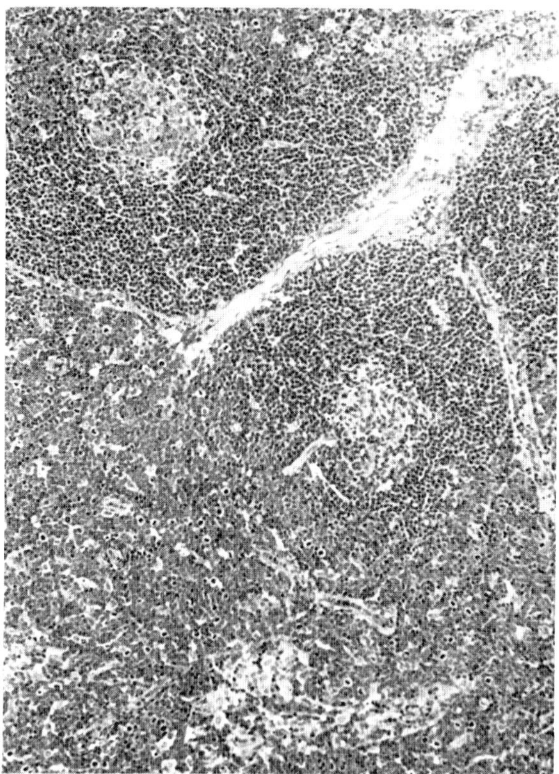

Fig. 11.14 Lymph node from a boy of 16 showing infiltration by T-lymphoblastic malignant lymphoma (lower field and top right). Note sparing of cortical follicles. The T-lymphoblasts are relatively small and do not contrast so strikingly with the residual normal lymphocytes. (H E × 120)

The neoplastic cells are appreciably smaller than those of the B-lymphoblastic lymphomas and because of this and their lack of cohesion, they are less readily identified as 'blast' cells. High power examination, however, often reveals a much greater degree of pleomorphism and variation in cell size than was apparent at first sight and the high mitotic rate then becomes obvious (Fig. 11.17). Large areas of necrosis are unusual, but as with all high grade lymphomas, individual cell necrosis is common and macrophages are frequently prominent, sometimes even giving a 'starry sky' pattern, though this is seldom as marked a feature as it is in the Burkitt-type lymphomas. Scattered eosinophils are sometimes seen.

Close study of the individual tumour cells shows these to have relatively large nuclei and a very

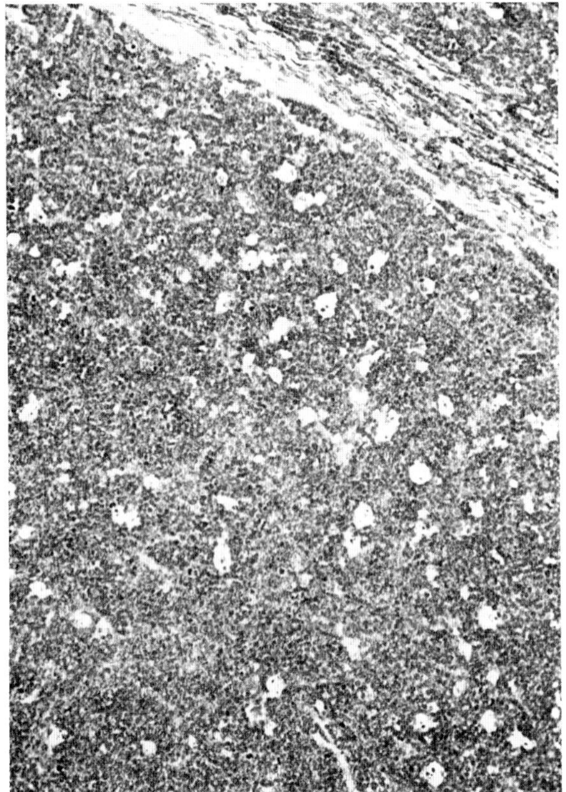

Fig. 11.15 Lymph node from a boy of 9 showing diffuse infiltration by T-lymphoblastic lymphoma. Note capsular and extra-capsular infiltration (top right). Abundant macrophages in this case give a starry sky appearance and this feature led initially to a mistaken diagnosis of Burkitt's lymphoma. (H E × 120)

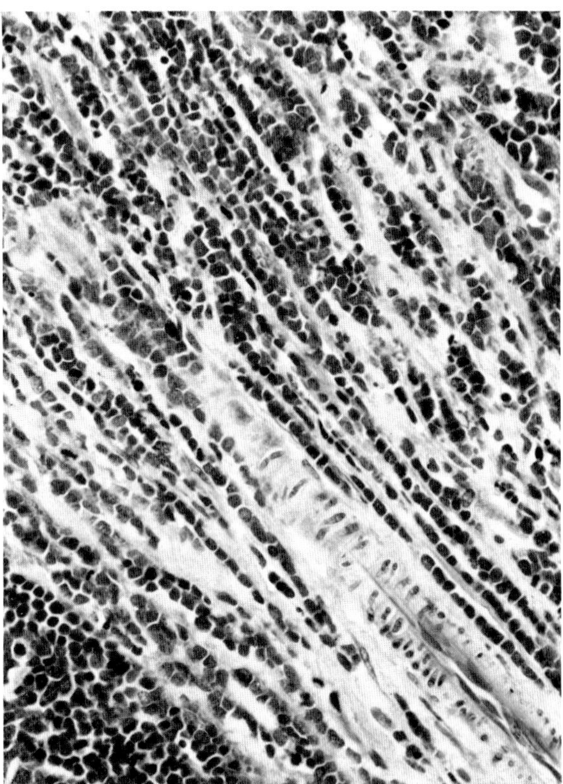

Fig. 11.16 Another case of T-lymphoblastic lymphoma showing characteristic pattern of infiltration of a lymph node trabecula (note central arteriole). Parallel arrays of neoplastic cells lie between the collagen bundles of the trabecula. (H E × 300)

scanty, moderately basophilic and pyroninophilic cytoplasm. The nuclear chromatin is finely dispersed, which at once distinguishes the cells from lymphocytes, and the generally solitary nucleolus is small and inconspicuous. In conventional paraffin sections, 'convoluted' nuclei may be recognised by the 'chicken foot imprint' pattern of darker streaks traversing the nucleus (Lukes & Collins, 1975). In thin paraffin sections and, more particularly in semi-thin (1–2 μm) sections of resin-embedded tissue, the irregular, 'convoluted' outline of the nuclei is generally more obvious (Fig. 11.18). This feature is, however, quite variable and is sometimes seen only in a minority of cells and it may even be absent, the nuclei appearing round or oval with few indentations (Nathwani et al, 1976). Perhaps the most distinctive cytological feature, which is found in the majority of T-lymphoblastic lymphomas, is the presence of a sharply defined focus of acid phosphatase (or acid esterase) activity in the Golgi zone (Lennert et al, 1975). This cannot usually be demonstrated in frozen sections and is best shown in imprint preparations or cytocentrifuge preparations from pleural effusions (Fig. 11.19). These should be allowed to dry and remain on the bench for 2 or 3 days without fixation before staining (Lennert, 1978, p 394–395). Paraffin sections stained with PAS sometimes show a PAS positive spot in the same Golgi region of each cell, but glycogen granules in the cytoplasm may cause confusion in imprints or frozen sections.

Prognosis. Even with 'aggressive' chemotherapy the prognosis of T-lymphoblastic lym-

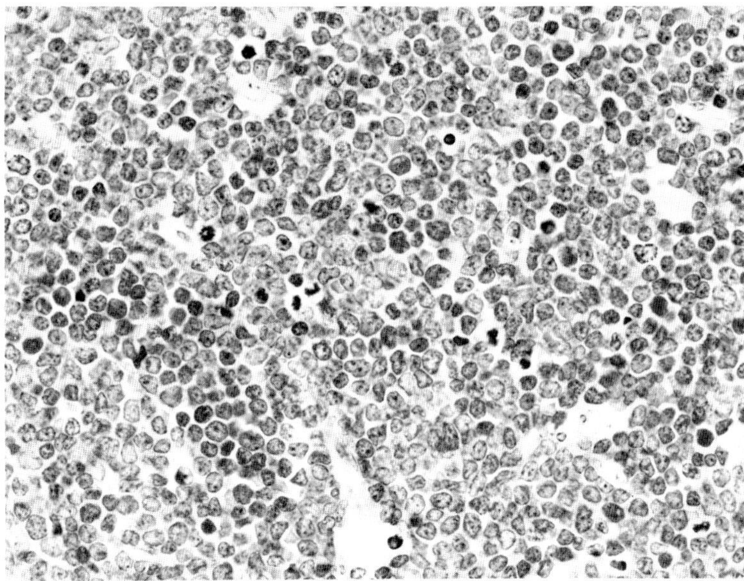

Fig. 11.17 Lymph node biopsy from a young adult showing typical features of T-lymphoblastic lymphoma. The cells are closely packed but not cohesive and they are smaller in size than the cells of Burkitt's lymphoma (see Fig. 11.11). Note the convoluted outline of many of the nuclei, the fine chromatin structure and inconspicuous nucleoli. Mitoses are numerous. (Giemsa × 470)

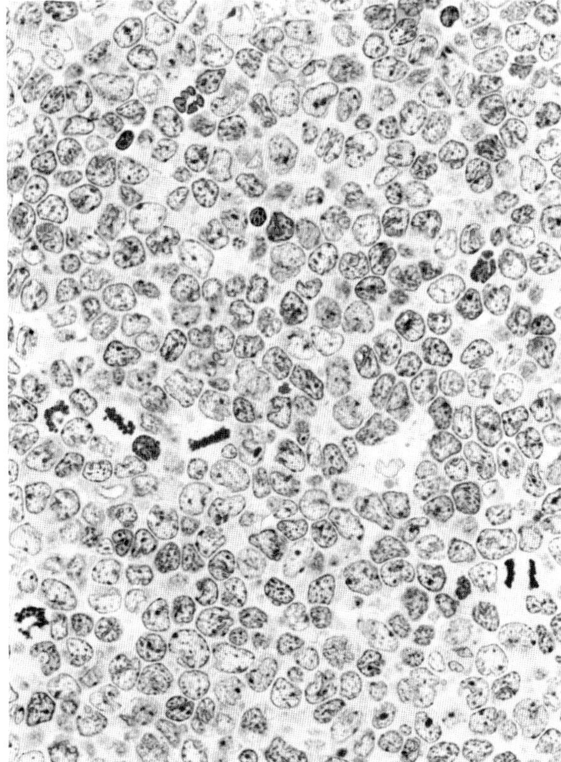

Fig. 11.18 T-lymphoblastic lymphoma (same case as Fig. 11.15), high power view to show details of nuclei. Note many mitoses. Resin embedding. (H E × 590)

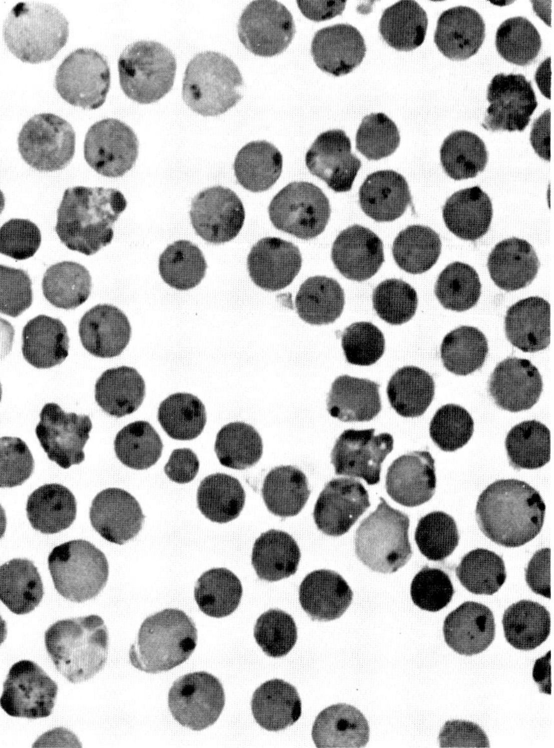

Fig. 11.19 Cytocentrifuge preparation of pleural fluid, from the same case as Figs 11.15 and 11.18, stained to show focal acid phosphatase activity (black dots in illustration) (Gomori's acid phosphatase × 940)

phoma remains very grave. The mediastinal masses and lymph nodes generally melt away rapidly with radiotherapy and/or chemotherapy necessitating the administration of allopurinol to prevent renal complications. However, relapse of the disease is the rule and there are few long term survivors in this type of lymphoma.

Differential diagnosis. In typical cases there is little likelihood of confusion of T-lymphoblastic lymphoma with other malignant lymphomas. The age of the subject, the presence of a mediastinal shadow on chest X-ray and the rapid growth of the tumour generally suggest the diagnosis before biopsy is undertaken. In the absence of such suggestive clinical evidence, it is possible to misinterpret the biopsy findings and to confuse the rather small 'convoluted' cells with 'cleaved' follicular centre cells (centrocytes) and thus arrive at an erroneous diagnosis of centrocytic lymphoma. With good quality sections and an adequate biopsy, this should rarely happen. The mitotic rate is generally much higher in the T-lymphoblastic lymphomas than in centrocytic lymphomas.

ML Lymphoblastic — Unclassified

There is a group of high-grade malignant lymphomas of lymphoblastic type which may present with lymphadenopathy, but in which the cells fail to mark either as T or B cells. Morphologically these neoplasms differ in certain respects from both the B and T lymphoblastic lymphomas, the cell characteristics often lying somewhere in between those of these two types. Some of these cases may be said to represent a 'tissue phase' of common acute lymphoblastic leukaemia (ALL), for the cells display the common ALL antigen and react with specific antibodies for this (e.g. J5). Furthermore, lymphadenopathy sometimes appears in the course of common ALL and may be the first sign of relapse in a patient who had gone into remission following treatment of the leukaemia. Tissue relapse in common ALL also occurs in other sites, like the testis or CNS, and sometimes the primary presentation is with a testicular or other extranodal tumour. Interestingly, a lymphoblastic lymphoma and/or leukaemia in which the cells exhibit the common ALL antigen may occur as a sequel of chronic myeloid leukaemia (see Ch. 13).

Not all unclassified lymphoblastic lymphomas are leukaemic, however, some presenting as a purely localised tumour, without ever developing signs of leukaemia and others showing only a limited 'spill-over' of neoplastic cells into the blood stream. When cases which are unclassifiable for technical reasons are included, it is apparent that this is a heterogeneous group and not a single, well defined entity. For this reason it is not possible to give a comprehensive description which is applicable to all cases of unclassified lymphoblastic lymphoma.

As might be expected, the *age incidence* overall shows a predominance of young patients, although there is quite a wide scatter in this regard. Most cases are found under the age of 50. The *presentation* varies as indicated above. Some patients present with lymphadenopathy, others with extranodal masses in the skin, gastrointestinal tract or elsewhere.

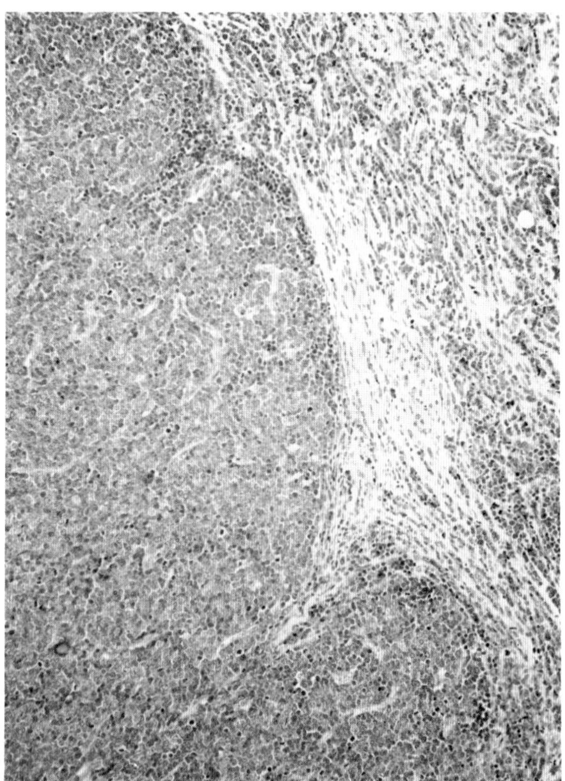

Fig. 11.20 Lymph node biopsy from a man of 22 with acute lymphoblastic leukaemia showing diffuse infiltration by lymphoblastic lymphoma with capsular and extracapsular spread. A starry sky pattern is not seen. (H E × 120)

Histology. In cases with a nodal presentation, the affected lymph nodes are generally widely infiltrated and often totally replaced by cells which are appreciably larger than any residual lymphocytes and have larger, more palely staining nuclei than the latter (Fig. 11.20). In common ALL, the lymphoblasts in tissue sections are similar in size to, or slightly smaller than, the cells of T-lymphoblastic lymphoma. In some other cases, however, the cells are definitely larger and approach the diameter of B-lymphoblasts. Although closely packed, the cells are not cohesive like those of Burkitt's lymphoma and a 'starry sky' pattern is seldom seen (Fig. 11.21). The nuclei generally show a fine chromatin structure and often one or several, small nucleoli. Mitoses are frequent (Fig. 11.22). The scanty cytoplasm is moderately basophilic and, in imprint preparations, glycogen may be demonstrated in the cytoplasm with PAS staining.

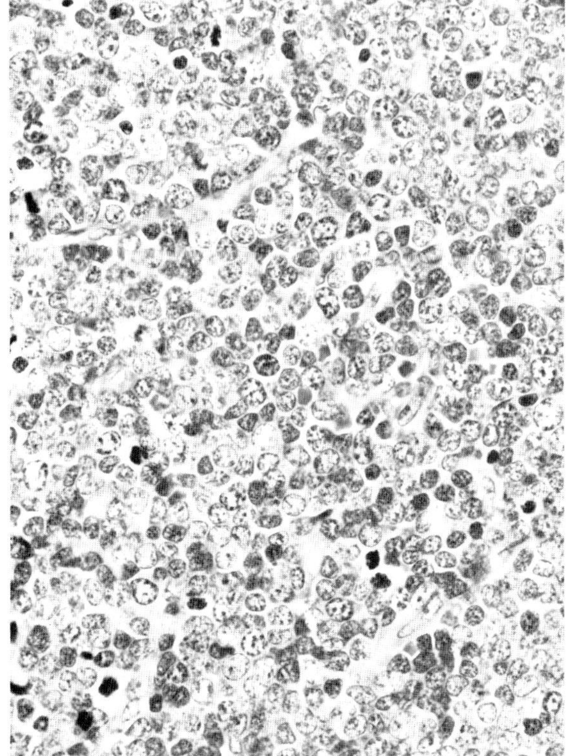

Fig. 11.21 Higher power view of same node as Fig. 11.20 to show details of cells. The nuclear characteristics are intermediate between those of B-lymphoblastic lymphoma and those of T-lymphoblastic lymphoma. (H E × 470)

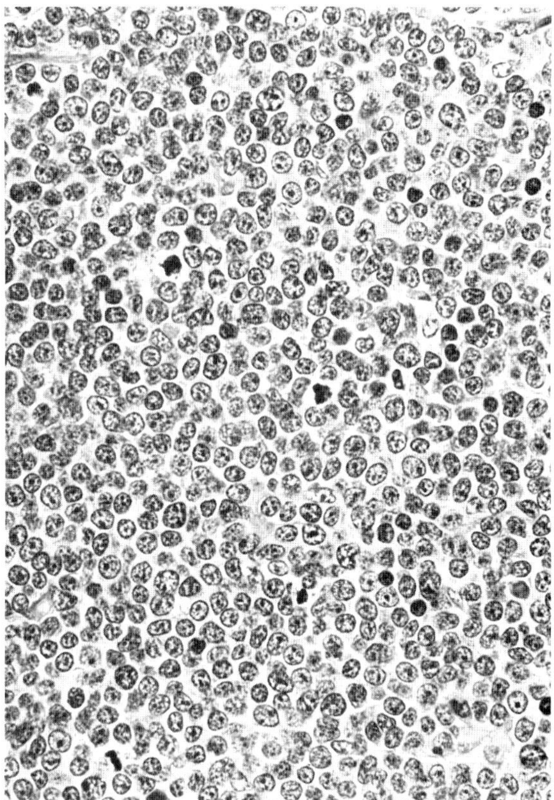

Fig. 11.22 Another case of lymphoblastic lymphoma of unclassified type in a man of 49, who developed acute lymphoblastic leukaemia (H E × 470)

In cases where ALL supervenes in chronic myeloid leukaemia (CML), the lymph nodes may show a confusing picture, with residual collections of myeloid leucocytes and megakaryocytes, especially towards the periphery of the node whilst the more central parts are infiltrated by lymphoblasts. The distinction of this 'lymphoid blast crisis' from a myeloblastic 'blast crisis' in CML cannot be reliably made on histological criteria and is dependent on the cytological characteristics of the transformed cells (see p. 339).

In leukaemic cases, a remarkably intimate infiltration of the tissues may be seen. In lymph nodes every crevice is filled with cells and there is often diffuse expansion and infiltration of capsule and trabeculae as in other types of acute leukaemia. In extranodal sites like the skin or ovary, where there is dense connective tissue, and occasionally also in lymph nodes, the infiltrating neoplastic cells lie in regular rows ('Indian file' formation) and the gyriform pattern so produced has been likened to watered silk (Fig. 11.23).

Prognosis. The general outlook for children with ALL of the 'common' type has improved markedly with the introduction of aggressive chemotherapy, combined with CNS prophylaxis and a close watch for relapse in sequestered sites, such as the testis in boys. In older patients, whether leukaemic or non-leukaemic, the prognosis is much worse.

Differential diagnosis. The picture has first to be distinguished from those of B-lymphoblastic and T-lymphoblastic lymphomas and this may be difficult, especially with thick or poor quality sections. Indeed it is certain that some unclassified lymphoblastic lymphomas would be reclassified as B- or T- if a better biopsy or ancillary data were available. Present evidence suggests that some, at least, of the 'null' lymphoblastic neoplasms are derived from 'pre-B' cells (Brouet et al, 1979).

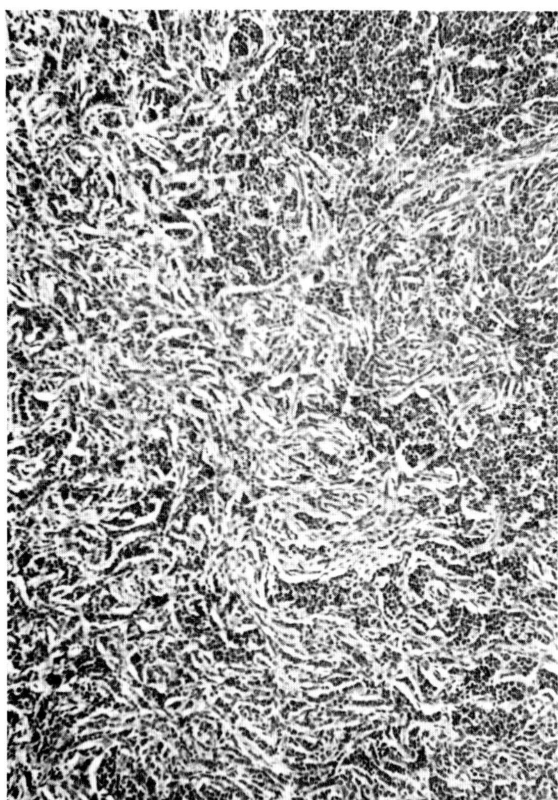

Fig. 11.23 Part of same lymph node as Figs 11.20 and 11.21 showing gyriform patterns of infiltration, sometimes seen in lymphoblastic lymphomas, especially in childhood (H E × 120)

In every case, it is a useful rule to perform the chloroacetate esterase stain (p. 35) to exclude, as far as possible, a diagnosis of myeloblastic sarcoma/leukaemia. If this is done routinely on all unclassified lymphoblastic lymphomas, the possibility of a myeloblastic neoplasm will not be overlooked, as it may otherwise be (see p. 339). The presence of scattered eosinophil myelocytes in the tumour may arouse suspicion of the latter, but they are not invariably present. Equally a negative result with the chloroacetate stain does not totally exclude a myeloblastic tumour. Cytological and cytochemical studies are generally a more reliable guide than histology.

The benign, self-limiting proliferation of lymphoid cells which takes place in infectious mononucleosis may be mistaken for a lymphoblastic lymphoma by the unwary (see p. 132). This mistake should not be made if the node (or tonsil) is examined carefully, for despite the widespread blastic transformation of lymphoid cells and mitotic activity, it is not a homogeneous cell population and many of the cells show unmistakeable signs of plasmacytoid differentiation.

Finally, malignant neoplasms of other types may sometimes be mistaken for lymphoblastic lymphomas. In children, such tumours include some small-celled rhabdomyosarcomas, neuroblastomas and Ewing's sarcoma. The large content of glycogen in the cells, revealed by PAS staining, generally serves to distinguish the last and there is often much glycogen too in the rhabdomyosarcomas. The vascular pattern, shown up by reticulin stains, is distinctive in neuroblastomas. Occasionally a small cell carcinoma of the bronchus may be mistaken for a lymphoblastic lymphoma (see Ch. 15). Such problems seldom arise if the biopsy is adequate and good sections are available.

ML IMMUNOBLASTIC (ML Ib)

Synonyms:
Histiocytic lymphoma, diffuse (some examples).
Undifferentiated diffuse lymphoma, large cell.
Reticulum cell sarcoma (old terminology).

This is a comparatively common group of high

grade malignant lymphomas in which the relatively large neoplastic cells generally mark as B-cells, infrequently as T-cells and sometimes as null cells. The B and T types cannot always be reliably distinguished morphologically, although the presence of obvious plasmacytoid or plasmablastic differentiation clearly points to a B-cell neoplasm. Since there is now evidence that many of the null cell tumours of this type are in fact of B-cell origin, these tumours will not be described separately and this account will deal only with the B-cell type of immunoblastic lymphoma. The T-cell type will be dealt with in the next chapter (p. 312).

ML Immunoblastic — B-type (ML Ib-B)

Synonyms:
Immunoblastic sarcoma (Lennert).
Immunoblastic sarcoma (Lukes & Collins).

The term 'immunoblastic sarcoma' is used both by Lennert and by Lukes & Collins, but in a slightly different sense by each. The Lukes & Collins' definition is narrower and includes only those neoplasms which show distinct plasmacytoid or plasmablastic features. Lennert's definition includes these cases, but also includes cases in which the neoplastic cells resemble immunoblasts, but do not show any features of plasma cells. Since the latter concept is that adopted in the Kiel classification, we shall adhere to it in this account.

Incidence and presentation

This is the commonest type of high grade, large cell, malignant lymphoma. It occurs most frequently in adults, with a peak incidence over the age of 50, although there is a wide age range and it is occasionally found in children. It is slightly commoner in males, but the sex difference is not great.

ML Ib-B may present *de novo* or as a result of transformation of a pre-existing, low grade, B-cell lymphoma — usually ML Cb-Cc, and less often a lymphoplasmacytoid lymphoma or even a lymphocytic lymphoma (B-CLL) (Richter's syndrome). In either event, these tumours most often occur as lymph node swellings, and these may crop up in almost any site. The existence of a previous, low grade neoplasm may or may not have been known, when the rapid enlargement of nodes in a single site draws attention to this tumour.

Extranodal tumours also occur in ML Ib-B and not only in sites such as Waldeyer's ring, spleen and gastrointestinal tract, but also in sites determined by the prior existence of an auto-immune lymphoid proliferation, for example, in the thyroid in association with Hashimoto's thyroiditis or in salivary glands in Sjögren's syndrome. In fact, B-immunoblastic lymphoma is much the most common type of malignant lymphoma to arise in immunodefective states (Lukes & Collins, 1974) and especially those which are acquired or result from immunosuppression (see p. 239). Most of the malignant lymphomas reported to have arisen in patients receiving immunosuppressive therapy following an organ transplantation appear to have been of this class. B-immunoblastic lymphomas of the gut arising in patients with α-chain disease may be cited as another example and perhaps the occasional occurrence of this same type of neoplasm in patients with Hodgkin's disease (see p. 219). High grade malignant lymphomas developing in patients with immunoblastic lymphadenopathy may also be of this type although few reported cases have been convincingly shown to be of B-cell origin.

A leukaemic presentation or the development of leukaemia in the course of the disease are both rare.

Lymph node changes

Macroscopic. There are no specific macroscopic features, but generally these fast growing tumours are soft and bulge out over the cut edge of the capsule when incised fresh. Foci of necrosis may be present and sometimes the entire node is necrotic.

Histology. The lymph node removed for biopsy is generally massively, if not totally, replaced by the large, palely staining cells of the neoplasm. The pattern of growth is diffuse, except in those instances where the tumour has arisen by transformation of a previous centroblastic-centrocytic lymphoma and where remnants of a follicular pattern persist in some parts (Fig. 11.24). It should be noted that when blast-cell transformation occurs in B-CLL (Richter, 1928), the resultant tu-

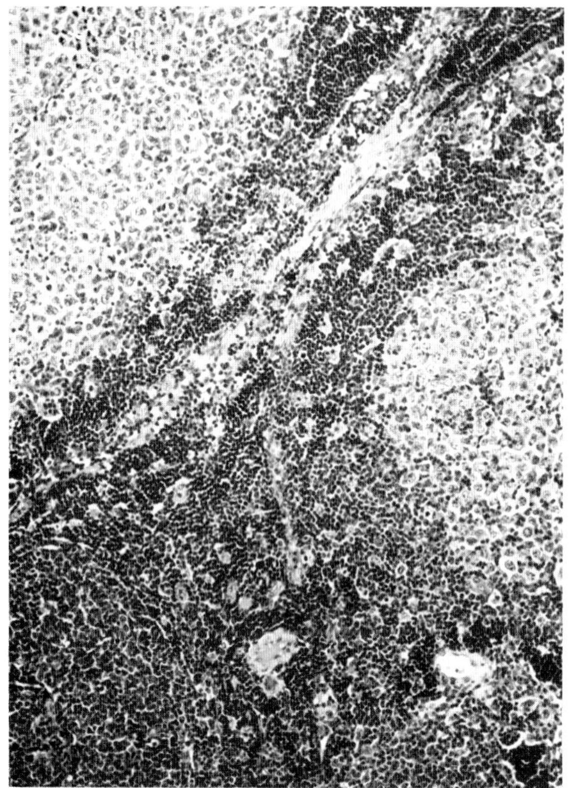

Fig. 11.24 Lymph node biopsy showing transformation of ML centroblastic-centrocytic, follicular (lower field) into ML immunoblastic. Two of the neoplastic follicles shown are overrun by immunoblastic lymphoma. (H E × 120)

Fig. 11.25 Diffuse malignant lymphoma of B-immunoblastic type which had resulted from transformation of ML Cb-Cc, follicular. A few of the blast cells resemble centroblasts, although most have the large, central nucleoli characteristic of immunoblasts. (Compare with Fig. 11.28 (H E × 470)

mour is morphologically an immunoblastic lymphoma, not a lymphoblastic lymphoma (see p. 236).

The cells in B-immunoblastic lymphomas are generally distinguishable from centroblasts in being larger, having rather more cytoplasm and showing a very large, prominent and often central nucleolus, in contradistinction to the multiple, smaller and generally peripheral nucleoli of the centroblast (Fig. 11.25). Having said that, however, it must be admitted that B-immunoblastic lymphomas, as a group, show much individual variation. The tumour may be strictly monomorphic, with every cell looking alike, or extremely pleomorphic, with many tumour giant-cells, often of bizarre configuration. The average cell size is equally variable, even in a single case, ranging from quite a small blast-type cell, little bigger than the B-lymphoblast of the Burkitt lymphoma, to cells of nearly twice that size (Fig. 11.26). The amount of cytoplasm varies with the size of the cells and although, in general, neoplastic immunoblasts are distinguishable by their greater volume of cytoplasm, this is not an invariable characteristic, furthermore the volume of cytoplasm may change in the course of the disease (Fig. 11.27). It needs to be remembered that the cell diameter, and especially that of the nucleus, may be exaggerated by poor fixation.

The blast cell nuclei are sometimes round, but are often irregular in shape, although gross irregularities and multilobed nuclei are more characteristic of some T-immunoblastic lymphomas (Fig. 11.28). The nucleus is classically described as 'vesicular' and indeed it often appears so through faulty fixation. The pale nuclear staining throws into relief the prominent nucleolus which may lie at the centre of the nucleus or extend from

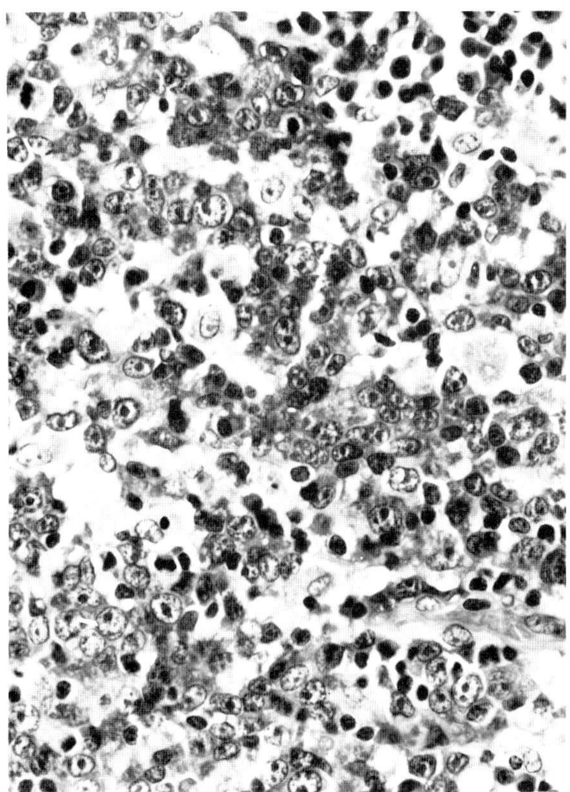

Fig. 11.26 Diffuse B-immunoblastic lymphoma in a man of 68 with a previous lymphoplasmacytoid lymphoma (Waldenström's disease). The neoplastic immunoblasts show marked variation in size. Note the presence of residual plasma cells. (H E × 470)

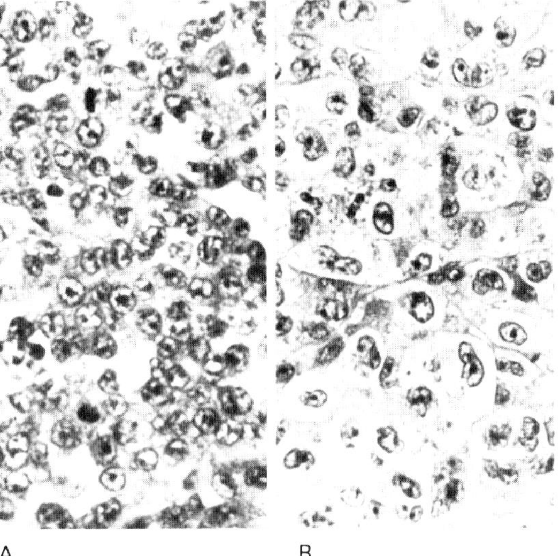

A B

Fig. 11.27 (a) and (b) (a) B-immunoblastic lymphoma of the terminal ileum in a boy of 13. The cells have large nuclei and scanty cytoplasm. (b) Recurrence of the tumour in the skin of the abdominal wall, 9 months later. The cells are larger and have voluminous cytoplasm. (Both H E × 600)

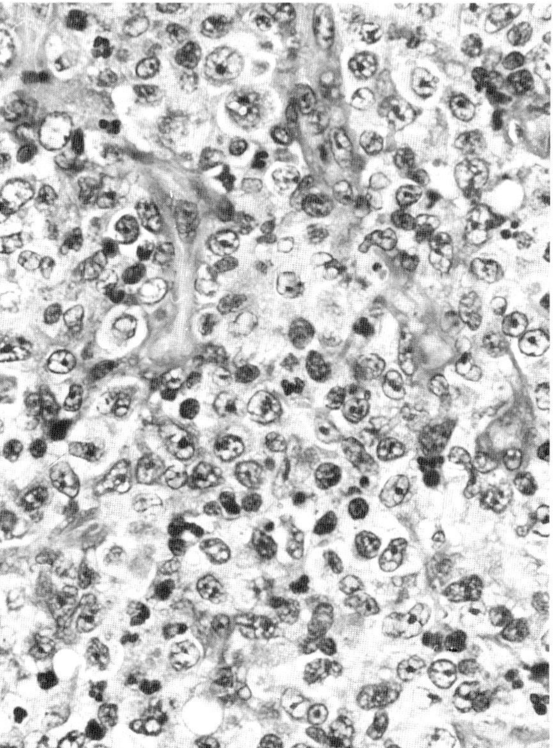

Fig. 11.28 T-immunoblastic lymphoma in a lymph node for comparison with B-immunoblastic lymphoma. The cells are very variable, often showing irregular nuclei and abundant, pale-staining cytoplasm. Note prominent venules. (Compare with Fig. 11.25) (H E × 470)

the nuclear membrane to the centre. This nucleolus is the most distinctive feature of the cells of this tumour. Not infrequently the nuclear membrane appears heavily outlined due to a peripheral condensation of chromatin and the nucleus may then bear an obvious resemblance to that of a plasmablast with its prominent central nucleolus (Figs 11.25, 11.26). The cytoplasm too, frequently shows evidence of plasmacytoid differentiation often staining strongly, even in an HE stained section, whilst it is strongly pyroninophilic when stained with methyl green-pyronin. Giemsa staining may show up not only the violet staining cytoplasm, but also a pale perinuclear *hof*, typical of a plasma cell. In a proportion of the cells the nucleus may be relatively smaller in size and eccentrically placed, even further emphasising the plasmacytoid characteristics of the tumour.

The degree of plasmacytoid or plasmablastic differentiation varies considerably, even in immunoblastic lymphomas of proven B-cell origin. At one end of the spectrum, there are uncommon tumours in which every cell bears such a striking resemblance to a plasmablast that it is justifiable to apply the term plasmablastic lymphoma (Figs 11.29, 11.30). At the opposite end, no evidence of such differentiation may be found and the cytoplasm, whilst moderately pyroninophilic, stains palely with H & E. The cytoplasmic staining is reflected in the ultrastructural features of the cell, those cells showing obvious plasmacytoid features having abundant rough endoplasmic reticulum (RER), whilst those without plasmacytoid features show many polyribosomes but little RER. Occasional tumours of this type show intracellular immunoglobulin, revealed as diastase-resistant, PAS-positive blocks or globules in the cytoplasm and sometimes there is a paraprotein of the same immunoglobulin class in the serum. It is important

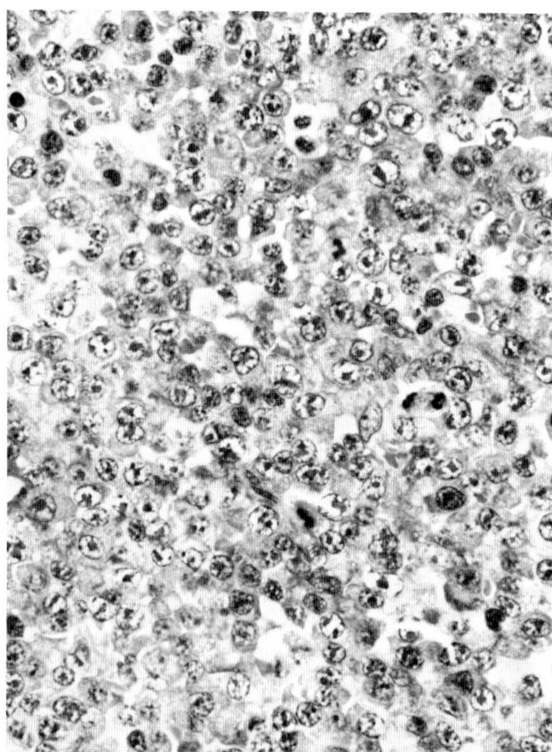

Fig. 11.29 Cervical lymph node biopsy from a woman of 65 showing B-immunoblastic lymphoma with plasmablastic features (H E × 470)

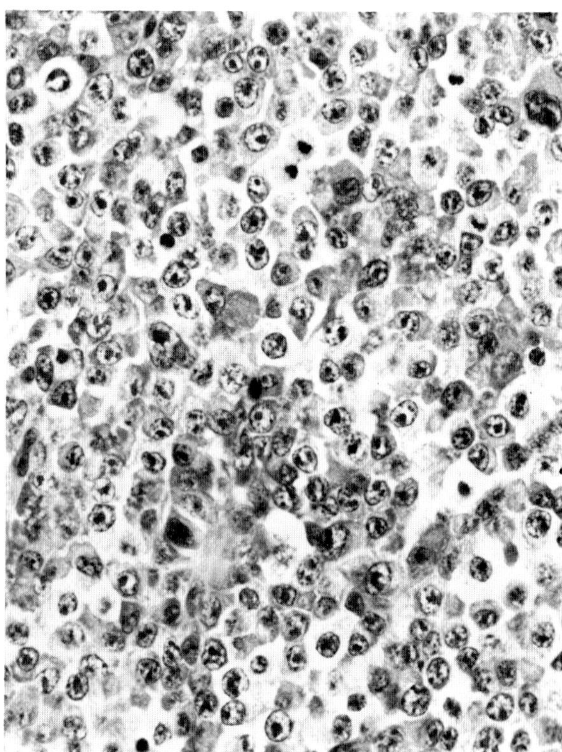

Fig. 11.30 Same node as Fig. 11.29. The plasmacytoid features are more apparent where there is some dissociation of the cells. (H E × 470)

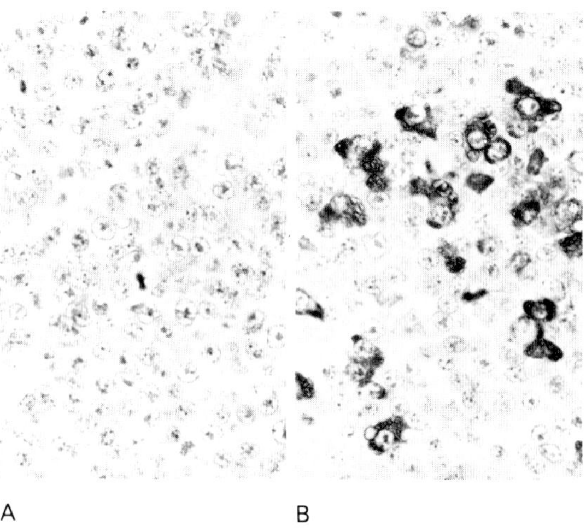

Fig. 11.31 (a) and (b) Same node as Figs 11.29 and 11.30 stained by the PAP method. (a) is negative for κ light chains, whilst (b) shows many cells staining positively for λ light chains. A similar result was obtained with antiserum to IgM. (Both PAP method × 470)

not to mistake PAS positive granules in macrophages for immunoglobulin deposits. Cytoplasmic immunoglobulin with class restricted light chains may also be demonstrated by the PAP method (Fig. 11.31).

B-immunoblastic lymphomas usually show a high mitotic rate and atypical mitoses are often seen, especially in the pleomorphic tumours containing many polyploid cells. Spontaneous necrosis is also a common feature, sometimes involving large areas of the tumour, but frequently occurring as individual cell necrosis throughout the tumour, when it is accompanied by a heavy infiltration of macrophages (Fig. 11.32). Macrophages are always abundant, but in the circumstances just described, they may be exceedingly numerous and active, sometimes outnumbering the tumour cells (Fig. 11.33). In such cases, it is important not to mistake the tumour for a histiocytic neoplasm. Epithelioid cells are not infrequently found, usually in the form of small clusters dispersed amongst the neoplastic cells rather than as larger granulomas. Where extensive necrosis has occurred collections of foamy macrophages may be found.

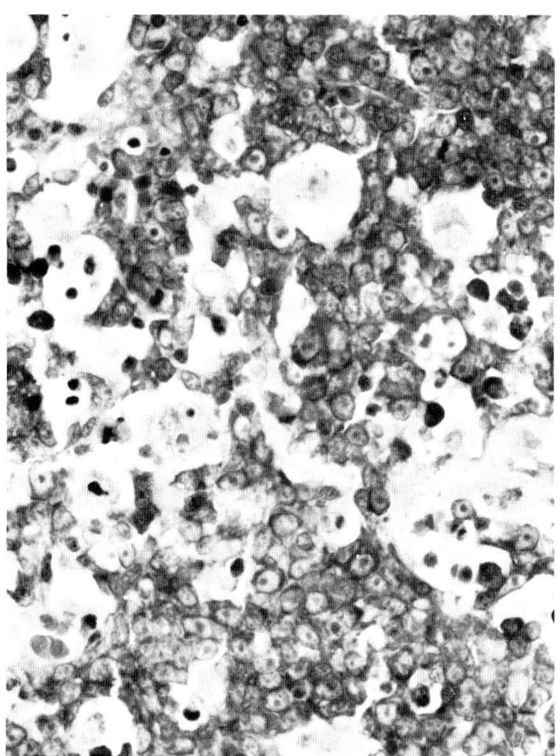

Fig. 11.32 B-immunoblastic lymphoma showing numerous macrophages containing nuclear debris. Note basophilia of the cytoplasm in the neoplastic cells. (Same case as Fig. 11.26.) (Giemsa × 470)

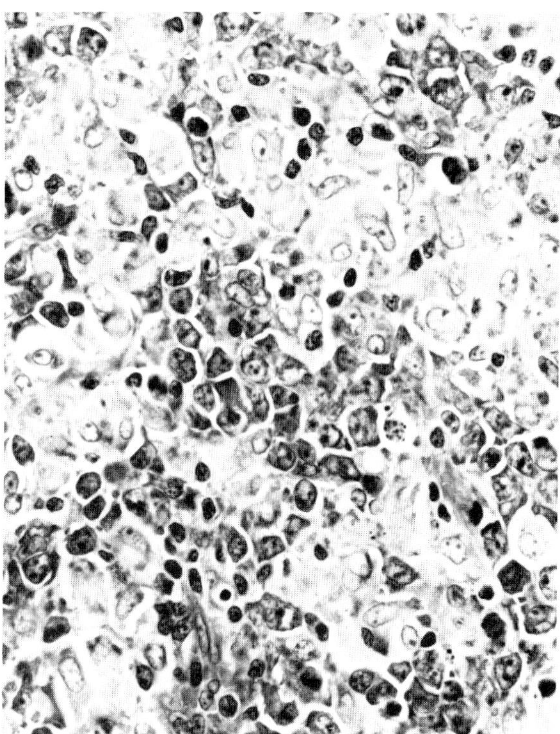

Fig. 11.33 Another case of B-immunoblastic lymphoma in which the neoplastic cells are almost outnumbered by large, active-appearing macrophages (Giemsa × 470)

On other occasions there may be a considerable admixture of inflammatory cells in tumours of this type. Neutrophils generally occur only in the presence of necrosis, but eosinophils are sometimes abundant, which may cause confusion with Hodgkin's disease. Reactive plasma cells of polyclonal type are often present in small numbers and may of course be numerous in extranodal tumours occurring in association with autoimmune disorders.

In contrast with centroblastic-centrocytic lymphomas and large celled centrocytic lymphomas, these tumours are seldom associated with significant fibrosis and silver staining often shows a marked reduction of reticulin fibres within the tumour. A characteristic coarse network of argyrophil fibres may be found in the plasmablastic variant, as in other plasma cell tumours (Fig. 11.34).

Prognosis. The prognosis of ML Ib-B is considerably worse than it is today with either centroblastic or large-cell centrocytic lymphomas (Strauchen et al, 1978). The outlook is better than it is with T-lymphoblastic lymphoma and is probably marginally better also than in T-immunoblastic lymphoma. There does appear, however, to be much variation in the response to treatment in the B-immunoblastic lymphomas.

Differential diagnosis. B-immunoblastic lymphoma cannot be reliably distinguished from T-immunoblastic lymphoma on morphology alone (Jaffe et al, 1982). Points of distinction are discussed in the next chapter. In addition, ML Ib-B may be confused at times with other large-cell malignant lymphomas — ML centroblastic (p. 278) and ML centrocytic, large-cell type (p. 258). The distinction between the polymorphic sub-type of centroblastic lymphoma and B-immunoblastic lymphoma is not sharp and awaits clarification from further studies on such tumours. The large-celled centrocytic lymphoma is only likely to be mistaken for B-immunoblastic lymphoma if poor fixation has caused 'ballooning' of the nuclei. However, the small size of the nucleoli in the former should suggest that these are not blast cells and this is confirmed by the weak staining of the cytoplasm with Giemsa or MGP.

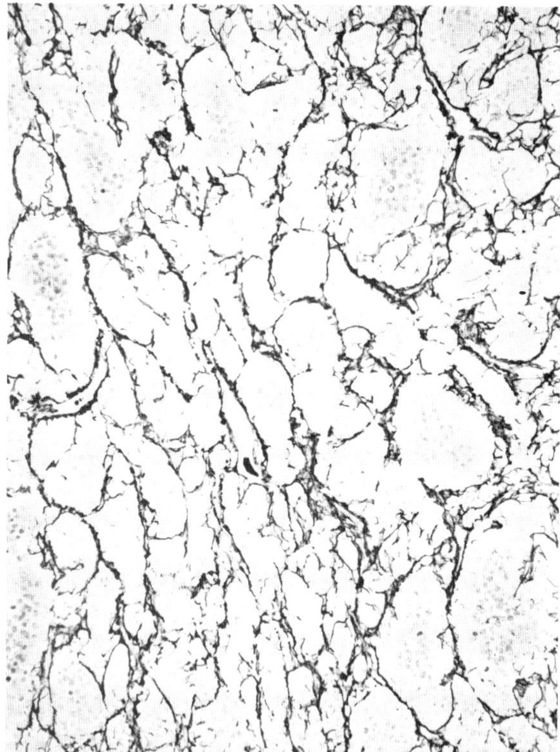

Fig. 11.34 Characteristic reticulin pattern in plasmablastic lymphoma (compare with Fig. 10.33, p. 250). (Same case as Figs 11.29 — 11.31.) (Gordon and Sweets reticulin × 120)

In the polymorphic sub-type of ML lymphoplasmacytoid, there may be sufficient immunoblasts present to cause confusion with ML immunoblastic, but the mixed population of B-cells present in the former generally serves to make the distinction. (It should be remembered that one may transform into the other.)

There may occasionally be difficulty in deciding between a B-lymphoblastic and a B-immunoblastic lymphoma and the boundary between these two is probably not quite as sharp as might be supposed.

True histiocytic tumours may pose a problem where these tumours are poorly differentiated and the cells possess prominent nucleoli (see p. 376). Myeloblastic sarcoma can usually be separated by the result of a chloroacetate esterase stain (p. 333). The distinction between pleomorphic B-immunoblastic lymphoma and Hodgkin's disease of reticular type (Hodgkin's sarcoma) may be difficult and may sometimes be a matter of semantics (p. 216). Finally, there may sometimes be difficulty in distinguishing immunoblastic lymphoma from undifferentiated malignant tumours of other types, especially nasopharyngeal or tonsillar carcinoma (lymphoepithelioma), amelanotic melanoma, and the recently described Merkel cell tumour (see Ch. 15). In doubtful cases, reticulin staining often helps to resolve the problem; in carcinoma the reticulin fibres are characteristically pushed aside, whilst in malignant lymphomas the reticulin framework is often expanded, but individual fibres are less displaced. Most, if not all, of the tumours of the thyroid formerly regarded as small-celled undifferentiated carcinomas are, in fact, malignant lymphomas (Heimann et al, 1978). Many diagnostic problems are caused by inadequate biopsies, poor fixation, or thick sections.

REFERENCES

Barcos M P, Lukes R J 1975 Malignant lymphoma of convoluted lymphocytes: a new entity of possible T-cell type. In: Sinks L F, Godden J O (eds) Conflicts in Childhood Cancer. An Evaluation of Current Management. Liss, New York, Volume 4, p 147–178

Berard C, O'Conor G T, Thomas L B, Torloni H et al 1969 Histopathological definition of Burkitt's tumour. Bulletin of the World Health Organization 40: 601–607

Brouet J C, Preud'Homme J L, Penit C, Valensi F, Rouget P, Seligmann M 1979 Acute lymphoblastic leukemia with pre-B-cell characteristics. Blood 54: 269–273

Burkitt D 1958 A sarcoma involving the jaws in African children. British Journal of Surgery 46: 218–233

Burkitt D P, Kyalwazi S K 1967 Spontaneous remission of African lymphoma. British Journal of Cancer 21: 14–16

Collins R D, Waldron J A, Glick A D 1979 Results of multiparameter studies of T-cell lymphoid neoplasms. American Journal of Clinical Pathology 72: 699–707

Cullen M H, Lister T A, Brearley R L, Shand W S, Stansfeld A G 1979 Histological transformation of non-Hodgkin's lymphoma — a prospective study. Cancer 44: 645–651

Epstein M A, Achong B G, Barr Y M 1964 Virus particles in cultured lymphoblasts from Burkitt's lymphoma. Lancet 1: 702–703

Habeshaw J A, Catley P F, Stansfeld A G, Brearley R L 1979 Surface phenotyping, histology and the nature of non-Hodgkin lymphoma in 157 patients. British Journal of Cancer 40: 11–34

Heimann R, Vanninheuse A, DeSloover C, Dor P 1978 Malignant lymphomas and undifferentiated small cell carcinoma of the thyroid: a clinicopathological review in the light of the Kiel classification for malignant lymphomas. Histopathology 2: 201–213

Henle W, Henle G, Diehl V 1968 Relation of Burkitt's tumor-associated herpes-type virus to infectious mononucleosis. Proceedings of the National Academy of Sciences of the United States of America (Washington) 59: 94–101

Jaffe E S, Strauchen J A, Berard C W 1982 Predictability of immunologic phenotype by morphologic criteria in diffuse aggressive non-Hodgkin's lymphomas. American Journal of Clinical Pathology 77: 46–49

Lennert K, in collaboration with Mohri N, Stein H, Kaiserling E, Müller-Hermelink H K 1978 Malignant Lymphomas other than Hodgkin's Disease. Springer-Verlag, Berlin

Lennert K 1981 Histopathology of non-Hodgkin's lymphomas. Springer-Verlag, Berlin

Lennert K, Stein H, Kaiserling E 1975 Cytological and functional criteria for the classification of malignant lymphomata. British Journal of Cancer 31: Supplement II, 29–43

Levine P H, Cho B R, Connelly R R, Berard C W, O'Conor G T, Dorfman R F, Easton J M, De Vita V T 1975 The American Burkitt lymphoma registry: a progress report. Annals of Internal Medicine 83: 31–36

Levine P H, Kamaraju L S, Connelly R R, Berard C W, Dorfman R F, Magrath I, Easton J M 1982 The American Burkitt lymphoma registry: eight years experience. Cancer 49: 1016–1022

Lukes R J, Collins R D 1973 New observations on follicular lymphoma. In: Akazaki K, Rappaport H, Berard C W, Bennett J M, Ishikawa E (eds) Malignant Diseases of the Hematopoietic System. GANN monograph on Cancer Research. University of Tokyo Press, Tokyo, Vol 15, p 209–215

Lukes R J, Collins R D 1974 Immunologic characterization of human malignant lymphomas. Cancer 34: 1488–1503

Lukes R J, Collins R D 1975 New approaches to the classification of the lymphomata. British Journal of Cancer 31: Supplement II, 1–28

Magrath I T 1974 Burkitt's lymphoma: a B or T cell tumour? European Journal of Cancer 10: 83–88

Minowada J, Klein G, Clifford P, Klein E, Moore G E 1967 Studies of Burkitt lymphoma cells. I Establishment of a cell line (B35M) and its characteristics. Cancer 20: 1430–1437

Nathwani B N, Kim H, Rappaport H 1976 Malignant lymphoma, lymphoblastic. Cancer 38: 964–983

Rappaport H 1966 Tumors of the Hematopoietic System. Atlas of Tumor Pathology, Section 3, Fascicle 8. Armed Forces Institute of Pathology, Washington DC

Richter M N 1928 Generalized reticular cell sarcoma of lymph nodes associated with lymphatic leukemia. American Journal of Pathology 4: 285–299

Stein H, Petersen N, Gaedicke G, Lennert K, Landbeck G 1976 Lymphoblastic lymphoma of convoluted or acid phosphatase type — a tumour of T precursor cells. International Journal of Cancer 17: 292–295

Stein H, Tolksdorf G 1977 Unpublished data, cited in: Lennert K (ed) Malignant lymphomas other than Hodgkin's disease. 1978 Springer-Verlag, Berlin, part 6, p 629

Stein H, Tolksdorf G, Lennert K 1980 T-cell neoplasia in the perspective of normal T-cell differentiation. In: van den Tweel J A (ed) Malignant lymphoproliferative diseases, Boerhaave Series, Leiden University Press, The Hague, ch 24, p 315–329

Sternberg C 1890 Über leukosarcomatose. Wiener Klinische Wochenschrift 21: 475–480

Strauchen J A, Young R C, De Vita V T et al 1978 Clinical relevance of the histopathologic subclassification of diffuse 'histiocytic' lymphoma. New England Journal of Medicine 299: 1382–1387

Wright D H 1970 In: Burkitt D P and Wright D H (eds) Burkitt's Lymphoma. Livingstone, Edinburgh, ch 8, (Gross distribution and haematology), p 64

12

A.G. Stansfeld

Peripheral T-cell lymphomas

INTRODUCTION

Malignant lymphomas of T-cell origin may be subdivided into two main categories, first, those derived from primitive precursors of the T lymphocyte — either prothymocytes (T_0) or thymocytes (T_1) and secondly, those derived from 'mature' (adult) T-cells — post-thymocytes or peripheral T-lymphocytes (T_2). Neoplasms in the first category are sometimes referred to as 'central' and these correspond to the T-lymphoblastic lymphomas, mainly encountered in childhood and adolescence, which have been described in the last chapter (p. 288). The common presenting feature of a mediastinal tumour is further supporting evidence of the thymic origin of these tumours. There is very little overlap between the central and peripheral T-cell lymphomas and the latter do not tend to involve the thymus, just as the former seldom involve the skin.

Problems of classification

The peripheral T-cell lymphomas and leukaemias are a heterogeneous group of neoplasms and they have proved much more difficult to classify than the more familiar B-cell neoplasms. The reasons for this are threefold:

1. T-cell neoplasms are much less frequent than B-cell neoplasms.
2. T-cell neoplasms are very varied and are sometimes prone to rapid changes in morphology. Moreover, apparently distinct categories may display overlapping features.
3. Fresh cells or tissue are required for the study of the surface markers of T-cells, so that retrospective marker studies of these tumours are impossible, unless stored frozen tissue is available.

In recent years it has become evident that the peripheral T-cell lymphomas are much more frequent in Japan than they are in the West (Table 12.1). The difference may not be quite as great as these figures suggest, for much of the excess of T-cell lymphomas in Japan can be ascribed to the frequency there of a single type (adult T-cell leukaemia/lymphoma). It is also likely that the frequency of some peripheral T-cell lymphomas has been underestimated in the West. Increasing awareness of the characteristics of these tumours is already bringing more cases to light.

Table 12.1 Relative incidence of different immunological types of non-Hodgkin's lymphomas in Japan and the West (Suchi et al, 1979)

Series	Number of cases	B	T	U
Japanese Lymphoma Study Group	110	49%	38.2%	12.7%
Tajima (Japan)	111	44.1%	31.5%	24.3%
Lukes (USA)	384	66.7%	15.4%	17.9%
Lennert (Germany)	1997	79.3%	6.1%	14.5%

[U = undefined]

Traditionally, classification of the malignant lymphomas has been based, first and foremost, upon the morphology of the tumour, as revealed by light microscopy. In recent years the introduction of tests more or less specific for T-cell markers has uncovered the inadequacies of a purely morphological approach. It is now clear that many T-cell neoplasms cannot be reliably distinguished from B-cell neoplasms by morphology alone. Moreover, what may be judged a single class of T-cell tumour on other criteria may show a variety of morphological expressions. Enzyme histochemistry, the demonstration of E-rosettes and immunostaining using monoclonal antibodies have helped not only to distinguish T-cells from B-cells, but also to define subsets of T-cells. These techniques have proved of great value in confirming the T-cell nature of neoplasms suspected as belonging to this group. Confusingly, however, neoplasms of a single morphological type do not invariably show the same phenotypic expression and *vice versa*. A further warning should be added here, that even a gross excess of T-cells in a suspension phenotype from a known malignant lymphoma does not necessarily imply that the lymphoma is a T-cell neoplasm, for there may be a minority population of monoclonal B-cells, which constitute the true neoplastic element (see p. 58, 61) and the excess of T-cells may represent a passing phase in the evolution of the lesion. Progress in this area is handicapped by the absence of a method of recognising clonality in T-lymphocytes.

Classification

Whilst recognising that ideas are likely to change within the next few years, a provisional classification of the peripheral T-cell lymphomas, based primarily on morphological criteria, is given in Table 12.2. Subdivision of these neoplasms into monomorphic and pleomorphic groups (Hanaoka et al, 1979; Watanabe et al, 1981), whilst theoretically sound, is not entirely satisfactory in practice. First, it is necessary to adhere to a strict definition of pleomorphic (lit. = 'many shaped') as being descriptive of the cell nuclei. The term is not correctly applied to variations in cell size — a pleomorphic T-cell lymphoma may be composed of cells of uniform size, if the nuclei are highly irregular in shape*. On the other hand, it has to be acknowledged that pleomorphism is a relative term. Close examination of the nuclei in many monomorphic peripheral T-cell lymphomas reveals them to be more irregular in outline than the nuclei of most B-cell lymphomas. There is thus no absolutely hard and fast line between the mono-

* Many Japanese authors apply the term pleomorphic only when the cells vary markedly in size as well as in shape.

Table 12.2 Provisional classification of peripheral T-cell lymphomas/leukaemias

	Nuclei more or less regular in shape or all showing the same type of irregularity (Monomorphic)		Nuclei very irregular and variable in shape (Pleomorphic)*
Cells mainly uniform in size	Small cell (lymphocytic)	Cutaneous types Mycosis fungoides Sézary's syndrome	
		Chronic lymphocytic leukaemia — T-types	Small cell (intermediate cell)
	Medium-sized cell including:	Prolymphocytic leukaemia, T-cell type	Medium-sized cell
		Monomorphic type with 'Centrocyte-like' cells	
	Large cell including:	'Pale cell' variant	Large cell
		T-immunoblastic lymphoma	
		'Multilobated' type	
Cells of varying sizes		T-zone lymphoma	Mixed — medium and large cell type
		'Immunoblastic lymphadenopathy-like' type (AIL type)	
		Lymphoepithelioid type (Lennert's lymphoma)	

* Probably includes all HTLV positive lymphomas/leukaemias, but not all pleomorphic cases are HTLV+

morphic and pleomorphic groups. In both monomorphic and pleomorphic groups there are some types composed predominantly of uniform sized cells and others in which the neoplastic cells show much variation in size. As with nuclear shape, the distinction of two classes is relative, not absolute. In the pleomorphic variety marked variation in cell size accentuates the pleomorphism of the tumour.

Some of the categories included in Table 12.2 are universally recognised and probably of world-wide distribution, although their incidence in many countries is unknown. This applies particularly to the cutaneous types — mycosis fungoides (MF) and Sézary's syndrome (SS). Some types are less well defined, either because of their rarity or because of their variability. It is this last characteristic which makes it extremely difficult to know just how many distinct categories of peripheral T-cell lymphoma there are, especially when so few cases are included in most published reports.

The peripheral T-cell neoplasms are not readily separable into low grade and high grade categories on the basis of the degree of transformation of the neoplastic cells, as is the case with the B-cell lymphomas (see Ch. 10). The very wide range of behaviour in these neoplasms does however correlate to a certain degree with cell size, uniformity and degree of transformation. Thus the small lymphocytic, cutaneous types (MF and SS) and some cases of T-cell chronic lymphocytic leukaemia (T-CLL) tend to be indolent in behaviour, whilst medium-sized and larger cell types of peripheral T-cell lymphoma generally have a grave prognosis and respond poorly to treatment. However, the 'multilobated' type described by Pinkus et al (1979) is said to have a better prognosis than most large cell lymphomas. The pleomorphic types tend to have a very poor prognosis, even in cases where the cells are predominantly small.

Despite the wide range of morphological appearances displayed by the peripheral T-cell lymphomas, there are certain clinical and pathological features common to different members of the group, which may lead the pathologist to suspect a T-cell origin when he is confronted by a malignant lymphoma (Table 12.3). It should be emphasised that none of the features in Table 12.3 is specific by itself and most of these may be encountered from time to time with B-cell tumours.

Table 12.3 Features suggesting T-cell origin in malignant lymphoma

Clinical presentation	Skin or lung involvement Hypercalcaemia
Histological features	Paracortical infiltrate with sparing of follicles Prominent venules 'Compartmentalising' fibrosis
Cytological features (neoplastic cells)	Marked irregularity of nuclear outline (multilobed, cerebriform, convoluted) Abundant pale cytoplasm
Associated cells	Interdigitating reticulum cells Epithelioid cells Eosinophils Mature plasma cells (polyclonal)

Conversely it is not to be expected that every T-cell lymphoma will necessarily display any of these features. However, a combination of such characteristics does provide strong presumptive evidence of a peripheral T-cell lymphoma. It is of course necessary to confirm this impression with tests for T-cell surface markers, enzyme cytochemistry and absence of immunoglobulin synthesis by the neoplastic cells.

MONOMORPHIC TYPES

1. CELLS MAINLY OF UNIFORM SIZE

(a) T-cell lymphoma — small cell types
(ML Lymphocytic — T types)

There are at least two distinct types of T-lymphocytic lymphoma — one presenting with skin infiltration (cutaneous type — mycosis fungoides and Sézary's syndrome), the other with splenic, lymph node, bone marrow and peripheral blood involvement (chronic lymphocytic leukaemia — T-cell type — T-CLL). A chronic lymphocytic leukaemia is a feature of Sézary's syndrome too, just as skin involvement is common in T-CLL, but the two disorders are quite distinct, clinically and pathologically. For instance, marrow involvement is minimal in Sézary's syndrome, but is invariable in T-CLL. A third type of T-lymphocytic leukaemia is found in the 'adult T-cell leukaemia/lymphoma' of Japan and the Caribbean region (qv) but this disorder differs so markedly from the other two diseases in its clinical behaviour and in other features that it will not be further discussed at this point (see p. 324).

Cutaneous T-cell lymphoma — mycosis fungoides and Sézary's syndrome

There is now widespread support for the belief that these two disorders are fundamentally the same and that Sézary's syndrome (SS) is a leukaemic variant of mycosis fungoides (MF). The diffuse nature of the skin involvement in SS is probably attributable to the presence of circulating Sézary cells in the peripheral blood, which are generally lacking in MF. As noted above, skin involvement is a feature common to a variety of peripheral T-cell lymphomas, but whereas in other types skin lesions are generally an incidental feature in a patient with widespread lymphomatous or leukaemic infiltration*, in the cutaneous type the skin lesions are the primary and central feature of the disease. At least in the great majority of cases of cutaneous T-cell lymphoma, the cells have the phenotype of T-helper cells (Boumsell et al, 1981). Knowles & Halper (1982) found cells of a more primitive phenotype in those cases of cutaneous T-cell lymphoma with lymph node involvement at presentation.

Mycosis fungoides

Although commoner in males, both sexes are affected and the disease usually presents in middle aged or older subjects. In mycosis fungoides the cutaneous lesions are described as evolving in three stages — premycotic stage, mycotic or plaque stage, and tumour stage. The rate at which this evolution takes place is very variable, but progression may be very slow. In the earlier stages, the skin biopsy appearances may be distinguished from those of a non-specific chronic inflammatory process in the dermis by the predominantly superficial, 'band-like' lymphocytic infiltrate, amongst which atypical lymphocytes and occasional mitoses may be found. As the disease progresses, the number of atypical cells (now mostly T-cells) increases and 'epidermotropism' becomes more obvious. The lymphocytes penetrate into the overlying epidermis, often in ones and twos, but frequently forming clusters ('Pautrier microabscesses') (Fig. 12.1). At this stage, the pleomorphic character and nuclear irregularity of the infiltrating cells can often be seen on high power examination, but the 'cerebriform' convolutions of the nuclei can best be appreciated on electron microscopy (Fig. 12.2) or in thin sections of resin embedded tissue. Amongst the prevailing 'Lutzner cells' (Lutzner & Jordan, 1968; Lutzner et al, 1971) a few larger, more deeply staining 'mycosis' (MF) cells may be found, which show even more deeply incised nuclei than the Lutzner cells. The rapid

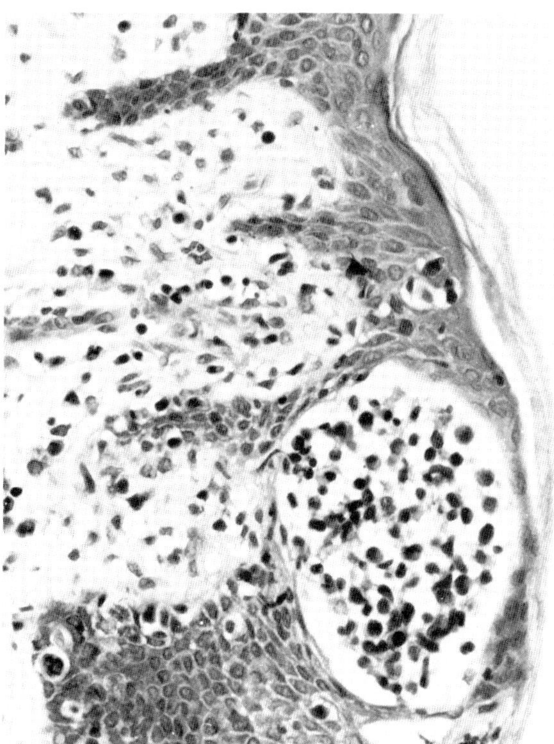

Fig. 12.1 Skin in mycosis fungoides showing epidermotropism of the Lutzner cells and a large Pautrier 'microabscess' within the epidermis. Note the pleomorphism and variation in size of the lymphoid cells. (H E × 300)

* This statement may need to be modified in the light of further experience. Van der Putte et al (1982) have described a form of cutaneous T-cell lymphoma characterised by 'papules, nodules and tumours' which 'slowly progressed in size and extent in one region of the skin'. Only one patient had regional lymph node involvement. The cells had 'multilobated' nuclei with marginal nucleoli, (see p. 313). These are clearly not the features of mycosis fungoides.

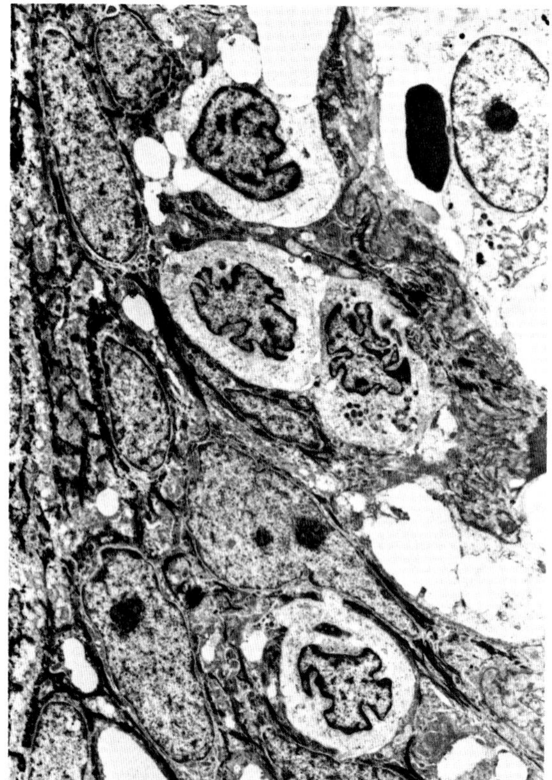

Fig. 12.2 Electron micrograph of skin in mycosis fungoides showing four Lutzner cells which have penetrated into the base of the epidermis. The convoluted nuclear outlines of these cells are well shown. A histiocyte is also present (upper right).

growth of the lesions, which characterises the tumour stage, is reflected not only in the massive accumulation of Lutzner cells but in their increasing anaplasia and mitotic activity. Bizarre neoplastic giant-cells may be found and transformation into a T-immunoblastic lymphoma has been recorded (Lennert, 1978; Knowles & Halper, 1982). In a survey of 45 autopsied cases of MF, Rappaport & Thomas (1974) found extracutaneous involvement in 71%.

Lymph node changes in MF

Lymphadenopathy is commonly observed in MF. It affects primarily the superficial node groups (especially inguinal and axillary) which drain involved areas of skin. The nodes are moderately to markedly enlarged, often rubbery in consistency and may show yellowish-brown mottling on the cut surface.

Histology. Very often a node biopsy shows only the changes of dermatopathic lymphadenitis (see p. 353). Careful search of the section, however, may reveal the presence in the paracortical areas of scattered atypical lymphocytes resembling the Lutzner cells of the skin infiltrate or even MF cells. Both types of cell mingle with the pale, interdigitating reticulum cells which characteristically make up the bulk of the paracortical infiltrate (Fig. 12.3). Lutzner cells are distinctly larger than ordinary small lymphocytes and, having a less dense nuclear chromatin, the irregularly shaped nuclei stain more palely. MF cells in conventional sections often have hyperchromatic nuclei (Fig. 12.4).

In course of time, increasing numbers of Lutzner cells occupy the T-zones displacing other types

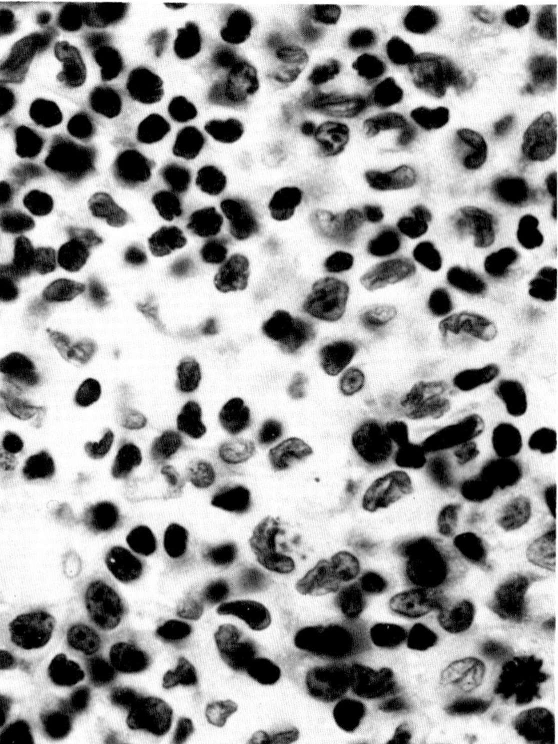

Fig. 12.3 Lymph node from a patient with mycosis fungoides. At low magnification the picture was typical of dermatopathic lymphadenitis, but close scrutiny shows the irregular outlines of the lymphocyte nuclei (upper left). Many interdigitating reticulum cells and some histiocytes are also present. Note mitosis (bottom right). (H E × 940)

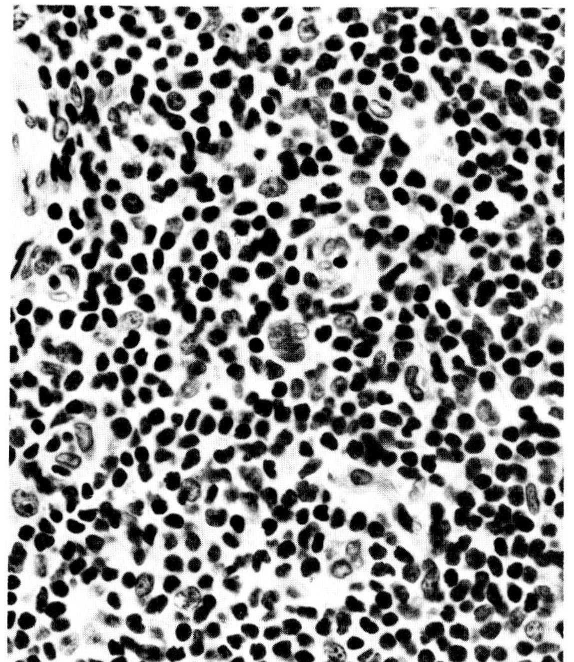

Fig. 12.4 Inguinal lymph node from another case of mycosis fungoides. The typical picture of dermatopathic lymphadenitis is not seen here, but instead an insidious infiltration of the T zones by small Lutzner cells. A large 'MF cell' with multilobed nucleus is seen at the centre of the field. (H E × 480)

of cell in these areas until the infiltrate consists principally of Lutzner cells, often showing mitotic figures (Fig. 12.5). The non-specific histological picture of dermatopathic lymphadenitis is thus progressively transformed into the specific picture of mycosis fungoides. Accompanying this transformation, the post-capillary venules assume greater prominence and the appearances may then resemble those of malignant lymphoma of T-zone type (see p. 315), especially when the follicles are still preserved, as is often the case (Fig. 12.6). Finally, even the follicles are overrun and the whole node is diffusely infiltrated by atypical T-cells of Lutzner type (Fig. 12.7), but showing varying degrees of anaplasia, with only isolated interdigitating reticulum cells remaining (Fig. 12.8).

Sézary's syndrome

In this variant of cutaneous T-cell lymphoma the skin lesion takes the form of a diffuse erythroderma ('homme rouge'), which may or may not be associated with ulcerated plaques or nodules. A skin biopsy shows histological features similar to those of MF, but the lymphoid infiltrate in the superficial dermis is often sparser and more diffuse, whilst the 'Sézary cells' generally appear smaller and more deeply staining than the Lutzner cells of MF. The denser nuclear chromatin makes it more difficult to distinguish the irregular outline of the nuclei. The remarkable nuclear convolutions can best be seen by electron microscopy or in a semi-thin section of resin embedded tissue. As in the case of MF, the cutaneous lesions may prove remarkably indolent.

Lymph node changes in Sézary's syndrome

In this disorder the superficial lymph nodes tend to be involved by the lymphomatous process at an earlier stage than in MF and a lymph node biopsy

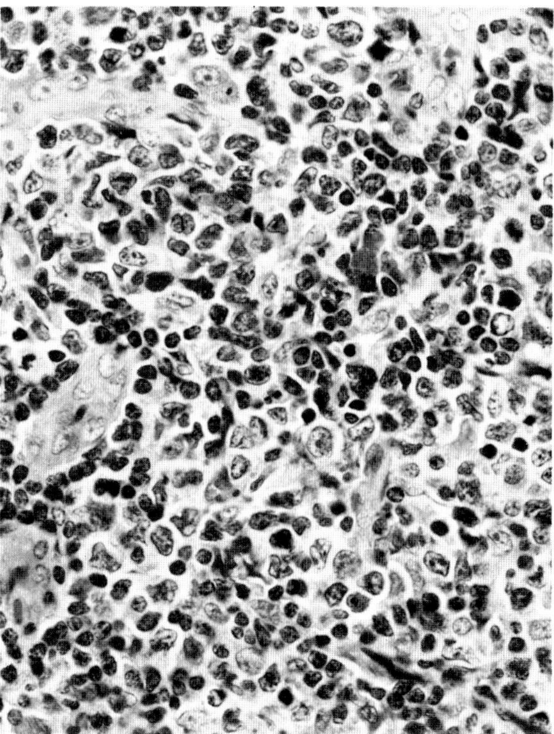

Fig. 12.5 Axillary lymph node biopsy in mycosis fungoides — later stage, showing mixed cellular infiltrate which includes many Lutzner cells, and prominent venules (same case as Fig. 12.1) (H E × 470)

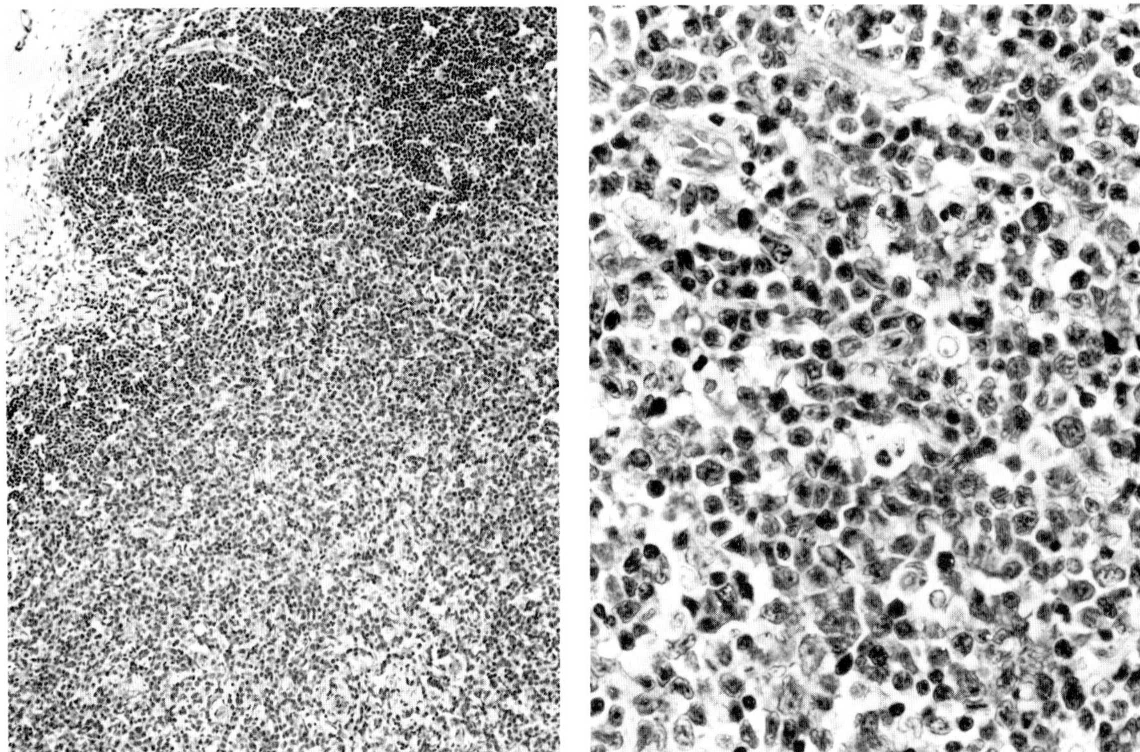

Fig. 12.6 Later lymph node biopsy from the same patient as Figs 12.1 and 12.5. A few cortical follicles remain (top and left), but the paracortex is diffusely infiltrated by Lutzner cells. (H E × 120)

Fig.12.7 High power view of paracortical infiltrate in same node as Fig. 12.6. The cells are almost entirely Lutzner cells with occasional 'blast' type cells. (H E × 470)

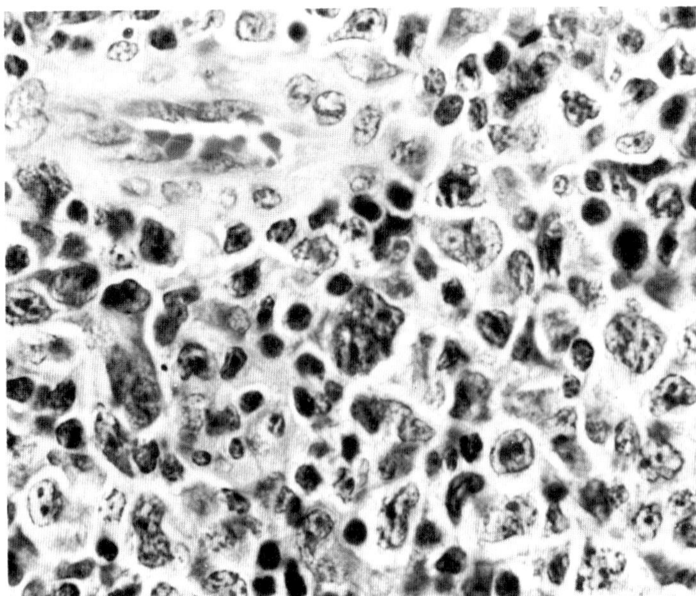

Fig. 12.8 Detail from same node as Fig. 12.5 showing a binucleate cell resembling a Sternberg-Reed cell. Such cells are commonly found in MF which may account for the confusion in the past between mycosis fungoides and Hodgkin's disease (H E × 750)

often shows widespread infiltration by Sézary cells rather than the picture of dermatophatic lymphadenitis with only scattered atypical T-lymphocytes. Apart from the slightly smaller size of the Sézary cells, the picture is basically similar to that seen in MF (Fig. 12.9).

Prognosis in cutaneous T-cell lymphoma. The slow progression of the disease has been referred to above. However, the tempo accelerates in the tumour stage and rapid deterioration in the patient's health may accompany generalisation of the disease, or blast cell transformation in the neoplasm.

Differential diagnosis. There is seldom much difficulty in recognising the nodal changes for what they are in these two conditions, since in most cases the skin lesions will have attracted attention first and the diagnosis will already have been established by skin biopsy. Two difficulties may, however, arise. The first of these concerns the early recognition of Lutzner cells in a node presenting the picture of simple dermatopathic lymphadenitis. It is often a problem to decide at what stage such a node may be said to be 'involved' by MF. Rarely the skin lesions may have been overlooked (this probably occurs most frequently in black patients), while the enlarged nodes attract attention. It is thus always important to look for atypical cells when the node biopsy appears to show nothing more than dermatopathic lymphadenopathy, especially when there is no obvious skin condition to account for the lymph node changes. The second difficulty lies in distinguishing the nodal changes of MF from those of T-zone lymphoma, as mentioned above. The latter neoplasm, however, rarely shows skin lesions and when these do occur their distribution in the dermis is quite different (see p. 315). Weisenburger et al (1982) have described a type of T-cell lymphoma in which the nodal infiltrate resembled that of MF although skin lesions were lacking. These may have been cases of T-zone lymphoma.

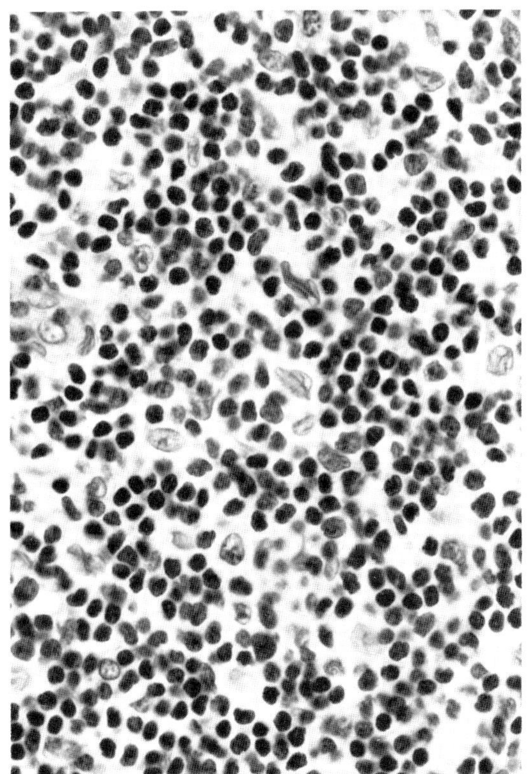

Fig. 12.9 Lymph node biposy in Sézary's syndrome. Nearly all the lymphocytes shown are Sézary cells, but only a few give a hint of nuclear convolution by conventional light microscopy. Note interdigitating reticulum cells with twisted-looking nuclei. (H E × 600)

Chronic lymphocytic leukaemia of T-cell type (T-CLL)

The T-cell types of chronic lymphocytic leukaemia are much rarer than B-CLL, but their precise incidence is still unknown. It appears that there are at least two distinct variants of T-CLL, as well as a rare prolymphocytic form, (Lennert et al, 1981). One type is evidently a neoplastic proliferation of T-suppressor cells whilst in the other type the cells show the characteristics of T-helper cells.

The first has been described by Brouet et al (1975) and by Costello et al (1980). The clinical and haematological features of this disease are sufficiently distinctive for the diagnosis to be suspected before corroborative tests have been performed (Brouet et al, 1975). In these authors' experience of nine cases, massive splenomegaly was common whilst lymphadenopathy was generally inconspicuous. Skin lesions and marked neutropenia were each seen in four patients, whilst blood and marrow infiltration were generally of moderate degree. In this variety the leukaemic cells are of 'mature type' and show distinct azurophilic granules in the cytoplasm by light microscopy. Most show a granular pattern of acid phosphatase activity in the cytoplasm and electron microscopy reveals distinctive parallel tubular arrays (Costello et al, 1980). The neoplastic cells stain positively with OKT8 and negatively with OKT4, thus confirming that they belong to a T-suppressor subset (Lennert et al, 1982). In the second type (Levine, 1981), the cells show irregular nuclear protrusions ('knobby' type), whilst cytoplasmic granules are absent. There is spot-like acid phosphatase activity in the leukaemic cells, which are OKT4 positive. The *prolymphocytic* type of T-cell leukaemia shows features similar to those of the commoner B-cell prolymphocytic leukaemia, presenting with massive splenomegaly and a high white cell count, which contrasts with the much lower counts generally found in T-CLL. The cells are somewhat larger than those of T-CLL and have a prominent nucleolus (Costello et al, 1980).

Lymph node changes

Lymphadenopathy is seldom a striking feature in this group of diseases. As in B-CLL, the normal architecture of the nodes is obscured by a diffuse infiltrate of small lymphocytes, but there are three notable differences in T-CLL: (1) proliferation centres are absent, although occasional blast cells with prominent central nucleoli may be seen; (2) venules are very much more prominent throughout (Fig. 12.10, 12.11) and tend to be lined by tall endothelium. Lymphocytes may be seen, sometimes in large numbers within the walls of venules (Fig. 12.12); (3) the cell nuclei in a well fixed preparation and especially in semi-thin sections

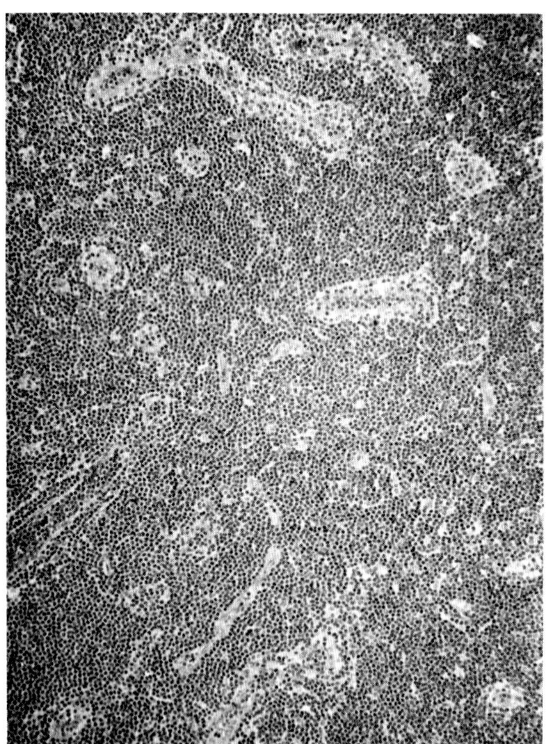

Fig. 12.10 Lymph node biopsy from a man of 55 with T-CLL. The picture at low power differs from that of B-CLL in the absence of proliferation centres and the prominence of venules. (This patient had diffuse skin involvement with erythroderma.) (H E × 120)

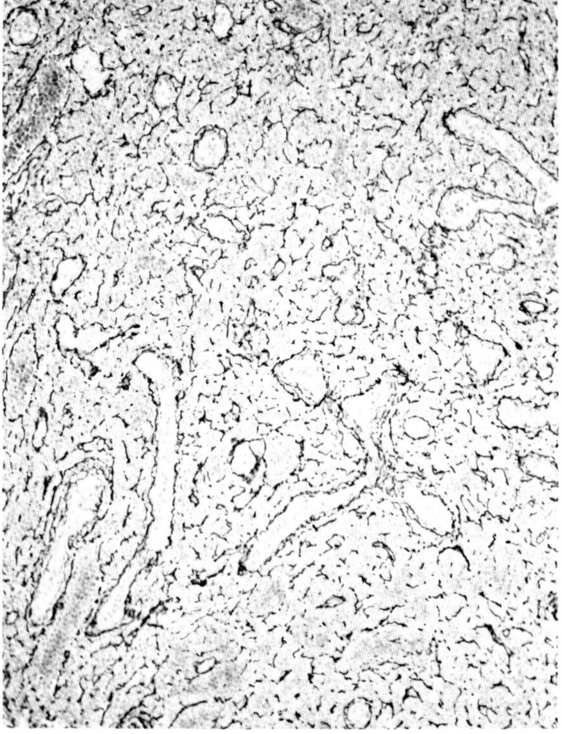

Fig. 12.11 Same node as Fig. 12.10. Reticulin staining emphasises the remarkable number and prominence of the venules (compare with Fig. 10.2, p. 234). (Gordon and Sweets reticulin × 120)

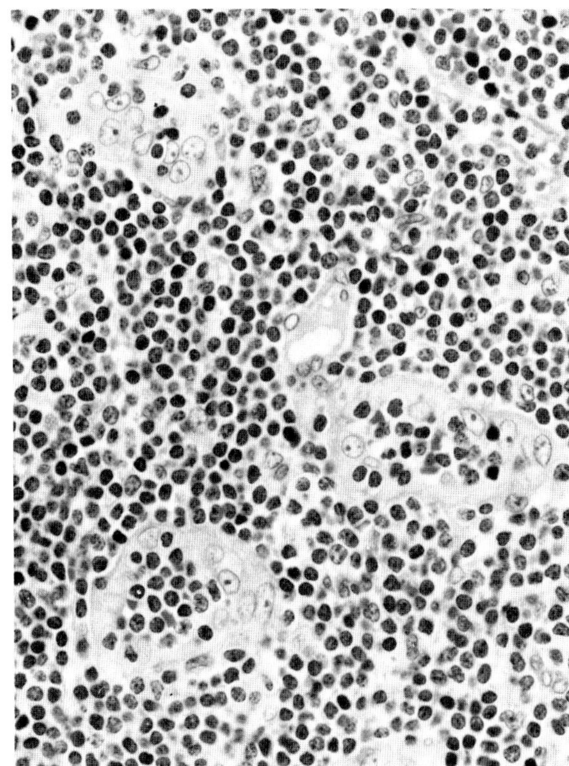

Fig. 12.12 Higher power view of same node as Figs 12.10 and 12.11, to show the 'high endothelial' venules with lymphocytes in their lumina and walls. The lymphocyte nuclei are less regular than those of B-CLL. (H E × 470)

after resin embedding, appear distinctly less regular in shape than the nuclei of B-cell CLL, so that there is an overall impression of less cellular uniformity.

(b) T-cell lymphoma of medium-sized cells

The T-cell variety of prolymphocytic leukaemia has been mentioned above. Other neoplasms in this group may present with lymphadenopathy or with cutaneous tumours. Leukaemia seems to be infrequent. These are uncommon neoplasms and it is uncertain at the present time whether or not they constitute a homogeneous category. Watanabe and co-workers (1981) distinguish two types: (1) a tumour composed of medium-sized cells with relatively small nuclei and abundant, pale cytoplasm (pale cell type) and (2) a type with highly irregular 'twisted' nuclei and scanty cytoplasm. From their description of this second type it seems properly to belong in the pleomorphic group. Approximately 50% of their cases of this type had leukaemia.

The 'clear cell' or 'pale cell' appearance of the first type of Watanabe et al seems to be a non-specific change occurring in 'activated' T-cells (see p. 310). It is not peculiar to a specific type of T-cell lymphoma. An example of a monomorphic peripheral T-cell lymphoma of this type is illustrated in Figure 12.13.

Some authors have described a monomorphic type of peripheral T-cell lymphoma composed of uniform, centrocyte-like cells with scanty cytoplasm, a type which is illustrated by the following case: a 48 year old male presented with enlarged

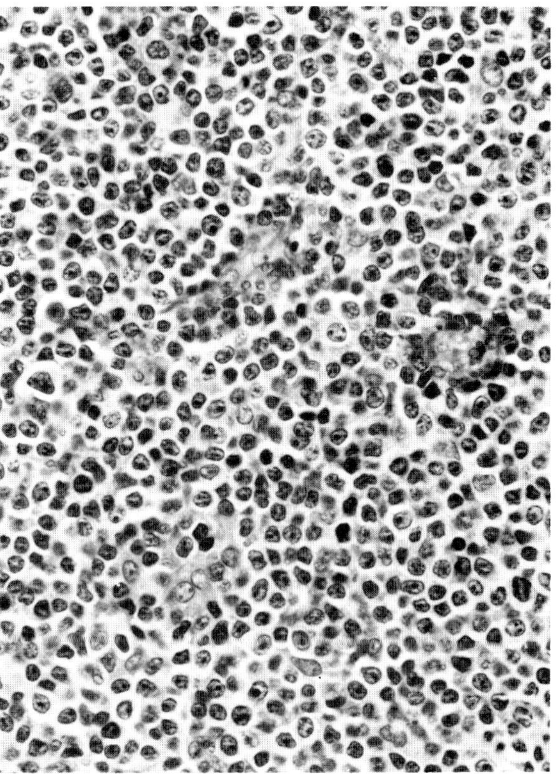

Fig. 12.13 Lymph node from a man of 56 showing a monomorphic T-cell malignant lymphoma of medium-sized (intermediate) cell type. Most of the cell nuclei appear regular in shape and the most distinctive feature is the halo of 'clear' cytoplasm which surrounds the nucleus. Early clear cell change is more readily appreciated under the microscope than in a photomicrograph in which the separation of the nuclei seems to suggest poor fixation. (H E × 470)

inguinal nodes of recent appearance and hepatosplenomegaly. There was neither leukaemia nor skin involvement. Biopsy showed diffuse effacement of the nodal architecture by a monomorphic malignant lymphoma composed exclusively of intermediate sized cells (intermediate between small and medium) with irregularly shaped nuclei and scanty cytoplasm (Figs 12.14, 12.15). The vessels in the node showed slight hyaline thickening of their walls and an erroneous diagnosis of centrocytic lymphoma was made (see p. 60). However, the suspension phenotype of the node convincingly showed that the neoplastic cells were T-cells of T-helper sub-type and B-cells were almost entirely absent. The tumour behaved in a highly aggressive manner and responded poorly to treatment.

(c) T-cell lymphoma — large cell types

Some peripheral T-cell lymphomas of monomorphic type are composed of large cells and these are not all true blast-cell neoplasms, although many may represent tumours which are in process of transformation. The *non-immunoblastic large cell lymphomas of T-type* may contain a small proportion of blast cells, but often the predominant cells have smaller, round nuclei, less leptochromatic than those of blast cells and with smaller nucleoli. The large size of these cells is due to an abundance of weakly staining cytoplasm. This 'clear cell' phenomenon, referred to in the last section, is apparently due to an imbibition of water by the cells and is a peculiarity of activated T-cells (p. 309). It is not specific for a single type of T-cell lymphoma, being met with also in T-zone lymphomas and in the 'immunoblastic lymphadenopathy-like' type. The relationship of these three types to one another needs to be clarified.

The large clear cells, whether present singly or in clusters, stand out very distinctly against the darker background of lymphocytes and plasma cells (Figs 12.16, 12.17, 12.18). Plasma cells are

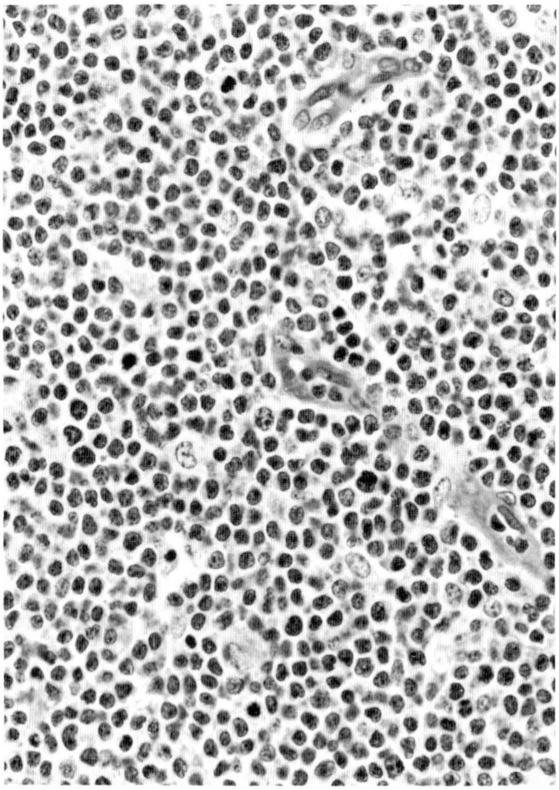

Fig. 12.14 Inguinal node biopsy from a man of 48 showing a monomorphic, medium-sized, T-cell lymphoma of centrocyte-like cells (H E × 470)

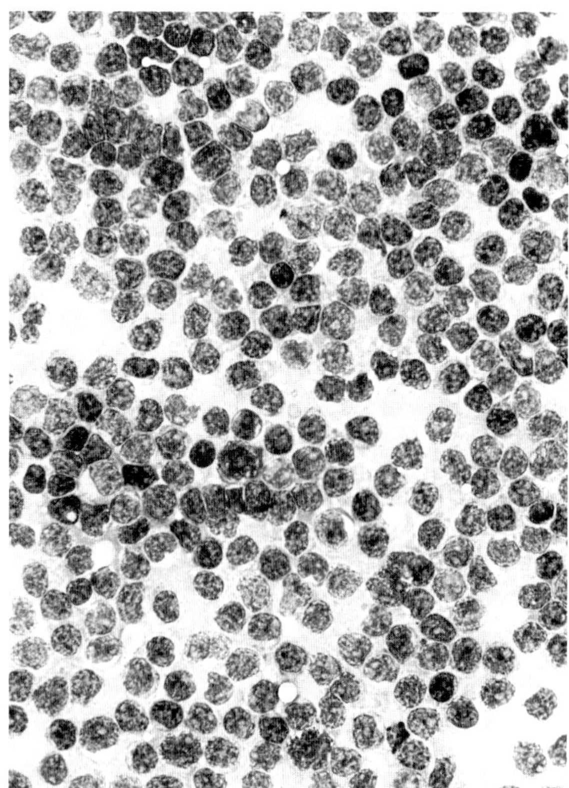

Fig. 12.15 Imprint of same node as shown in Fig. 12.14. The subtle nuclear convolutions are here more apparent than they are in a paraffin section. (May-Grünwald Giemsa × 470)

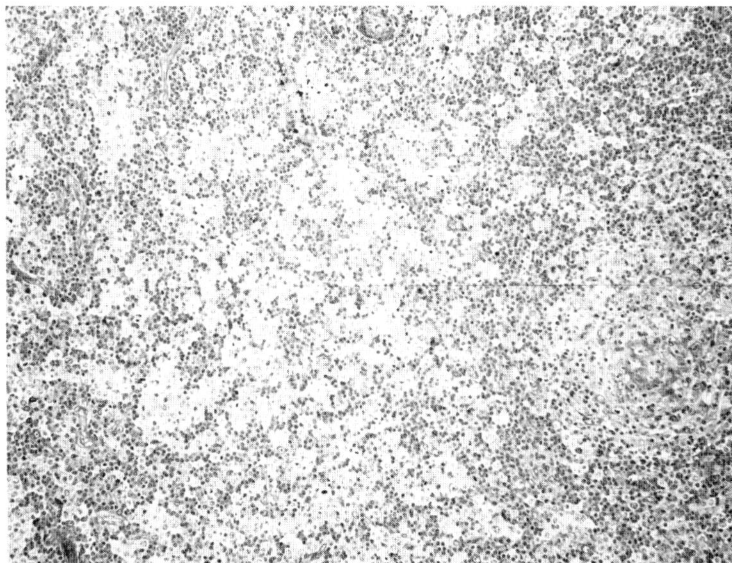

Fig. 12.16 Cervical lymph node biopsy from a woman of 49 with a peripheral T cell lymphoma showing pronounced 'clear-cell' change. The clusters of pale cells stand out sharply, producing a very distinctive picture. Remnants of a germinal follicle are seen (right). An earlier node biopsy from this patient showed a much less specific picture with vague loss of architecture, but without clear cell change. (Giemsa × 120)

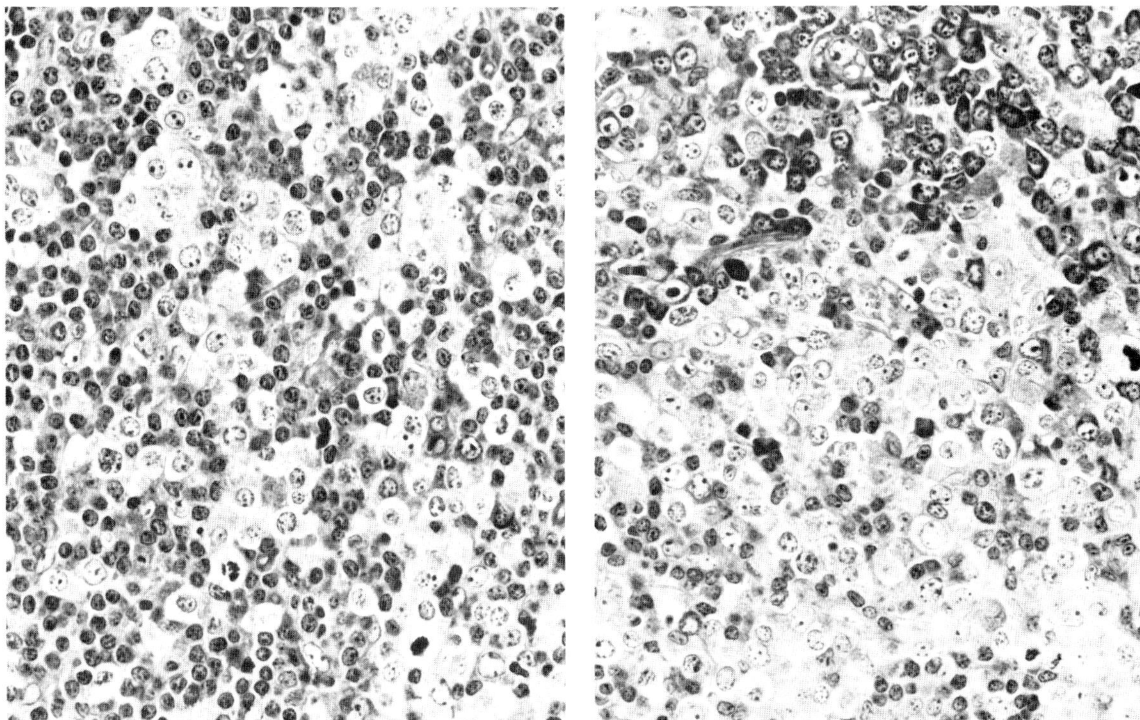

Fig. 12.17 Same node as Fig. 12.16 at a higher magnification to show large neoplastic cells with abundant pale cytoplasm against a background of lymphocytes and plasma cells. The clear cells probably represent partially transformed T cells. (H E × 470)

Fig. 12.18 Same node as Figs 12.16 and 12.17. A large cluster of clear cells (below) contrasts with darkly staining (polyclonal) plasma cells in relation to a venule (top of field). Epithelioid cell clusters (not shown) were also present in parts of this tumour. (Giemsa × 470)

often very numerous and, being of polyclonal type, their presence is ascribed to helper activity of the neoplastic T-cells. Epithelioid histiocytes may also be found in this type, sometimes in considerable numbers.

ML Immunoblastic — T-type (ML Ib-T)

These tumours are much less frequently encountered than B-immunoblastic lymphomas, at least in Western countries. They usually present as lymph node masses, but may occur in the tonsils and elsewhere. Like their B-cell counterparts, the T-immunoblastic lymphomas often arise as a result of blast-cell transformation of a previously 'low grade' T-cell neoplasm such as a T-zone lymphoma or even mycosis fungoides (Fig. 12.19).

The true immunoblastic lymphoma of T-cell type is composed, exclusively or predominantly, of cells with large 'vesicular' nuclei, prominent, usually central, nucleoli, and generally abundant cytoplasm which is basophilic with Giemsa staining (Fig. 12.20). The cells of T-immunoblastic lymphomas differ from those of B-immunoblastic lymphomas in having a paler staining cytoplasm, less basophilic and pyroninophilic, reflecting the smaller cytoplasmic content of organelles (Said & Pinkus, 1980). Naturally, T-immunoblastic lymphomas never show plasmacytoid or plasmablastic differentiation, but the distinction between B- and T-immunoblastic lymphomas is not always possible without surface marker studies. They are rapidly growing neoplasms and display a high mitotic rate, often with abnormal mitoses and sometimes with bizarre Sternberg-Reed-like giant-cells. The occasional presence of mature-appearing (polyclonal) plasma cells in such tumours should not be

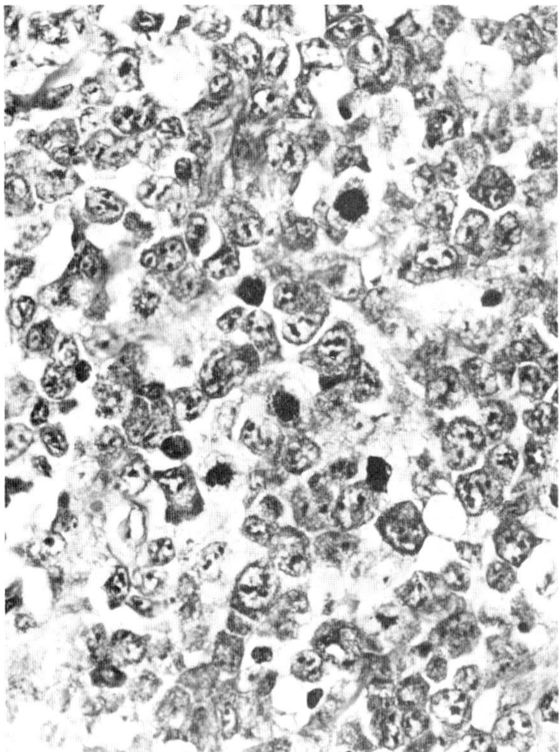

Fig. 12.19 Lymphnode showing diffuse malignant lymphoma of T-immunoblastic type which arose as a result of transformation of mycosis fungoides in a man aged 64 (H E × 750)

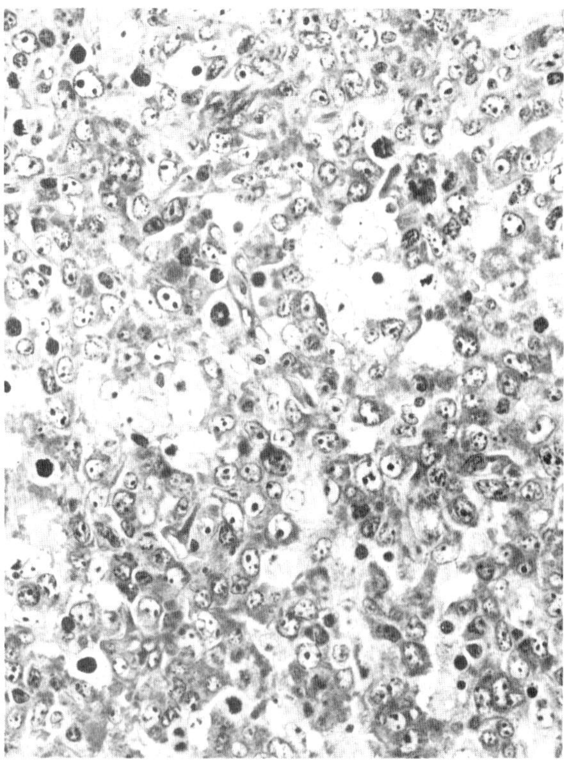

Fig. 12.20 Supraclavicular lymph node biopsy taken 3 months later from the same patient as Figs 12.16, 12.17 and 12.18. The tumour has now transformed fully into a T-immunoblastic lymphoma. Compare with Figs 12.17 and 12.18 and note the more prominent nucleoli and basophilic cytoplasm in the second biopsy. A few large clear cells still remain, but some of the pale cells are epithelioid cells. (Giemsa × 470)

misconstrued as evidence of a B-cell origin since in some instances the neoplastic cells have been shown to be of T-helper phenotype. Eosinophils are sometimes present and may be abundant. Reactive macrophages and epithelioid cells may also be numerous (Fig. 12.21).

Differential diagnosis. The distinction of T-immunoblastic lymphoma from other types of large T-cell lymphoma and from B-immunoblastic lymphoma has been discussed above. As with other large-cell malignant lymphomas, confusion may sometimes occur with histiocytic reticulosarcoma and malignant histiocytosis. Difficulties are most likely to arise with less well differentiated histiocytic neoplasms which lack the smaller nuclei and abundant eosinophilic cytoplasm of well differentiated neoplastic histiocytes. In such cases, surface markers, enzyme histochemical reactions or electron microscopy may be required to decide the nature of the tumour. Undifferentiated metastatic carcinoma, especially of tonsillar or nasopharyngeal origin needs also to be distinguished from T-immunoblastic lymphoma.

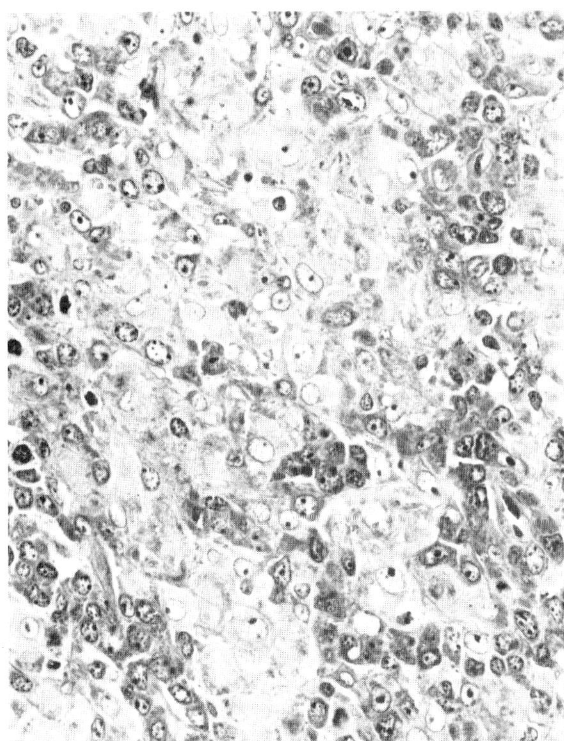

Fig. 12.21 Another field from the same biopsy as Fig. 12.20, showing large masses of epithelioid cells amongst the neoplastic cells. Epithelioid cells are commonly found in some varieties of peripheral T-cell lymphoma. (Giemsa × 470)

T-cell lymphoma with 'multilobated' nuclei

A third large cell type of peripheral T-cell lymphoma, in which the cells are characterised by large, 'multilobated' nuclei, was described by Pinkus et al (1979). An extranodal presentation was found in three out of the four cases originally described by these authors, with involvement of skin, subcutaneous tissue and bone as common characteristics. Lymphadenopathy occurred in all, but was the dominant feature in only one patient. Histologically, the tumour was characterised by the dominance of large cells with 'markedly irregular multilobated nuclei having relatively fine nuclear chromatin and small to inconspicuous nucleoli'. Abundant, pale staining cytoplasm was present. These cells marked specifically as T-cells. Despite widespread involvement, the prognosis seemed to be better than that of many T-cell lymphomas, three of the four patients being alive without evidence of disease $1\frac{1}{2}$ to 5 years from the onset.

In a further, retrospective study from the same group, (Weinberg & Pinkus, 1981), ten patients were identified as having a similar type of neoplasm, but since identification depended upon morphology alone, no reliance can be put on the findings. Others have shown that similar nuclear characteristics may sometimes be found in B-cell lymphomas (Lennert, 1983).

It is not yet clear how specific this variety of T-cell lymphoma is. One out of three cutaneous T-cell lymphomas described by Van der Putte et al (1982) was thought to belong to this category. A single case of a 'large-cell, T-cell lymphoma with hypersegmented nuclei' has been described from Sweden (Pallesen et al, 1981). However, further studies are necessary to define the entity more clearly.

An example of a 'multilobated' T-cell lymphoma is illustrated in Figure 12.22. Although the cells have distinctive multilobed, and therefore irregular, nuclei, the tumour is monomorphic in the sense that all the cells look alike.

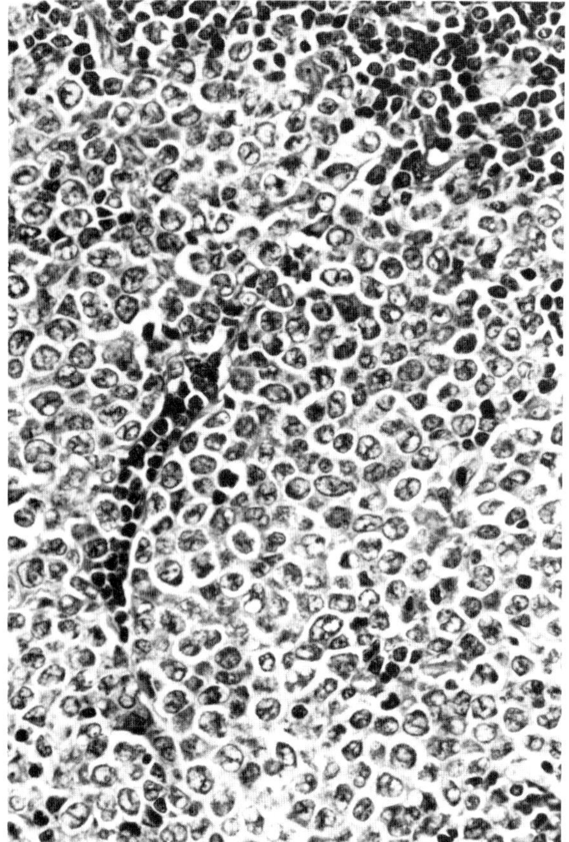

Fig. 12.22 Lymph node showing a peripheral T-cell lymphoma of large cell, multilobated type. Clefts can be seen between the individual lobes of each nucleus. Mitoses are scanty. Compare the size of the neoplastic cells with that of the residual lymphocyte population. (Giemsa × 470)

2. CELLS OF VARYING SIZES

T-zone lymphoma (Lennert, 1978)

Synonyms:
ML lymphocytic — T zone type.
? Immunoblastic sarcoma — T cell type (Lukes, 1979).
? Node-based T-cell lymphoma (Collins et al, 1979).
? Peripheral T-cell lymphoma (Waldron et al, 1977).

Question marks have been placed against the three terms listed above since it is not certain whether these are strictly synonymous although it seems from the descriptions given that each of these authors is describing fundamentally the same tumour. Each term has been used for a peripheral T-cell lymphoma with a distinctive cell picture which includes small and medium-sized T-lymphocytes and blast cells in varying proportions. The term T-zone lymphoma was proposed by Lennert (1978), not only to emphasise the specific localisation of the neoplastic infiltrate within the T-zones of the affected lymph node, but to draw attention to the participation of all the elements of the T-zones — T-lymphocytes, interdigitating reticulum cells and post-capillary venules — in the neoplasm. In the initial stages at least, the follicles (B-zones) are preserved and Lennert postulated that T-zone lymphoma represents the converse of the situation seen in follicular B-cell lymphoma, in which the follicular cells are the neoplastic element and the interfollicular T-zones are reactive. Lennert has further pointed out that even when the follicles are entirely overrun by the neoplasm and are no longer visible in an ordinary section, their position can still be shown by immunostaining with a monoclonal antibody to dendritic reticulum cells (Lennert, 1981). Other authors have tended to place less emphasis on follicular preservation in tumours of apparently similar type. Although T-zone lymphoma is an uncommon neoplasm (about 1% of all NHL in Germany and Holland — Lennert, 1981), it is possibly more frequent than is generally believed. It does not appear to be any more frequent in Japan (Watanabe et al, 1981).

Clinical features

In a series of 25 cases of T-zone lymphoma observed by Lennert (1978), the clinical features included the following. The patients were adults and the incidence was approximately equal in the two sexes. Fever and weight loss were common. Lymphadenopathy was almost invariable and developed rapidly. Superficial node groups were mainly affected. Splenomegaly and/or hepatomegaly were noted in 50% of patients. Tonsillar and lung involvement were seen in a minority. In contrast with the findings in the pleomorphic type, bone marrow infiltration and leukaemia were exceptional at presentation, but marked eosinophilia

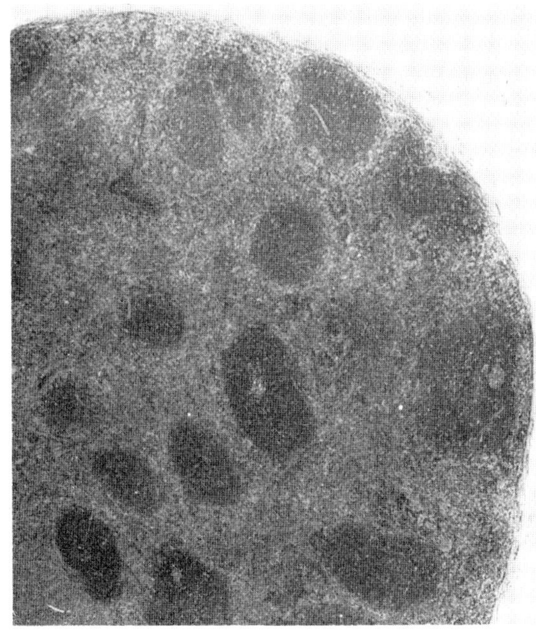

Fig. 12.23 Cervical lymph node biopsy from a man of 52 showing the characteristic pattern of T-zone lymphoma. Well preserved follicles (B-zone) are seen against the paler background of T-zone infiltrate. A few follicles have small germinal centres. (H E × 47)

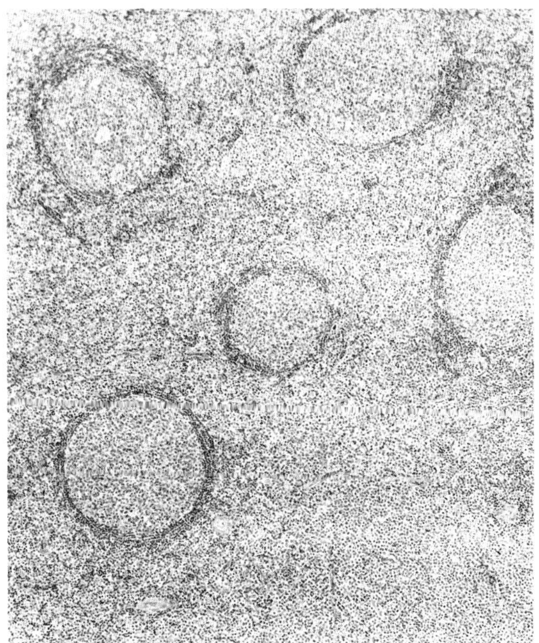

Fig. 12.24 Another case of T-zone lymphoma in a woman of 80. Here the follicles show large, reactive germinal centres, each outlined by a mantle zone of B lymphocytes. The intervening T-zone is expanded. (H E × 120)

was noted in several instances. Some patients had polyclonal hyperglobulinaemia.

We have seen one patient with skin deposits which lay deep in the dermis, sparing the papillary zone and epidermis. In the small series reported by Waldron et al (1977) many of the features were similar to those described by Lennert, and although bone marrow infiltration was uncommon at the outset, it was noted in all six patients later in the disease. Pulmonary and pleural involvement were also common.

Pathological features

Macroscopically the affected nodes show no specific features.

Histology. The most striking feature at a low magnification is the preservation of lymph follicles which stand out clearly against the paler staining background of the infiltrated and usually expanded interfollicular pulp (Figs 12.23, 12.24). The small, darkly staining B-lymphocytes of the follicles have a normal appearance and there may or may not be active germinal centres. In contrast the paracortical areas contain a characteristically pleomorphic cellular infiltrate consisting mainly of T-lymphocytes exhibiting a range of sizes and appearances and showing fairly frequent mitoses (Figs 12.25, 12.26). Smaller cells usually predominate, but even these are perceptibly larger than the residual B-lymphocytes and a proportion of them have irregular, sometimes elongate, sometimes cerebriform, nuclei. Clear cell change, described in the previous two sections, is not infrequent and may be a striking feature (Fig. 12.27). It often affects small groups of T-cells, scattered throughout the tumour. Intermingled with the T-lymphocytes there is a smaller but variable population of blast type cells with larger, often rounded nuclei and prominent nucleoli. At times even these large transformed cells have irregularly shaped nuclei and bizarre, multinucleate cells resembling Sternberg-Reed cells may be found on occasions. The resemblance to Hodgkin's disease is further heightened by the frequent presence of eosinophils, sometimes in considerable numbers. Interdigitating reticulum cells are often seen, as well as small groups of epithelioid cells (Fig. 12.28). Typical plasma cells are sometimes found in small

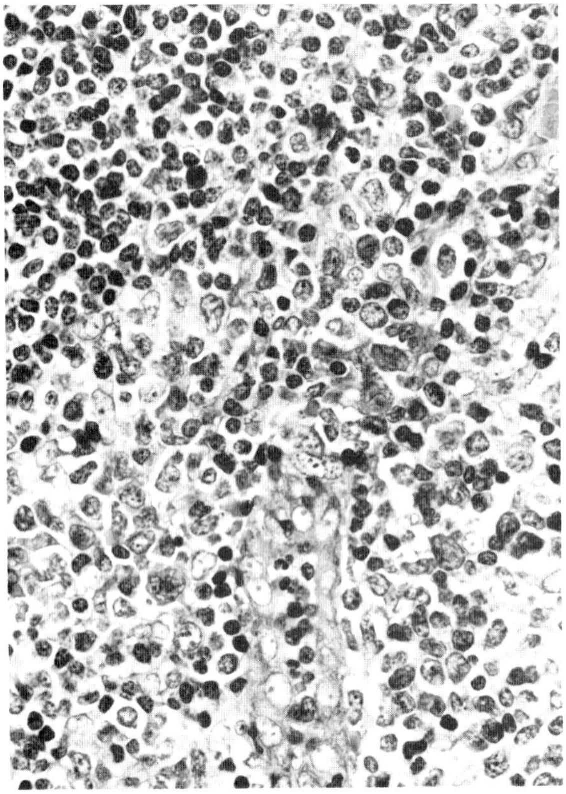

Fig. 12.25 Same node as Fig. 12.23 at a higher magnification to show the mixed T-zone infiltrate and a prominent venule lined by plump endothelial cells. The edge of a follicle is seen (top left). (Giemsa × 470)

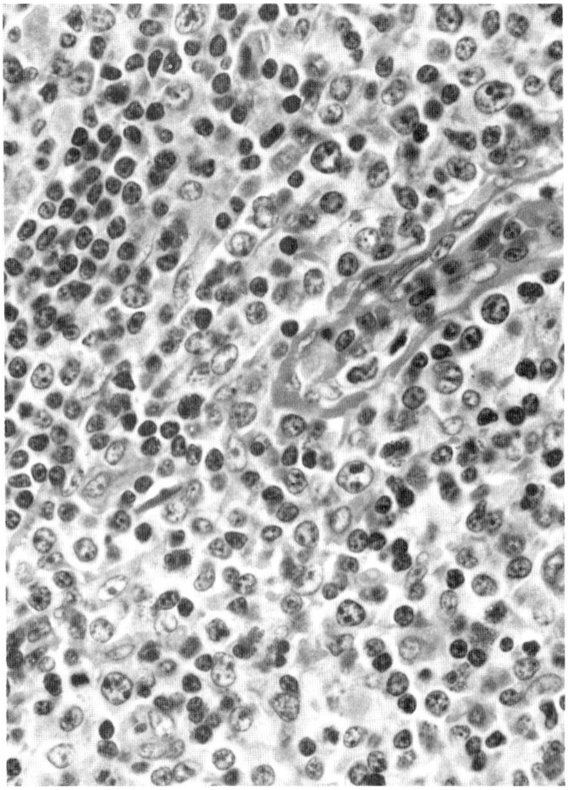

Fig. 12.26 Same node as Fig. 12.24 to show detail of the cellular infiltrate which includes some T-immunoblasts, along with T-lymphocytes, eosinophils, histiocytes and inconspicuous interdigitating reticulum cells. The edge of a reactive follicle is also shown (top left). (H E × 470)

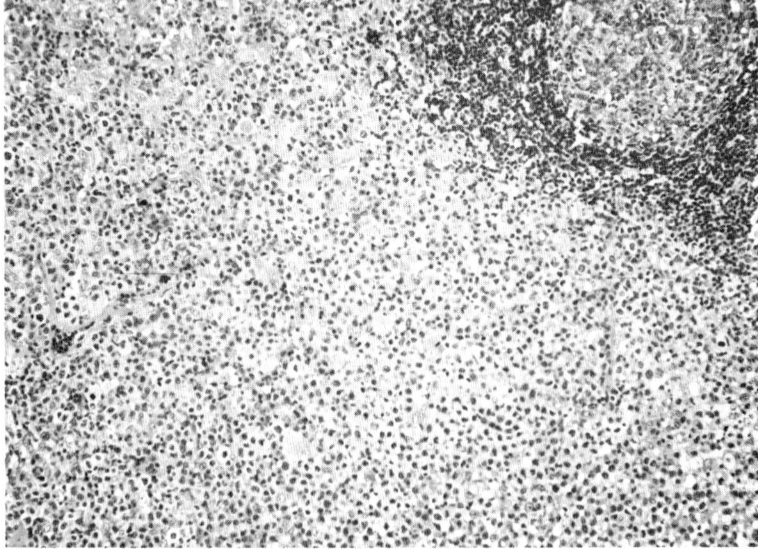

Fig. 12.27 Lymph node from another case of T-zone lymphoma in a woman of 65, showing the clear-cell phenomenon in many of the neoplastic T-cells (H E × 120)

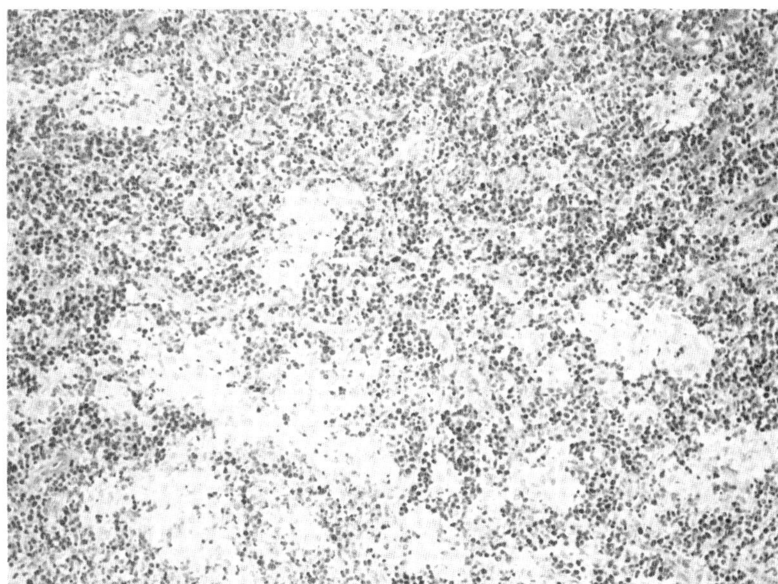

Fig. 12.28 T-zone lymphoma showing prominent clusters of pale-staining epithelioid cells in the neoplastic infiltrate (same node as Figs 12.23 and 12.25) (H E × 120)

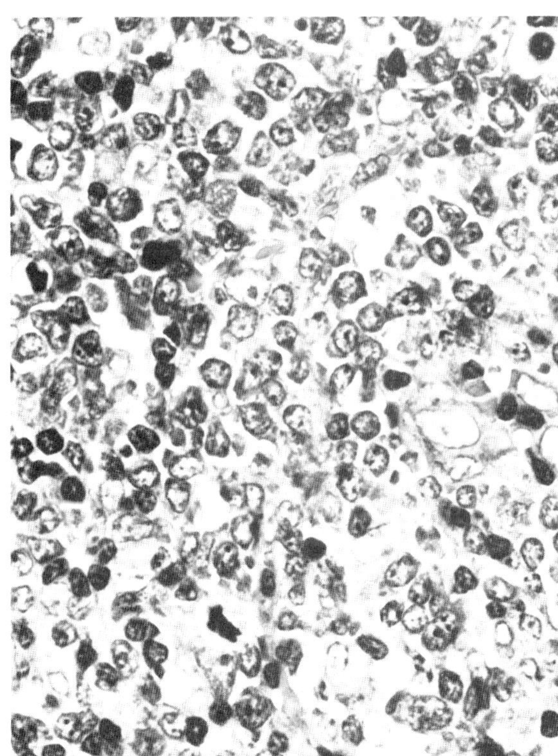

Fig. 12.29 Another field of the same node as Figs 12.23, 12.25 and 12.28, at a high magnification, showing many plasmacytoid T-cells (centre of field) (Giemsa × 750)

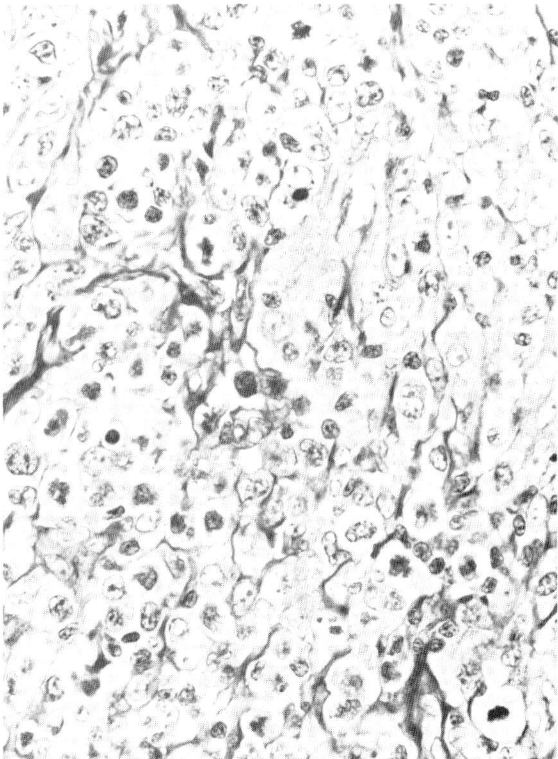

Fig. 12.30 Same node as Fig. 12.27 showing fine, 'compartmentalising' sclerosis. Note that the large clear cells of the neoplastic infiltrate do not contain glycogen. Several mitoses are present. (P A S × 470)

numbers amongst the prevailing T-cells, their presence being attributed to the helper-cell activity of the neoplastic T-lymphocytes. In addition there are often groups of the smaller 'plasmacytoid T-cells' (Lennert, 1978), with round nuclei like those of a true plasma cell but with less cytoplasm (Fig. 12.29).

A particularly distinctive feature of this tumour is the prominence of the venules which appear to be increased both in size and number and which generally show marked swelling of the lining endothelium (see Figs 12.25, 12.26). Waldron et al (1977) drew attention to the characteristic 'compartmentalisation' of the tumour by delicate collagenous strands — a feature which may be seen in some other peripheral T-cell lymphomas (Fig. 12.30). More extensive fibrosis and capsular thickening are sometimes seen.

Later in the disease, the initially paracortical neoplastic infiltrate overruns the follicles and the distinctive pattern of the T-zone lymphoma is lost. This progression is generally accompanied by an increase in the number of blast cells and the picture may merge into that of a T-immunoblastic lymphoma.

Prognosis. In common with the pleomorphic types of peripheral T-cell lymphoma, the response to treatment is generally short lived and the median survival is about 12 months (Lennert, 1981).

Differential diagnosis. T-zone lymphoma is most likely to be confused with Hodgkin's disease (HD), in which also persistent reactive follicles are associated with a pleomorphic paracortical infiltrate, often containing eosinophils. Venules may show increased prominence in HD, but seldom to the same degree as in T-zone lymphoma. The presence of occasional Sternberg-Reed-like cells in T-zone lymphoma may strengthen the impression of HD, but on detailed examination of the prevailing mononuclear cells, the bizarre nuclear shapes of the small and medium-sized cells will be apparent. Although the lymph nodes in Hodgkin's disease may contain a high proportion of T-lymphocytes the morphology of these is quite different, the cells being smaller and more regular.

Erythrophagocytic T-cell lymphoma

Two cases of an apparently identical type of T-cell lymphoma were described by Kadin et al (1981). The presentation was with fever, night sweats, jaundice and hepatosplenomegaly. Lymphadenopathy was slight. The authors drew attention to the clinical similarity between this disease and histiocytic medullary reticulosis, a similarity which was carried further by the demonstration that a minority of the neoplastic T-cells exhibited erythrophagocytosis. The distribution of the cellular infiltrate within the nodes resembled that of a T-zone lymphoma, but in the spleen the infiltrate involved mainly the red pulp. Whereas most cases of T-zone lymphoma that have been investigated have shown a T μ phenotype, in these two patients the neoplastic cells had a T γ phenotype and the authors speculated that the neoplasm may have originated in the spleen in which cells of this phenotype are common.

'Immunoblastic lymphadenopathy-like' T-cell lymphoma (AIL type)

Recently Japanese authors (Shimoyama et al, 1979; Watanabe et al, 1980) have described a type of peripheral T-cell lymphoma with clinical and histological features 'indistinguishable from those of immunoblastic (angioimmunoblastic) lymphenopathy'. The five adult patients described all had hyperglobulinaemia and their lymph node biopsies showed 'focal proliferation of monotonous pale cells and foci composed of polymorphic large, medium and small cells'. Vascular proliferation, eosinophil infiltration and small histiocytic aggregates were also present. Cells of all sizes formed E-rosettes and had T-cell surface antigens. One of the two fatal cases had widespread extension of the tumour with intestinal involvement at autopsy. The authors believed all five cases to be malignant on clinical and pathological grounds; karyotypic abnormalities were demonstrated in two.

There is now widespread agreement on the existence of the 'AIL type' of T-cell lymphoma which has many features in common with published descriptions of angioimmunoblastic lymphadenopathy (AIL) (see p. 175). Phenotyping of cell suspensions in cases of AIL has often shown a high content of T-cells and 'clear cells' have been noted in such cases by several observers (Nathwani et al, 1978; Cullen et al, 1979). Prominent clusters of epithelioid cells and numerous eosinophils are common in both conditions, as well as an often notable population of immunoblasts and polyclonal plasma cells. The presence of the last may be due to helper activity on the part of the T-cells. Vascular proliferation, which is such a striking feature of the histological picture of AIL, is also a characteristic of many peripheral T-cell lymphomas.

Transformation of AIL into T-zone lymphoma has been recorded (Lennert, 1981) and it is likely that some of the immunoblastic lymphomas arising in AIL patients are of T-cell type. These observations prompt the question as to whether 'angioimmunoblastic lymphadenopathy', as currently conceived, represents more than one disease entity. Possibly those cases of AIL reported as showing clusters of clear cells or many epithelioid cells as prominent features are in reality instances of this type of T-cell lymphoma. Further studies are necessary to clarify the issue before any definitive statement can be made.

Clinical features

As indicated above, the presentation of this disease is similar to that of angioimmunoblastic lymphadenopathy (p. 175). The patients are adults, of either sex, who generally present with a recent onset of widespread lymphadenopathy often accompanied by hepatosplenomegaly, fever, malaise and skin rashes. Investigation may disclose polyclonal hyperglobulinaemia and an autoimmune haemolytic anaemia.

Pathological features

These are again similar to those of AIL, as outlined above. In the initial stages, the nodal architecture is not totally effaced; the peripheral sinus is often patent, despite capsular and extracapsular infiltration by a polymorphous infiltrate. There may also be remnants of lymph follicles and, at an early stage when many small lymphocytes are still present, diagnosis may be very difficult. Partial effacement of the normal pattern, accompanied by increased prominence of blood vessels and the appearance of small clusters of 'pale' or 'clear' cells may attract attention and lead to a suspicion of AIL. The clear cells generally have relatively small, round, pachychromatic nuclei and abundant clear cytoplasm, which is negative for glycogen with PAS staining. Mitoses are regularly seen and may be quite numerous. The clear cells are easily overlooked when present in small numbers, but further biopsies will often show increasing numbers of these cells until the greater part of the node is filled with masses of clear cells, interspersed with prominent venules and capillaries which are often surrounded by plasma cells (Figs 12.31, 12.32). Eosinophils and clusters of epithelioid cells are frequently seen at this stage, although in variable numbers. Although clear cells are often the most distinctive feature of the cellular infiltrate in the AIL type of T-cell lymphoma, they are not confined to this type (see p. 310) nor are they invariably found in this type. The numbers of immunoblasts and the mitotic rate both tend to increase with the passage of time.

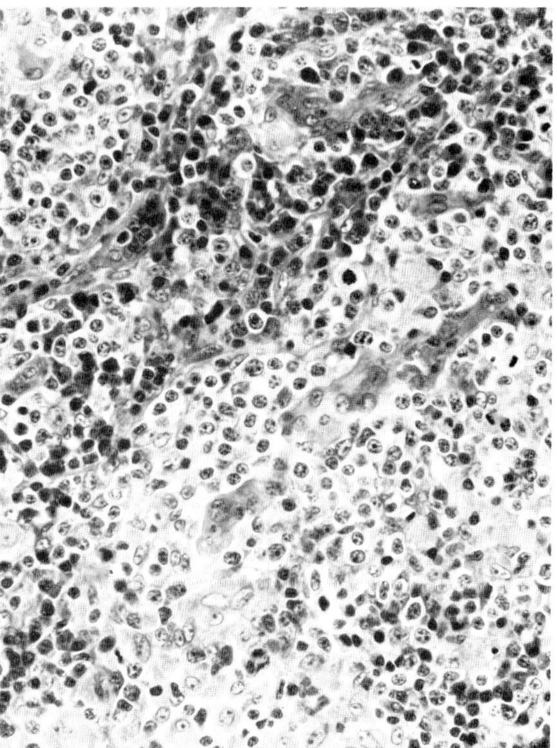

Fig. 12.31 Lymph node biopsy from a man of 63 showing 'immunoblastic lymphadenopathy-like' peripheral T-cell lymphoma. Prominent clear cells are interspersed with many plasma cells, often in relation to the proliferating vessels. Some epithelioid cells are present (bottom of field). The patient had hyperglobulinaemia. (H E × 300)

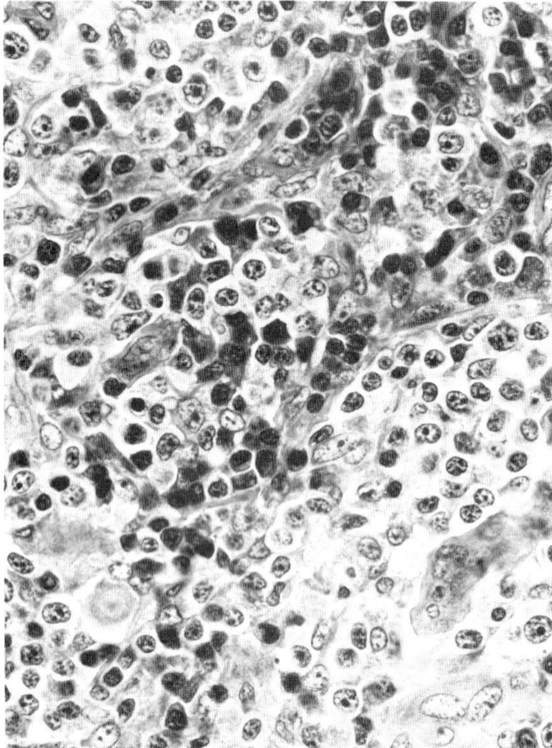

Fig. 12.32 Higher power view of the centre of the field in Fig. 12.31 to show detail of cellular infiltrate and arborising vessels (H E × 470)

Prognosis. The prognosis is slightly better than that of T-zone lymphoma or the pleomorphic T-cell lymphoma in terms of duration of survival, though apparently no better in regard to long term survival.

Differential diagnosis. The lymph node lesion in the early stages may easily be mistaken for an inflammatory process, but it should be noted that even when some lymph follicles persist, these do not have prominent germinal centres. Later on, the main differential diagnosis is with angioimmunoblastic lymphadenopathy. The problem of the identity or otherwise of these two conditions has been discussed above.

Overlapping features such as the presence of clear cells, prominent venules, eosinophils and epithelioid cells may cause confusion with other types of peripheral T-cell lymphoma — notably T-zone lymphoma and lymphoepithelioid lymphoma. The distinction is more of academic than practical importance. Confusion with Hodgkin's disease may occasionally arise.

Lymphoepithelioid T-cell lymphoma

Synonyms:
Epithelioid cellular lymphogranulomatosis.
Lennert's lymphoma.

Lennert & Mestdagh (1968) were the first to describe an uncommon but distinctive histopathological lesion in lymph nodes characterised by diffusely distributed small clusters of epithelioid cells. In the belief that this was a variant of Hodgkin's disease, the authors named the condition epithelioid cellular lymphogranulomatosis, but despite similarities to Hodgkin's disease, Sternberg-Reed cells were absent or very scanty. The condition affected elderly subjects and had a poor prognosis. Since the original account, there have been a number of further publications on what has become widely known as Lennert's lymphoma (Burke & Butler, 1976). One of the reasons for the continued debate on the nature of this unusual tumour is that there are several different disorders which may be mistaken for one another (see differential diagnosis below), but there are good grounds for regarding the classical Lennert's lymphoma as a distinct variety of peripheral T-cell lymphoma. This lesion has several histopathological features in common with other varieties of T-cell lymphoma already described. Vascular prominence is often seen, although the proliferation of blood vessels is seldom as striking as in the AIL type. Epithelioid histiocytes, as noted already, are a feature of several types of T-cell lymphoma, but none more so than the lymphoepithelioid lymphoma. Eosinophils are sometimes seen, but less consistently so than in the AIL type or T-zone lymphoma.

We have seen one case in which T-lymphocytic leukaemia developed during the course of the disease. The cells in the peripheral blood showed granular acid phosphatase activity.

Clinical features

This type of peripheral T-cell lymphoma is a disease of elderly people and shows a slight preponderance in women (Lennert, 1981). There may be widespread or localised lymphadenopathy at presentation, sometimes with hepatosplenomegaly, and tonsillar involvement was found at the outset in no less than one-quarter of Lennert's cases. Fever and loss of weight are commonly seen.

Pathological features

The most obvious feature of the histological picture is the presence of huge numbers of epithelioid histiocytes distributed throughout a node in which the normal architecture is effaced. The process begins in the paracortex and a few lymph follicles may remain for a time, but it is important to note that these show, at most, only small, inactive-looking germinal centres. The epithelioid cells lie singly or more often in uniform, small clusters which are at times so numerous as to virtually coalesce throughout large areas of the node (Fig. 12.33). The appearance of these conspicuous cells varies from case to case. Sometimes they resemble large rounded macrophages with abundant eosinophilic cytoplasm, having well defined cell boundaries and standing out sharply from their surroundings. More often, however, they have assumed the features of epithelioid cells with often vacuolated, eosinophilic cytoplasm and ill defined cell boundaries when they may appear to 'melt into the background' (Fig. 12.34). The nuclei may appear large and active with prominent nucleoli and a few mitoses are often seen amongst these cells. Multinucleate giant-cells of the same type are sometimes found. Dense masses of epithelioid cells may ensheath the larger blood vessels of the node and, in cases where the tumour has spread through the capsule, these same cells may infiltrate the sur-

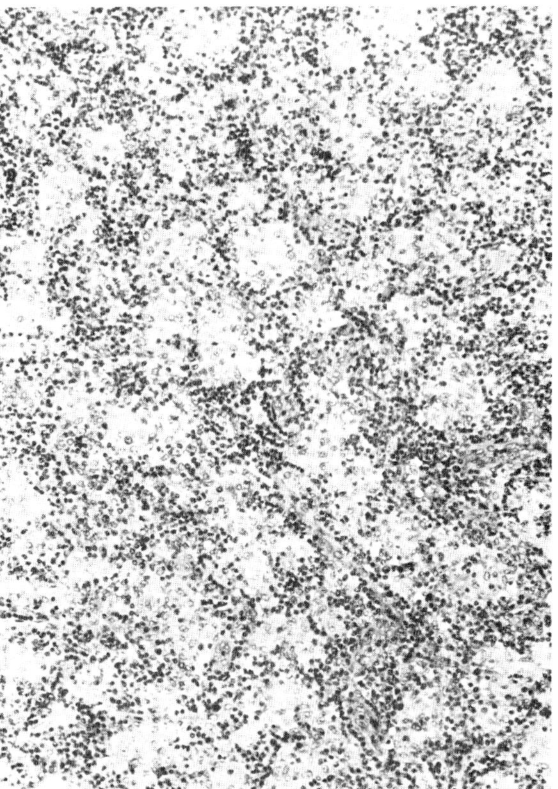

Fig. 12.34 Same node is Fig. 12.33 at a slightly higher magnification to show indistinct epithelioid cell clusters typical of the lymphoepithelioid cell lymphoma (H E × 120)

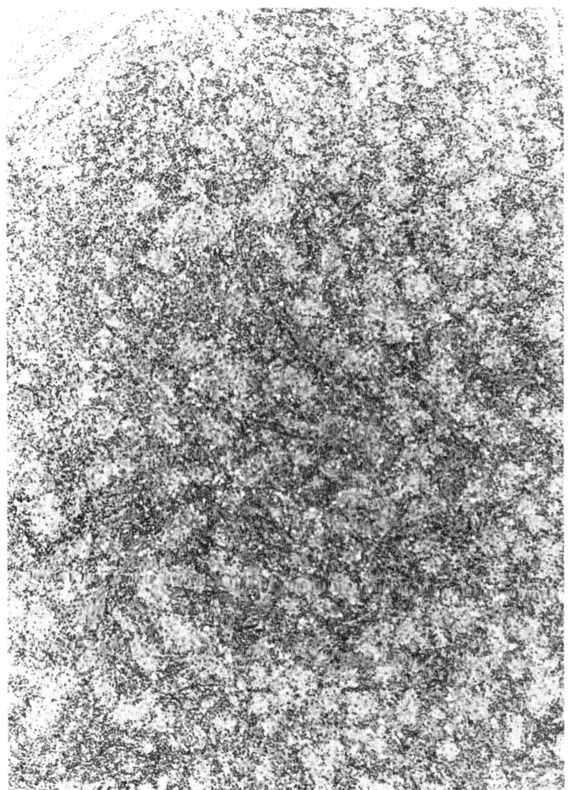

Fig. 12.33 Lymph node biopsy showing the lymphoepithelioid type of peripheral T-cell lymphoma (Lennert's lymphoma). Small clusters of pale-staining epithelioid cells are uniformly distributed throughout the node which shows loss of normal architecture with disappearance of follicles. (H E × 50)

rounding tissues. Venules may not be very noticeable in a routine-stained section, but PAS or reticulin staining will often reveal striking vascular proliferation (Fig. 12.35).

The essential cells of the neoplasm are intermingled with the reactive epithelioid cells. These consist of a dual population of small lymphocytes with irregular, angular nuclei and larger, blast-type cells, often showing some mitoses (Fig. 12.36). Occasional large, bizarre blast cells with a certain resemblance to Sternberg-Reed cells may also be found (Fig. 12.37). Plasma cells are absent or infrequent, but eosinophils are often present in small numbers.

The accumulation of epithelioid cells has been ascribed to the production of a lymphokine by the T-lymphocytes (Lennert, 1981). Their numbers appear to fluctuate in this, as in other peripheral T-cell lymphomas and their total disappearance at post-mortem has been observed (Kim et al, 1978).

Prognosis. The prognosis in these often elderly patients is poor and survival beyond 1–2 years from diagnosis is unusual.

Differential diagnosis. Lymphoepithelioid lymphoma (LEL) is liable to be confused with a variety of other lesions in which epithelioid cells are a prominent component. Most inflammatory disorders — notably toxoplasmosis and secondary syphilis, can be immediately excluded by the absence of follicular hyperplasia. In sarcoidosis the epithelioid cell groups are much larger, forming distinct granulomas.

The lesions which present the greatest difficulty in diagnosis are: (1) Hodgkin's disease with a large content of epithelioid cells; (2) some cases of lymphoplasmacytoid lymphoma (immunocytoma) which also present this feature: and (3) some cases of angioimmunoblastic lymphadenopathy (lympho-

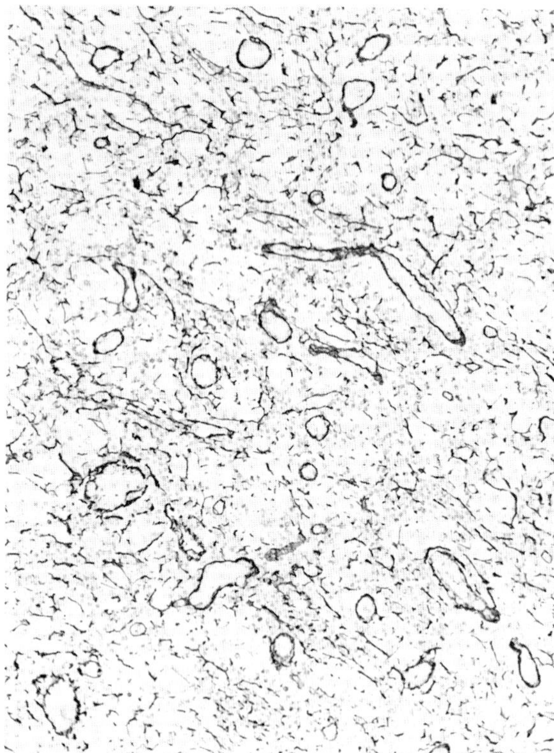

Fig. 12.35 Same node as Figs 12.33 and 12.34 stained for reticulin to show abundant venules (Gordon and Sweets reticulin × 120)

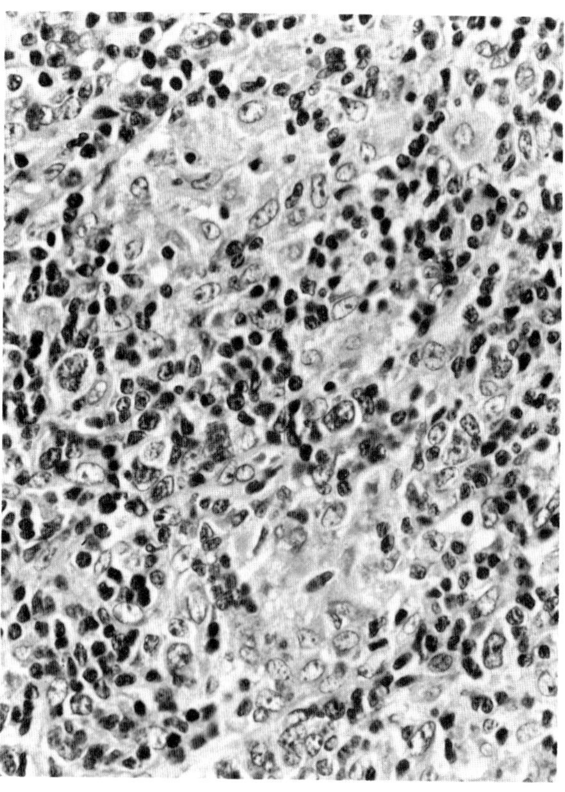

Fig. 12.36 Lymph node from a man of 58 showing, at a higher magnification, details of the cellular infiltrate in lympho-epithelioid lymphoma. Groups of epithelioid cells are seen, interspersed with T-lymphocytes and scattered, large, 'blast' cells. This patient subsequently developed a T-cell leukaemia of suppressor T-cell phenotype. (H E × 470)

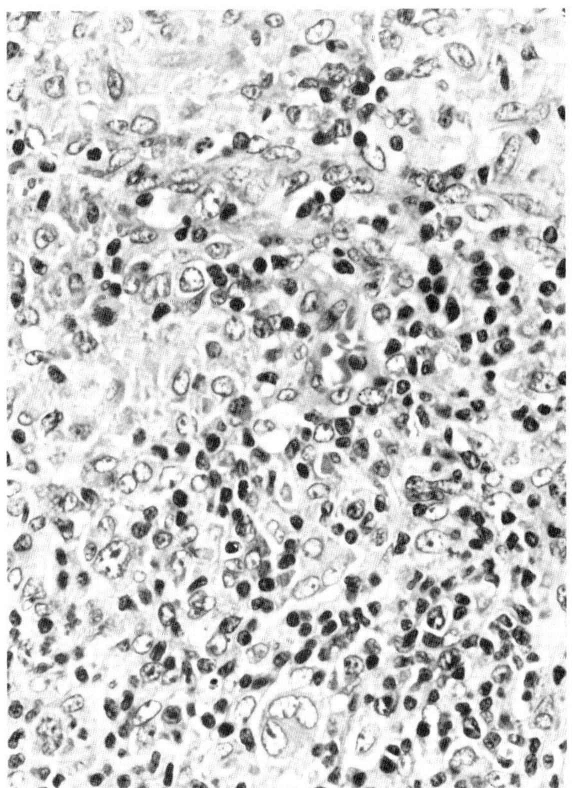

Fig. 12.37 Another field from the same node as Fig. 12.36, showing (below) a bizarre giant-cell resembling a Sternberg-Reed cell (H E × 470)

granulomatosis X) and/or the peripheral T-cell lymphoma of 'AIL type' (see p. 318). In each of the above the normal architecture is lost, and epithelioid cells may be seen in numbers comparable with those found in LEL. The differential diagnosis therefore depends upon a close and critical examination of the accompanying cells.

In Hodgkin's disease with a high content of epithelioid cells, the latter commonly form larger, more irregularly distributed aggregates or definite granulomas, but it has to be acknowledged that one occasionally sees the same, small, evenly distributed clusters of epithelioid cells in cases of unmistakeable Hodgkin's disease. As a rule Sternberg-Reed cells are found in this form of HD without too much difficulty, whilst Sternberg-Reed-like blast cells are much fewer in LEL and are generally smaller in size. Necrosis is more characteristic of HD, but is not invariable. The patients with HD are usually younger.

Some lymphoplasmacytoid lymphomas present similar histological features to those of Lennert's lymphoma. Loss of normal architecture is accompanied by vascular proliferation (less marked than in LEL) and prominent clusters of epithelioid cells throughout the node. However, the high content of plasma cells and lymphoplasmacytoid cells (monotypic for light chain) distinguish these tumours from a T-cell lymphoma. At times malignant lymphomas of immunoblastic type (either T or B) may show considerable numbers of epithelioid cells, but the large nuclei and prominent central nucleoli of the prevailing blast cells will generally make the distinction easy. As indicated in the last section, the AIL type of T-cell lymphoma has again many features in common with LEL, clear cells do not, however, apparently occur in Lennert's lymphoma whilst they are common in T-zone lymphoma and the AIL type. Plasma cells of polyclonal type also favour one of the latter diagnoses.

PLEOMORPHIC TYPES

The necessity for a strict definition of *pleomorphism* has been emphasised on page 301 but, as noted above, pleomorphism can only be a relative term when applied to the peripheral T-cell lymphomas, for irregularity of nuclear outline is commonly seen as a feature of many 'monomorphic' T-cell lymphomas too. It is just that nuclear pleomorphism is most extreme in the T-cell lymphomas of the pleomorphic group, whether or not the neoplastic cells show appreciable variation in size. Even in the pleomorphic tumours, however, there is much variation in the degree of nuclear pleomorphism from case to case. Perhaps the main justification for distinguishing this variable group of pleomorphic T-cell lymphomas is that it includes the virus-associated lymphomas and leukaemias found in endemic areas in Japan, the Caribbean basin and possibly elsewhere. Despite the variable morphology of these virus-associated T-cell neoplasms, they seem to form a homogeneous group in respect of their behavioural characteristics and very bad prognosis. It is not, however, always possible to distinguish morphologically virus-positive cases of peripheral T-cell lymphoma from similar tumours occurring sporadically in patients who show no evidence of virus infection (Lennert et al, 1985). It is therefore necessary to recognise the occurrence of rare instances of pleomorphic T-cell lymphoma, which do not appear to be associated with human T-lymphoma/leukaemia virus (HTLV)*. Failure to distinguish morphologically between virus positive and virus negative cases does not of course imply that such neoplasms are identical in all respects except for the presence or absence of HTLV and the natural history of the HTLV negative cases may well prove to be different.

Japanese pleomorphic type (Suchi et al, 1979)

Synonyms:
Adult T-cell leukaemia (JATL).
Caribbean T-cell lymphoma/leukaemia (CaTL).

This type of T-cell neoplasm has roused considerable interest in the past few years, initially in Japan, where it is the commonest type of peripheral T-cell neoplasm (Kikuchi et al, 1979, and others) and more recently in the West, with the discovery than an apparently identical disease occurs among blacks born in the Caribbean basin (Catovsky et al, 1982). In Japan this highly aggressive neoplasm is virtually confined to Japanese born in the Southernmost major island of Japan — Kyushu. The strict localisation of the disease to these two areas led to the discovery by Gallo and colleagues of a distinctive Type C retrovirus (HTLV) in Caribbean patients (Poiesz et al, 1980) and the later identification of the same virus in Japanese patients. Extensive epidemiological surveys are now in progress to discover the extent of HTLV infection, both within and outside endemic areas. It is clear from the discovery of antibodies to HTLV in healthy individuals that not every person harbouring the virus develops a malignant lymphoma. The situation may thus be analogous to the role of the EB virus in Burkitt's lymphoma. The mode of transmission is still unknown, but the virus is probably acquired early in life, possibly in utero, and the risk of developing the disease has been shown to be related to the place of birth, not that of subsequent residence (Catovsky et al, 1982).

Clinical and pathological descriptions of adult T-cell lymphoma/leukaemia in Japanese patients and in Caribbean patients are close enough to suggest that the disease is identical in the two endemic areas, wide as is the range of morphological appearances in these neoplasms.

Clinical features

JATL is a neoplasm of adult life, age range 16–78 (mean 52.7 ± 2.5) and sex ratio is 1 ♂:3 ♀ (Tajima et al, 1982). The age and sex incidence in the Caribbean cases are probably similar, though fewer have been studied.

The presentation is variable — leukaemia is present in over 80% of cases (Kikuchi et al, 1979), lymphadenopathy is common and at least 30% of patients are found to be hypercalcaemic. In a recent study of Caribbean adult lymphoma/leukaemia, all four patients had hypercalcaemia (Swerdlow et al, 1984). One patient in this series presented with appendiceal perforation due to lymphomatous involvement of the appendix. Overt evidence of bone disease is rare, but there is commonly diffuse or patchy marrow infiltration and a bone biopsy will frequently show enhanced osteoclastic activity. The latter has been attributed to the production of an osteoclast-activating factor by the neoplastic cells and this is probably responsible for the hypercalcaemia (Grossman et al, 1981). Skin involvement is reported to be common in Japanese patients, although it has not as yet been a significant feature of Caribbean cases.

Pathological features

The following account is based on a personal study of cases of Caribbean T-cell lymphoma/leukaemia presenting in London and on a later study of Japanese cases. An account of the histopathological features in Caribbean cases has also been published by O'Brien et al (1983). One of the remarkable characteristics of this neoplasm is the variation in the cytological and histological appearances between one case and another — a variation which

* Now known as HTLV 1, to distinguish this from other, more recently discovered, human T-lymphotropic viruses HTLV 2 and HTLV 3. The last has been identified as the probable cause of acquired immunodeficiency syndrome (AIDS).

may reflect rapid alterations in the morphology of the neoplasm in a single patient.

Macroscopically, there is nothing distinctive about the involved nodes.

Histologically, affected nodes show a variable degree of architectural effacement. Small nodes may show preservation of follicles, at least to some degree, and patent lymph sinuses, so that close examination may be needed to observe that the pulp and sinuses are infiltrated by variable-sized lymphocytes with highly irregular, often cerebriform or multilobed nuclei (Fig. 12.38). It is these 'cloverleaf' cells which commonly appear in the blood stream, sometimes in considerable numbers, in the leukaemic phase (Fig. 12.38, inset).

However, the cytological features of this distinctive type of leukaemia are not necessarily reflected in the lymph node biopsy, for the latter may show varying degrees of transformation of the lymphoma cells — sometimes partial (Fig. 12.39), sometimes total (Fig. 12.40). Successive lymph node biopsies from one patient, taken 6 weeks apart, showed a striking increase in the number of blasts and in the degree of anaplasia of the neoplastic cells over this short space of time (Fig. 12.41a & b). The larger blast-type cells may or may not show the irregular nuclear shapes that are characteristic of the smaller and medium-sized

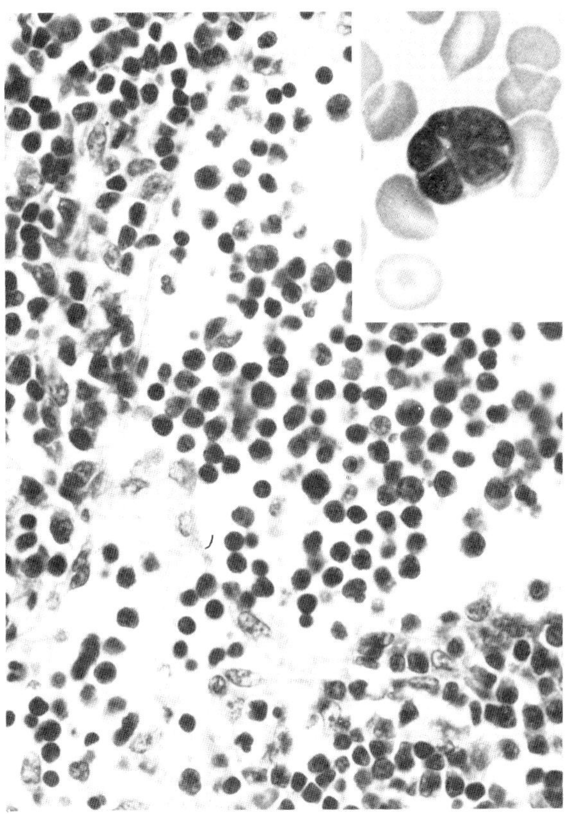

Fig. 12.38 Mesenteric lymph node from a young West Indian woman who presented with hypercalcaemia and abdominal pain. At laparotomy perforation of an infiltrated appendix was found. She was then discovered to have leukaemia which advanced rapidly despite aggressive treatment until her death a few weeks later. (Case referred to in text on page 324. HTLV-positive). The figure shows a dilated lymph sinus filled with variable-sized lymphocytes many having highly irregular, multilobed nuclei. There are few transformed cells. (H E × 120) Inset: Lymphoid cell with 'cloverleaf' nucleus typical of the cells in the peripheral blood of this patient. Note abnormal red cells. (May-Grünwald Giemsa × 1175)

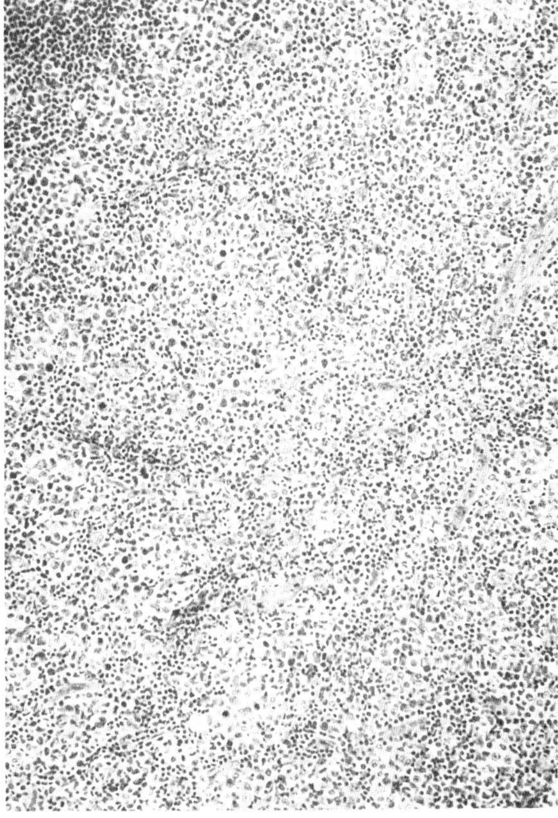

Fig. 12.39 Pleomorphic T-cell lymphoma (HTLV-positive). Lymph node biopsy in an adult Japanese patient showing characteristic variation in cell size with partial transformation. Part of a surviving follicle is seen (top left). Note prominent venules in the tumour. This patient did not have leukaemia, although leukaemia was present in a Caribbean patient whose node biopsy presented a similar picture. (H E × 120)

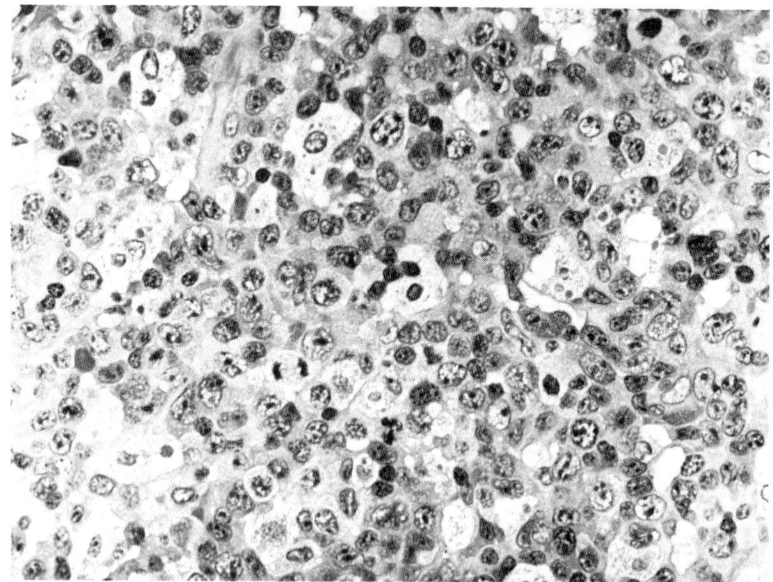

Fig. 12.40 Pleomorphic T-cell lymphoma (HTLV-positive, with leukaemia and hypercalcaemia) in a West Indian woman of 22. The initial lymph node biopsy (shown here) shows a diffuse infiltrate composed entirely of transformed cells interspersed with many macrophages (paler staining). The cells in the peripheral blood were not 'blast' cells. (H E × 470)

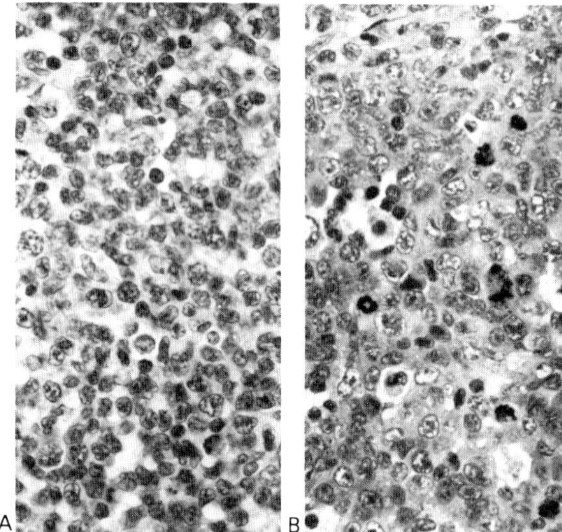

Fig. 12.41 (a) and (b) Two lymph node biopsies, taken 6 weeks apart, from a West Indian woman of 49 showing rapid transformation in a pleomorphic T-cell lymphoma (HTLV-positive, with leukaemia and hypercalcaemia). (a) The first biopsy shows only small numbers of transformed cells although the nuclear irregularity of the medium-sized lymphocytes can be clearly seen. (b) In the second biopsy the cells are much larger and more variable with enhanced mitotic activity and many atypical mitoses. (Both H E × 470)

cells. However, in the cases of mixed, medium and large cell type, the nuclear pleomorphism reaches its zenith and cells of all sizes tend to exhibit bizarre nuclear shapes. Often deep indentations are seen along one side of the nucleus which has a smooth, convex outline on the other side, resulting in shapes likened to a jellyfish, an embryo or a bunch of bananas (Fig. 12.42). The nuclear chromatin is often coarsely clumped and irregular mitoses are frequently seen. Sternberg-Reed-like cells are common (Fig. 12.43), but these are less characteristic of the Japanese pleomorphic T-cell lymphoma than are large blast-type cells with convoluted nuclei and smaller nucleoli (Kikuchi, 1983).

Cases showing this extreme degree of pleomorphism generally prove to be HTLV-positive, but not all virus positive cases are like this. Some are composed predominantly of much more uniform cells of medium or large size (Fig. 12.40) and in these cases morphology is a poor guide to the presence or absence of virus.

Prognosis. The prognosis of adult T-cell lymphoma/leukaemia is extremely grave and most patients are dead within one year, although a few have survived for longer periods. Some patients go

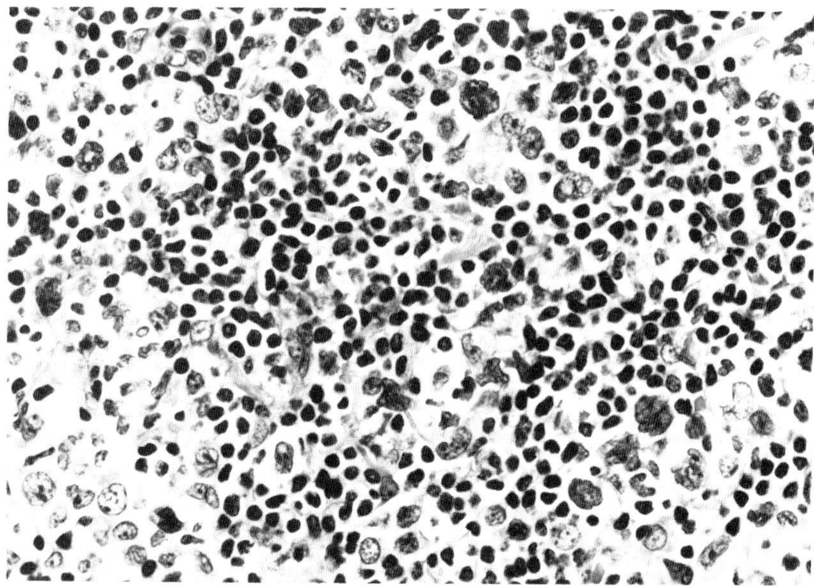

Fig. 12.42 Japanese pleomorphic T-cell lymphoma (same case as Fig. 12.39). Higher magnification shows the degree of nuclear pleomorphism, especially evident here in some of the larger cells. The large cells at top right are characteristic. (H E × 470)

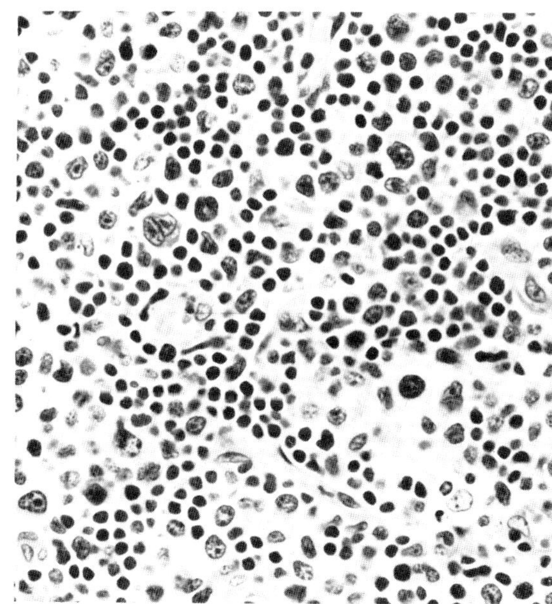

Fig. 12.43 Lymph node biopsy from another Caribbean patient with a pleomorphic T-cell lymphoma (HTLV-positive, leukaemia present). The bizarre nuclear shapes are less evident here than in Fig. 12.42 but the variation in cell size is well shown. A Sternberg-Reed-like cell is present in this field (left upper quadrant). (H E × 470)

into remission with aggressive chemotherapy, but as a rule remissions are of brief duration. Death commonly results from infection or hypercalcaemia.

Differential diagnosis. Hypercalcaemia is a rare event in other types of malignant lymphoma or leukaemia, and its occurrence in any patient with a lymphoproliferative disorder should arouse a suspicion of adult T-cell lymphoma/leukaemia, especially in a West Indian or Japanese patient. The polymorphic cell picture and the presence of Sternberg-Reed-like cells may lead to a suspicion of Hodgkin's disease, but the picture as a whole differs from that of HD in the extreme pleomorphism of the nuclei in cells of all sizes — small as well as large. In leukaemic cases, the distinctive morphology of the lymphoid cells in the blood or marrow will help to confirm the diagnosis, as will the presence of antibodies to HTLV.

However, there are rare instances of HTLV-negative pleomorphic T-cell lymphomas, which occur in Europe and other non-endemic areas (see next section). Such patients do not as a rule have hypercalcaemia and leukaemia is much less frequent than it is in HTLV-positive cases, but morphologically their tumours may be indistinguishable. It should be noted that although these pleo-

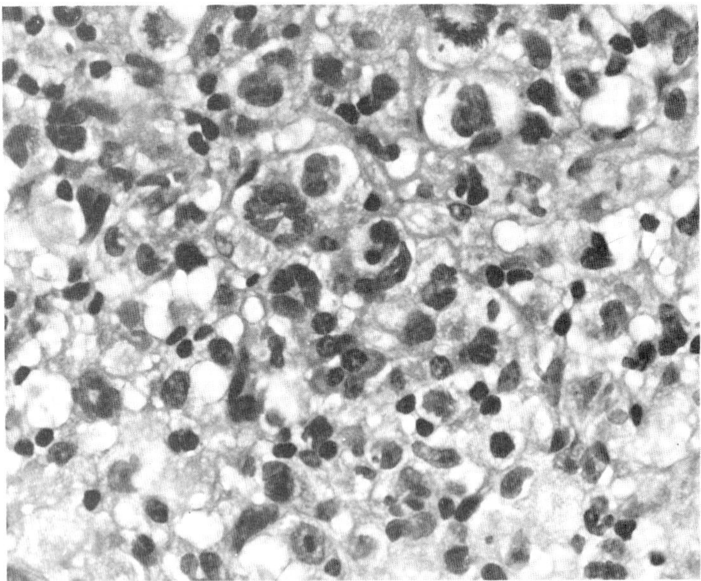

Fig. 12.44 European case of pleomorphic T-cell lymphoma (HTLV-negative: leukaemia absent). The field shows typical nuclear pleomorphism with a group of bizarre cells at the centre and reactive plasma cells below. (H E × 470)

morphic T-cell lymphomas may show prominent venules, this is not such a striking feature as it is in the case of the monomorphic types. Moreover, interdigitating reticulum cells, epithelioid cells and eosinophils are generally absent or inconspicuous.

Non-endemic pleomorphic type

As mentioned above, sporadic instances of pleomorphic T-cell lymphoma may occasionally be met with in Europe and probably elsewhere. Although such tumours may closely resemble the Japanese and Caribbean pleomorphic T-cell lymphomas in their morphology (Fig. 12.44), the cases are HTLV negative and leukaemia appears to be a less frequent accompaniment than it is in HTLV positive cases.

Within the next few years, some clarification of the peripheral T-cell lymphomas may occur, but it is likely that these will always remain a difficult group of neoplasms for the histopathologist for the reasons set out at the beginning of this chapter.

REFERENCES

Boumsell L, Bernard A, Reinherz E L, Nadler L M, Ritz J, Coppin H et al 1981 Surface antigens on malignant Sézary and T-CLL cells correspond to those of mature T cells. Blood 57: 526–530

Brouet J C, Flandrin G, Sasportes M, Preud'homme J L, Seligmann M 1975 Chronic lymphocytic leukaemia of T-cell origin. Immunological and clinical evaluation in 11 patients. Lancet 2: 890–893

Burke J S, Butler J J 1967 Malignant lymphoma with a high content of epithelioid histiocytes (Lennert's lymphoma). American Journal of Clinical Pathology 66: 1–9.

Catovsky D, Greaves M F, Rose M et al 1982 Adult T-cell lymphoma-leukaemia in blacks from the West Indies. Lancet 1: 639–643

Collins R D, Waldron J A, Glick A D 1979 Results of multiparameter studies of T-cell lymphoid neoplasms. American Journal of Clinical Pathology 72: 699–707

Costello C, Catovsky D, O'Brien M, Morilla R, Varadi S 1980 Chronic T-cell leukaemias I Morphology, cytochemistry and ultrastructure. Leukaemia Research 4: 463–476

Cullen M H, Stansfeld A G, Oliver R T D, Lister T A, Malpas J S 1979 Angioimmunoblastic lymphadenopathy: report of ten cases and review of the literature. Quarterly Journal of Medicine 48 No 189: 151–177

Grossman B, Schechter G P, Horton J E, Pierce L, Jaffe E, Wahl L 1981 Hypercalcemia associated with T-cell

lymphoma-leukaemia. American Journal of Clinical Pathology 75: 149–155
Hanaoka M, Sasaki M, Matsumoto H, Tankawa H, Yamabe H, Tominoto K et al 1979 Adult T cell leukemia — histological classification and characteristics. Acta Pathologica of Japan 29: 723–738
Kadin M E, Kamoun M, Lamberg J 1981 Erythrophagocytic Tγ lymphoma — a clinicopathologic entity resembling malignant histiocytosis. New England Journal of Medicine 304: 648–653
Kikuchi M, Mitsui T, Matsui N, Sato E, Tokunaga M, Hasui K et al 1979 T-cell malignancies in adults: histopathological studies of lymph nodes in 110 patients. Japanese Journal of Clinical Oncology 9 (supplement): 407–422
Kikuchi M 1983 Personal communication
Kim H, Jacobs C, Warnke R A, Dorfman R F 1978 Malignant lymphoma with a high content of epithelioid histiocytes — a distinct clinicopathological entity and a form of so-called Lennert's lymphoma. Cancer 41: 620–635
Kim H, Nathwani B N, Rappaport H 1980 So-called 'Lennert's lymphoma' — is it a clinicopathologic entity? Cancer 45: 1379–1399
Knowles D M, Halper J P 1982 Human T-cell malignancies: correlative clinical, histopathologic, immunologic and cytochemical analysis of 23 cases. American Journal of Pathology 106: 187–203
Lennert K 1981 Histopathology of non-Hodgkin's lymphomas (based on the Kiel classification). Springer-Verlag, Berlin
Lennert K, Mestdagh J 1968 Lymphogranulomatosen mit konstant hohem Epithelioidzellgehalt. Virchows Archiv (Pathol Anat) 344: 1–20
Lennert K in collaboration with Mohri N, Stein H, Kaiserling E, Müller-Hermelink H K 1978 Malignant lymphomas other than Hodgkin's disease. Springer-Verlag, Berlin
Lennert K, Stein H, Feller A C, Gerdes J 1983 Morphology, cytochemistry and immunohistology of T cell lymphomas. In: Vitetta E S (ed) B and T cell tumors: UCLA Symposium on Molecular and Cellular Biology No 24, p 9–28
Lennert K, Kikuchi M, Feller A C, Sato E, Müller-Hermelink H K, Stansfeld A G, Suchi T 1985 ATLV-positive and negative T-cell lymphomas. Morphological and immunohistochemical differences. International Journal of Cancer (in press)
Levine A 1981 In: Proceedings of the Second International Lymphoma Conference, Athens, Greece, April 5–10, 1981
Lukes R J 1979 The immunologic approach to the pathology of malignant lymphomas. American Journal of Clinical Pathology 72: 657–669
Lutzner M A, Jordan H W 1968 The ultrastructure of an abnormal cell in Sézary's syndrome. Blood 31: 719–726
Lutzner M A, Hobbs J W, Horvath P 1971 Ultrastructure of abnormal cells in Sézary syndrome, mycosis fungoides, and parapsoriasis en plaque. Archives of Dermatology 103: 375–386
Nathwani B N, Rappaport H, Moran E M, Pangalis G A, Kim H 1978 Malignant lymphoma arising in angioimmunoblastic lymphadenopathy. Cancer 41: 578–606
O'Brien C, Lampert I A, Catovsky D 1983 The histopathology of adult T-cell lymphoma/leukaemia in blacks from the Caribbean. Histopathology 7: 349–364
Pallesen G, Madsen M, Hastrup J 1981 Large-cell T-lymphoma with hypersegmented nuclei. Scandinavian Journal of Haematology 26: 72–79
Pinkus G S, Said J W, Hargreaves H 1979 Malignant lymphoma, T-cell type — a distinct morphologic variant with large multilobated nuclei, with a report of four cases. American Journal of Clinical Pathology 72: 540–550
Poiesz B J, Ruscetti F W, Gazdar A F, Bunn P A, Minna J D, Gallo R C 1980 Detection and isolation of type C retrovirus particles from fresh and cultured lymphocytes of a patient with cutaneous T-cell lymphoma. Proceedings of the National Academy of Sciences of the United States of America 77: 7415–7419
Rappaport H, Thomas L B 1974 Mycosis fungoides: the pathology of extracutaneous involvement. Cancer 34: 1198–1229
Said J W, Pinkus G S 1980 Immunoblastic sarcoma of the T-cell type — an ultrastructural study of five cases. American Journal of Pathology 101: 515–526
Shimoyama M, Minato K, Saito H, Takenaka T, Watanabe S, Nagatani T, Naruto M 1979 Immunoblastic lymphadenopathy (IBL)-like T-cell lymphoma. Japanese Journal of Clinical Oncology 9 (Supplement 1): 347–356
Suchi T, Tajima K, Nanba K, Wakasa H, Mikata A, Kikuchi M et al 1979 Some problems on the histopathological diagnosis of non-Hodgkin's malignant lymphoma — a proposal of a new type. Acta Pathologica of Japan 29: 755–776
Swerdlow S H, Habeshaw J A, Rohatiner A Z S, Lister T A, Stansfeld A G 1984 Caribbean T-cell lymphoma leukaemia. Cancer 54: 687–696
Tajima K, Tominaga S, Suchi T 1982 Clinico-epidemiological analysis of adult T cell leukemia. GANN Monograph on Cancer Research 28: 197–210
van der Putte S C J, Toonstra J, de Weger R A, van Unnik J A M 1982 Cutaneous T-cell lymphoma, multilobated type. Histopathology 6: 35–54
Waldron J A, Leech J H, Glick A D, Flexner J M, Collins R D 1977 Malignant lymphoma of peripheral T-lymphocyte origin. Cancer 40: 1604–1617
Watanabe S, Nakajima I, Shimosato Y, Shimoyama M, Minato K 1979 T-cell malignancies: subclassification and interrelationship. Japanese Journal of Clinical Oncology 9 (Supplement): 423–442
Watanabe S, Shimosato Y, Shimoyama M, Minato K, Suzuki M, Abe M, Nagatani T 1980 Adult T-cell lymphoma with hypergammaglobulinemia. Cancer 46: 2472–2483
Watanabe S, Shimosato Y, Shimoyama M 1981 Lymphoma and leukemia of T-lymphocytes. Pathology Annual 16 (Part 2): 155–203
Weinberg D S, Pinkus G S 1981 Non-Hodgkin's lymphoma of large multilobated cell type — a clinicopathologic study of ten cases. American Journal of Clinical Pathology 76: 190–196
Weisenburger D D, Nathwani B N, Forman S J, Rappaport H 1982 Noncutaneous peripheral T-cell lymphoma histologically resembling mycosis fungoides. Cancer 49: 1839–1847

13

J. A. L. Ames

Lymph nodes in primarily haematological disorders

This chapter considers those conditions which are generally looked upon as the province of the haematologist, although often having implication for the histopathologist in the interpretation of a lymph node biopsy. The major part of the chapter will concentrate on the leukaemias, excluding chronic lymphocytic leukaemia and prolymphocytic leukaemia which have been discussed in connection with lymphocytic lymphoma in Chapter 10. Myeloid metaplasia and mastocytosis will also be considered.

Haematologists make a diagnosis by combining knowledge of the clinical state of the patient, the peripheral blood count, blood film morphology and, where necessary, examination of the bone-marrow aspirate and trephine sections. However, the final diagnosis may require close liaison between the haematologist and histopathologist. The haematologist may also be helped in the interpretation of the bone-marrow aspirate by examining a lymph node imprint.

A Romanowsky technique is used for the routine staining of the peripheral blood film and bone-marrow aspirate. Haematoxylin and eosin (H E) and a silver impregnation stain are usually used in the examination of the bone-marrow trephines. The use of additional cytochemical stains will be discussed in the appropriate sections of the chapter.

LEUKAEMIA

Introduction

In 1845, Virchow, when describing the blood of a patient with hepatosplenomegaly and an increased number of white bodies in the blood used the term 'Weisses Blut'. In a paper 2 years later he introduced the term leukaemia (white blood). This term, however, failed to specify the site of the basic pathological condition. The importance of the bone-marrow in the production of blood cells in health and disease was demonstrated by Neumann in 1870. A full historical background to leukaemia has been set out in a review by Gunz & Baikie (1974).

The leukaemias might best be described as a group of malignant diseases of the blood-forming organs. In their typical evolution there is a progressive replacement of normal bone-marrow and lymphatic tissues by either myeloid or lymphoid leucocytes with varying degrees of maturity. In rare instances the predominant proliferating cells may be erythroid or megakaryocyte precursors. The abnormal cells are usually found in the peripheral blood. Patients with malignant lymphomas commonly have blood and bone-marrow involvement. However, this group of diseases is not usually considered under the general heading of leukaemia.

The leukaemias are divided into acute and chronic types. These terms were initially used to denote the survival of the untreated patient. However, the haematologist now uses 'acute' to describe the leukaemias where the predominant cells in the bone-marrow are blasts and, 'chronic' where the main cells are mature granulocytes, monocytes or lymphocytes. The acute leukaemias will be first considered and within this section chloroma and mastocytosis will be discussed.

ACUTE LEUKAEMIAS

The acute leukaemias are characterised by the replacement of normal bone-marrow elements by blast cells or immature leucocytes, e.g. promyelocytes or 'promonocytes'. This usually leads to a decrease in the normal cells and the appearance of blast cells in the peripheral blood. The diagnosis is made from the blood film and bone-marrow aspirate. In the majority of patients, examination of the blood and bone-marrow slides, stained by a Romanowsky technique, leads to the division of the acute leukaemias into two main groups, myeloblastic and lymphoblastic. The use of cytochemical stains, particularly the myeloperoxidase or sudan black B stains, which are positive in acute myeloblastic leukaemia (AML), aid the recognition of these groups. The French-American-British (FAB) Co-operative Group (Bennett et al, 1976) have suggested six main morphological types of AML (M1–M6) (Table 13.1) and three morphological types of acute lymphoblastic leukaemia (L1–L3).

Table 13.1 Morphological classification of acute myeloblastic leukaemia (FAB Co-operative Group)

	Acute myeloblastic leukaemia (AML)	Characteristic cell
M1	Myeloblastic leukaemia without maturation	Myeloblast
M2	Myeloblastic leukaemia with maturation	Myeloblast with maturation beyond the promyelocyte
M3	Promyelocytic leukaemia	Promyelocyte
M4	Myelomonocytic leukaemia	Myeloblast with differentiation to mature monocytes
M5	Monoblastic leukaemia	Monoblast
M6	Erythroleukaemia	Myeloblasts and proerythroblasts
*	Megakaryoblastic leukaemia	

* No FAB classification

In the L1 type the blast cells are typically small and homogeneous in appearance, in L2 the blasts are large and heterogeneous and in L3 the blasts are those seen with Burkitt's lymphoma. The L1 type represents the acute lymphoblastic leukaemia (ALL) most commonly seen in childhood.

The Romanowsky stained films continue to be the mainstay in the diagnosis of acute leukaemias. However, the combination of morphology, chromosome analysis and membrane and enzyme markers has helped in the recognition of important subtypes. For example, the Philadelphia chromosome is present in as many as 25% of adult patients presenting with ALL (Bloomfield et al, 1978). The FAB classification of ALL does not allow definite differentiation between common ALL (non-B, non-T), T-ALL and B-ALL, although many of the former are of L1 morphology and the latter of L3 type. The acid phosphatase reaction is positive in the blast cells of the majority of cases of T-derived ALL, with typical localisation in a small paranuclear area (Catovsky et al, 1974a; Brouet et al, 1976). However, most information has been gained by the investigation of cell surface antigens and other cell enzymes. The techniques that are used in the diagnosis of acute leukaemia have recently been reviewed by Catovsky et al (1981).

Lymph node changes

Enlargement of the superficial lymph nodes, liver and spleen occurs commonly in acute leukaemia. At presentation lymphadenopathy is present in approximately 80% of ALL and 50% of AML (Boggs et al, 1962). When tissue is biopsied from a patient with acute leukaemia then fresh imprints should be made and stained using a Romanowsky technique. Failure to do this may lead to misinterpretation of the lymph node histology.

Macroscopically the lymph nodes are discrete and slightly to moderately enlarged; usually their consistency shows no appreciable deviation from the normal.

Histology. The characteristic changes in all acute leukaemias consist of extensive replacement of the normal cellular elements of the lymph node by a diffuse proliferation of primitive cells (Figs 13.1 and 13.2). This infiltration appears to begin at the centre of the node and to extend peripherally, so that collections of lymphocytes at the periphery of the cortex (not necessarily representing complete follicles) often remain when the rest of the node has been overrun. Adult nodes, which had previously shown central fatty involution, tend to show leukaemic infiltration of the hilar fat. Massive infiltration of the perinodal fat, with practically complete obliteration of the capsule, is often evident, especially in childhood T-ALL. In all but the rare L3 (Burkitt's) type the cells have delicate,

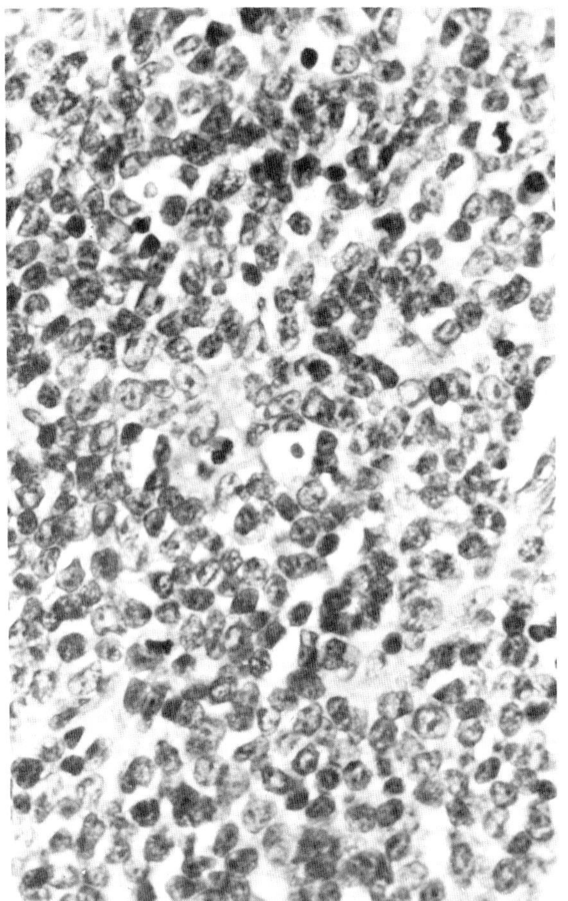

Fig. 13.1 Lymph node involvement in acute myeloblastic leukaemia. Most of the infiltrating myeloblasts have fairly small and often multiple nucleoli. (H E × 500)

Fig. 13.2 Lymph node involvement in acute lymphoblastic leukaemia of common type (H E × 500)

evenly distributed chromatin and small rather inconspicuous nucleoli.

Although in the two examples illustrated (Figs 13.1, 13.2) the cells appear quite distinct, the differentiation of AML from ALL is often difficult. It depends primarily upon the identification of cells that show evidence of early granulocytic or monocytic differentiation. The latter can be distinguished by their indented and lobulated nuclei (Forkner, 1934). Early granulocytic differentiation may be most easily detected in the perivascular infiltrates in the hilar region or along the trabeculae. Here the cells are often less tightly packed and it is easier to observe that a proportion of the neoplastic cells show an appreciable increase of somewhat eosinophilic cytoplasm. When eosinophil myelocytes are present these readily attract attention. The chloroacetate esterase stain is positive in the granulocytic series, its reactivity increasing with cell maturity (Figs 13.3, 13.4). It should be remembered, however, that positivity will also be present if there is extramedullary haematopoiesis and that mast cells are also strongly positive. A negative result does not necessarily exclude myeloblastic leukaemia, if the cells are all of undifferentiated type. The introduction of immunostaining with monoclonal antibodies will refine the diagnosis of these disorders. These techniques have been discussed in Chapters 3 and 4.

Chloroma

Synonyms: chloromyeloma, chloromyelosarcoma,

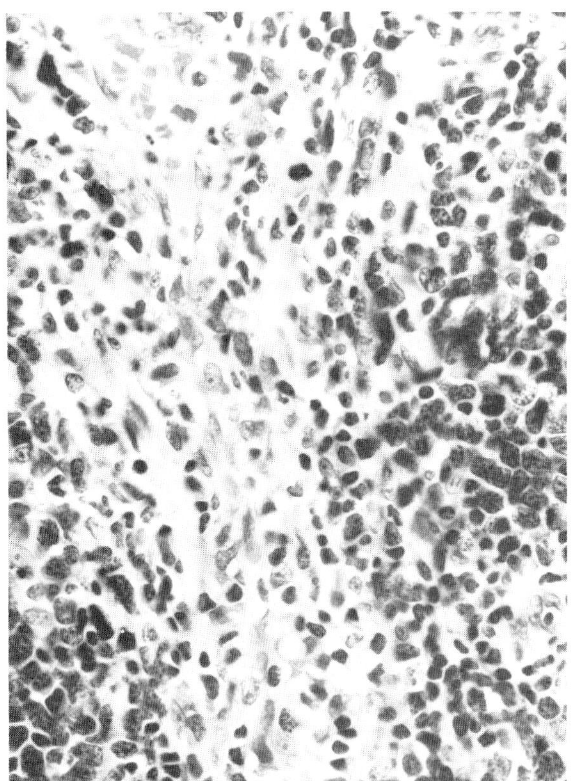

Fig. 13.3 Lymph node in myeloblastic leukaemia showing some maturation of the infiltrating cells around a trabecular vessel, in contrast with the undifferentiated myeloblasts throughout most of the node pulp (H E × 470)

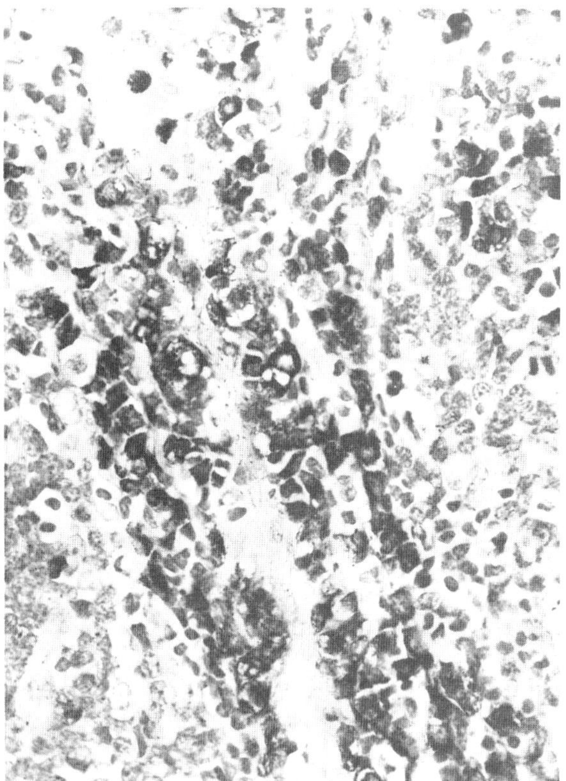

Fig. 13.4 Same field as Fig. 13.3 stained by the α-naphthyl chloroacetate esterase method showing a positive reaction in many of the slightly more mature cells. The granules which have appear black, show up a bright red by this method. (CAE × 470)

granulocytic leukosarcoma, granulocytic sarcoma, myeloblastic sarcoma, myeloblastoma, myelocytoma and myelosarcoma.

This may be considered as a variant of AML. It is characterised by the formation of invasive and destructive tumour masses that are usually green in appearance to the naked-eye and are composed of immature cells of the granulocytic series. The name is derived from the observation that the cut surface of such tumours transiently turns green when exposed to light, a phenomenon that probably reflects the myeloperoxidase content of the cellular lysosomes (Schultz & Schwartz, 1956).

In some patients chloromas appear before there is evidence of AML on examination of the blood and marrow (Krause, 1979). Moreover, generalised AML may not become evident for up to 3 years (Brugo et al, 1977; Mason et al, 1973). Chloromas usually occur in bone, often presenting subperiostally, but almost any organ may be affected. A tumour of the orbit is the classical presentation (Ross, 1955), however the site of initial disease is quite variable: including lymph nodes, stomach, ileum, breast, tonsil, pericardium, skin and spinal epidural area (Brugo et al, 1977; Krause, 1979; Long & Mihm, 1977; Mason et al, 1973). It is not known why a minority of cases of myeloblastic neoplasia present with a localised, destructive tumour, whilst most show only diffuse, nondestructive, 'leukaemic' infiltration.

Histology. Chloromas are firm to hard in consistency. As in the development of 'localised blast crisis' of chronic myeloid leukaemia (p. 339) the chloroma may be mistaken for a lymphoma or even an undifferentiated carcinoma (Long & Mihm, 1977). In questionable cases the use of tis-

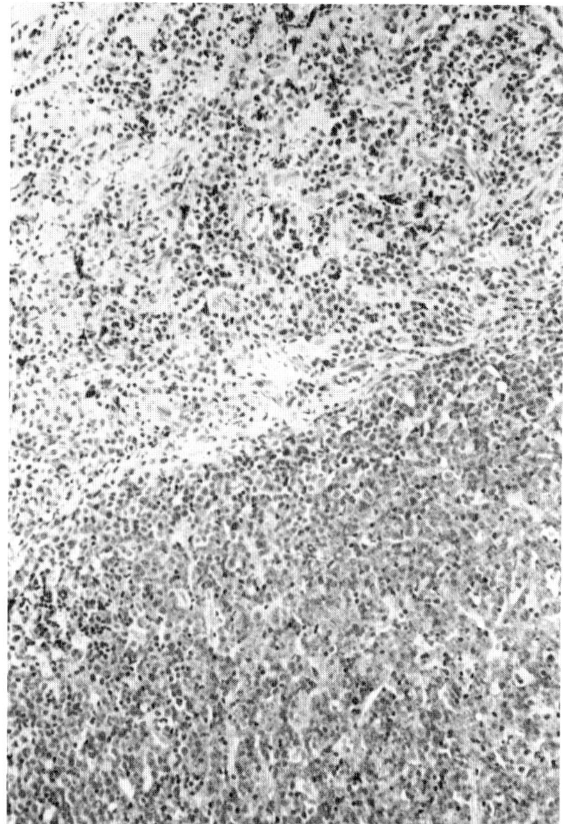

Fig. 13.5 Chloroma (myeloblastic sarcoma) in a lymph node, showing capsular invasion (top). A few residual lymphocytes are seen in the cortex (left). (H E × 120)

sue imprints and special stains, such as the chloroacetate esterase method, will lead to the correct diagnosis (Krause, 1979; Seo et al, 1977). Chloromas are usually composed of myeloblasts (Figs 13.5, 13.6), however, the granulocytic nature of the proliferation becomes more apparent when myelocytes accompany the blastic proliferation; even more mature cell forms are sometimes observed. The aggressive nature of the neoplasm is microscopically apparent not only from its unrestrained growth through such tough and resistant tissue as the periosteum but also from its massive and destructive infiltration of non-haemopoietic organs.

Mastocytosis

It seems appropriate to include this disorder under the general heading of AML, since there is evidence that the mast cell is derived from the pluripotent myeloid stem cell (Turpin et al, 1978), and there are rare instances of an overlap between mastocytosis and AML. Mastocytosis denotes an increased number of normal or abnormal mast cells in various tissues. The most common form of mastocytosis is a cutaneous disease, urticaria pigmentosa (Nettleship, 1869). This is usually a benign, self-limiting condition in children; however, when multiple lesions develop in adults this usually signifies the beginning of a chronic or progressive systemic disease (Berlin, 1955; Caplan, 1963). In systemic mastocytosis mast cells infiltrate the lymph nodes, liver, lungs, bones, bone-marrow, spleen or any organ which contains mesenchymal tissue (Sagher & Even-Paz, 1967). Skin involvement is not invariable in such cases and, when present, may take the form of localised tumour nodules rather than diffuse pigmented le-

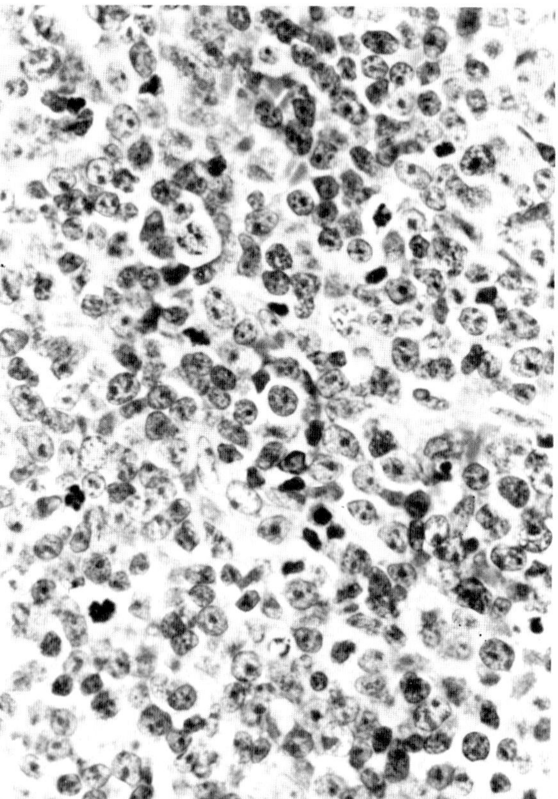

Fig. 13.6 Higher magnification of same node as Fig. 13.5 to show details of cells (H E × 500)

sions. In extreme cases of systemic mastocytosis, large numbers of mast cells are found in the blood, leading some authors to apply the term mast cell leukaemia (Coser et al, 1980; Daniel et al, 1975; Parker, 1976).

Increased numbers of mature mast cells are found in the bone-marrow of elderly women with skeletal demineralisation and in particles of marrow aspirated from patients with aplastic anaemia (Frame & Nixon, 1968), hypoplastic anaemia and mature cell lymphoproliferative diseases (Nixon, 1966). None of these, however, represents a premalignant mast cell proliferation and the mast cells in these conditions are diffusely dispersed, not aggregated together in masses.

Histology. In systemic mastocytosis most organs and tissues show varying degrees of infiltration by tissue mast cells. In mild cases, mature, fully granulated mast cells are dispersed through the tissue in increased numbers. These oval or rounded cells in an HE stained section resemble large eosinophils, in that the abundant cytoplasm is filled with eosinophilic granules. The nucleus, however. is different and the granules stain less brightly that those of an eosinophil leucocyte. More massive infiltrates generally contain a high proportion of more immature cells with few or no cytoplasmic granules (Fig. 13.7). These cells are spindle-shaped, resembling fibroblasts or histiocytes in routinely stained sections, though often showing a rather distinctive, 'clear' cytoplasm. The association of such cells with mature, granulated mast cells, and with eosinophil leucocytes as well, may lead to a suspicion of mastocytosis; the diagnosis can be confirmed by the use of more-specific staining methods. The granules are well shown by staining with alcian blue at a pH 2, as in the combined Unna Pappenheim-alcian blue method (p. 40). Toluidine blue or Giemsa staining will show the metachromasia of the granules (Fig. 13.7) and they are positive also for chloroacetate esterase (unlike eosinophil granules). There is often some degree of collagen deposition in association with these solid infiltrates of mastocytosis and in long-standing cases fibrosis may be very extensive, overshadowing the mast cell infiltration. Bone-marrow infiltration may be focal, diffuse or both; marrow fibrosis and sclerosis are commonly present. The pathological features of mast cell disease have been well reviewed by Lennert & Parwaresch (1979).

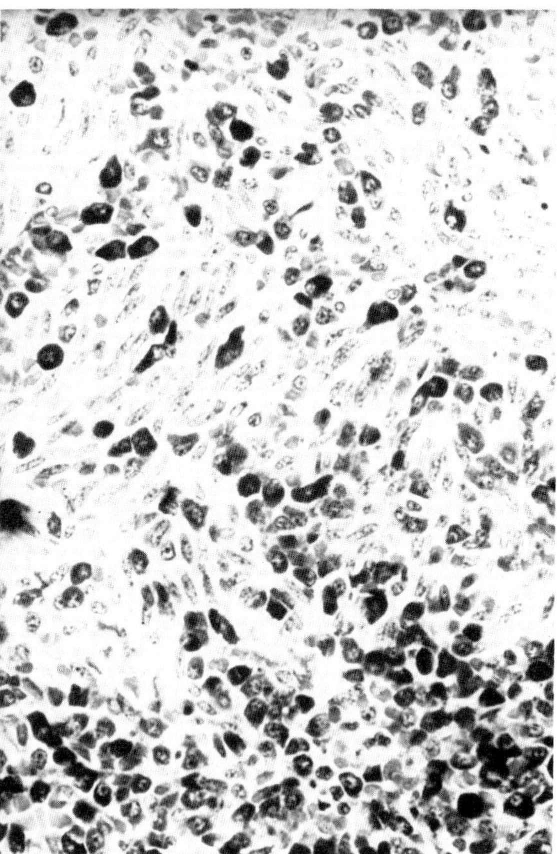

Fig. 13.7 Mastocytosis in the spleen. The field shows mast cells of varying maturity, from heavily granulated mature cells (black in figure) to pale-staining, spindle-shaped immature cells. (Giemsa × 375)

Lymph node changes

Lymphadenopathy is occasionally a presenting feature, though lymph node biopsy is seldom required for diagnosis. Affected nodes may be massively infiltrated by mast cells with extension through the capsule and into the perinodal fat (Fig. 13.8) or infiltration may be more limited, being sometimes confined to the sinuses. As in other tissues, the mast cell infiltrate is generally composed of mast cells of varying degrees of maturity. Even when the cells are predominantly of

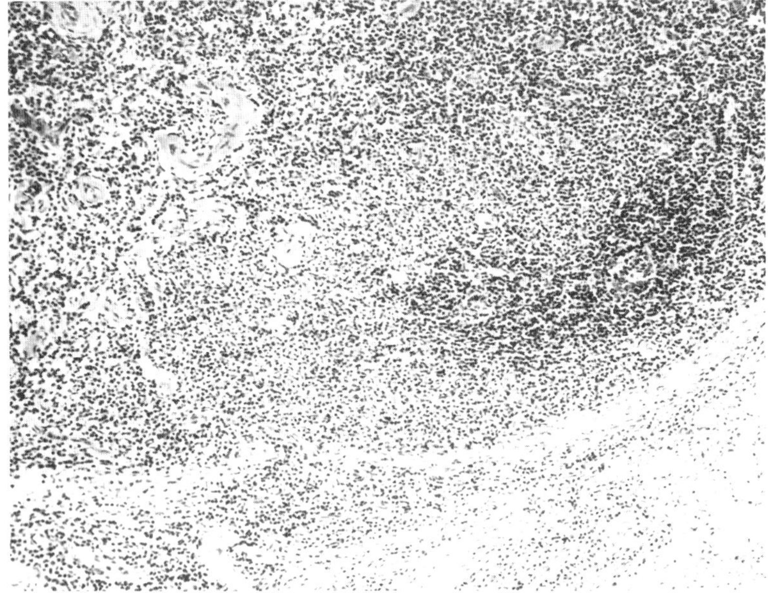

Fig. 13.8 Mastocytosis in a lymph node showing capsular and extracapsular infiltration. A residual collection of lymphocytes is seen (centre right). (H E × 120)

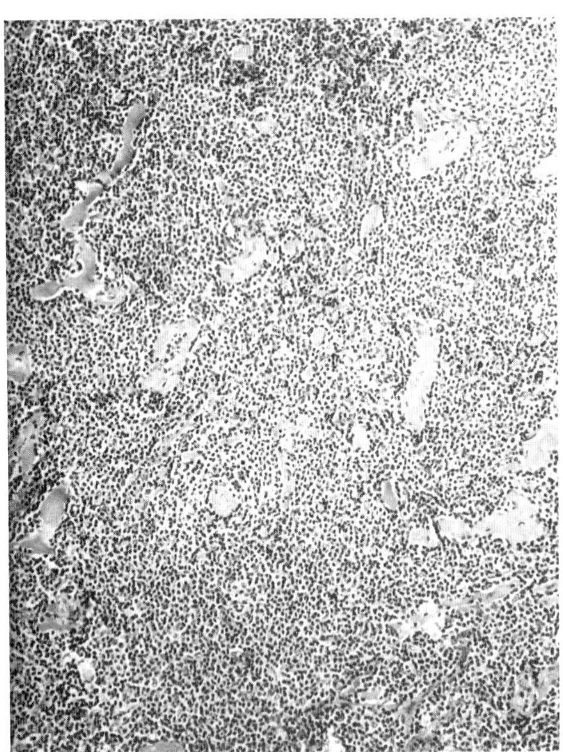

Fig. 13.9 Mastocytosis in a lymph node showing diffuse infiltration by mainly immature mast cells. Note hyalinisation of vessels. (H E × 120)

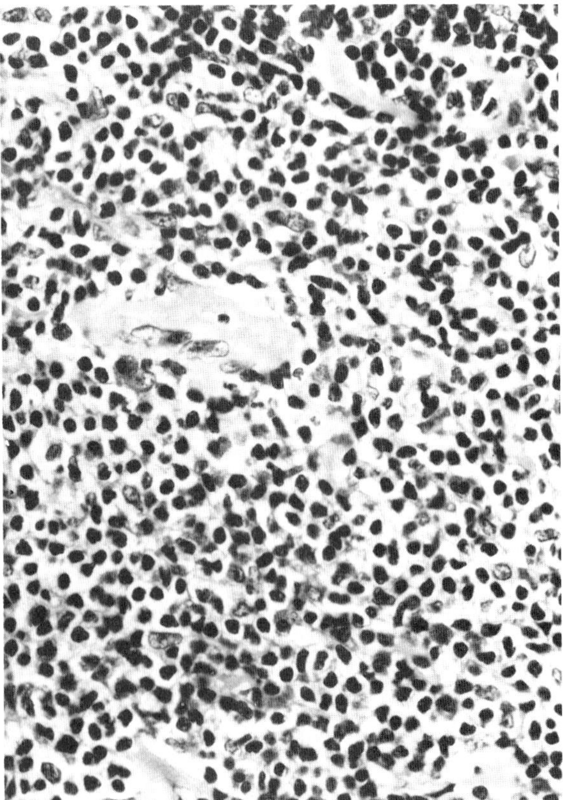

Fig. 13.10 Same case as Fig. 13.9 at higher magnification. A few residual lymphocytes are seen at the top. (H E × 470)

immature, non-granulated type, they have a quite distinctive appearance, being ovoid or spindled in shape and having a characteristic clear cytoplasm so that they stand out against the smaller, more darkly staining residual lymphocytes in the node. The presence of scattered, more mature, granulated mast cells will of course assist in the recognition of the disease. A further diagnostic pointer is the presence of hyalinisation in the walls of small vessels (Figs 13.9, 13.10) and in chronic cases hyalinisation may be very extensive (Fig. 13.11).

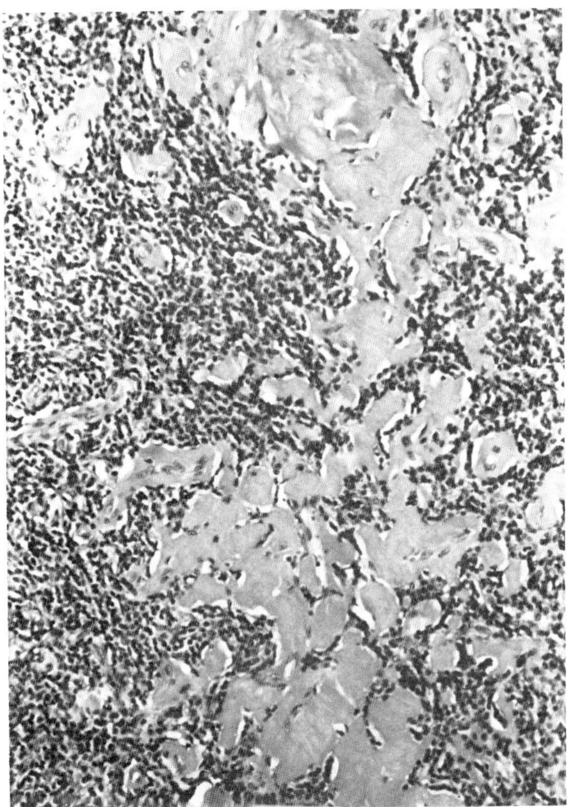

Fig. 13.11 Advanced hyalinisation of lymph node in chronic mastocytosis (H E × 120)

CHRONIC LEUKAEMIAS

The term chronic refers to the prognosis as compared with untreated acute leukaemia. The two main types are chronic myeloid leukaemia (CML) and chronic lymphocytic leukaemia (CLL). The latter has been discussed in Chapter 10 with the less common prolymphocytic leukaemia. Hairy cell leukaemia will be considered in this section. CML can be divided into Philadelphia chromosome positive and negative types. There are also morphological variants of CML (chronic eosinophilic, chronic basophilic and chronic neutrophilic leukaemia) which have been reviewed by Gunz & Baikie (1974). Chronic myelomonocytic leukaemia is probably best considered separately and is well described by Geary et al (1975).

Chronic myeloid leukaemia

The peripheral blood findings are diagnostic in most cases. The leucocyte count is higher than 100 $\times 10^9/1$ in a majority of patients. All stages of the neutrophilic series from myeloblasts to segmented neutrophils usually are present. Neutrophils are the most common type of cells, followed by metamyelocytes and myelocytes, promyelocytes and myeloblasts. Promyelocytes and myeloblasts make up only a small percentage of the total number of cells until blast crisis supervenes (see below). Basophils and eosinophils are increased in absolute number in most patients. Anaemia is present at the time of diagnosis in a majority of patients but is often mild. The platelet count is raised in approximately 50% of patients; severe thrombocytopenia is rare in typical CML at the time of diagnosis.

The diagnosis is made from the above peripheral blood findings. Marrow examination is usually of little diagnostic help except for the material it provides for cytogenetic studies. Marrow aspiration and biopsy reveal marked granulocyte hyperplasia. The Philadelphia (Ph^1) chromosome has been reported to be present in 70 to 90% of patients with CML (Ezdinli et al, 1970; Whang-Peng et al, 1968; Witts et al, 1968). The patients with Ph^1 chromosome negative CML have a poorer prognosis than those with Ph^1 chromosome. They also tend to present with lower leucocyte and platelet counts (Ezdinli et al. 1970; Whang-Peng et al, 1968). Infants and young children with the juvenile type of CML do not have the Ph^1 chromosome (Hardisty et al, 1964; Reisman & Trujillo, 1963).

Blast crisis is the prime cause of death in CML patients (Boggs, 1976; Karanas & Silver, 1968). As the crisis develops, an increased number of blasts are seen in the peripheral blood and marrow. Eventually, a picture similar to acute leukaemia develops. The haematological picture may be either that of AML or ALL, however, in some patients a mixed population of blasts occurs (Boggs, 1974; Janossy et al, 1979; Rosenthal et al, 1977). A few patients first appear in blast crisis without an initial period of symptomatic CML (Beard et al, 1976; Catovsky, 1979; Peterson et al, 1976).

Lymph node changes

The lymph nodes are rarely enlarged in patients with typical CML (Duvall et al, 1967). The development of lymphadenopathy suggests that the disease is no longer in the chronic phase. However, in the juvenile type of CML greater lymph node involvement is found (Hardisty et al, 1964; Reisman & Trujillo, 1963).

Histology. The characteristic histological feature in the lymph nodes of patients in the chronic phase is the development of myeloid metaplasia (extramedullary haematopoiesis), even though it is predominantly granulocytic in type (Fig. 13.12). Starting centrally, the granulocytic proliferation gradually replaces the lymphatic tissue (Fig. 13.13). Peripheral sinuses and occasional small follicles may be preserved. The capsule usually remains intact. The presence of eosinophilic myelocytes and occasional megakaryocytes, in a section stained with H E, help in the diagnosis. The presence of basophilic granulocytes, as seen with a Giemsa stain, is also characteristic.

When CML transforms into a more accelerated phase or blast crisis then the primary site of this

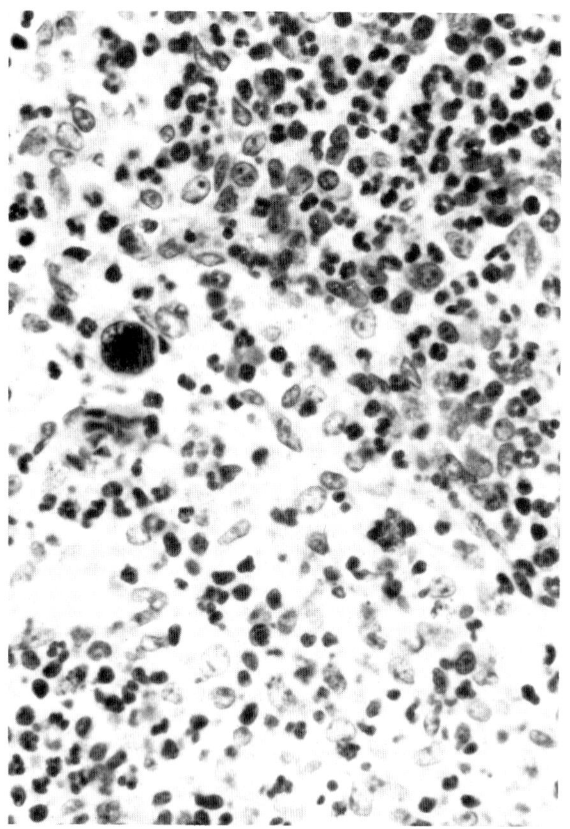

Fig. 13.12 Lymph node involvement by chronic myeloid leukaemia, showing extramedullary haematopoiesis (H E × 500)

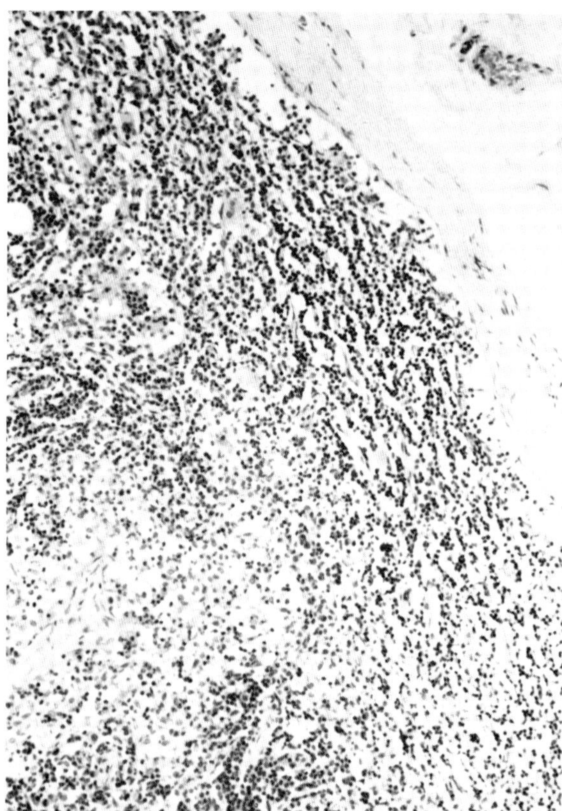

FIg. 13.13 Same node as Fig. 13.12 showing residual subcapsular lymphoid tissue (H E × 120)

change may be extramedullary (Rosenthal et al, 1977). Lymph nodes probably are the most common site for the manifestation of localised blast crisis (Boggs, 1976). In the past, these extramedullary sites of involvement have been mistaken for second malignancies (Garfinkel & Bennett 1969; Pascoe, 1970). This confusion can be avoided if imprints are made from any excised tumour from a patient with leukaemia. The imprinted cells, after staining by a Romanowsky technique, should be correctly identified.

Histologically, most of the lymph node is replaced by blasts showing frequent mitoses and the picture may be indistinguishable from that seen in acute leukaemia (Fig. 13.14). If the existence of CML was unsuspected before lymph node biopsy the change in the node may be misinterpreted as indicating a high grade malignant lymphoma. The presence of scattered eosinophil myelocytes or megakaryocytes amongst the blast cells should point to the correct diagnosis (Fig. 13.15). The nature of the blasts can be assessed by using cytochemical stains, e.g. a chloroacetate esterase stain for granulocytic cells. If the blast crisis appears lymphoid then the cells of the lymph node can be further studied for their surface marker characteristics (Bernheim et al, 1981; Janossy et al, 1976). Recently, a T-lymphoblastic transformation of CML in a lymph node was reported (Palutke et al, 1982).

In Ph^1 positive CML this chromosome abnormality, with rare exceptions, is a constant feature, being found in overt disease, during clinical and haematological remissions, and in the terminal stages. Ph^1 positive cells may become established in the spleen (Spiers & Baikie, 1965) and other extramedullary sites (Duvall et al, 1967). In some patients the Ph^1 chromosome is the only karyo-

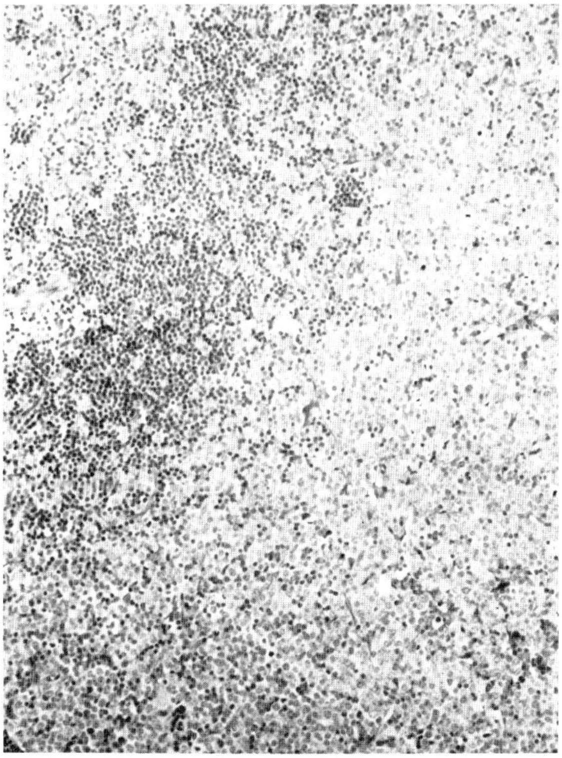

Fig. 13.14 Blast crisis of chronic myeloid leukaemia manifest in a lymph node biopsy. Compare residual lymphoid tissue at top left. (H E × 120)

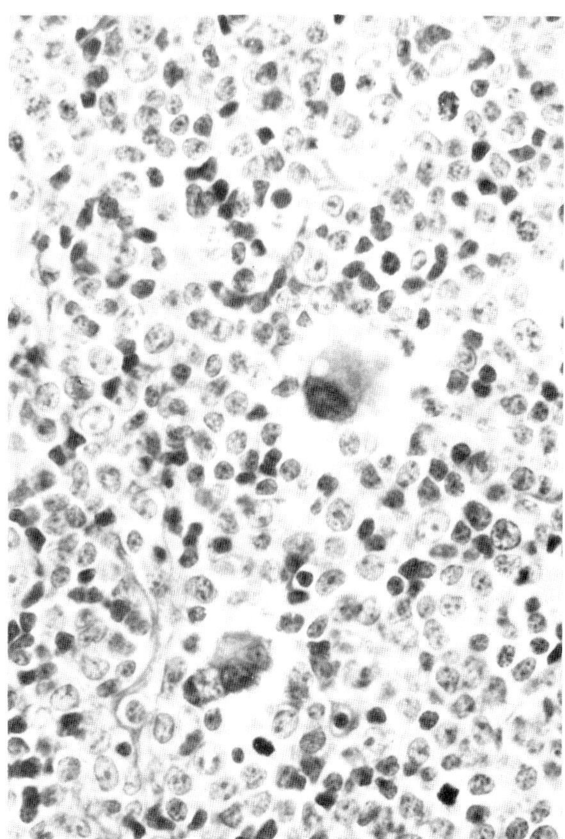

Fig. 13.15 Lymph node involvement by the blast crisis of chronic myeloid leukaemia, showing residual megakaryocytes (H E × 500)

typic abnormality detectable throughout the course of the disease. However, additional cytogenetic abnormalities may appear as the patient enters the terminal stage. These include changes in the number of chromosomes, the appearance of 'marker' chromosomes, and the presence of cells containing two Ph^1 chromosomes (Whang-Peng et al, 1968). Clonal evolution may not only occur in the bone-marrow but also extramedullary sites such as the spleen (Gomez et al, 1975).

Hairy cell leukaemia
Synonym:
Leukaemic reticuloendotheliosis

Hairy cell leukaemia (HCL) was considered to be a rare disorder until Bouroncle et al published a report of 26 patients in 1958 and, subsequently, even larger series have been published (Flandrin et al, 1973). Yam et al demonstrated in 1972 that in hairy cell leukaemia the cells contain tartrate-resistant acid phosphatase. Subsequent studies have confirmed this to be a useful characteristic, although not specific for HCL. The term 'hairy cell' was suggested by Schrek & Donnelly in 1966. The disease should be suspected in patients with peripheral blood pancytopenia and massive splenomegaly. It occurs in adults of both sexes, and in the majority of cases typical hairy cells can be seen in the blood film or buffy coat. However, on occasions, the 'hairs' may be inconspicuous or even absent.

Hairy cells, on Romanowsky-stained films, have relatively abundant cytoplasm. The cytoplasmic membrane appears irregular and serrated and the nucleus resembles that of a medium-sized lymphocyte. The hair-like projections are more easily seen with phase-microscopy or by electron-microscopy (Fig. 13.16) than by standard light microscopy.

The hairy cell has most often been characterised as a B-lymphocyte (Burns et al 1978; Catovsky et al, 1974c; Golde et al, 1977; Zidar et al, 1977; Lennert, 1978). However, other patients, seemingly, have cells with typical characteristics of T-lymphocytes (Cawley et al, 1978) or monocyte-macrophages (Reyes et al, 1978). In still others, 'hybrid' characteristics of B- and T-lymphocytes (Burns et al, 1978; Zidar et al, 1977), B-lymphocytes and monocytes (Cohen et al, 1979; Utsinger et al, 1977), or B- and T-lymphocytes and monocyte-macrophages (Boldt et al, 1977; Burns et al, 1977) have been reported. If HCL represents a pluripotent stem cell disorder, similar to CML, then a variable phenotypic expression is possible. Cawley et al (1980) showed that cells of individuals with HCL can change their phenotype. In addition, a markedly dyserythropoietic population of erythroblasts associated with two populations of blood erythrocytes, one of which was markedly macrocytic, was reported in one patient (Berkowitz et al, 1980) and platelets with multiple functional abnormalities have been noted in another (Rosove et al, 1980).

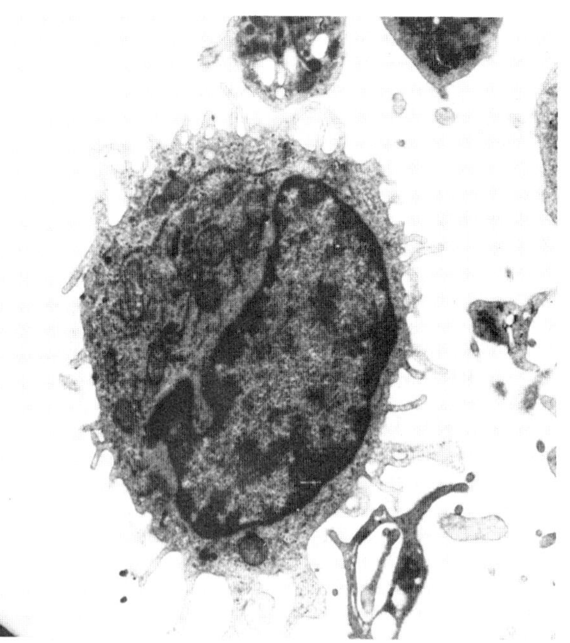

Fig. 13.16 Electron micrograph of a hairy cell from a case of hairy cell leukaemia

Histology. Bone-marrow aspirate often yields a 'dry-tap'. However, sections from a bone-marrow trephine are usually diagnostic (Bouroncle 1979; Golomb et al, 1978). Increased reticulin fibres with or without frank myelofibrosis are noted in almost all patients. Diagnosis from the bone-marrow trephine is based on infiltration with moderately large, uniform cells which, due to their abundant cytoplasm, leave a greater space between cell nuclei than is seen in other malignant lymphomas. This very distinctive feature can be appreciated in a well-fixed preparation under the low power of the microscope.

Lymph node changes

In contrast with the massive infiltration generally found in the spleen, lymphadenopathy is not prominent in HCL. Katayama & Finkel (1974) found that only splenic hilar lymph nodes were involved, never peripheral lymph nodes. Occasionally, at post-mortem the para-aortic lymph nodes are found to be enlarged (Catovsky et al, 1974b).

Macroscopic findings. The involved lymph nodes are seldom much enlarged. They exhibit a delicate smooth capsule and a homogeneous, fleshy, pale grey cut surface (Naeim & Smith, 1974).

Histology. The histological changes in the lymph nodes have been well described (Bouroncle et al, 1958; Burke et al, 1974; Catovsky et al, 1974b; Naeim & Smith, 1974; Lennert et al, 1978). In contrast to the massive hairy cell infiltration of the spleen, lymph nodes become infiltrated relatively late, if at all, in the disease. The hairy cells first settle in the B-cell region, often leaving the T-cell region intact. The most typical primary site of localisation in affected lymph nodes is the lymphatic tissue beneath the marginal sinus. There the hairy cells establish themselves in small nodules or in broad bands (Fig. 13.17). In the small nodules there is sometimes a bizarre fibre network that probably comes from small vessels. Only in late phases are the entire lymphatic parenchyma, the capsule and trabeculae infiltrated. In general, the marginal sinus remains intact.

The infiltrating cells are usually monomorphic and somewhat larger than typical lymphocytes. The nuclei are often slightly bean-shaped. Characteristically, the hairy cells are distinguished by a

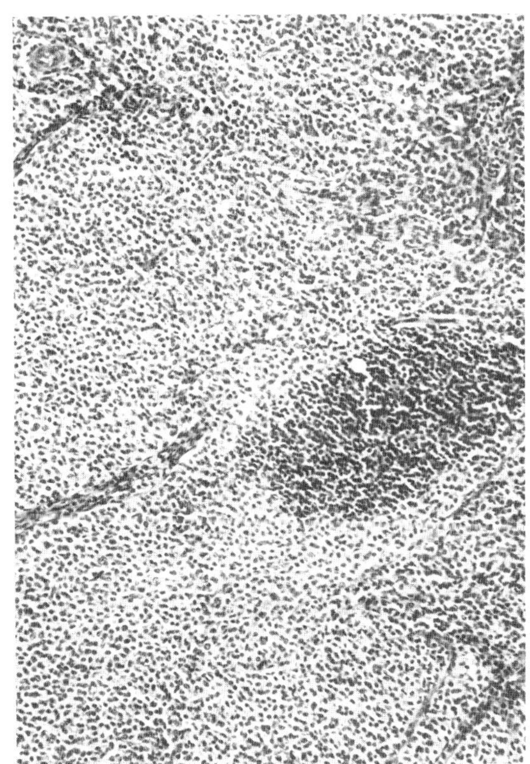

Fig. 13.17 Lymph node in hairy cell leukaemia. The pale cytoplasm of the hairy cells makes them conspicuous in comparison with the residual focus of lymphocytes. (H E × 120)

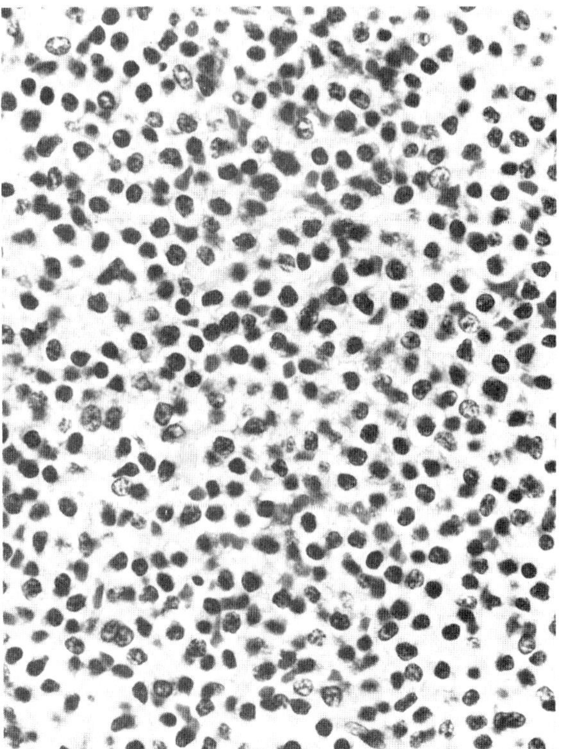

Fig. 13.18 Hairy cells in lymph node at a higher magnification. The pale cytoplasm and well defined cell walls give them a 'plant-cell'-like quality. (H E × 470)

relatively broad rim of pale-staining cytoplasm; the nuclei appear fairly far apart for this reason (Fig. 13.18). Lennert et al (1978) have described three patients with HCL where the lymph node biopsy has shown an increase in plasma cells. In addition, in two lymph node biopsies extramedullary haematopoiesis was found. An increase in plasma cells is often seen in the spleen of patients with HCL.

Myeloid metaplasia

Synonym:
Extramedullary haematopoiesis

The term myeloid metaplasia refers to extramedullary haematopoiesis, i.e. the finding of erythroblasts, granulocyte precursors and megakaryocytes in varying numbers in sites outside the bone-marrow. The most common sites of extramedullary haematopoiesis are the liver, spleen and lymph nodes.

This finding may be present in a variety of disease processes. These include the myeloproliferative disorders, bone-marrow infiltration by tumours and haemolytic anaemias (Rappaport & Crosby, 1957). There are frequently erythroblasts and immature leucocytes in the circulation — a leucoerythroblastic blood picture (Vaughan, 1936).

Extramedullary haematopoiesis is invariably present in idiopathic myelofibrosis but is less marked in CML and polycythaemia rubra vera. The haematopoietic islands may contain only one type of blood cell precursor, or erythropoiesis, granulopoiesis and megakaryocytopoiesis may be found in the same area. There may be small foci of cells or large tumours of haematopoietic tissue (Glew et al, 1973).

Lymph node findings

In idiopathic myelofibrosis the lymph node sinuses contain clusters of erythroblasts, immature granulocytes and megakaryocytes. Prominent atypical megakaryocytes and a scarcity of mature cells will suggest that the myeloid metaplasia is part of a systemic myeloproliferative disease rather than a compensatory extramedullary haematopoiesis (Fig. 13.19). In CML, as previously mentioned, granulopoiesis is most prominent, whereas small clusters of erythroid cells are most likely with polycythaemia rubra vera.

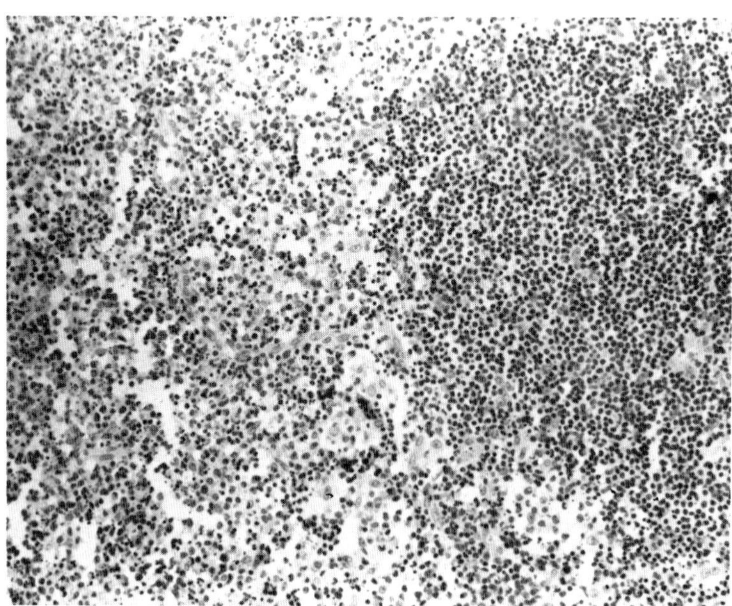

Fig. 13.19 Extramedullary haematopoiesis in a lymph node biopsy from a patient with myelofibrosis. Note residual lymphocytes on right of field (H E × 120)

REFERENCES

Beard M E J et al 1976 Blast crisis of chronic myeloid leukaemia (CML) I Presentation simulating acute lymphoblastic leukaemia (ALL). British Journal of Haematology 34: 167–178

Bennett J M et al 1976 Proposals for the classification of the acute leukaemias (FAB co-operative group). British Journal of Haematology 33: 451–458

Berlin C 1955 Urticaria pigmentosa as a systemic disease. Archives of Dermatology (Chicago) 71: 703–712

Berkowitz L R, Ross D W, Orringer E P 1980 Hairy cell leukaemia with acquired dyserythropoiesis. Archives of Internal Medicine 140: 554–555

Bernheim A, Berger R, Preud'Homme J I, Labaume S, Bussel A, Barot-Ciorbaru R 1981 Philadelphia chromosome positive blood B lymphocytes in chronic myelocytic leukaemia. Leukaemia Research 5: 331–339

Bloomfield C D, Lindquist L L, Brunning R D, Yunis J J, Coccia P F 1978 Philadelphia chromosome in acute leukaemia. Virchows Archiv B Cell Pathology 29: 81–91

Boggs D R 1974 Hematopoietic stem cell theory in relation to possible lymphoblastic conversion of chronic myeloid leukaemia. Blood 44: 449–453

Boggs D R 1976 The pathogenesis and clinical pattern of blast crisis of chronic myeloid leukaemia. Seminars in Oncology 3: 289–296

Boggs D R, Wintrobe M M, Cartwright G E 1962 The acute leukaemias. Analysis of 322 cases and review of the literature. Medicine 41: 163–225

Boldt D H, Speckart S F, MacDermott R P, Nash G S, Valeski J E 1977 Leukaemic reticuloendotheliosis. 'Hairy cell leukaemia', functional and structural features of the abnormal cell in a patient with profound leukocytosis. Blood 49: 745–757

Bouroncle B A 1979 Leukaemic reticuloendotheliosis (Hairy cell leukaemia). Blood 53: 412–436

Bouroncle B A, Wiseman B K, Doan C A 1958 Leukaemic reticuloendotheliosis. Blood 13: 609–639

Brouet J-C, Valensi F, Daniel M-T, Flandrin G, Preud'Homme J-L, Seligmann M 1976 Immunological classification of acute lymphoblastic leukaemia: evaluation of its clinical significance in a hundred patients. British Journal of Haematology 33: 319–328

Brugo E A, Marshall R B, Riberi A M, Pautasso O E 1977 Preleukaemic granulocytic sarcomas of the gastrointestinal tract. Report of two cases. American Journal of Clinical Pathology 68: 616–621

Burke J S, Byrne G E, Rappaport H 1974 Hairy cell leukaemia (leukaemic reticuloendotheliosis) 1. A clinical pathologic study of 21 patients. Cancer 33: 1399–1410

Burns G F, Nash A A, Worman C P, Barker C R, Hayhoe F G J, Cawley J C 1977 A human leukaemic cell expressing hybrid membrane phenotypes. Nature 268: 243–245

Burns G F et al 1978 Multiple heavy chain isotypes on the surface of the cells of hairy cell leukaemia. Blood 52: 1132–1147

Caplan R M 1963 The natural course of urticaria pigmentosa. Archives of Dermatology (Chicago) 87: 146–157

Catovsky D 1979 Ph[1]-positive acute leukaemia and chronic granulocytic leukaemia: one or two diseases? British Journal of Haematology 42: 493–498

Catovsky D (ed) 1981 The leukaemic cell — methods in haematology, volume 2. Churchill Livingstone, Edinburgh

Catovsky D, Galetto J, Okos A, Miliani E, Galton D A G 1974a Cytochemical profile of B and T leukaemic lymphocytes with special reference to acute lymphoblastic leukaemia. Journal of Clinical Pathology 27: 767–771

Catovsky D, Pettit J E, Galton D A G, Spiers A S D, Harrison C V 1974b Leukaemic reticuloendotheliosis ('hairy' cell leukaemia) a distinct clinico-pathological entity. British Journal of Haematology 26: 9–27

Catovsky D, Pettit J E, Galetto J, Okos A, Galton D A G 1974c The B-lymphocyte nature of the hairy cell of leukaemic reticuloendotheliosis. British Journal of Haematology 26: 29–37

Cawley J C, Burns G F, Nash A A, Higgy K E, Child J A, Roberts B E 1978 Hairy-cell leukaemia with T-cell features. Blood 51: 61–69

Cawley J C, Burns GF, Worman C P, Roberts B E, Hayhoe F G. 1980 Clinical and hematologic fluctuations in hairy-cell leukaemia: a sequential surface-marker analysis. Blood 55: 784–791

Cohen H J, George E R, Kremer W B 1979 Hairy cell leukaemia: cellular characteristics including surface immunoglobulin dynamics and biosynthesis. Blood 53: 764–775

Coser P, Quaglino D, De Pasquale A, Colombetti V, Prinoth O 1980 Cytobiological and clinical aspects of tissue mast cell leukaemia. British Journal of Haematology 45: 5–12

Daniel M–T, Flandrin G, Bernard J 1975 Leucemie aigue a mastocytes. Etude cytochimique et ultrastructurale, a propos d'une observation. Nouvelle Revue Francaise Haematologie 15: 319–332

Duvall C P, Carbone P P, Bell W R, Whang J, Tjio J H, Perry S 1967 Chronic myelocytic leukaemia with two Philadelphia chromosomes and prominent peripheral lymphadenopathy. Blood 29: 652–666

Ezdinli E Z, Sokal J E, Crosswhite B S, Sandberg A A 1970 Philadelphia-chromosome -positive and -negative chronic myelocytic leukaemia. Annals of Internal Medicine 72: 175–182

Flandrin G, Daniel M-T, Fourcade M, Chelloul N 1973 Leucemie a tricholeucocyte (hairy cell leukaemia). Etude clinique et cytologique de 55 observations. Nouvelle Revue Francaise Haematologie 13: 609–640

Forkner C E 1934 Clinical and pathologic differentiation of the acute leukaemias with special reference to acute monocytic leukaemia. Archives of Internal Medicine 53: 1–34

Frame B, Nixon R K 1968 Bone-marrow mast cells in osteoporosis of ageing. New England Journal of Medicine 279: 626–630

Garfinkel L S, Bennett D E 1969 Extramedullary myeloblastic transformation in chronic myelocytic leukaemia simulating a coexistent malignant lymphoma. American Journal of Clinical Pathology 51: 638–645

Geary C G et al 1975 Chronic myelomonocytic leukaemia. British Journal of Haematology 30: 289–302

Glew R H, Haese W H, McIntyre P A, 1973 Myeloid metaplasia with myelofibrosis. The clinical spectrum of extramedullary haematopoiesis and tumour formation. John Hopkins Medical Journal 132: 253–270

Golde D W, Stevens R H, Quan S G, Saxon A 1977 Immunoglobulin synthesis in hairy cell leukaemia. British Journal of Haematology 35: 359–365

Golomb H M, Catovsky D, Golde D W 1978 Hairy cell leukaemia, a clinical review based on 71 cases. Annals of Internal Medicine 89: 677–683

Gomez G, Hossfeld D K, Sokal J E 1975 Removal of abnormal clone of leukaemic cells by splenectomy. British Medical Journal 2: 421–423

Gunz F, Baikie A G 1974 Leukaemia, 3rd end. Grune and Stratton, New York

Hardisty R M, Speed D E, Till M 1964 Granulocytic leukaemia in childhood. British Journal of Haematology 10: 551–566

Janossy G, Robetts M, Greaves M F 1976 Target cell in chronic myeloid leukaemia and its relationship to acute lymphoid leukaemia. Lancet 2: 1058–1061

Janossy G et al 1979 Relation of 'lymphoid' phenotype and response to chemotherapy incorporating vincristine — prednisolone in the acute phase of Ph^1 positive leukaemia. Cancer 43: 426–434

Karanas A, Silver R T 1968 Characteristics of the terminal phase of chronic granulocytic leukaemia. Blood 32: 445–459

Katayama I, Finkel H E 1974 Leukaemic reticuloendothelosis. A clinico-pathological study with a review of the literature. American Journal of Medicine 57: 115–126

Krause J R 1979 Granulocytic sarcoma preceding acute leukaemia. A report of six cases. Cancer 44: 1017–1021

Lennert K, in collaboration with Mohri N, Stein H, Kaiserling E, Müller-Hermelink H K 1978 Malignant lymphomas. Springer-Verlag, Berlin

Lennert K, Parwaresch M R 1979 Mast cells and mast cell neoplasia: a review. Histopathology 3: 349–365

Long J C, Mihm M C 1977 Multiple granulocytic tumors of the skin. Report of 6 cases of myelogenous leukaemia with initial manifestations in the skin. Cancer 39: 2004–2016

Mason T E, Demaree R S, Margolis C I 1973 Granulocytic sarcoma (chloroma), two years preceding myelogenous leukaemia. Cancer 31: 423–432

Naeim F, Smith G S 1974 Leukaemic reticuloendotheliosis. Cancer 34: 1813–1821

Nettleship E 1869 Rare forms of urticaria. British Medical Journal 2: 323–324

Neumann E 1870 Ein fall von leukamie mit erkrankung des knockenmarkes. Arch Heilk 11: 1

Nixon R K 1966 The relation of mastocytosis and lymphomatous disease. Annals of Internal Medicine 64: 856–860

Palutke M, Eisenberg L, Nathan L 1982 Ph^1-positive T lymphoblastic transformation of chronic granulocytic leukaemia in a lymph node. Lancet 2:1053

Parker C 1976 Systemic mastocytosis. American Journal of Medicine 61: 671–680

Pascoe H R 1970 Tumours composed of immature granulocytes occurring in the breast in chronic granulocytic leukaemia. Cancer 25: 697–704

Peterson L C, Bloomfield C D, Brunning R B 1976 Blast crisis as an initial or terminal manifestation of chronic myeloid leukaemia: a study of twenty-eight patients. American Journal of Medicine 60: 209–220

Rappaport H, Crosby W H 1957 Auto-immune hemolytic anaemia. II Morphologic observations and clinicopathologic correlations. American Journal of Pathology 33: 429–457

Reisman L E, Trujillo J M 1963 Chronic granulocytic leukaemia of childhood. Clinical and cytogenetic studies. Journal of Paediatrics 62: 710–723

Reyes F, Gourdin M F, Farcet J P, Dreyfus B, Breton-Gorius J 1978 Synthesis of a peroxidase activity by cells of hairy cell leukaemia: a study by ultrastructural cytochemistry. Blood 52: 537–550

Rosenthal S, Canellos G P, Whang-Peng J, Gralnick H R 1977 Blast crisis of chronic granulocytic leukaemia. Morphologic variants and therapeutic implications. American Journal of Medicine 63: 542–555

Rosove M H, Naeim F, Harwig S, Zighelboim J 1980 Severe platelet dysfunction in hairy cell leukaemia with improvement after splenectomy. Blood 55: 903–906

Ross R R 1955 Chloroma and chloroleukaemia. American Journal of Medicine 18: 671–676

Sagher F, Even-Paz Z 1967 Mastocytosis and the mast cell. Karger, Basel.

Schrek R, Donnelly W J 1966 'Hairy' cells in blood lymphoreticular neoplastic disease and 'flagellated' cells of normal lymph nodes. Blood 27: 199–211

Schultz J Schwartz S 1956 The chemistry of experimental chloroma. Cancer Research 16: 565–574

Seo I S, Hull M T, Pak H Y 1977 Granulocytic sarcoma of the cervix as a primary manifestation. Case without overt leukaemic features for 26 months. Cancer 40: 3030–3037

Spiers A S D, Baikie A G 1965 Chronic granulocytic leukaemia: demonstration of the Philadelphia chromosome in cultures of spleen cells. Nature 208:497

Turpin F, Lejeune F, Vilde J L, Le Coq D, Lotholary P, Paraf A 1978 Deficit en peroxydase des granulocytes neutrophiles au cour d'une mastocytose difuse. Nouvelle Revue Francaise Haematologie 20: 77–97

Utsinger P D, Yount W J, Fuller C R, Logue M J, Orringer E P 1977 Hairy cell leukaemia: B-lymphocyte and phagocytic properties. Blood 49: 19–27

Vaughan J M 1936 Leuco-erythroblastic anaemia. Journal of Pathology and Bacteriology 42: 541–564

Virchow R 1845 Weisses Blut. Froriep's Notzien 36:151

Whang-Peng J, Canellos G P, Carbone P P, Tjio J H 1968 Clinical implications of cytogenetic variants in chronic myelocytic leukaemia (CML). Blood 32: 755–766

Witts L J et al 1968 Chronic granulocytic leukaemia: comparison of radiotherapy and busulphan therapy. Report of the Medical Research Council's Working Party for Therapeutic Trials in Leukaemia. British Medical Journal 1: 201–208

Yam L T, Li C-Y, Finkel H E 1972 Leukaemic reticuloendotheliosis. The role of tartrate-resistant acid phosphatase in diagnosis and splenectomy in treatment. Archives of Internal Medicine 130: 248–256

Zidar B L et al 1977 Hairy cell leukaemia: seven cases with probable B-lymphocytic origin. British Journal of Haematology 37: 455–465

Histiocytosis and histiocytic neoplasms

The other main component of the lymphoreticular tissues beside the lymphoid cells is a system of reticulum (reticular) cells, which includes the histiocytes of the mononuclear phagocyte system, but is not restricted to them (see Ch. 5, p. 78). Whilst the true histiocyte is an avidly phagocytic cell, becoming a macrophage in its active state, none of the other varieties of reticulum cell (dendritic, interdigitating and fibrocytic) is phagocytic in the full sense, although the first two are capable of retaining complexed antigen (see Ch 1, p. 5). These other types of reticulum cell display different enzyme activities from true histiocytes (Table 5.1, p. 79) and two have different and largely specific locations within lymphoreticular tissues. They apparently respond to different stimuli and they look different from one another when studied ultrastructurally. Nevertheless, the different types of reticulum cell cannot be reliably distinguished from one another by light microscopy, especially when viewed singly in paraffin sections of conventional thickness. When seen in the mass, the rather subtle morphological distinctions become obvious and one can then readily distinguish, for example, interdigitating cells from histiocytes.

In earlier chapters, we have seen how an increase of histiocytes and other types of reticulum cell is a common feature of reactive states and also of neoplasms in lymph nodes. In this chapter, we shall consider those situations in which an increase of histiocytes (histiocytosis) or interdigitating reticulum cells is the primary event or the central feature of the histological picture. Inevitably there will be some overlap with Chapter 6 in which some granulomatous reactions have been discussed (p. 89).

The conditions to be discussed here include:

(1) reactive histiocytosis and allied disorders,
(2) 'Histiocytosis X', and (3) malignant histiocytosis and histiocytic reticulosarcoma.

REACTIVE HISTIOCYTOSIS

Increased numbers of histiocytes are seen in lymph nodes in response to a variety of stimuli. These accumulations show two main patterns, involving predominantly either the sinus-lining histiocytes or the histiocytes of the dense pulp of the node.

Sinus histiocytosis

In this pattern of reactive histiocytosis lymph node sinuses become progressively filled with histiocytes. There is usually little tendency for the sinus histiocytes to encroach on the adjacent dense pulp and this causes a striking contrast in a conventionally stained section between the dark lymphoid tissue of the node and the pale cellular mass in the sinuses. The histiocytes show large, oval or indented nuclei of uniform size and shape, with delicate chromatin and small central nucleoli. The uniformity of the histiocytes, the rarity of mitoses and the absence of nuclear atypia immediately distinguish reactive sinus histiocytosis from malignant histiocytosis. Although the sinus infiltrate is predominantly histiocytic, there is commonly a variable proportion of lymphocytes and neutrophils or eosinophils as well. Occasional histiocytes may contain phagocytosed red cells or lymphocytes, although this never reaches the proportions seen in 'sinus histiocytosis with massive lymphadenopathy' (see below).

Simple sinus histiocytosis is very common and usually without significance (Fig. 14.1). It arises in nodes draining tissues infiltrated by large numbers of histiocytes, and is thus the result of any chronic inflammatory process within the drainage area of the nodes. It is commonly seen in axillary nodes draining a carcinoma of the breast, for example, and some studies have claimed that the better prognosis in breast cancer patients whose axillary nodes exhibit this change is directly attributable to the defensive role of the sinus histiocytes (Black et al, 1953). The fallacies in this study have been exposed by Berg (1956). The histiocytes frequently contain pigment or lipid engulfed in the peripheral tissue; they may stain intensely for iron in nodes draining an area of haemorrhage or after extravasation into the lymph sinuses of the node. In haemochromatosis and haemosiderosis, the abdominal nodes often show dark brown pigmentation of the sinus-lining histiocytes. Other particulate material (e.g. micro-organisms) may be taken up by these avidly phagocytic cells (Fig. 14.2)

Small quantities of lipid are commonly seen in sinus histiocytes, indeed, foamy macrophages are normally present in the coeliac and mesenteric nodes and are commonly found in the cystic node in the presence of gall bladder disease. In appropriate circumstances, large, lipid-filled macrophages in the sinuses may suggest a lipid storage disease. In *Gaucher's disease*, the bulk of the accumulated lipid is stored in spleen, liver and bone marrow and the lymph nodes are seldom significantly enlarged. On histological examination of abdominal nodes, however, one commonly sees small numbers of Gaucher's cells in the pulp adjacent to the lymph sinuses (Fig. 14.3). These cells are so large and have such abundant, pale, streaky cytoplasm, that even when present in small numbers, they are easily spotted. In *Niemann-Pick's*

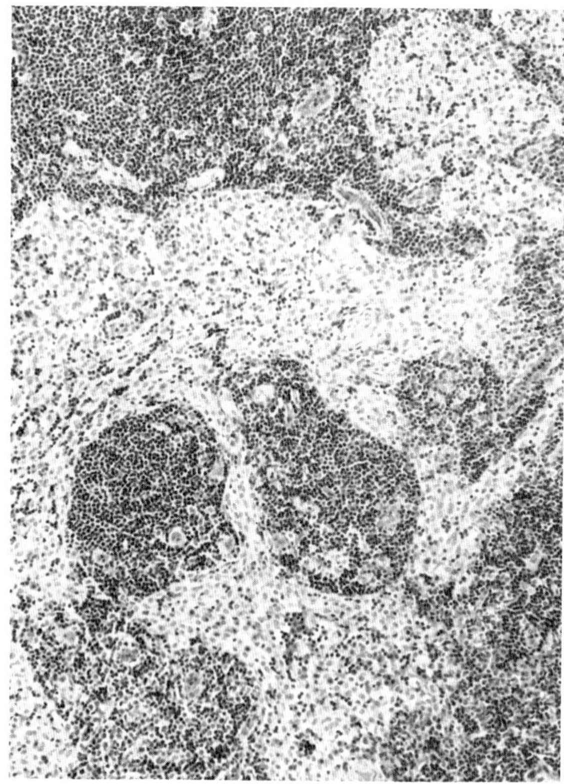

Fig. 14.1 Simple sinus histiocytosis in an adult axillary lymph node (H E × 120)

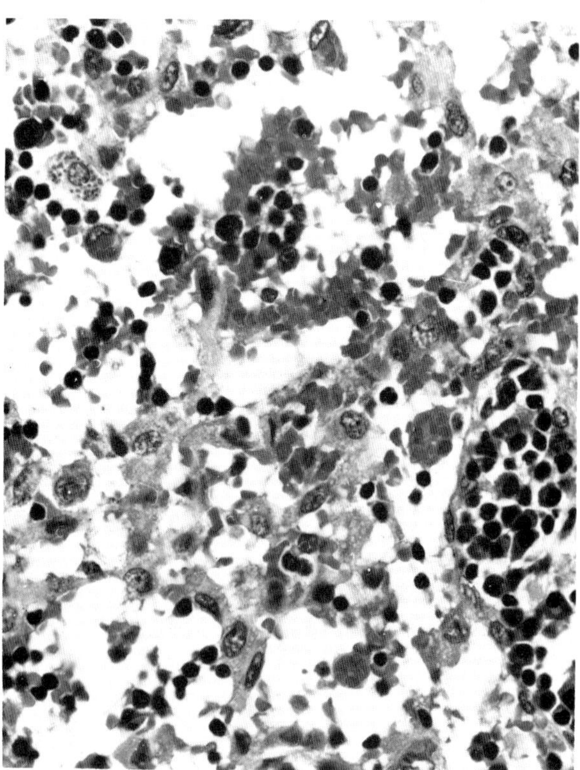

Fig. 14.2 Abdominal lymph node from a child with visceral leishmaniasis showing active sinus histiocytosis with phagocytosis of L-D bodies (top left) (H E × 470)

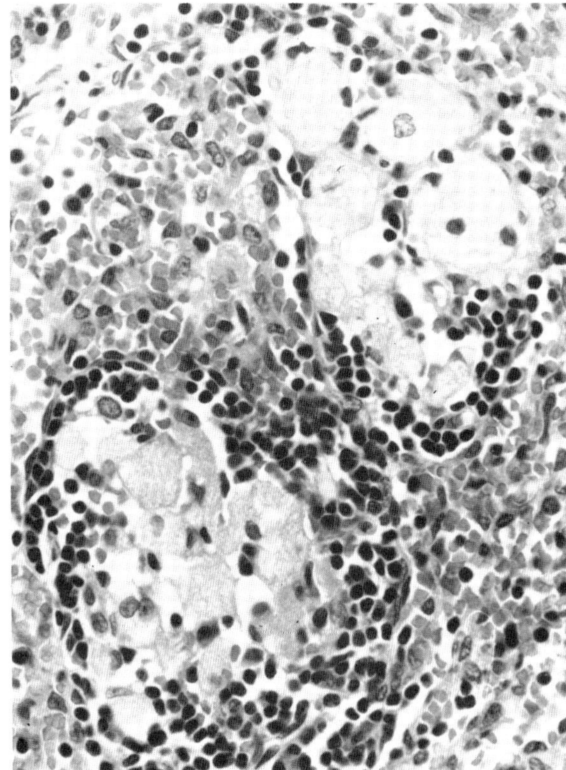

Fig. 14.3 Abdominal lymph node from a child with Gaucher's disease showing groups of Gaucher cells in the pulp adjacent to a lymph sinus. The 'streaky' cytoplasm of these large cells is characteristic. (H E × 470)

disease the cytoplasmic lipid appears in in the form of fine droplets, resembling neutral fat in appearance.

A quite distinctive form of sinus histiocytosis is seen in *Whipple's disease*. The same, large, pale-staining macrophages, as are present in huge numbers in the small intestinal mucosa, are also found in the lymph sinuses of the draining lymph nodes (Figs 14.4, 14.5). Although these macrophages are present in largest numbers in the abdominal nodes, they may also be found sometimes in inguinal, axillary and cervical nodes and the correct diagnosis may occasionally be made on a superficial lymph node biopsy in a patient with an obscure febrile illness, without overt evidence of intestinal disease. The macrophages in Whipple's disease are mostly mononuclear with relatively small nuclei and abundant pale, faintly basophilic cytoplasm, which can appear granular or finely vacuolated. The cytoplasm is strikingly PAS-positive, giving a much stronger and more diffuse reaction than that ordinarily seen in macrophages (Fig. 14.6). In abdominal nodes, globules of fat may also be found in the lymph sinuses and, at a later stage, secondary fibrosis may develop in these nodes. The distinctive macrophages are then much less obvious. The aetiology of Whipple's disease is still obscure, despite the demonstration of bacterial remains in the macrophage cytoplasm by electron microscopy (Fig. 14.7).

The above conditions must, of course, be distinguished from the appearances seen in lymph nodes following *lymphangiography* (see Figs 14.8, 14.9). Clear globules of the oil-contrast medium may be seen filling the lymph sinuses and sometimes spilling into the dense pulp of the node as well. The globules in the sinuses are often surrounded by mononuclear and multinucleate macrophages, sometimes with a transient polymorph infiltration, but there is no granulomatous reaction or secondary fibrosis, such as may be provoked by more irritant oils, and the oil shows little tendency to break up into very fine droplets, even after several months.

In *malakoplakia* of the bladder or other organs, draining lymph nodes are occasionally involved. Affected nodes initially show sinus histiocytosis (Fig. 14.10). At a later stage the characteristically large, rounded macrophages containing Michaelis-Guttmann bodies may be found also in the dense pulp. Plasma cell infiltration is usual and progressive destruction of the nodes may occur with subsequent fibrosis.

In so-called '*immature sinus histiocytosis*' the sinuses are focally filled with uniform cells which have less cytoplasm than the cells of simple sinus histiocytosis, and nuclei with denser chromatin, containing larger nucleoli. Although the infiltrate is predominantly sinusoidal, the demarcation between the sinusoidal infiltrate and the pulp is less clear than in simple sinus histiocytosis, the cells tending to infiltrate the adjacent lymphoid tissue (see Fig. 6.51, p. 117). Despite their monocytoid appearance the cells do not show phagocytosis. They were earlier thought to be 'immature' histiocytes, but there is good evidence that they are stimulated lymphocytes. These cells are a feature of several diseases associated with the presence of

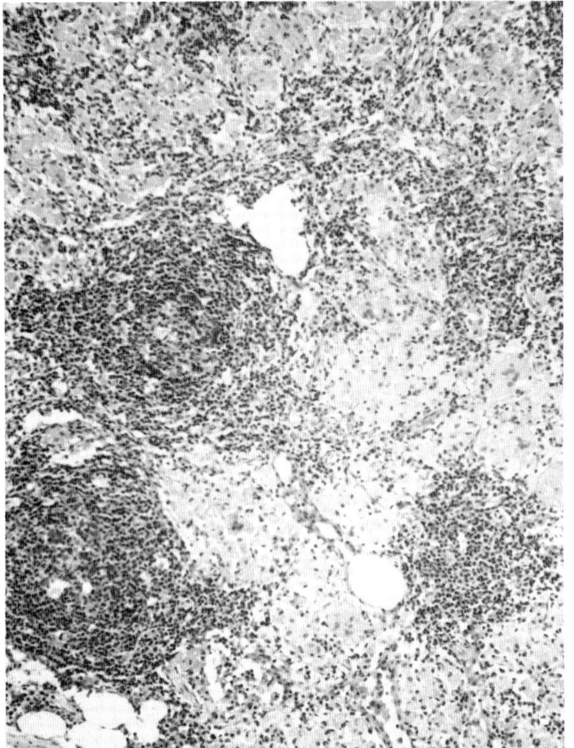

Fig. 14.4 Mesenteric lymph node in Whipple's disease showing the characteristic sinus histiocytosis. Note fat globules in sinus. (H E × 120)

Fig. 14.5 Same node as Fig. 14.4 at a higher magnification showing a multinucleate macrophage (H E × 470)

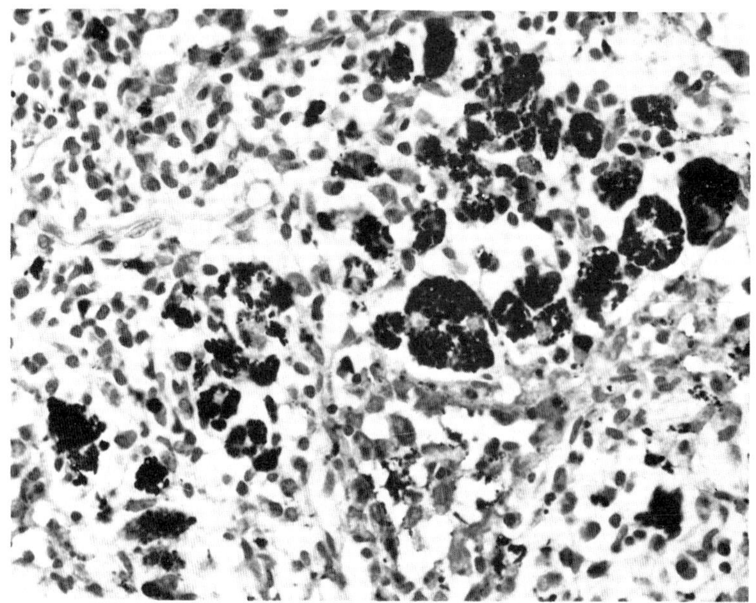

Fig. 14.6 Same node as Figs 14.4 and 14.5 showing strong PAS positivity of macrophages (PAS × 470)

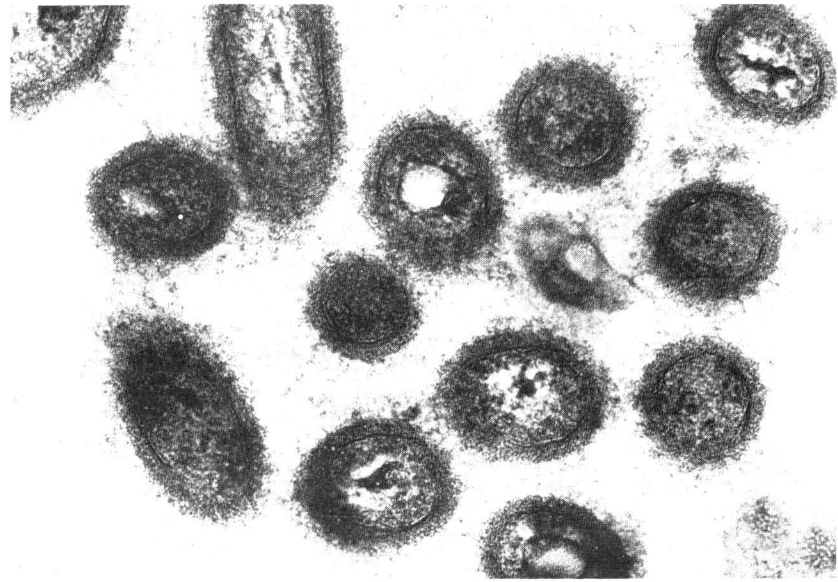

Fig. 14.7 Electron micrograph showing bacterial bodies in the cytoplasm of a macrophage in Whipple's disease

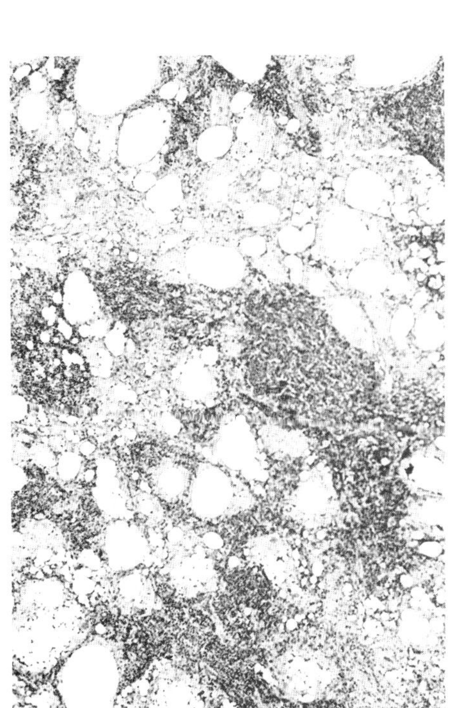

Fig. 14.8 Para-aortic lymph node showing characteristic appearances following lymphangiography. The empty holes represent globules of the oily contrast medium. (H E × 47)

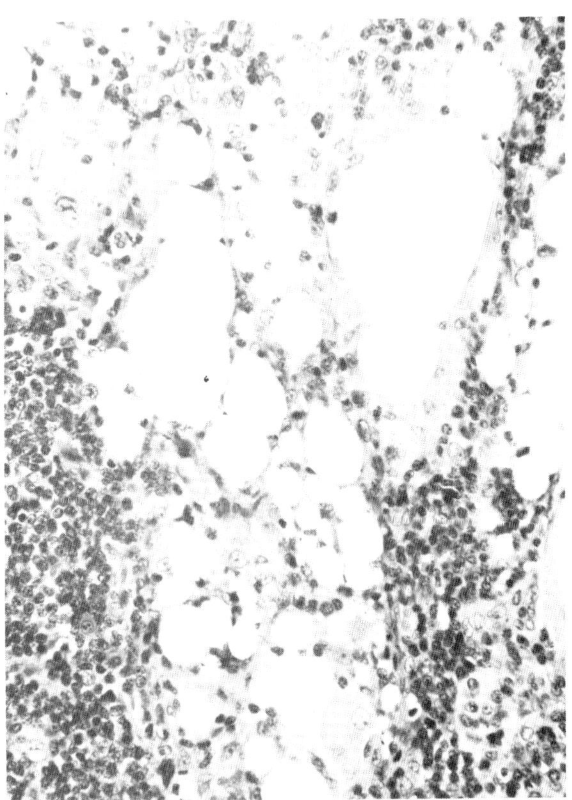

Fig. 14.9 Same node as Fig. 14.8 at a higher magnification to show macrophage reaction to the oil droplets (H E × 300)

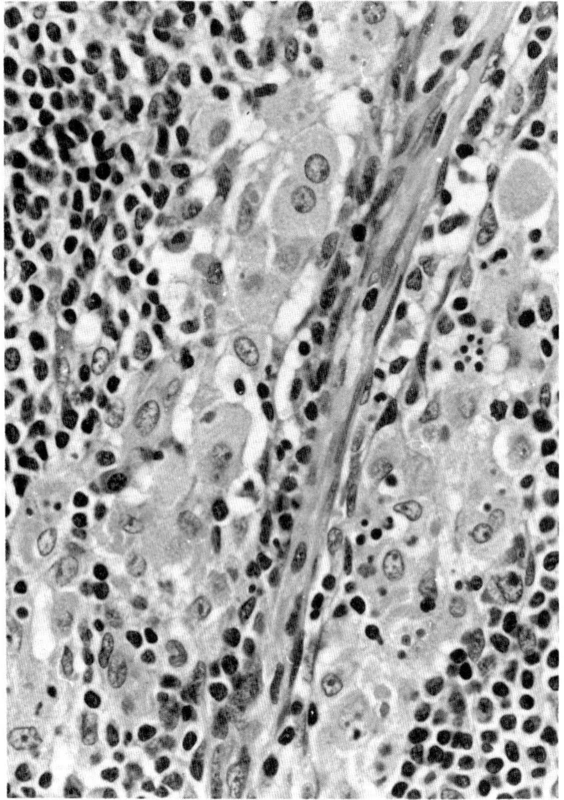

Fig. 14.10 Pelvic lymph node showing large sinus macrophages from a case of malakoplakia of the bladder. The darkly staining, haematoxyphil bodies, sometimes surrounded by a pale halo, are Michaelis-Guttmann bodies. (H E × 470)

circulating atypical mononuclear cells. Thus 'immature sinus histiocytosis' is seen characteristically in infectious mononucleosis, post-vaccinial lymphadenitis, cat scratch disease and toxoplasmosis. It may occur in some other infections, and has been noted in brucellosis. Although generally indicative of a benign reactive process, the phenomenon may rarely be seen in Hodgkin's disease.

Sinus histiocytosis with massive lymphadenopathy

Sinus histiocytosis with massive lymphadenopathy (SHML) is a rare condition outside Africa and has been recognised only recently as a distinct clinicopathological entity (Rosai & Dorfman, 1969, 1972). It has the morphological features of a greatly exaggerated reactive process. The lymph nodes may reach an enormous size, and may remain persistently enlarged, in the absence of a demonstrable aetiological agent, for many years. The aetiology is quite unknown, but the histological picture is so distinctive that the process is easily recognised, even when it arises in an extranodal site.

Clinical features. The disease seems to affect Negroes more commonly than whites, but it is not confined to any particular race or geographical area. It usually presents in the first decade of life, but may also present in adulthood. It is characterised by massive, painless, generally bilateral, cervical lymphadenopathy (Fig. 14.11) with relatively minor involvement of other groups of nodes in most instances. About a quarter of the patients have involvement of extranodal sites (especially the upper respiratory tract, salivary glands, orbit and testis) and lesions at these sites or in the skin may present before the appearance of lymphadenopathy (Foucar et al, 1978). Patients usually have moderate pyrexia, with a neutrophil leucocytosis, a raised ESR and polyclonal hyperglobulinaemia. The natural history of the disease is persistence of

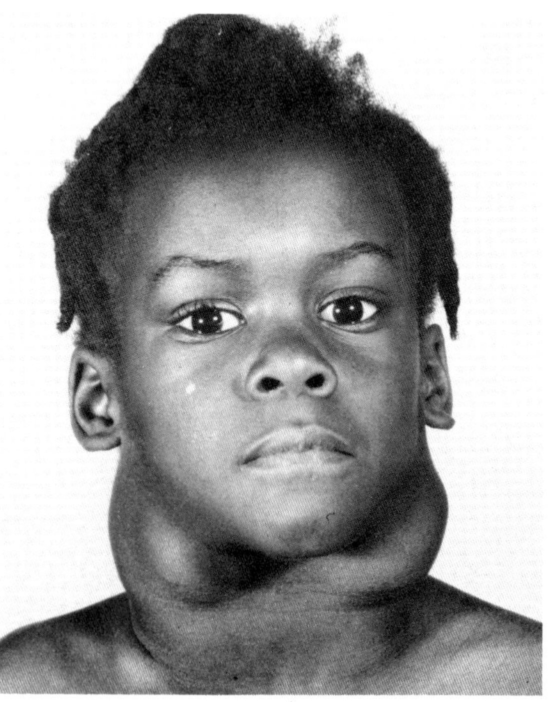

Fig. 14.11 Sinus histiocytosis with massive lymphadenopathy (SHML) in a five and a half year old West Indian girl

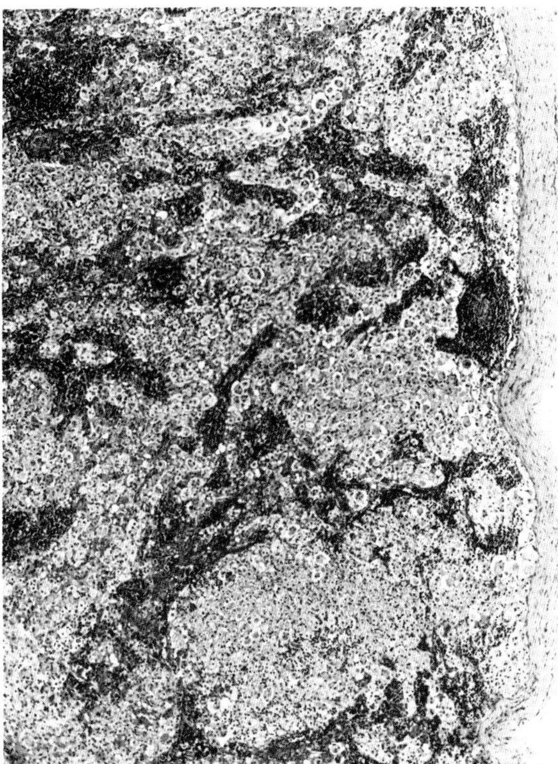

Fig. 14.12 Lymph node biopsy from the child shown in Fig. 14.11. The lymph sinuses are distended by large, pale-staining macrophages with compression of the intervening pulp. A single lymph follicle is seen (right). (H E × 47)

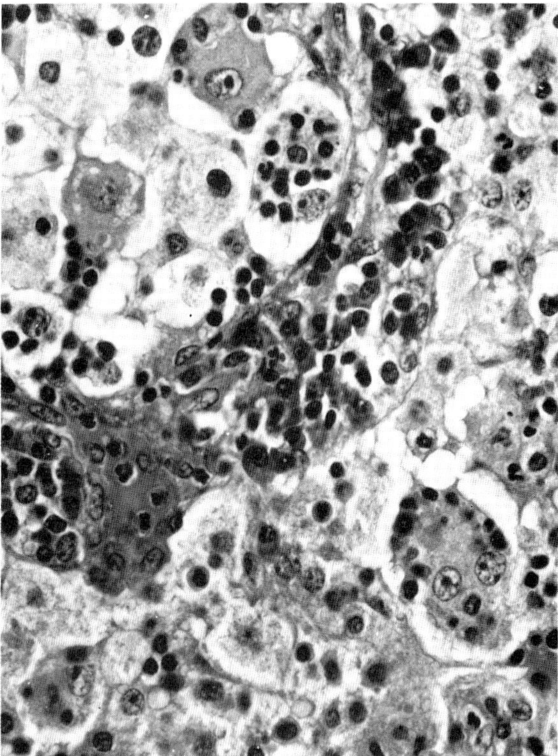

Fig. 14.13 Higher power view of the same lymph node as that shown in Fig. 14.12 to show detail of macrophages, many of which contain engulfed cells or nuclear debris. The thin strand of tissue between the expanded sinuses is stuffed with plasma cells. (H E × 470)

lymphadenopathy for months or years, sometimes with intermittent recession and resurgence, followed eventually by complete resolution. No form of therapy has been shown to be of any benefit. Of the 34 patients in the series of Rosai & Dorfman (1972), one died of renal amyloidosis, another after cytotoxic therapy.

Histology. Affected lymph nodes show marked and often gross dilatation of sinuses by a mixed population of cells, with very large histiocytes predominating over lymphocytes, plasma cells and neutrophils (Figs 14.12, 14.13). In the fully developed lesion, this infiltrate compresses the intersinusoidal lymphoid tissue which may be reduced to thin columns of tissue between the expanded sinuses and may eventually disappear altogether with consequent diffuse infiltration of the node pulp (Fig. 14.14). The most conspicuous element of the sinusoidal infiltrate is a very large histiocyte of distinctive appearance which is quite unlike the normal sinus-lining cell. These cells have large, vesicular, round or oval nuclei and abundant pale granular or finely vacuolated cytoplasm which contains only small quantities of finely divided fat. Occasional multinucleated cells of the same type are present. Some of the histiocytes may show mild nuclear atypia, with pleomorphism, hyperchromatism and large nucleoli (Fig. 14.15). However, mitoses amongst these cells are rare. A constant and characteristic finding in this disease is the presence of phagocytosed cells within the giant histiocytes (Fig. 14.13). The ingested cells are predominantly lymphocytes, but neutrophils, plasma cells and red cells are sometimes also ingested. There may be many such cells in a single histiocyte, giving rise to an unusual impression under low magnification of clusters or rosettes of cells. The surviving intersinusoidal tissue consists

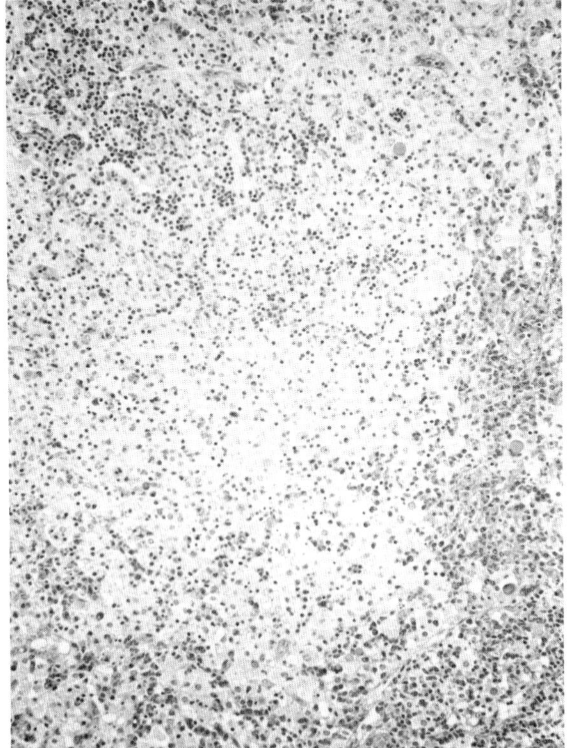

Fig. 14.14 Lymph node biopsy from a West Indian male of 33 who claimed to have had cervical lymphadenopathy for 18 years. Sinuses are no longer discernible and the macrophage infiltrate has spread diffusely through the node pulp. The clustering of lymphocytes (upper field) is due to their containment within macrophages. (H E × 120)

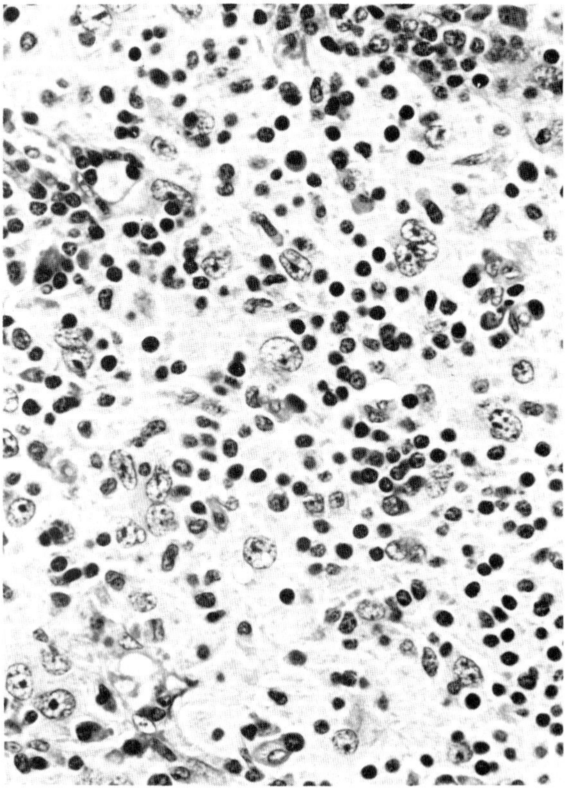

Fig. 14.15 Same node as Fig. 14.14 to show some macrophages with atypical nuclei and prominent nucleoli. These should not be mistaken for malignant cells. (H E × 470)

of small lymphocytes with a variable, often large, number of plasma cells, some of which show Russell bodies. Lymph follicles and germinal centres are inconspicuous or absent. Eosinophils are not a feature and there are no granulomas or areas of necrosis. There is often marked capsular and pericapsular fibrosis as the disease progresses and, in long-standing cases, some fibrosis may develop in the node itself.

Differential diagnosis. Although the clinical and histological features of SHML may appear alarming to those unfamiliar with the disease, the histological appearance of the nodes is so characteristic that it is not likely to be confused with other conditions by anyone who has once seen it. In malignant histiocytosis (p. 368) the sinus histiocytes show much more obvious nucleocytoplasmic atypia and mitotic activity. In familial haemophagocytic reticulosis (p. 371) most of the cells engulfed by sinusoidal macrophages are erythrocytes rather than lymphocytes. Storage diseases can be excluded by the absence of significant amounts of lipid, carbohydrate or mucopolysaccharide in the histiocytes. There is no real justification for mistaking SHML for Hodgkin's disease, although the mistake has been made.

Pulp histiocytosis

As we have seen, the highest concentration of phagocytic cells in a lymph node resides in the lymph sinuses and it is thus natural that many reactions, in which phagocytosis of lymph-borne material is occurring, should show a sinus pattern. In some circumstances the scattered histiocytes of the dense pulp are engaged as well and, in other

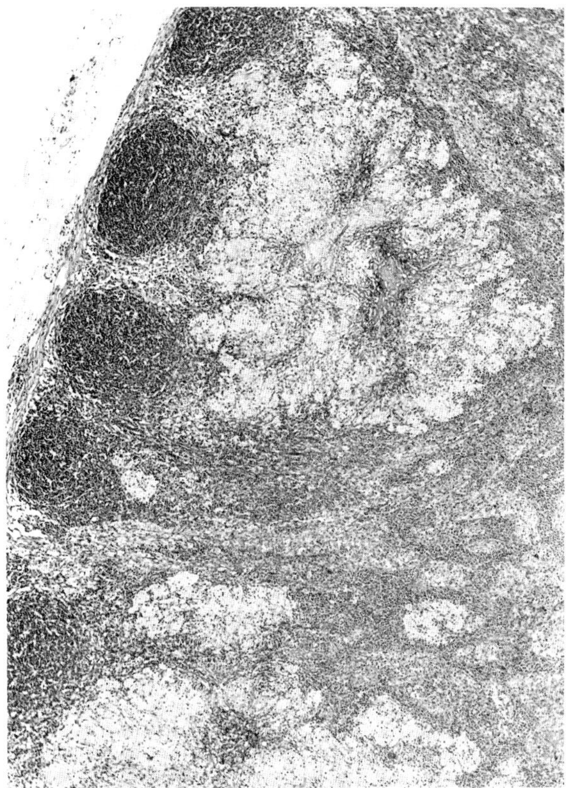

Fig. 14.16 Coeliac lymph node from a woman of 36 which was found to be enlarged in the course of a cholecystectomy operation and was removed. There is a striking pulp histiocytosis, the cause of which was not discovered. (H E × 47)

Fig. 14.17 Same node as Fig. 14.16 at a higher magnification showing large pale histiocytes, some of multinucleate type (H E × 375)

instances, a sinus histiocytosis is hardly apparent and the reaction is concentrated in the dense pulp of the node (Fig. 14.16, 14.17). This is often seen, for example, in the massive accumulation of dust-containing macrophages in bronchopulmonary and mediastinal lymph nodes of individuals who live or work in a dusty atmosphere. In the presence of fibrogenic dusts (especially those containing silica) the macrophage population may be progressively replaced by dense acellular collagen, with or without the supervention of necrosis in the tissue.

Dermatopathic lymphadenopathy (dermatopathic lymphadenitis: lipomelanic reticulosis)

A special instance of pulp histiocytosis, in which there is often a massive accumulation of interdigitating reticulum cells, is seen in dermatopathic lymphadenopathy. Patients with chronic skin disorders, particularly exfoliative dermatitis, but sometimes psoriasis or other conditions, commonly develop enlargement of the superficial lymph node groups, mainly axillary and inguinal. Since a reason for the lymphadenopathy is often apparent, lymph node biopsy is only likely to be performed when the nodes attract attention and the skin condition is overlooked or when there is doubt about the nature of the lymph node enlargement. The condition is undoubtedly much more frequent than the number of positive biopsies submitted to the laboratory would suggest.

Macroscopically, the nodes are seldom more than 2 cm in diameter unless some other condition (e.g. mycosis fungoides) is superimposed. The cut surface of the node may show a distinct yellow-brown mottling, but is usually unremarkable.

Histologically, the picture is distinctive and often diagnostic, even when no history of a skin disorder is given. The cortical follicles are generally well preserved, with sharply defined edges, and sometimes contain prominent germinal centres. The enlargement of the node is, however, due to striking expansion of the paracortex which becomes progressively filled up with pale-staining mononuclear reticulum cells, displacing the lymphocyte population. In the initial stages, small clusters of these cells are scattered through the paracortex but, as the condition progresses, more and more accumulate until they form coalescent sheets which appear as festoons around the contrasting follicles when the section is examined with a hand lens (Fig. 14.18). Detailed examination of the paracortical infiltrate reveals a scattering of plasma cells and eosinophils amongst the reticulum cells. A minority of the latter appear to be histiocytes (mononuclear phagocytes) and these often contain granules of melanin pigment or lipid. Most of these pale-staining cells are, however, non-phagocytic and show the enzyme histochemical and electron microscopic features of interdigitating reticulum cells (Fig. 14.19). In a good quality section, it is possible to make out the curiously shaped, 'folded' nuclei of the interdigitating cells by light microscopy (Fig. 14.20). On electron microscopy, the interlocking plasma membranes are strikingly revealed. The origin of these cells is still uncertain, but it has been suggested that they may be derived from Langerhans cells of the epidermis, which have migrated in the lymph stream to the nodes.

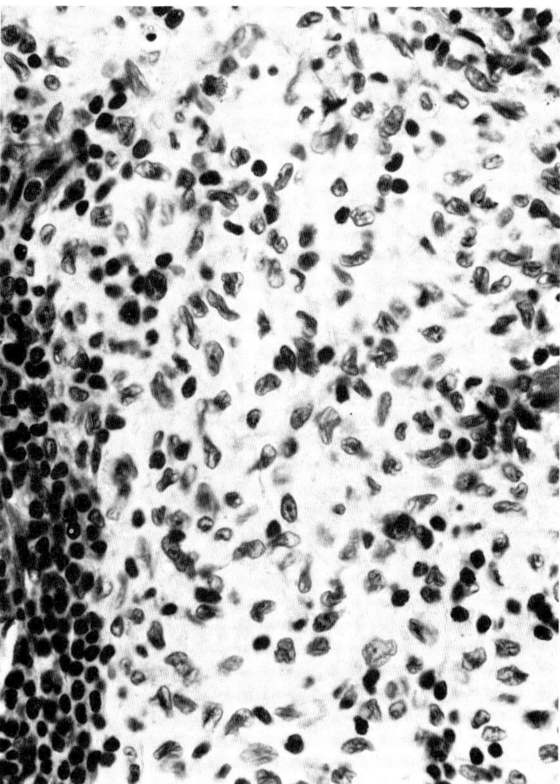

Fig. 14.19 Same node as Fig. 14.18. The well defined edge of a follicle (left) contrasts with the paracortical infiltrate consisting mainly of interdigitating reticulum cells with a few histiocytes and some eosinophils. (H E × 470)

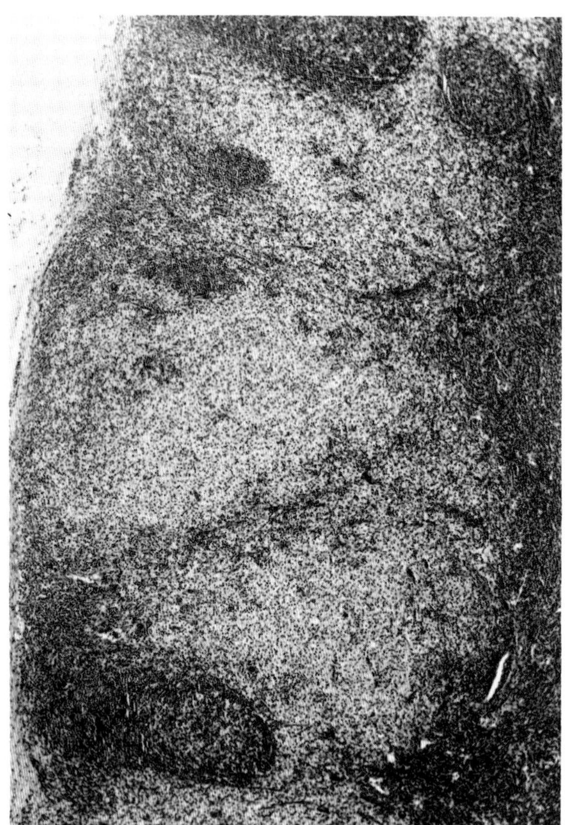

Fig. 14.18 Axillary lymph node from a man of 60 with chronic exfoliative dermatitis showing typical features of dermatopathic lymphadenitis. The expanded paracortex is filled with sharply defined masses of pale reticulum cells whilst the cortical follicles are preserved. (H E × 47)

Dermatopathic lymphadenopathy is of itself a benign, reactive condition. It is, however, import-

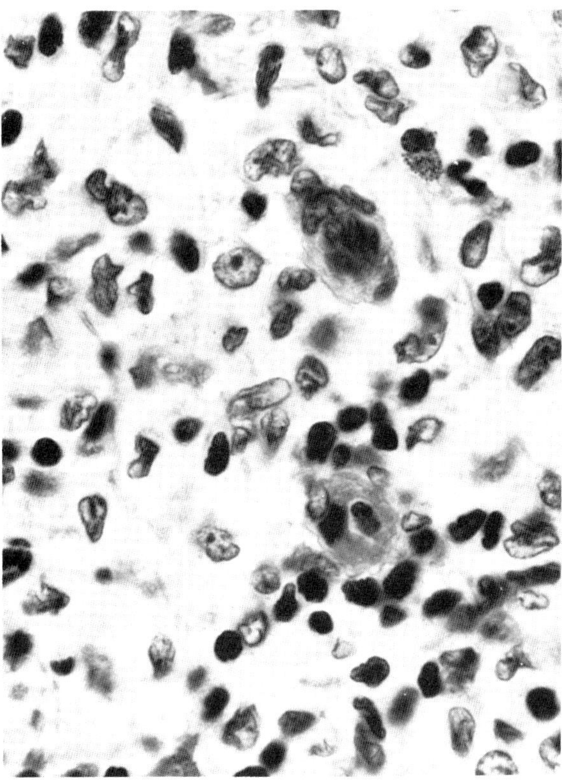

Fig. 14.20 Same node as Figs 14.18 and 14.19 to show detail of interdigitating reticulum cells. Note the curiously shaped nuclei and abundant pale cytoplasm of the latter. An eosinophil is seen (upper right) and a histiocyte (left of vessel) with prominent central nucleolus. (H E × 940)

ant to remember that the skin disorder which elicited this reaction may be neoplastic, i.e. mycosis fungoides (or Sézary syndrome). It is, therefore, not uncommon to see lymph nodes in which a neoplastic lymphoid cell infiltrate is superimposed upon the changes of a long-standing dermatopathic lymphadenopathy (see p. 304–5).

Granulomatous lesions

In some circumstances, the macrophages which accumulate in the node retain the capacity for active phagocytosis, whether they persist as large, rounded cells or appear elongate and irregular. However, in circumstances which are not fully understood, some or all of the cells lose their phagocytic potency and become transformed into epithelioid cells (Spector, 1974) In this transformation process, the cells take on the character of secreting cells with alteration of their ultrastructural features. They also tend to adhere together to form small clusters or larger 'granulomas', often attended by the formation of multinucleate giant-cells or polykaryons. Small epithelioid cell clusters or larger granulomas are a feature of the histological picture in many infective processes in lymph nodes which have already been discussed in Chapter 6 (p. 89). In this section we shall discuss some granulomatous lesions which are not obviously infective in origin.

Sarcoidosis

The *aetiology* of this strange granulomatous disorder is still unknown although there have been many speculations. The close resemblance of the histological picture to that of non-caseating tuberculosis and the occasional development of overt tuberculosis in patients who have had an initial diagnosis of sarcoidosis, have led some to believe that sarcoidosis is a form of tuberculosis, perhaps caused by ultramicroscopic sub-units of *M. tuberculosis*, for absence of demonstrable organisms has hitherto been a *sine qua non* for the diagnosis. The regular finding of a negative Mantoux reaction in sarcoidosis has been held to support the theory of tuberculosis without hypersensitivity, but others have pointed to a general depression of T-lymphocyte function in this disease. This observation and others (e.g. the Kveim reaction) have been cited in support of the belief that sarcoidosis does not have a single cause, infective or otherwise, but is basically an immunological disturbance, in which a variety of stimuli may evoke a granulomatous response. Whatever the true nature of sarcoidosis may be, there are some phenomena, such as the distribution of the lesions and the occurrence of hypercalcaemia, which are difficult to explain.

Incidence. The disease is common throughout Northern Europe, including Britain, and occurs in many other parts of the world. Although sarcoidosis occurs commonly, and often in florid form, amongst blacks in the USA and in the W. Indies, it does not seem to be prevalent in Africa. It is principally a disease of adults, but shows a wide age range. The sexes are affected equally.

Presentation. The diverse sites of presentation of the disease — salivary glands, skin, eyes, lungs, lymph nodes and bones — account for the fact that different manifestations of the disease were described originally as separate diseases and it was years before the essential unity of these varied phenomena was appreciated. In all the above sites and in other organs too, for the disease has been described in practically every organ of the body, the underlying lesion is the same — a small, non-caseating, tuberculoid granuloma.

Lymphadenopathy is common in sarcoidosis and the presence of bilateral hilar node enlargement in a chest radiograph is one of the commonest findings, especially in young adults with the disease. Such lymph node swellings may be attended by malaise and cough or may be asymptomatic. The diagnosis can be confirmed by biopsy of a superficial enlarged node or a scalene node in the presence of lung involvement. The Mantoux test is negative and in doubtful cases a positive Kveim test is confirmatory.

Macroscopically, affected lymph nodes are a pinkish buff or sometimes a pale tan colour. The consistency varies, from soft to moderately firm, depending upon the duration of the disease. Individual nodes are seldom more than 2–3 cm in diameter.

Histology. Typically the node is filled with small non-caseating granulomas with or without multinucleate giant-cells (Fig. 14.21). The residual lymphoid tissue shows little evidence of immunological stimulation and although the follicles are often spared at first, the germinal centres remain small and non-reactive. Likewise, there are no immunoblasts and few or no plasma cells.

The individual sarcoid granulomas are small in size and initially they are neatly circumscribed and discrete, consisting of a large cluster of epithelioid cells (Fig. 14.22). Later the granulomatous foci

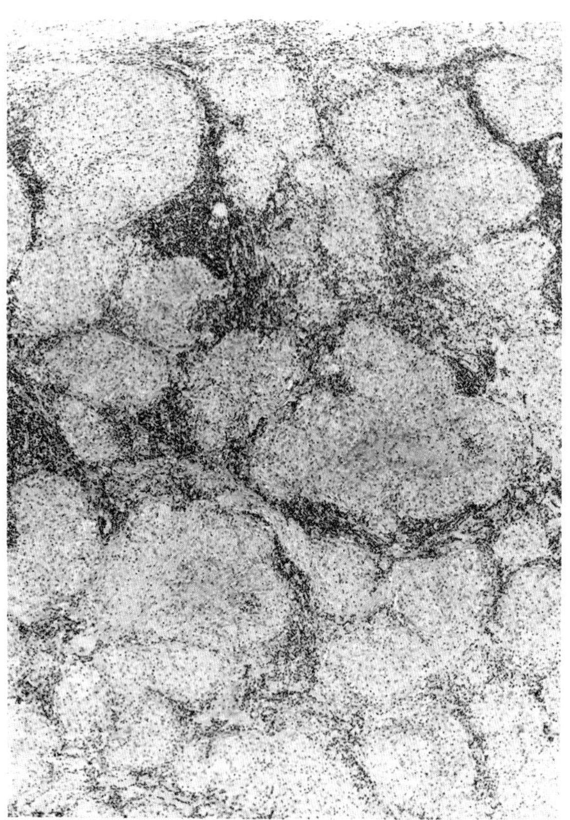

Fig. 14.21 Lymph node filled with typical granulomas of sarcoidosis (H E × 47)

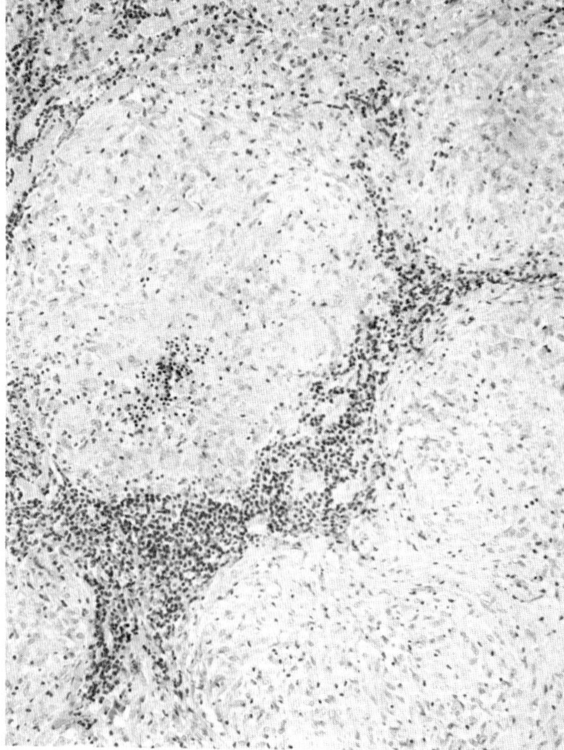

Fig. 14.22 Same node as Fig. 14.21 at a higher magnification. The granulomatous foci are compact and sharply defined. There is early fibrosis around the confluent granulomas (bottom right). (H E × 120)

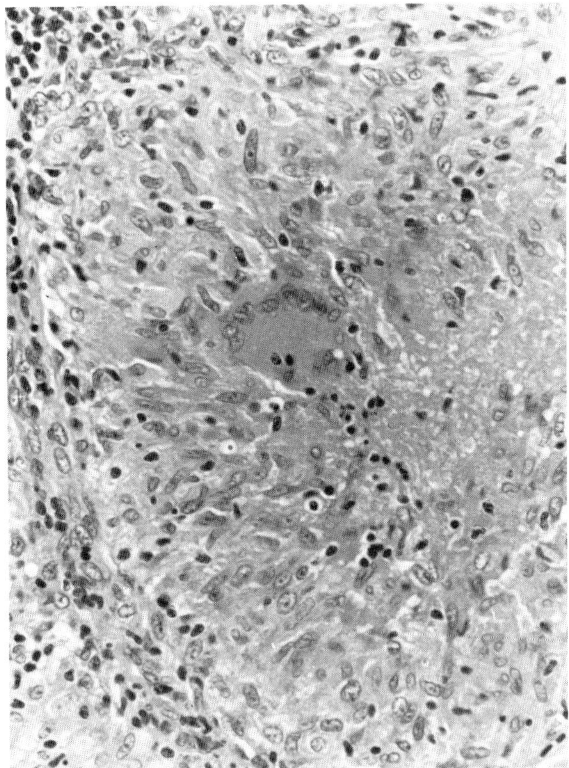

Fig. 14.23 Margin of a sarcoid granuloma showing a multinucleate giant-cell among the epithelioid cells and central necrosis of the lesion. (Same node as Figs 14.21 and 14.22.) (H E × 300)

coalesce, but, as in tuberculosis, the individual 'units' remain clearly visible. The centres of the coalescent foci often show necrosis and stain brightly with eosin, but there is no caseation (Fig. 14.23).

Multinucleate giant-cells are a variable feature: they may be entirely absent from the granulomas, on the other hand, they can be numerous. They are seldom such a conspicuous feature as the giant-cells in tuberculosis and classical Langhans type giant-cells are uncommon. Two types of inclusion may be found in the giant-cells: (1) strongly haematoxyphil, laminated or 'conchoidal', Schaumann bodies. These consist often of an outer shell of amorphous calcific material enclosing central, doubly refractile, non-staining, crystals of calcite (Fig. 14.24). (2) Asteroid bodies, consisting of a star-shaped, slightly refractile, but isotropic body, lying in a cytoplasmic vacuole. Neither of these

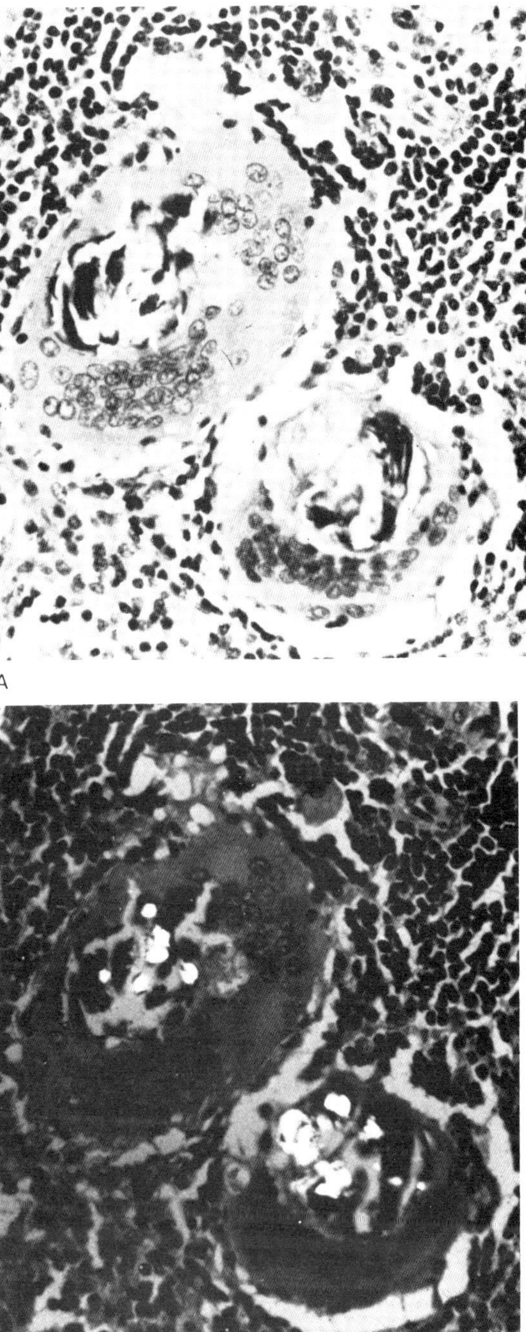

Fig. 14.24 (a) and (b) Another lymph node in sarcoidosis showing two large multinucleate giant-cells without surrounding epithelioid cells. (a) Each giant cell contains a laminated calcified conchoidal body (Schaumann body). (b) The same field viewed by polarised light showing birefringent calcite crystals within the Schaumann bodies. (H E × 300)

structures is peculiar to sarcoidosis — Schaumann bodies may be found in giant-cells in chronic tuberculosis, whilst asteroid bodies are commonly seen in foreign-body type giant-cells.

In the initial stages the granulomas show remarkably little reticulin with silver impregnation but, in course of time, they are gradually replaced by collagen and amorphous protein, eventually becoming extensively hyalinised or even calcified (Fig. 14.25). A few epithelioid cells and sometimes giant-cells may persist, however, for a very long time.

Differential diagnosis. Points of distinction from chronic tuberculosis have been discussed above and on page 105. As already indicated, this distinction is not always possible on histological grounds and in these circumstances it may be deemed wise to treat the patient (if treatment is indicated) with steroids administered concurrently with anti-tuberculous drugs. The absence of immunological reactivity in the lymphoid tissue of the node distinguishes sarcoidosis from a number of other infective processes in which a granulomatous reaction is seen, e.g. toxoplasmosis. In most of these and in Hodgkin's disease too, the granulomatous foci tend to be smaller, less uniform and less neatly circumscribed than the granulomas of sarcoidosis.

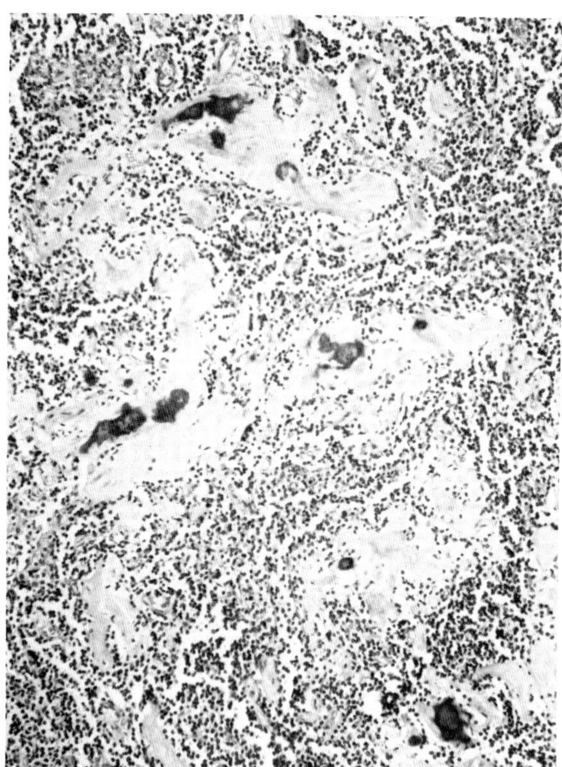

Fig. 14.25 Lymph node showing 'burnt out' sarcoidosis. The granulomas have been replaced by hyaline collagen with focal calcification. (H E × 120)

It is important to appreciate that granulomas of identical type may be found in a variety of different circumstances, e.g. in berylliosis or in association with malignant disease. Some of the most important of these 'sarcoid-type reactions' will be discussed below. In general, the granulomas found in lymph nodes in sarcoid-type reactions are less numerous and thus less crowded than the granulomas of sarcoidosis.

Sarcoid-type reactions associated with 'foreign' material

A variety of mineral and other substances have been reported as eliciting a sarcoid-type granulomatous reaction in tissues and notably in lymph nodes. Perhaps the most important condition in this category is *berylliosis*. Granulomatous lesions closely resembling those of sarcoidosis may develop in the lymph nodes (generally axillary) draining the site of entry of beryllium salts through the skin. Such lesions were more commonly seen before the danger of handling beryllium products was appreciated. *Talc* introduced into the tissues, and formerly widely used as glove powder, also evokes a granulomatous reaction of sarcoid-type. As with beryllium salts and with siliceous granulomas, there is commonly a long latent period (sometimes several years) between the time of first exposure and the local swelling which leads to the discovery of granulomas. The talc particles, being comparatively large, are less likely to be transported to draining lymph nodes. They are also more readily detected, especially if the section is examined by polarised light — a practice which is to be recommended in all cases where a granulomatous reaction of this type is seen. *Zirconium* salts which have been used in antiperspirant preparations are also said to be capable of exciting a sarcoid-type reaction.

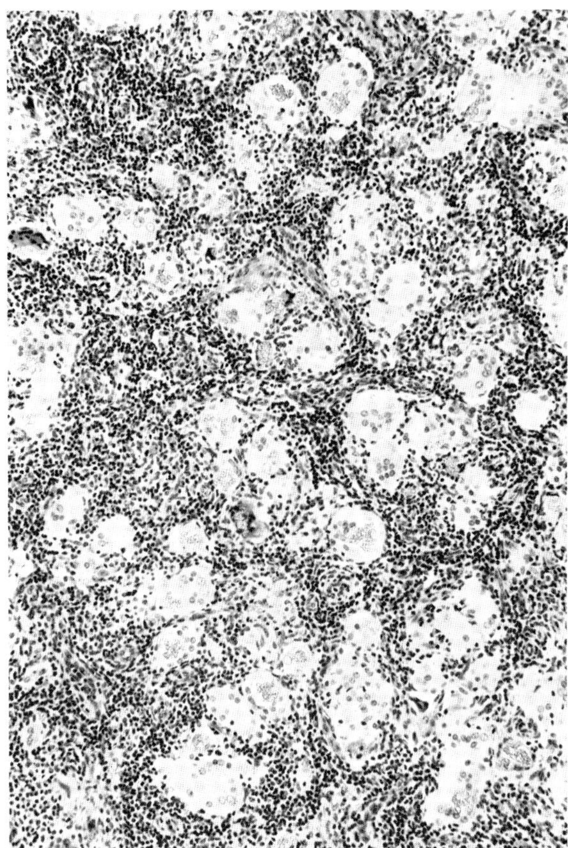

Fig. 14.26 Inguinal lymph node biopsy from a young woman, who had previously had a 'silastic' implant in the foot, showing numerous foreign-body type giant-cells, some containing non-birefringent foreign material. Sarcoid-type granulomas were found in another part of the same node. (H E × 120)

Fig. 14.27 Same node as Fig. 14.26 at a higher magnification, to show the typical features of silicone lymphadenopathy. Foreign material, which was demonstrated by electron probe analysis to consist principally of silicon, can be seen in several of the giant-cells. An asteroid body can be seen in the giant-cell to the left of centre. (H E × 300)

Other exogenous materials, introduced into the tissues in a variety of ways and for a variety of reasons, may find their way into regional lymph nodes and there evoke a 'foreign-body' reaction (Fig. 14.26, 14.27). Sometimes this reaction elicits granulomas with a striking resemblance to sarcoid lesions, at other times the clustered macrophages (with or without giant-cells) remain discrete and do not transform into epithelioid cells. Such is usually the case with *polyvinylpyrrolidone* (PVP), a substance which has been widely used in Continental Europe as a plasma expander and a vehicle for parenteral injections. This almost inert material is taken up by macrophages throughout the reticuloendothelial system and is often stored in lymph nodes, resulting in a picture not unlike that of lepromatous leprosy (p. 107). The two conditions can be distinguished by appropriate stains for lepra bacilli or for PVP (Pearse, 1972). The pathologist should always consider the possibility of a reaction to foreign material before making a confident diagnosis of sarcoidosis.

Other sarcoid-type granulomas

Small non-caseating granulomas, more or less closely resembling those of sarcoidosis may also be found in Crohn's disease, in primary biliary cirrhosis and in association with various types of malignant disease. In *Crohn's disease* the granulomas are found both in the bowel lesion and in the draining (generally ileocolic) lymph nodes (Fig. 14.28). They may be scarce or plentiful in these sites, but are seldom very numerous in the nodes. The aggregates of epithelioid cells are generally less compact than those of sarcoidosis and there is seldom any difficulty in making the distinction. In *primary biliary cirrhosis* granulomas may be found in upper abdominal lymph nodes as well as in the liver. Again such lesions are unlikely to be confused with sarcoidosis, being generally more variable in size and less well circumscribed than sarcoid granulomas.

Sarcoid-type granulomas which may closely resemble those of sarcoidosis, are uncommonly found in *lymph nodes draining carcinomas* in a variety of sites. Such lesions are most frequently seen in axillary nodes in association with carcinoma of the breast and rarely the primary tumour shows a similar granulomatous reaction. As a rule the nodes showing this reaction, are themselves free of secondary carcinoma, but this is by no means invariable (Figs 14.29, 14.30). In cases of nasopharyngeal carcinoma and seminoma a granulomatous reaction in the draining nodes may be associated with metastatic tumour and the latter sometimes shows evidence of spontaneous regression (see Ch. 15). In most other instances, however, there is no evidence that the presence of nodal granulomas is of prognostic significance.

The occurrence of a granulomatous reaction in lymph nodes in association with *malignant lymphomas* has been discussed earlier (p. 247). It is worth noting that a granulomatous reaction of similar type is a conspicuous feature in some cases of immunoblastic lymphadenopathy (p. 180). In non-Hodgkin's lymphomas such granulomas are usually found in nodes involved by the tumour,

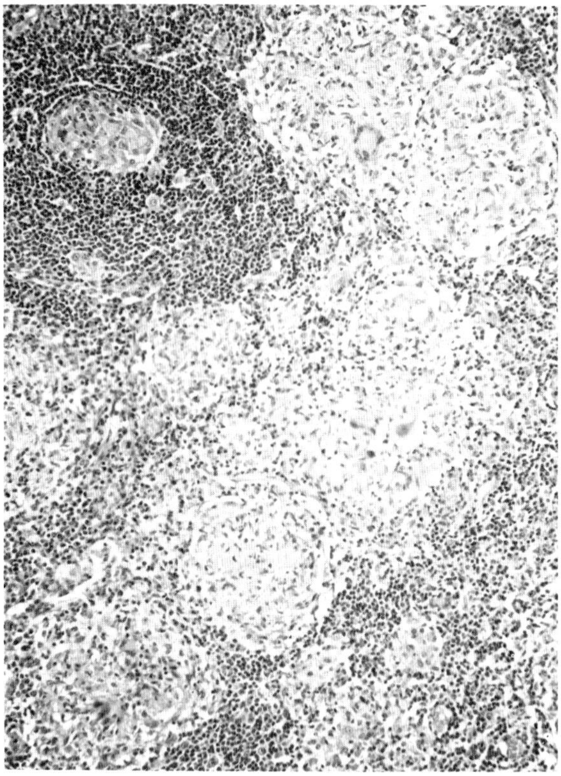

Fig. 14.28 Ileo-colic lymph node from a patient with Crohn's disease showing multiple, small, non-caseating granulomas. These are often less compact than the granulomas of sarcoidosis. Granulomas in this condition are sometimes found within germinal centres (top left). (H E × 120)

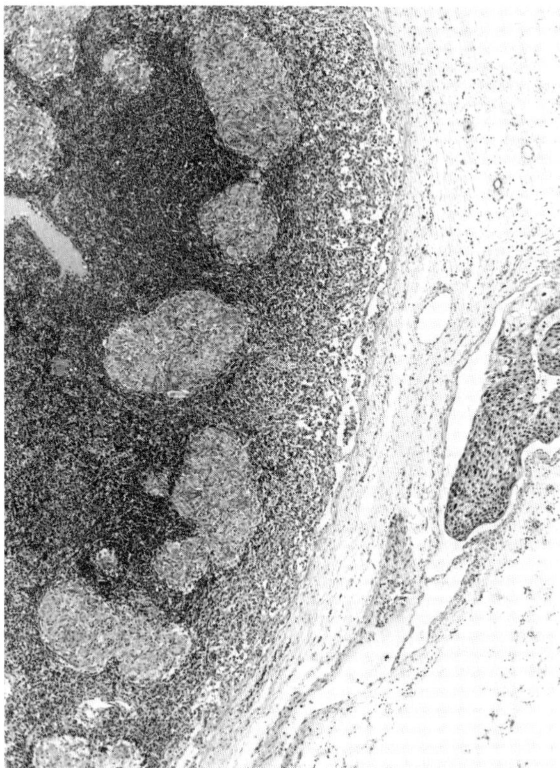

Fig. 14.29 Cervical lymph node draining a carcinoma of oesophagus in a man of 71. A plug of poorly differentiated squamous carcinoma can be seen within an afferent lymphatic (right) and in the node there are multiple, sarcoid-type granulomas. (H E × 47)

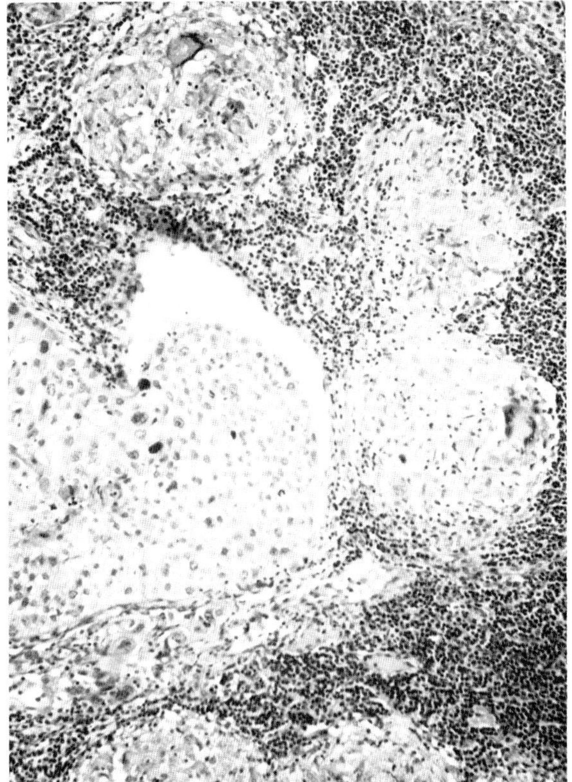

Fig. 14.30 Same node as Fig. 14.29. In this field carcinoma is present in a dilated lymph sinus (left) with granulomas in the surrounding node pulp. (H E × 120)

but in *Hodgkin's disease* granulomas may be found in abdominal lymph nodes, as in the spleen, liver and bone marrow, in the absence of Hodgkin's infiltration in these sites (see p. 219–220).

Finally, it must be said that isolated or occasionally multiple granulomas are sometimes found in lymph nodes taken for biopsy, when there is no other evidence of sarcoidosis and no explanation for their presence is found.

'HISTIOCYTOSIS X'

'Histiocytosis X' is a term introduced by Lichtenstein (1953) to include a group of diseases which had been previously described individually as eosinophilic granuloma of bone, Hand-Schüller-Christian disease and Letterer-Siwe disease. These disorders are linked by shared clinicopathological features: all show accumulations of cells which are, by light microscopy, well-differentiated, cytologically benign 'histiocytes' (see below). Although the more benign variants tend to contain an admixture of eosinophils and more fat-laden cells than the more aggressive Letterer-Siwe disease, the diseases cannot be reliably distinguished by histology alone (Daneshbod & Kissane, 1978). It was also proposed that the diseases represent points on a continuous spectrum (between single lesions and systemic accumulations) across which the disease might move in an individual patient (Engelbreth-Holm et al, 1944). The evidence for a transition was never universally accepted. Although the literature is full of reports describing 'transitions' from a single to multiple bony lesions (eosinophilic granuloma to Hand-Schüller-Christian disease), several recent large series show no evidence for progression of these 'localised' forms of the disease to the systemic, Letterer-Siwe disease (Lieberman et al, 1969; Newton & Hamoudi, 1973; Daneshbod & Kissane, 1978). Thus there appear to be two distinct clinical patterns of disease: a generalised (Letterer-Siwe disease), and a 'localised' (eosinophilic granuloma and Hand-Schüller-Christian disease).

In the generalised form there is diffuse infiltration of the reticuloendothelial system and other organs by 'histiocytes'. The patient (an infant) is ill at presentation, with a characteristic skin eruption, hepatosplenomegaly, generalised lymphadenopathy and impaired bone marrow function. The prognosis is poor whatever the treatment. In the 'localised' form the age range is much broader, the general condition of the patient is good, the lesions are self-healing and the disease does not require cytotoxic therapy. There are localised accumulations of 'histiocytes' and eosinophils involving one or more bones, either at one time or in sequence. The occurrence of cutaneous and localised lymph node involvement does not affect the prognosis. Bone marrow and liver function are undisturbed. Only the rare occurrence of diffuse pulmonary infiltration is of serious import, since this may lead to one form of 'honeycomb lung'. The natural history of the disease is gradual regression of the infiltrates, accompanied by fibrosis and callus formation in bony lesions. In older lesions foamy macrophages appear and cholesterol accumulates. Local radiation therapy or curettage accelerates healing. Hand-Schüller-Christian disease, with the triad of numerous osseous defects, proptosis and diabetes insipidus, is in fact a polyostotic eosinophil granuloma involving the orbital bones and the body of the sphenoid. Polyostotic and monostotic eosinophilic granuloma have the same course, prognosis and histological appearances. Neither progresses to a systemic disease. Disseminated 'histiocytosis' (Letterer-Siwe) is a diffuse disease from the outset; it does not start as monostotic or polyostotic eosinophilic granuloma.

Nature of 'Histiocytosis X'

The cells which accumulate in lesions of the 'Histiocytosis X' group, and which have traditionally been regarded as histiocytes, can in fact be readily distinguished from true histiocytes, even by light microscopy, especially when seen in the mass. Morphologically they resemble the interdigitating reticulum cells (IRC) of the T-zones in their nuclear features, for they have a similarly 'twisted-looking' nucleus with folds in the nuclear membrane. The cytoplasm, however, often stains more strongly and the cell boundaries are sharper since these cells do not interdigitate to the same degree. By electron microscopy they have been found to contain Langerhans granules (Basset & Turiaf, 1965; Nézelof & Jaubert, 1978), which are specific for an antigen-presenting, non-phagocytic bone marrow-derived cell which circulates to peripheral tissues such as epithelia before migrating to lymph nodes. From its systemic nature, Letterer-Siwe disease might represent either a neoplasm (with tissue distribution reflecting the environmental preferences of the normal counterpart) or a reactive accumulation of these cells (in response to an unknown aetiological agent or as part of an immunological defect) (Cederbaum et al, 1974). The self-limiting pattern of behaviour, seen in the localised forms of 'histiocytosis X', is unlike that of a neoplastic disease, and suggests that a local environmental stimulus (e.g. an infective agent) might be causing an accumulation of normal Langerhans-like cells.

Letterer-Siwe disease

Synonym:
Acute reticuloendotheliosis of infancy

Clinical features. This rare disease seldom, if ever develops in individuals of more than 3 years of age. Patients are febrile and ill on presentation, and the majority show a characteristic scaly, brown-red eczematoid or seborrhoeic skin eruption. Generalised lymphadenopathy and hepatosplenomegaly are present and numerous areas of osseous rarefaction may be seen on X-ray of skull, pelvis and long bones. Chest X-ray often shows miliary nodular infiltrates. Although recovery has occasionally been reported, the usual outcome is death within a few months. This is caused either by intercurrent infection or pancytopenia, the result of bone marrow replacement by 'histiocytes'.

Pathological features. Lymph nodes, taken for biopsy, are grey-red in colour and may show necrosis and haemorrhage on the cut surface. Like all other affected tissues they show extensive accumulation of cytologically uniform large cells with abundant eosinophilic cytoplasm, and an oval or indented, sometimes 'twisted' nucleus (Figs 14.31, 14.32). Nucleoli are inconspicuous and mitoses are generally infrequent. Multinucleate giant-cells of the same type are sometimes present. Eosinophils are scanty, if present at all, and neutrophils are only found in the presence of necrosis. Phagocytosis of red cells is rarely seen, but some accumulation of lipid in the 'histiocytes' may be found which tends to increase with the duration of illness, and may become sufficiently pronounced to cause confusion with eosinophilic granuloma. In the lymph nodes, 'histiocytes' accumulate first in the sinuses, but soon spread into the dense pulp, crowding out the normal lymphoid cells, although follicles may persist for some time (Fig. 14.31).

Sections from tumour-like masses in bone show extensive accumulation of identical cells, much bone destruction, and minimal bone regenerative activity. In skin biopsies the focal aggregates of uniform 'histiocytes' are characteristically limited to the upper dermis, although sometimes the biopsy only shows non-specific chronic inflammation. In the spleen there is diffuse accumulation

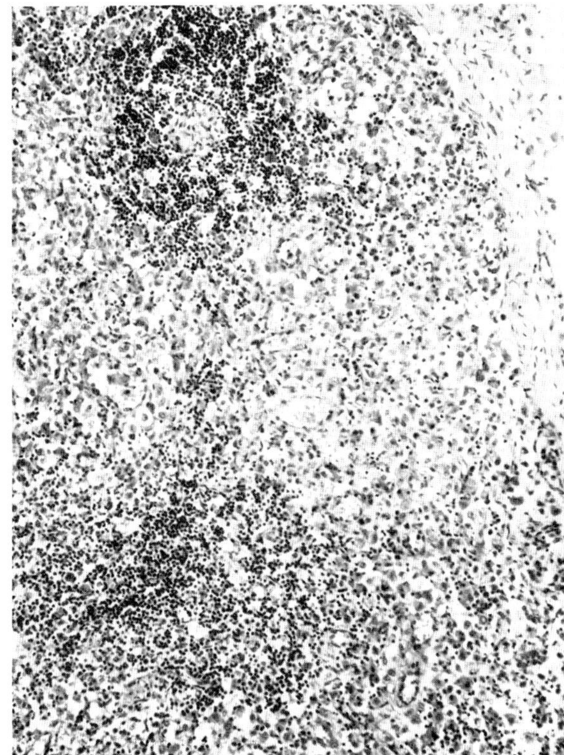

Fig. 14.31 Post-mortem lymph node from an infant aged 8 months with Letterer-Siwe disease. The sinuses and pulp are diffusely infiltrated by large 'histiocytic' cells. A preserved germinal follicle is seen (top). (H E × 120)

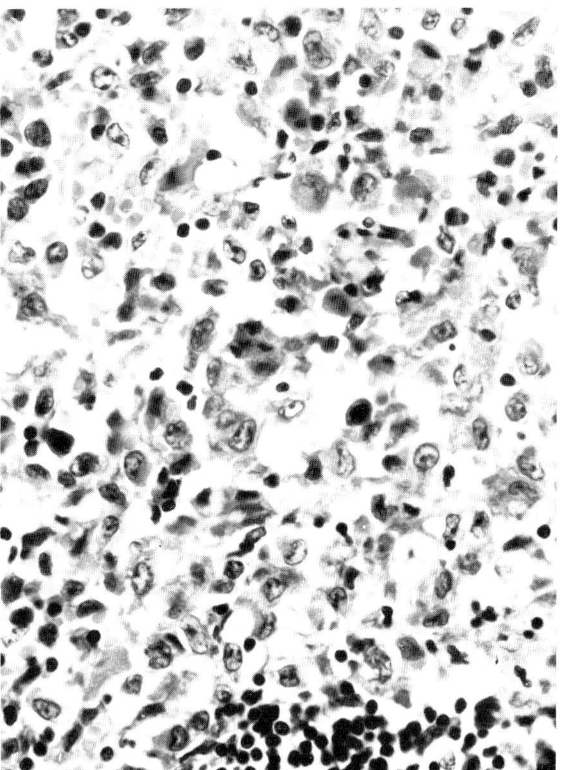

Fig. 14.32 Same node as Fig. 14.31 at a higher magnification, to show cellular detail. The characteristic 'histiocytes' have abundant eosinophilic cytoplasm and elongate, indented or twisted-looking nuclei. (H E × 470)

of 'histiocytes' appearing first in the red pulp but gradually encroaching upon the white pulp.

Differential diagnosis. Histiocytic medullary reticulosis, which can occur in infants, may clinically simulate Letterer-Siwe disease, including the occurrence of a skin eruption. The cellular infiltrates of histiocytic medullary reticulosis always show more atypia, however. In addition, the pattern of skin infiltration differs: in histiocytic medullary reticulosis the histiocytes accumulate deep in the dermis, around skin appendages, and in the subcutis; in contrast to Letterer-Siwe disease they do not involve the subepidermal (Grenz) zone. Rarely, a reactive histiocytosis, such as that sometimes produced by *Mycobacteria* (p. 105) has been mistaken for Letterer-Siwe diseaase, but the clinical features are so different in the two, that confusion is unlikely to arise.

Eosinophilic granuloma

Synonym:
Eosinophil granuloma of bone

Clinical features. Although eosinophilic granuloma occurs most commonly in childhood, it is not limited to infants and children, but can present at any age. The disease is usually characterised by focal destructive lesions of bone, which present either by the pain and swelling they cause, or by local effects such as diabetes insipidus, exophthalmos, or vertebral collapse. A single bone defect may precede the appearance of multiple lesions, or multiple bone lesions may be apparent when the patient is first observed. Sometimes patients also have localised skin infiltrations (e.g. on vulva), with or without regional lymphadenopathy. Lymphadenopathy may be the mode of presen-

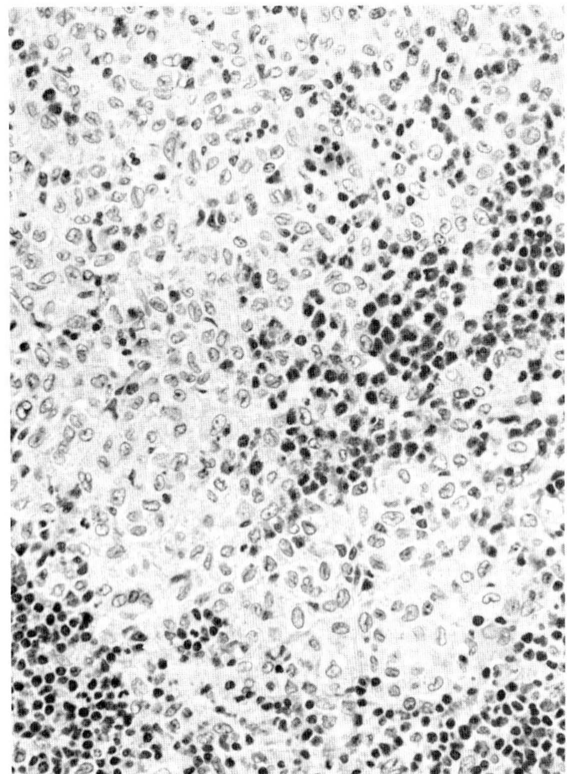

Fig. 14.33 A solitary focus of eosinophilic granuloma which was an incidental finding in an axillary lymph node biopsy removed from a man of 60 who had a previous history of Hodgkin's disease. The characteristic pale-staining reticulum cells with ovoid, grooved nuclei are unmistakable. (H E × 300)

Fig. 14.34 Cervical lymph node from a boy of 6 with eosinophilic granuloma. The lymph sinuses are distended by 'histiocytes' but there is little infiltration of the pulp. Note the paucity of fibres amongst the 'histiocytes'. (Gordon and Sweets reticulin × 47)

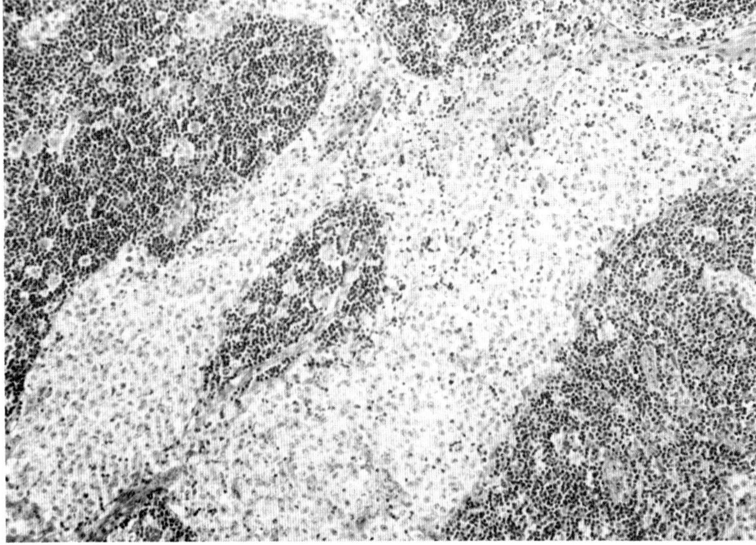

Fig. 14.35 Same node as Fig. 14.34 showing sharply outlined lymph sinuses filled by cells typical of eosinophilic granuloma (H E = 120)

tation of eosinophilic granuloma and sometimes lymph nodes are the only tissue showing evidence of involvement (Motoi et al, 1980). A history of recurrent lymphadenopathy may be obtained, sometimes associated with episodic fever and constitutional disturbance (Williams & Dorfman, 1979). At other times, small foci of eosinophilic granuloma have been an incidental finding in lymph nodes involved by malignant lymphoma (Kjeldsberg & Kim, 1980) or in otherwise normal lymph nodes removed from lymphoma patients (Fig. 14.33).

Pathological features. In lymph node presentation of eosinophilic granuloma, the nodes are seldom more than 2 cm in diameter. Sometimes they are friable due to necrosis and may be mistaken at operation for tuberculous nodes. They can show yellowish patches on the cut surface when much lipid is present.

Histologically the infiltrating cells are found primarily and principally in the sinuses which may be grossly distended (Figs 14.34, 14.35). Follicles and intersinusoidal pulp are preserved in varying degrees. The characteristic 'histiocytes' have indented and often 'folded' nuclei with fine chromatin structure and inconspicuous nucleoli (Fig. 14.36). Mitoses are generally scanty. The cytoplasm is abundant and weakly eosinophilic. There is no evidence of phagocytosis by these cells. Multinucleate cells of the same type are often present and are sometimes numerous (Figs 14.37, 14.38). Lipid droplets may be visible in the cytoplasm of both mononuclear and multinucleate cells, but lipid is rarely present in large amounts. When seen in closely packed masses in the lymph sinuses, these 'histiocytes' are highly distinctive and do not resemble ordinary macrophages. Furthermore they are accompanied by mature eosinophil leucocytes in variable, but often large,

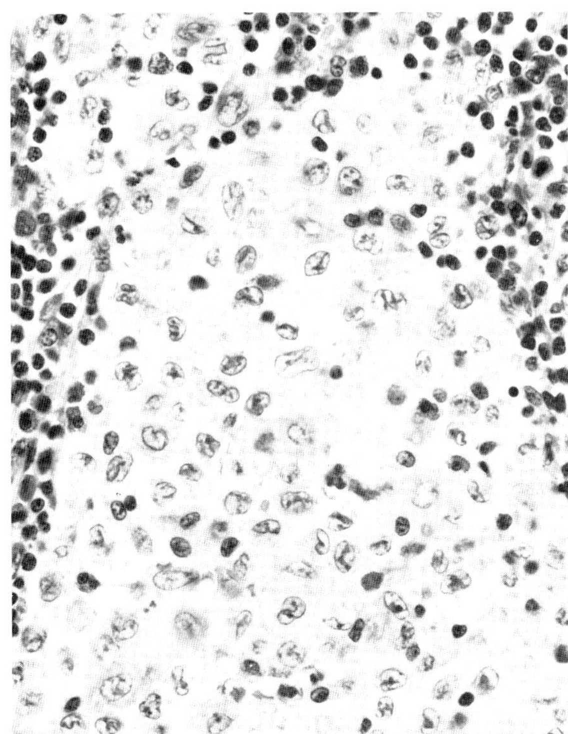

Fig. 14.36 Same node as Figs 14.34 and 14.35 showing details of cells. The grooved or folded nuclei of the 'histiocytes' are well shown. Eosinophils are scanty in this field. (H E × 470)

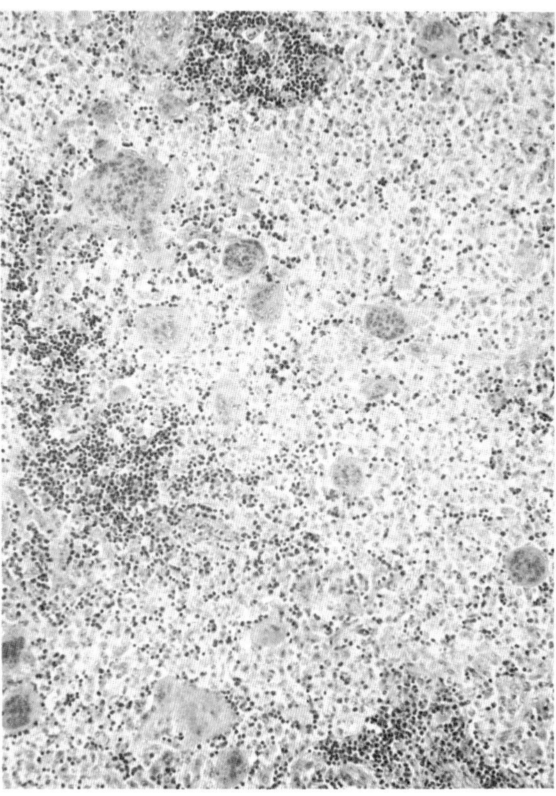

Fig. 14.37 Lymph node biopsy from another case of eosinophilic granuloma in a child showing numerous multinucleate giant-cells. The infiltrate has spread into the node pulp. Most of the darkly staining cells in the infiltrated areas are eosinophils. (H E × 120)

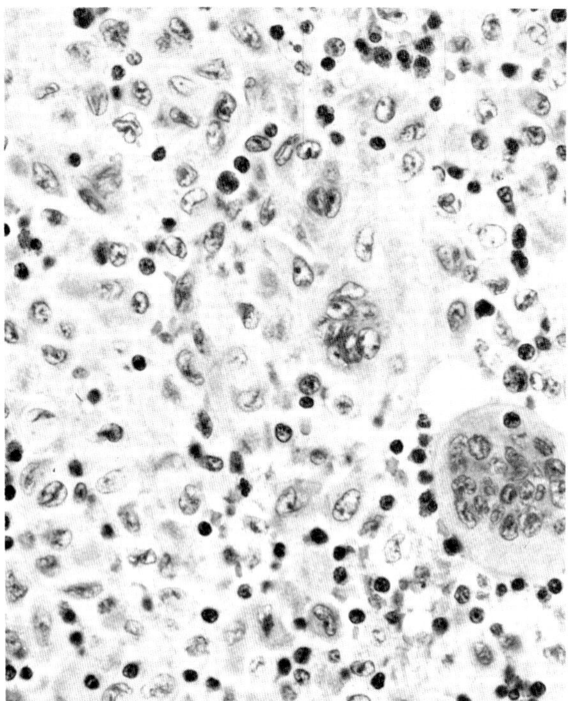

Fig. 14.38 Same node as Fig. 14.37 at a higher magnification to show details of cells. The nuclei of many of the mononuclear cells resemble those of interdigitating reticulum cells (compare with Figs 14.19 and 14.20). (HE × 470).

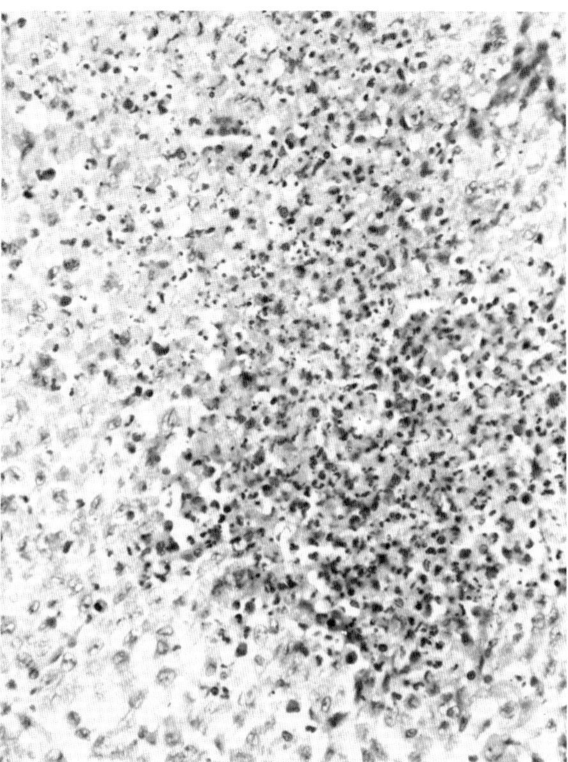

Fig. 14.39 Same node as Figs 14.37 and 14.38. Eosinophilic granuloma showing a focus of necrosis crowded with eosinophils ('eosinophilic abscess'). (H E × 300)

numbers. The foci of necrosis, which are commonly seen, may be strongly eosinophilic when eosinophils are numerous ('eosinophilic abscesses') (Fig. 14.39).

The lesions of eosinophilic granuloma in bone and other sites are similar, but here the specific infiltrates of 'histiocytes' and eosinophils are often mingled with or surrounded by lymphocytes and plasma cells, especially in regressing lesions. Some fibrosis of the lesions is also common. No doubt fibrosis also occurs in time in affected lymph nodes, but lesions in lymph nodes are seldom seen at this stage.

Differential diagnosis. The histological picture may at times closely resemble that of Letterer-Siwe disease and it is this which had led to the belief that one disease may lead into the other. Many cases of symptomatic eosinophilic granuloma in infancy have been wrongly diagnosed as Letterer-Siwe disease. Multinucleate 'histiocytes', numerous eosinophils and conspicuous necrosis are all more characteristic of eosinophilic granuloma than of Letterer-Siwe disease.

Confusion with Hodgkin's disease has occasionally arisen due to the tissue eosinophilia and the presence of giant-cells, but attention to the other cellular ingredients should prevent such errors occurring.

HISTIOCYTIC NEOPLASMS

Introduction

That cells of the mononuclear phagocyte system are capable of undergoing neoplasia is beyond question and none would dispute that acute monoblastic and monocytic leukaemia exemplify this. There has, however, been controversy in recent years about whether neoplasms can arise from tissue histiocytes, which are regarded by cell biologists as differentiated, end-stage cells with only limited powers of replication. Unquestionably there has been in the past far too uncritical an acceptance of the histiocytic origin of many tumours, in which today the histogenesis would be challenged. Nevertheless there undoubtedly exist uncommon neoplasms composed of cells which have not only the light microscopic characteristics of histiocytes, but also the ultrastructural features, the enzyme histochemical properties, the surface marker characteristics, and sometimes a capacity for phagocytosis. To argue that such lesions are (a) not neoplasms or (b) not derived from histiocytes, is to fly in the face of the evidence.

It is, however, necessary to exercise caution before concluding that a given neoplasm is of histiocytic origin and to bear in mind the following points:

1. Reactive histiocytes (macrophages) are present in practically all malignant tumours, whatever their origin. The numbers of such reactive cells may increase by recruitment to a point where they outnumber the neoplastic cells, as not infrequently happens when the latter show a tendency to undergo spontaneous necrosis. This is particularly seen in some high-grade malignant lymphomas (see p. 297).
2. Active macrophages in these circumstances, may have large and 'atypical' nuclei, even though mitoses may be infrequent. Small samples of a tumour of this kind submitted to electron microscopic examination, may easily give a false impression of a malignant histiocytic neoplasm.
3. Avid phagocytosis of red cells by macrophages is much more likely to indicate an abnormality in the red cells than a neoplasm of the macrophages. But the presence of abnormal red cell surface antigens will attract large numbers of macrophages, the 'active' appearance of which may be misconstrued as evidence of neoplasia. Whilst erythrophagocytosis is undoubtedly seen in some malignant histiocytic tumours (as in a variety of other malignant tumours) it is seldom a noteworthy feature. As is to be expected, the phagocytic capacity of neoplastic histiocytes is reduced rather than enhanced.

For the above reasons it is always necessary to ask two questions before making a diagnosis of a histiocytic neoplasm — (1) is the lesion definitely a neoplasm or could it be a reactive accumulation of monocyte/macrophage cells? (2) If unquestionably neoplastic, are the *neoplastic cells* definitely of histiocytic origin?

Two classes of 'histiocytic' neoplasm can immediately be rejected:

1. The 'histiocytic' types of malignant lymphoma as defined by Rappaport (1966). It is now generally acknowledged that the vast majority of tumours to which this designation has been applied are tumours of transformed lymphoid cells (see p. 277).
2. The 'fibrous histiocytomas' — benign or malignant. The concept of histiocytes as facultative fibroblasts (Ozello et al, 1963) was formulated before the existence of the mononuclear phagocyte system was established, on the basis of observations which even the original group now concede were wrongly interpreted (Fu et al, 1975). All the available evidence shows that macrophages cannot differentiate into collagen-producing cells and collagen-producing cells cannot give rise to macrophages. These tumours probably arise from a fibroblast-type connective tissue cell and the malignant tumours of this class behave like other soft tissue sarcomas.

Classification of histiocytic neoplasms

It is widely accepted that histiocytic neoplasms are uncommon, although their exact frequency in relation to lymphoid neoplasms is still unknown. Their infrequent occurrence and different criteria for their recognition are each partly responsible for the lack of an agreed classification of these neoplasms. Whilst some variants can be diagnosed with reasonable certainty on morphological criteria alone, other, less well differentiated examples cannot be reliably distinguished from high-grade malignant lymphomas without the aid of cytochemical or immunocytochemical tests.

Histiocytic neoplasms can be divided into two more or less distinct categories:

1. *Malignant histiocytosis* — a diffuse, apparently multifocal, and often systematised proliferation of atypical histiocytes and their precursors.

Localised tumours are exceptional, but occasionally develop.

2 *Histiocytic reticulosarcoma* — localised tumours of histiocytes, presenting in lymph nodes, skin or elsewhere. Those cases presenting with nodal masses are clinically indistinguishable from cases of malignant lymphoma.

Malignant histiocytosis

The term malignant histiocytosis (MH) was introduced by Rappaport (1966) to describe a systemic, progressive, invasive proliferation of morphologically atypical histiocytes and of their precursors. Rappaport drew a distinction between MH and the 'differentiated histiocytoses' (histiocytosis X). In more recent years the term MH has been widely used as a synonym for histiocytic medullary reticulosis (HMR) (Scott & Robb-Smith, 1939) in which systematised proliferation of neoplastic histiocytes is accompanied by fever and constitutional symptoms. A similar pattern of behaviour by malignant histiocytes, although in a totally different setting, was described by Isaacson & Wright (1978) in the small intestines of patients with long standing malabsorption. Since the term malignant histiocytosis is equally applicable to each of these two syndromes, it would seem desirable to revert to the use of the term HMR for the more specific syndrome and to apply the term MH only in a generic sense.

Histiocytic medullary reticulosis (HMR)

In 1939 Scott and Robb-Smith described four patients whose illness was characterised by 'fever, wasting and generalised lymphadenopathy associated with splenic and hepatic enlargement and, in the final stages, purpura, anaemia and profound leukopenia'. The disease was attributed to a systematised proliferation of atypical histiocytes and precursor cells. Little has been added to the clinicopathological description since.

Clinical features. This uncommon disease appears to occur at all ages, and to be commoner in males than females. Almost all patients have fever, widespread lymphadenopathy and hepatosplenomegaly. Anaemia, leukopenia and thrombocytopenia are common. Jaundice is often present in the terminal stages. A few patients develop a localised soft tissue mass or skin nodules (Warnke et al, 1975). A papular or frankly purpuric skin rash is sometimes observed. Atypical histiocytes can often be found in the bone marrow and peripheral blood (Lampert et al, 1978), but frank leukaemia is rare.

Pathological features. Both the enlarged spleen and affected lymph nodes may be blotched with areas of haemorrhage and necrosis, but the infiltration appears diffuse and localised tumour nodules are rarely observed in spleen or liver. The marrow infiltration too is often diffuse and haemorrhagic.

Histologically, the pattern of nodal infiltration is distinctive, typically starting in the lymph sinuses which become distended by large histiocytic cells. Soon, however, the pulp of the node is invaded and destroyed, although remnants of follicles may persist for some time. Eventually the whole node is replaced and extranodal extension then commonly occurs (Figs 14.40, 14.41).

The degree of pleomorphism is variable. Sometimes the cells appear relatively monomorphic and when present in close-packed, apparently cohesive clusters, the appearances may mimic metastatic carcinoma in the lymph sinuses. However, at the infiltrating edge the histiocytic cells are often separated from one another and their true nature is then more readily appreciated. At other times there is marked pleomorphism and then cells resembling histiocytes, having relatively small ovoid or indented nuclei and abundant eosinophilic cytoplasm, are interspersed with atypical histioblast-like cells having large irregular nuclei with coarse nuclear chromatin, prominent nucleoli and scantier, basophilic cytoplasm (Fig. 14.42). Lombardi et al (1978) in a histological and ultrastructural study of the lymph nodes in six cases of HMR found in every case histiocytes of varying grades of differentiation and atypia. It is important to stress that at least a proportion of the histiocytes in HMR is always atypical and shows features of malignancy (see differential diagnosis below).

In pleomorphic cases tumour giant-cells are often present, which may show a superficial resemblance to Sternberg-Reed cells. Mitoses may be numerous and are often atypical. Necrosis and haemorrhage are commonly seen. Plasma cells commonly accompany the histiocytic infiltrate and

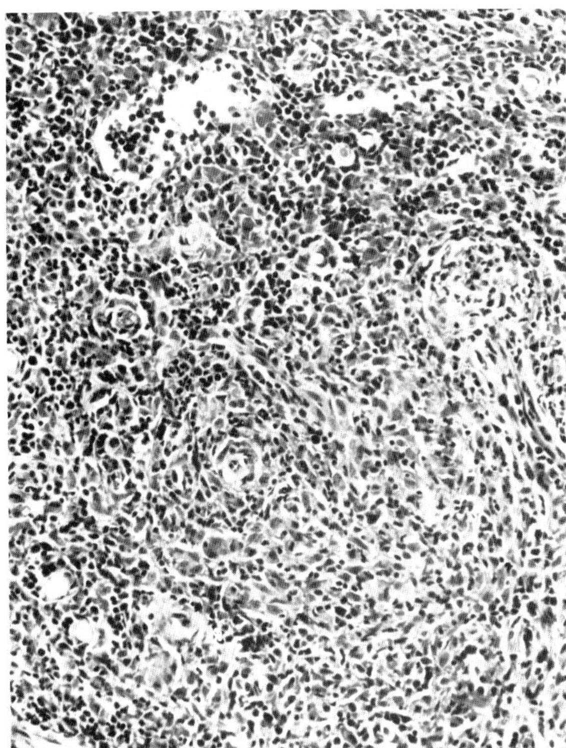

Fig. 14.40 Lymph node biopsy in histiocytic medullary reticulosis (HMR) showing the pleomorphic cell picture. Note neoplastic cells in a widely patent sinus (top). (H E × 150)

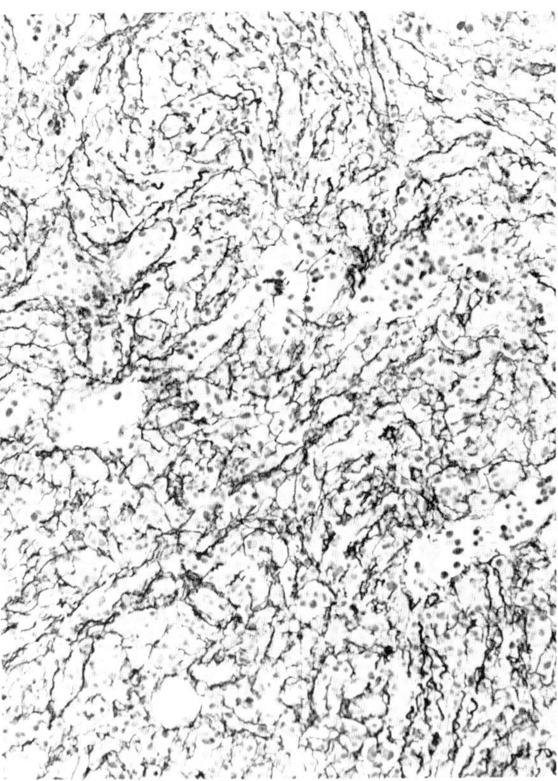

Fig. 14.41 Same node as Fig. 14.40 with silver impregnation. Note dense reticulin in the infiltrated pulp and patent sinuses filled with neoplastic histiocytes. (Gordon and Sweets reticulin × 150)

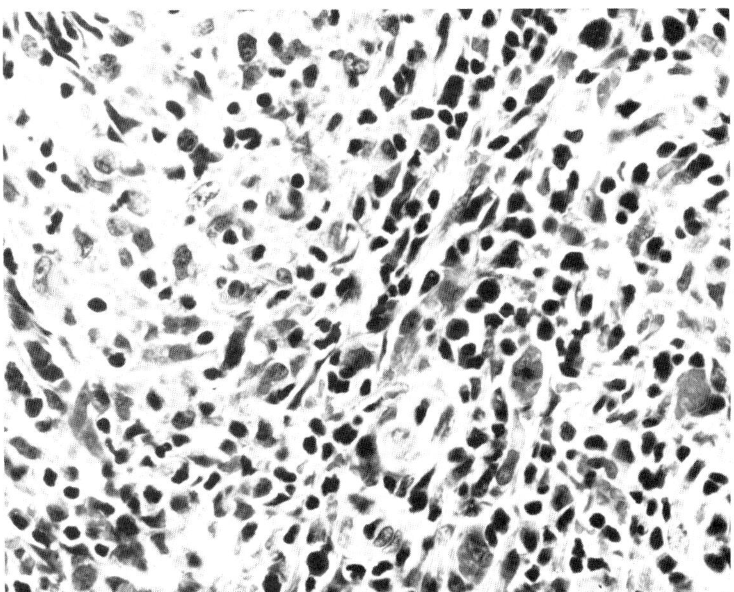

Fig. 14.42 Same node as Figs 14.40 and 14.41 at a higher magnification. The cells are a mixture of primitive histiocytes ('histioblasts') and mature appearing histiocytes. (H E × 470)

a few cases show abundant eosinophils (Warnke et al, 1975).

Erythrophagocytosis receives much attention in the literature on this subject, but is not usually a conspicuous feature and, when present, the engulfed red cells are generally seen within mature appearing histiocytes which may well be reactive. Evidence of phagocytosis by the neoplastic appearing cells is more often seen in imprint preparations of nodes or marrow smears than in sections (Fig. 14.43). The ingested material may include pyknotic nuclei, haemosiderin and fat as well as red cells (Marshall, 1956; Hauswirth & Rosenow, 1952).

In the spleen, the infiltration is centred on the red pulp, often infiltrating the sinuses (Figs 14.44, 14.45) and ultimately destroying the white pulp also. In the liver atypical histiocytes appear in the sinusoids and the Kupffer cells may appear to be involved in the process.

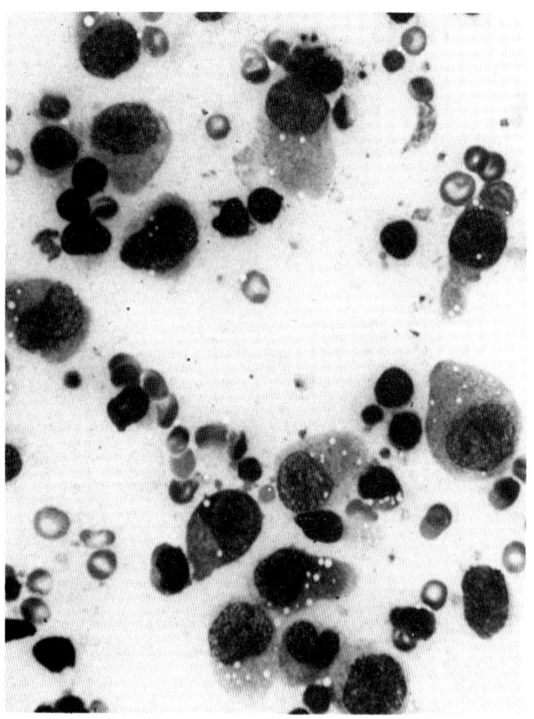

Fig. 14.43 Imprint of lymph node from a girl aged two and a half with malignant histiocytosis (HMR). Note abundant finely vacuolated cytoplasm of malignant histiocytes. One cell (top) contains phagocytosed nuclear particles. (Giemsa × 1200)

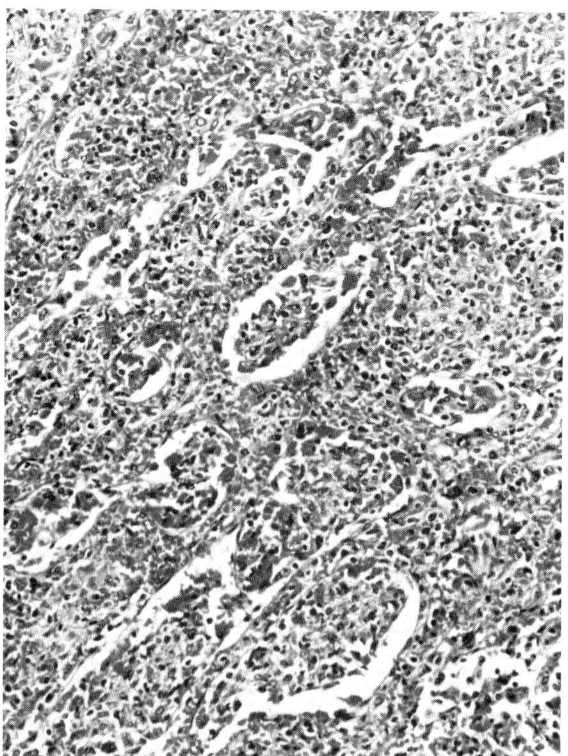

Fig. 14.44 Spleen from another case of HMR showing diffuse neoplastic infiltration of the red pulp with invasion of the venous sinuses (H E × 150)

The diagnosis is often more readily established with imprints, on which cytochemical tests may be performed. The cells are positive for acid phosphatase and non-specific esterase, the strength of the reaction depending upon the degree of differentiation of the cells. Immunohistochemistry can be carried out retrospectively on paraffin sections, employing the immunoperoxidase method with antisera against muramidase (lysozome) or alpha-l-antitrypsin. According to Isaacson et al (1981), a granular paranuclear reaction for alpha-l-antitrypsin is the most consistently reliable test for neoplastic histiocytic cells.

Prognosis. The median survival time in untreated patients is 6 months. In those patients who have survived long enough for chemotherapy to be effective, the median survival time is about 12 months (Warnke et al, 1975). With treatment there are a few long term survivors.

Differential diagnosis. Although it has been stated that histiocytic medullary reticulosis is

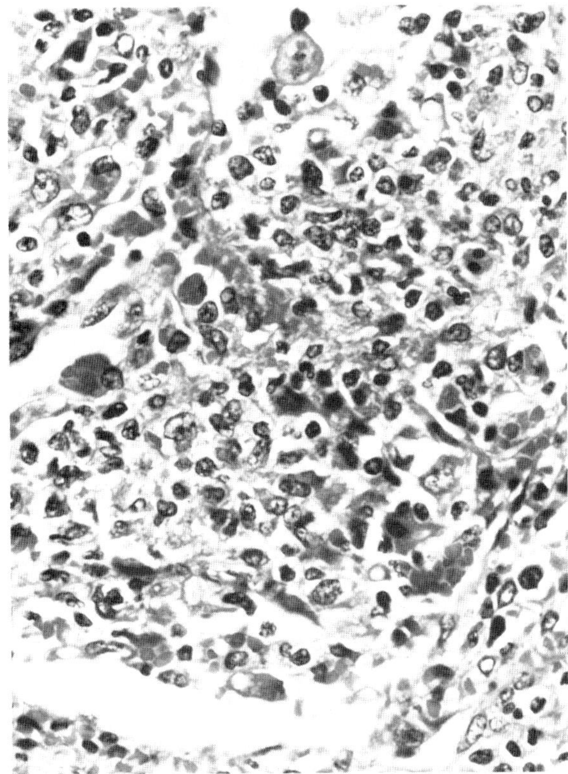

Fig. 14.45 Same spleen as Fig. 14.44 to show detail of infiltrating cells in a sinus. Some of the larger cells show phagocytic activity. (H E × 470)

probably commoner than the number of case reports would suggest (e.g. Lampert et al, 1978), the reverse is more likely to be true since in many published reports the diagnosis is open to question. As already stressed earlier, large reactive histiocytes are a prominent feature of many infectious lesions and many non-histiocytic neoplasms and sometimes erythrophagocytosis may be observed in such cases.

A special instance seems to be the occurrence of a HMR-like syndrome reported in two cases of T-cell lymphoma by Kadin et al (1981). Both patients presented with fever and hepatosplenomegaly; lymphadenopathy was inconspicuous. Phagocytosed red cells were seen, not only in large histiocytic cells, but also in the lymphoma cells which were demonstrated to be T gamma cells. It was surmised that the lymphoma might have originated in the spleen, in which T gamma cells are normally plentiful. Kadin (1981) was led to speculate on the nature of the association in several previously published cases of HMR following in the wake of 'acute lymphocytic leukaemia'. In all three cases studied the leukaemic cells were found to be T cells, but whether the erythrophagocytic histiocytes which appeared in these cases were neoplastic or merely reactive remains unproven.

Some of the pitfalls of misinterpreting sinus histiocytic proliferations or accumulations, as malignant histiocytosis have been cited above. The lack of cellular atypia at once distinguishes simple sinus histiocytosis, however active, from MH. Again sinus histiocytosis with massive lymphadenopathy (p. 351) has such distinctive histological features that confusion should not occur. Infiltration of the lymph sinuses by other kinds of neoplasm may sometimes give rise to diagnostic difficulty, especially with undifferentiated, large-cell carcinomas in which the nodal infiltration is confined to the sinuses (see Ch. 15). Non-Hodgkin's lymphomas (Osborne et al, 1980) and rarely even Hodgkin's disease may how a sinus pattern of infiltration which can cause confusion, despite the cytological differences. The differentiation of Letterer-Siwe disease from MH has been discussed on page 363 and the localised forms of histiocytosis X are distinctive both clinically and pathologically (p. 363). The rare condition of 'familial haemophagocytic reticulosis' (Farquhar & Claireaux, 1952) which occurs in siblings, is thought by some to be identical with HMR (Warnke et al, 1975), though their identity is denied by others (Marshall, 1956).

Probably the most important differential diagnosis of HMR is the virus-associated haemophagocytic syndrome (VAHS) described by Risdall and co-workers (Risdall et al, 1979; McKenna et al, 1981). This disease may closely mimic HMR both clinically and pathologically. It affects infants and children, following in the wake of an acute viral infection (mainly herpes-type viruses), or older individuals who have been on immunosuppressive therapy. The disease is characterised clinically by fever, constitutional symptoms, hepatosplenomegaly and lymphadenopathy and sometimes by a skin rash and diffuse pulmonary infiltrates. Pathologically, all patients showed anaemia and pancytopenia associated with marrow depression and marrow infiltration by histiocytes showing active erythrophagocytosis. VAHS has a mortality rate of 30–40%, but the surviving patients recovered completely (McKenna et al, 1981). In comparing the pathological features of VAHS with those of three cases of HMR, the authors concluded that the only real distinction lay in the degree of maturity of the infiltrating histiocytes. In VAHS the histiocytes were all of mature type and erythrophagocytosis was much more conspicuous than it was in HMR, where 'minimal phagocytosis' was 'identified in the poorly differentiated malignant histiocytes'. In a number of accounts in the literature purporting to describe cases of HMR, stress is laid on the 'deceptively benign' appearance of the histiocytes and the prominence of erythrophagocytosis. It is probable that many of the patients reported to have recovered and some of those who died from 'HMR', in fact had VAHS.

Malignant histiocytosis of the intestine (MHI)

A small minority of patients with coeliac disease develop an illness of sudden onset with weight loss, diarrhoea and abdominal pain. These patients previously labelled 'ulcerative jejunitis' are now considered to have developed a malignant histiocytosis of the intestine (Isaacson & Wright, 1978). The neoplastic histiocytes are thought to arise in the gut mucosa and rapidly spread to produce a systematised pattern of tissue infiltration similar to that seen in HMR.

Pathological features. The initial lesions may occur in any part of the small intestine, most commonly the jejunum. They may present as multiple ulcers, or strictures, large plaques or nodules, or areas of diffuse mural thickening. Histological features of involved mucosa are also highly variable, consisting either of monomorphic infiltrates of mature or immature histiocytes, or mixed populations of histiocytes and other inflammatory cells which may cause the lesions to be mistaken for an inflammatory condition, especially when the neoplastic cells are scarce. Multiple blocks may be required, and it is sometimes more fruitful to search for these atypical cells in other tissues, such as mesenteric nodes, liver, spleen or bone marrow, rather than amidst the heavily reactive infiltrate of the ulcer bases. Uninvolved mucosa invariably shows villous atrophy and crypt hyperplasia with a heavy plasmacytic infiltrate of the lamina propria.

The neoplasm is usually disseminated at the time of diagnosis and the prognosis is very bad. At laparotomy the intestinal lesion may not be visible but mesenteric lymph nodes are often enlarged and, on microscopy, they show sinus infiltration by atypical histiocytes which eventually extend into the medullary cords and replace the lymph node (Fig. 14.46). Involvement of spleen, liver and bone marrow is extremely common but easily missed without careful examination. Although the spleen is often reduced in size, as it usually is in coeliac disease, atypical histiocytes, sometimes showing erythrophagocytosis, may be

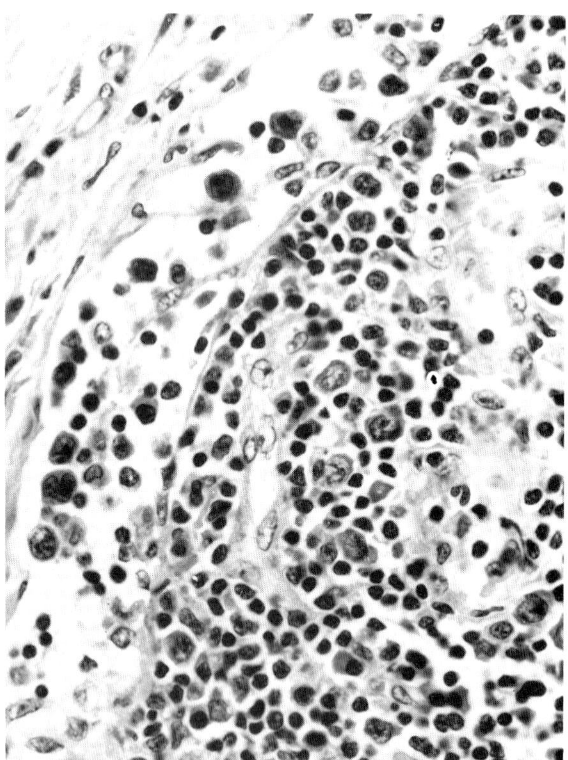

Fig. 14.46 Mesenteric lymph node biopsy from a woman of 55 with malignant histiocytosis of the intestine. Malignant histiocytes can be seen in the marginal sinus and isolated cells of the same type have infiltrated the underlying dense pulp. The patient gave a long history of steatorrhoea with recent diarrhoea and the surviving mucosa was flat in the resected segment of small intestine, which also showed widespread ulceration and infiltration by the neoplasm. (H E × 470)

seen in the red, and later the white pulp. The liver shows infiltrates of atypical histiocytes, first in portal triads, later within sinusoids. As in HMR, bone marrow aspirates may show bizarre phagocytic cells.

The histiocytic nature of the cells in this disorder has been confirmed cytochemically and by immunohistochemistry in three cases with widely divergent macroscopic and histological features (Isaacson et al, 1982).

Histiocytic reticulosarcoma

Synonyms:
Histiocytic sarcoma.
'True'histiocytic lymphoma.

By this term we understand a malignant neoplasm of histiocytes which arises initially in a single focus and presents as a localised tumour, rather than as a diffuse systematised and possibly multifocal proliferation, as is seen in malignant histiocytosis. Histiocytic reticulosarcoma appears to arise most commonly in lymph nodes, but presents sometimes in the skin and, less frequently, elsewhere. Presenting with lymphadenopathy, that is, in a manner indistinguishable from that of a malignant lymphoma, it may be thought unreasonable not to class these tumours with the malignant lymphomas, as 'histiocytic lymphomas' or 'malignant lymphomas of histiocytic type'. However, these terms have been used in the Rappaport classification for tumours of a different nature, most of which are clearly not derived from histiocytes and usage of the same terms can therefore only lead to confusion. Putting the word histiocyte into inverted commas, as has been done by some authors using Rappaport's classification, is merely perpetuating an erroneous terminology. It is absurd to talk about 'true' histiocytic lymphomas to distinguish those lymphoreticular tumours which are of histiocytic origin from those which are not and it therefore seemed best to the authors of the Kiel classification to take the histiocytic neoplasms out of the malignant lymphomas and put them, where they properly belong, in a separate category (Gérard-Marchant et al, 1974).

At the present time it remains to be determined whether histiocytic reticulosarcoma (HRS) represents a single class of neoplasm, differing only in the degree of differentiation of its constituent cells or whether two or more different types of tumour are included under this heading. There is also a divergence of opinion on the frequency of HRS, which hinges on the recognition of poorly differentiated tumours as being of histiocytic origin. There is no dispute about the well differentiated examples of HRS, in which the neoplastic cells can be recognised as histiocytes even by light microscopy and in which their histiocytic nature can be readily confirmed by histochemical and immunohistochemical tests.

Clinical features. Histiocytic reticulosarcomas apparently arise at all ages, although our experience has been that (at least in the differentiated tumours) the peak incidence is in childhood and adolescence. The sexes are apparently affected equally. The disease may present with peripheral lymphadenopathy, indistinguishable clinically from that of a high grade malignant lymphoma, or with a localised skin nodule, or both sites may be involved simultaneously. In those patients with a nodal presentation, skin lesions may appear later or in relapse, and skin involvement is much commoner than it is in most malignant lymphomas (excluding T-cell types). Skin lesions in HRS may take the form of scattered nodules or reddish papules. Van der Valk et al (1981) found a high incidence of bone involvement.

Pathological features. The macroscopic features of affected lymph nodes in HRS are not distinctive.

Histologically, the normal architecture of the node is partly or wholly effaced by a diffuse infiltrate of rather large, uniform-appearing cells, with relatively small nuclei and abundant cytoplasm. The latter feature accounts for the paler staining of the tumourous areas, which contrast strikingly with residual follicles or other elements of the original node (Fig. 14.47). At a higher magnification, the cells appear less uniform, but in the better differentiated examples, their histiocytic nature is obvious (Fig. 14.48). Erythrophagocytosis is seldom observed in sections, but may be seen in imprints or marrow smears when the latter becomes infiltrated. The nuclei may be round but are often reniform or irregular with a fairly fine chromatin pattern, and sometimes a prominent central

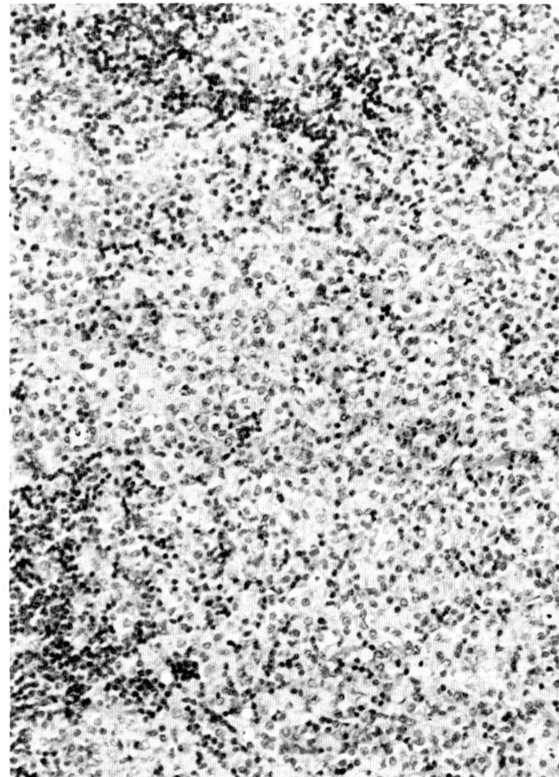

Fig. 14.47 Cervical lymph node biopsy from a 17 year old youth showing the low power features of histiocytic reticulosarcoma. The pale staining histiocytic cells with their abundant cytoplasm contrast strongly with the residual lymphocytes of the node. (H E × 150)

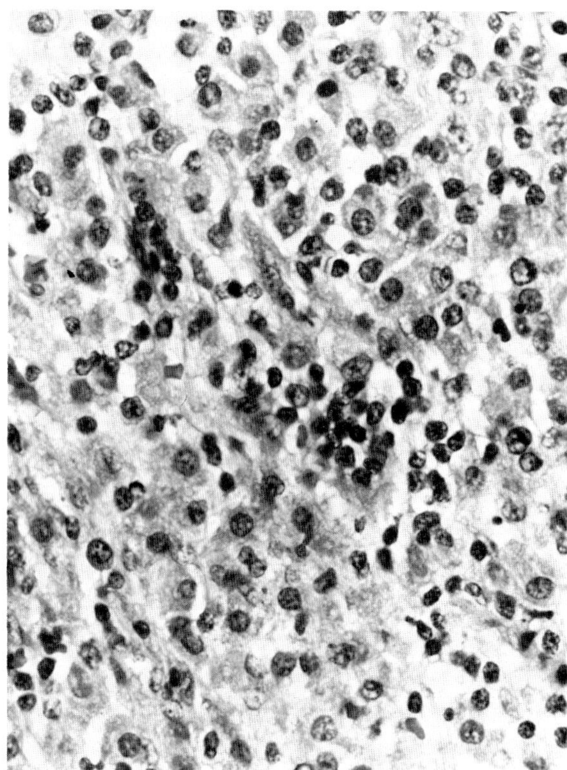

Fig. 14.48 Same node as Fig. 14.47 showing detail of neoplastic histiocytes. Cell boundaries are indistinct except where dissociation has occurred through faulty fixation (above). The copious eosinophilic cytoplasm appears finely vacuolated. Note scattered plasma cells. (H E × 470)

nucleolus. Mitoses are generally fairly frequent. The copious cytoplasm is pale, eosinophilic and commonly appears vacuolated, occasionally containing phagocytosed material. Cell boundaries may appear well or poorly defined. Giant-cells are absent or scarce, although in some instances there may be marked variation in cell size (Fig. 14.49). Plasma cells of polyclonal type are commonly found amongst the tumour cells and eosinophils are occasionally present. Silver impregnation shows a dense network of argyrophil fibres in the tumour, which is in striking contrast to the pattern usually seen in malignant lymphomas (Fig. 14.50). Necrosis is sometimes observed and in ischaemic areas the cell nuclei may appear shrunken, pyknotic and rounded.

As is the case with many other malignant neoplasms, the cells of HRS may enlarge and become more anaplastic with the passage of time (Figs. 14.51, 14.52). It is naturally more difficult to recognise the histiocytic nature of the less well differentiated tumours of this group. The cells are generally larger and more pleomorphic, with large nuclei and a coarser chromatin structure. The cytoplasm is relatively reduced in amount and becomes more basophilic and pyroninophilic, so that the morphological distinction of a poorly differentiated histiocytic reticulosarcoma from ML immunoblastic may sometimes be difficult (Fig. 14.52). Even in undifferentiated tumours, however, some distinctive characteristics of HRS may remain (Fig. 14.53). Histochemical and cytochemical tests for histiocytes (acid phosphatase, non-specific esterase) which give clear cut, positive results with the better differentiated cases of HRS, may give equivocal results in the less well differ-

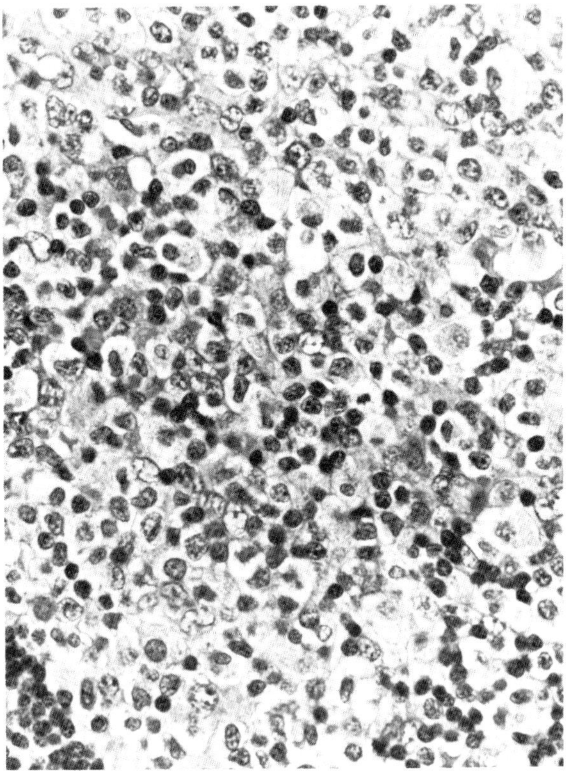

Fig. 14.49 Lymph node biopsy from another case of histiocytic reticulosarcoma in a girl aged 12. In this instance the cells are much more variable in size and cell boundaries are clearly seen. Many of the larger cells have copious, pale and finely vacuolated cytoplasm. (H E × 470)

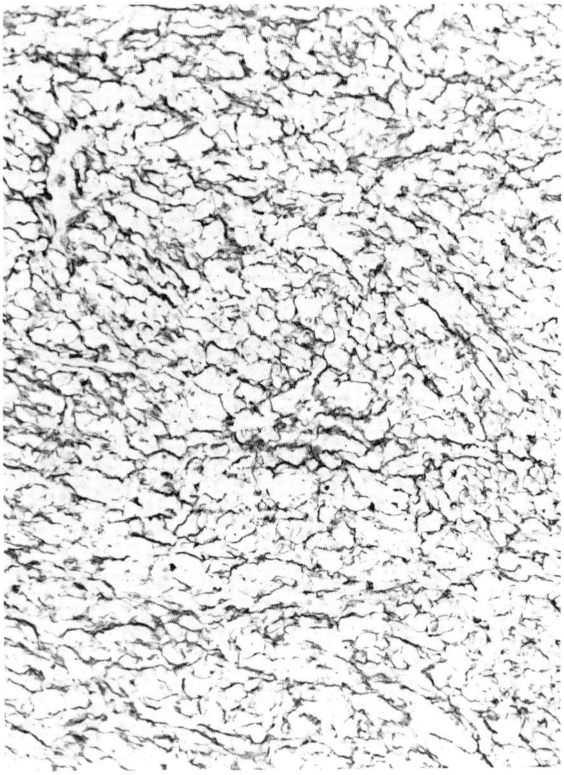

Fig. 14.50 Lymph node from a 16 year old boy showing the dense reticulin network in a histiocytic reticulosarcoma (Gordon and Sweets reticulin × 150)

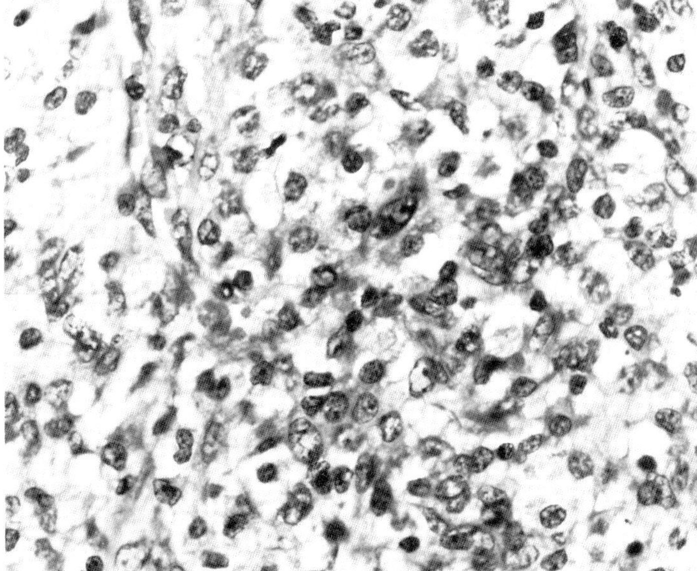

Fig. 14.51 Same node as Fig. 14.50 at a higher magnification showing the characteristic cellular features of a well differentiated HRS. Morphologically these cells are unmistakably histiocytes and do not resemble lymphoid cells. (H E × 470)

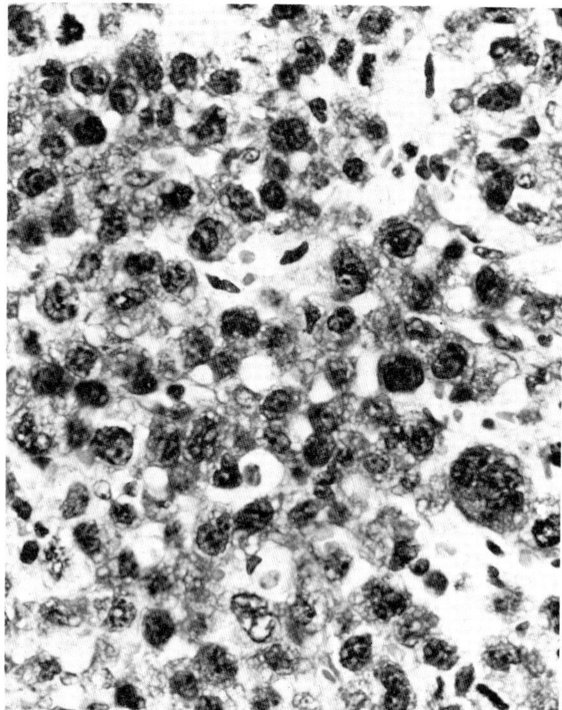

Fig. 14.52 Later lymph node biopsy, taken from the same patient as Figs 14.50 and 14.51, in relapse 14 months after complete remission had been achieved with chemotherapy. The cells are now much larger and more anaplastic than they were originally. (Compare with Fig. 14.51.) (Giemsa × 470)

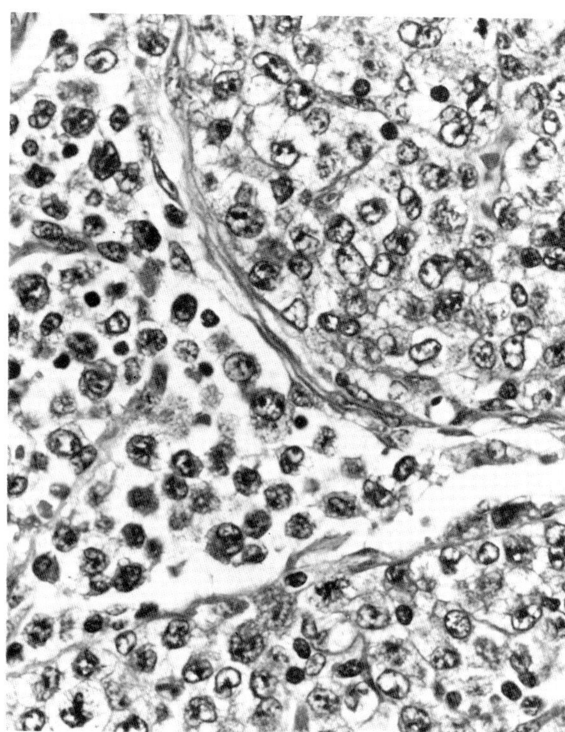

Fig. 14.53 Lymph node biopsy from a woman of 26 with multiple rapidly enlarging nodes. Despite the lack of differentiation, the tumour retains some of the characteristics of a histiocytic reticulosarcoma, including a patent lymph sinus filled with free neoplastic cells. (H E × 470)

entiated examples. More reliance has therefore to be placed on immunocytochemical and immunohistochemical tests, but even here interpretation may be difficult. A paranuclear granular reaction in the immunoperoxidase test, employing antiserum to alpha-1-antitrypsin, is probably the most reliable test for histiocytes (Isaacson et al, 1981).

Prognosis. The prognosis seems to be rather variable in the histiocytic reticulosarcomas. Some of the patients with a cutaneous presentation, even with regional node involvement, have been cured by radiotherapy. Other patients, presenting with lymph node swellings, have gone into remission with aggressive chemotherapeutic treatment, but some have relapsed with widespread disease in skin, lymph nodes, spleen, liver and bone marrow and have then failed to respond to further treatment. The variations in response have again raised the question as to whether HRS is a single entity.

Differential diagnosis. The very different types of presentation of HRS serve to distinguish these tumours from malignant histiocytosis, whether HMR or MHI. Furthermore, the sinus pattern of nodal infiltration seen in MH is lacking in HRS. There is generally little difficulty in deciding between HRS and Letterer-Siwe disease, despite a superficial similarity of the lymph node picture in the two. The latter disease occurs only in young infants and is disseminated at the outset.

The greatest problem is in distinguishing less well differentiated HRS from some T-cell lymphomas (see p. 313) and from high grade B-cell lymphomas, especially those of the large centrocytic and immunoblastic types (pp. 259, 298) Cells with abundant pale-staining cytoplasm are a feature of some peripheral T-cell lymphomas and these cells with their irregular, often indented, nuclei may be mistaken for histiocytes. Epithelioid

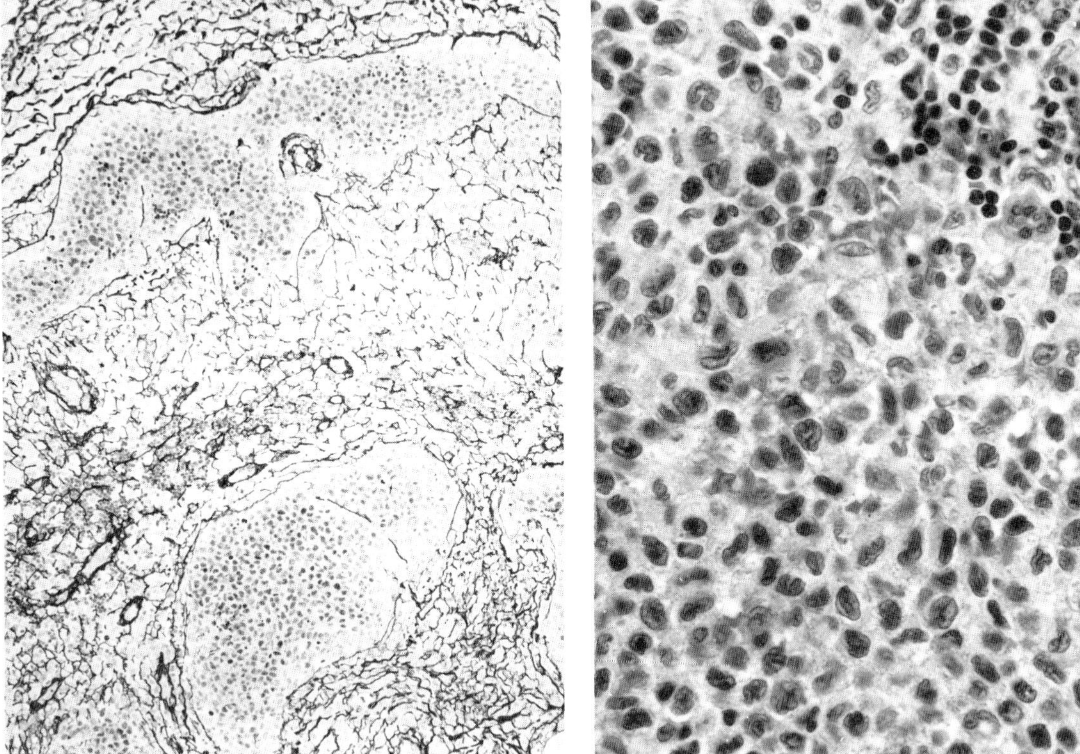

Fig. 14.54 Lymph node biopsy from a man of 55 with an interdigitating cell reticulosarcoma which arose in the small intestine and metastasised widely. The sinus infiltration shown here was a characteristic feature of the nodal involvement. (Gordon and Sweets reticulin × 120)

Fig. 14.55 Interdigitating cell reticulosarcoma. Higher power view of same node as Fig. 14.54 showing the irregular, convoluted nuclei of the neoplastic cells. (H E × 470)

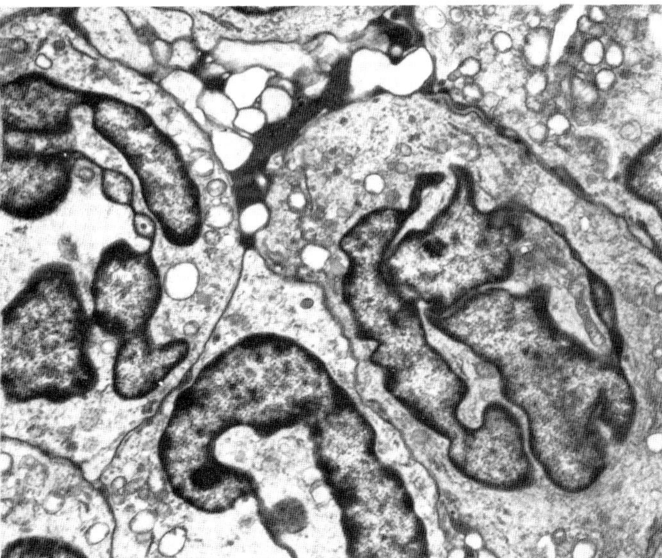

Fig. 14.56 Electron micrograph of interdigitating cell reticulosarcoma showing bizarre nuclei and interlocking cell processes (top). (Same case as Figs 14.54 and 14.55).

cells are also an ingredient of many T-cell lymphomas and fine sclerosis of such tumours has also been observed. The morphological resemblance of poorly differentiated 'histioblasts' to B-immunoblasts has already been mentioned. As indicated above, it is in this area that disagreement exists over the interpretation of individual tumours and hence the frequency of histiocytic reticulosarcoma as a whole. The problem will no doubt be resolved in time, perhaps with the use of monoclonal antibodies. The caveat about active histiocytes in non-histiocytic tumours (p. 367) is applicable here, as it is with all other histiocytic neoplasms.

Reticulosarcoma of other types

Without a doubt, neoplasms arise far more frequently from histiocytes than from other reticulum cells of the lymphoreticular tissues. Authentic cases of reticulosarcoma arising from dendritic reticulum cells appear to be exceedingly rare (van der Valk et al, 1982). Likewise there are very few published examples of interdigitating cell reticulosarcoma (Feltkamp et al, 1981). We have personally seen one example of this rare tumour, which presented in the gut in a 55 year old man (Figs 14.54, 14.55, 14.56). Lennert (1978) records an instance of interdigitating cell reticulosarcoma supervening in mycosis fungoides.

REFERENCES

Basset F, Turiaf J 1965 Identification par la microscopie electronique de particules de nature probablement virale dans les lesions granulomateuses d'une histiocytose X pulmonaire. Comptes Rendu des seances de l'Academie des Sciences, Serie III (Paris) 261: 3701–3703

Berg J W 1956 Sinus histiocytosis: a fallacious measure of host resistance to cancer. Cancer 9: 935–939

Black M M, Kerpe S, Speer F D 1953 Lymph node structure in patients with cancer of the breast. American Journal of Pathology 29: 505–521

Cederbaum S D, Niwayama G, Stiehm E R et al 1974 Combined immunodeficiency presenting as Letterer-Siwe syndrome. Journal of Pediatrics 85: 466–471

Daneshbod K, Kissane J M 1978 Idiopathic differentiated histiocytosis X. American Journal of Clinical Pathology 70: 381–389

Engelbreth-Holm J, Teilum G, Christensen E 1944 Eosinophil's granuloma of bone — Schüller-Christian's disease. Acta Medica Scandinavica 118: 292–312

Farquhar J W, Claireaux A E 1952 Familial haemophagocytic reticulosis. Archives of Disease in Childhood 27: 519–525

Feltkamp C A, van Heerde P, Feltkamp-Vroom T M, Koudstaal J 1981 A malignant tumor arising from interdigitating cells; light microscopical, ultrastructural, immuno- and enzyme-histochemical characteristics. Virchow's Archiv A (Pathol Anat) 393: 183–192

Foucar E, Rosai J, Dorfman R F 1978 Sinus histiocytosis with massive lymphadenopathy. Archives of Otolaryngology 104: 687–693

Fu Y, Gabbiani G, Kaye G I, Lattes R 1975 Malignant soft tissue tumors of probable histiocytic origin (malignant fibrous histiocytomas): general considerations and electron microscopical and tissue culture studies. Cancer 35: 176–198

Gérard-Marchant R, Hamlin I, Lennert K, Rilke F, Stansfeld A G, van Unnik J A M 1974 Classification of non-Hodgkin's lymphomas. Lancet 2: 406–408 (letter to the Editor)

Hauswirth L, Rosenow G 1952 Intravitam diagnosis of malignant reticulosis. Acta Haematologica 8: 293–304

Isaacson P, Wright D H 1978 Intestinal lymphoma associated with malabsorption. Lancet 1: 67–70

Isaacson P, Jones D B, Millward-Sadler G H, Judd M A, Payne S 1981 Alpha-l-antitrypsin in human macrophages. Journal of Clinical Pathology 34: 982–990

Isaacson P, Jones D B, Sworn M J, Wright D H 1982 Malignant histiocytosis of the intestine: report of three cases with immunological and cytochemical analysis. Journal of Clinical Pathology 35: 510–516

Kadin M E 1981 T gamma cells: a missing link between malignant histiocytosis and T cell leukemia-lymphoma? Human Pathology 12: 771–772

Kadin M E, Kamoun M, Lamberg J 1981 Erythrophagocytic Tγ lymphoma — a clinicopathologic entity resembling malignant histiocytosis. New England Journal of Medicine 304: 648–653

Kim H, Jacobs C, Warnke R A, Dorfman R F 1978 Malignant lymphoma with a high content of epithelioid histiocytes. Cancer 41: 620–635

Kjeldsberg C R, Kim H 1980 Eosinophilic granuloma as an incidental finding in malignant lymphoma. Archives of Pathology and Laboratory Medicine 104: 137–140

Lampert I A, Catovsky D, Bergier N 1978 Malignant histiocytosis: a clinicopathological study of 12 cases. British Journal of Haematology 40: 65–77

Lennert K, in collaboration with Mohri N, Stein H, Kaiserling E, Müller-Hermelink H K 1978 Malignant lymphomas other than Hodgkin's disease. Springer-Verlag, Berlin, part 4, p 465

Lichtenstein L 1953 Histiocytosis X: integration of eosinophilic granuloma of bone, 'Letterer-Siwe disease' and 'Schüller-Christian disease' as related manifestations of a single nosological entity. Archives of Pathology 56: 85–102

Lieberman P H, Jones C R, Dargeon H W K, Begg C F 1969 A reappraisal of eosinophilic granuloma of bone,

Hand-Schüller-Christian syndrome and Letterer-Siwe syndrome. Medicine 48: 375–400
Lombardi L, Carbone A, Pilotti S, Rilke F 1978 Malignant histiocytosis: a histological and ultrastructural study of lymph nodes in six cases. Histopathology 2: 315–328
McKenna R W, Risdall R J, Brunning R D 1981 Virus associated hemophagocytic syndrome. Human Pathology 12: 395–398
Marshall A H E 1956 Histiocytic medullary reticulosis. Journal of Pathology and Bacteriology 71: 61–71
Motoi M, Helbron D, Kaiserling E, Lennert K 1980 Eosinophilic granuloma of lymph nodes — a variant of histiocytosis X. Histopathology 4: 585–606
Newton W A Jr, Hamoudi A B 1973 Histiocytosis: a histological classification with clinical correlation. Perspectives in Pediatric Pathology 1: 251–283
Nézelof C, Jaubert F 1978 Histiocytic and/or reticulum cell neoplasias. In: Mathé G, Seligmann M, Tubiana M (eds) Recent results in cancer research, vol 64. Springer-Verlag, Berlin
Osborne B M, Butler J J, Mackay B 1980 Sinusoidal large cell (histiocytic) lymphoma. Cancer 46: 2484–2491
Ozello L, Stout A P, Murray M R 1963 Cultural characteristics of malignant histiocytomas and fibrous xanthomas. Cancer 16: 331–344
Pearse A G E 1972 Histochemistry — theoretical and applied, 3rd edn Churchill Livingstone, Edinburgh. Vol 2, p 1162
Rappaport H 1966 Tumors of the hematopoietic system. Atlas of Tumor Pathology, Section III, Fascicle 8, AFIP Washington DC
Risdall R J, McKenna R W, Nesbit M E, Krivit W, Balfour H H, Simmons R L, Brunning R D 1979 Virus associated hemophagocytic syndrome: a benign histiocytic proliferation distinct from malignant histiocytosis. Cancer 44: 993–1002
Rosai J, Dorfman R F 1969 Sinus histiocytosis with massive lymphadenopathy. A newly recognised benign clinicopathological entity. Archives of Pathology 87: 63–70
Rosai J, Dorfman R F 1972 Sinus histiocytosis with massive lymphadenopathy: a pseudolymphomatous benign disorder. Cancer 30: 1174–1188
Scott R B, Robb-Smith A H T 1939 Histiocytic medullary reticulosis. Lancet 2: 194–198
Spector W G 1974 The macrophage: its origins and role in pathology. In: Ioachim H L (ed) Pathobiology Annual, Appleton-Century-Crofts, New York, p 33–64
Valk P van Der, Te Velde J, Jansen J, Ruiter D J, Spaander P J, Cornelisse C J, Meijer C J L M 1981 Malignant lymphoma of true histiocytic origin: histiocytic sarcoma. A morphological, ultrastructural, immunological, cytochemical and clinical study of 10 cases. Virchow's Archiv A (Pathol Anat)391: 249–265
Valk P van der, Ruiter D J, Den Ottolander G J, Te Velde J, Spaander P J, Meijer C J L M 1982 Dendritic reticulum cell sarcoma? Four cases of a lymphoma probably derived from dendritic reticulum cells of the follicular compartment. Histopathology 6: 269–287
Warnke R A, Kim H, Dorfman R F 1975 Malignant histiocytosis (histiocytic medullary reticulosis) I Clinicopathological study of 29 cases. Cancer 35: 215–230
Williams J W, Dorfman R F 1979 Lymphadenopathy as the initial manifestation of histiocytosis X. American Journal of Surgical Pathology 3: 405–421

15

A.J. Blackshaw

Metastatic tumours in lymph nodes

The problems associated with metastatic lesions in lymph nodes can be grouped into three categories:

1. Differentiation of metastatic malignancy from primary lymphoreticular tumours.
2. Determination of the possible site of origin of metastatic tumour.
3. Differentiation of benign, mainly epithelial lymph node inclusions from metastatic malignant tumour.

DIFFERENTIATION OF METASTATIC MALIGNANCY FROM PRIMARY LYMPHORETICULAR NEOPLASMS.

The histological distinction of metastatic tumour in a lymph node from primary lymphoreticular malignancy has an extremely important bearing on the possible treatment of patients. The course of further investigations and the modes of therapy are profoundly influenced by the pathologist's decisions. It is therefore of the utmost importance that the diagnosis should be correct.

The types of metastatic tumour which may mimic primary lymphoreticular malignancy are relatively few and all are undifferentiated tumours composed of round or polygonal cells. These types of tumour will be discussed individually after some general remarks about the separation of primary from secondary malignancy in lymph nodes.

A malignant process which occupies only part of a lymph node and leaves the remainder with a normal architecture is more likely to be a metastatic deposit than a primary lymphoreticular tumour. This rule, like all rules, cannot be rigidly applied. Hodgkin's disease is quite often observed to involve only part of a node. Even non-Hodgkin's lymphomas, when arising in an extranodal site and spreading to regional nodes, can partially occupy a lymph node in a fashion which is often thought to be characteristic of metastatic non-lymphoid malignancy.

Malignant histiocytosis sometimes displays a distinctive pattern of invasion in nodes with extensive permeation of sinuses but little involvement of the pulp. The sinusoidal pattern of invasion of malignant histiocytosis, which is a rare condition, is often displayed also by metastatic carcinoma, which is very much commoner (Fig. 15.1). Neither does this pattern of lymph node invasion exclude a diagnosis of malignant lymphoma (Osborne et al, 1980). Some types of metastatic carcinoma can also mimic the granulomatous pattern of histiocytic proliferations (Fig. 15.2) and others may have a genuinely granulomatous stromal reaction (e.g. seminoma and nasopharyngeal carcinoma (Fig. 15.3)).

In well fixed sections metastatic carcinoma shows a cohesiveness of the cells which is generally lacking in malignant lymphomas. Reticulin staining can be most helpful in making this distinction. The groups of cells in a carcinoma are sharply demarcated by reticulin, which tends to be pushed aside by the expanding tumour mass. Within the cell groups reticulin is very sparse or absent. In contrast, lymphoreticular tumours show a more intricate intermingling of reticulin fibre with the tumour cells, a feature displayed by sarcomas in general. The expansile pattern is seldom seen in lymphoreticular tumours. The density of reticulin fibre reaches its zenith in some examples of histiocytic malignancy where the fibre network tends to be pericellular. In respect of its reticulin pattern,

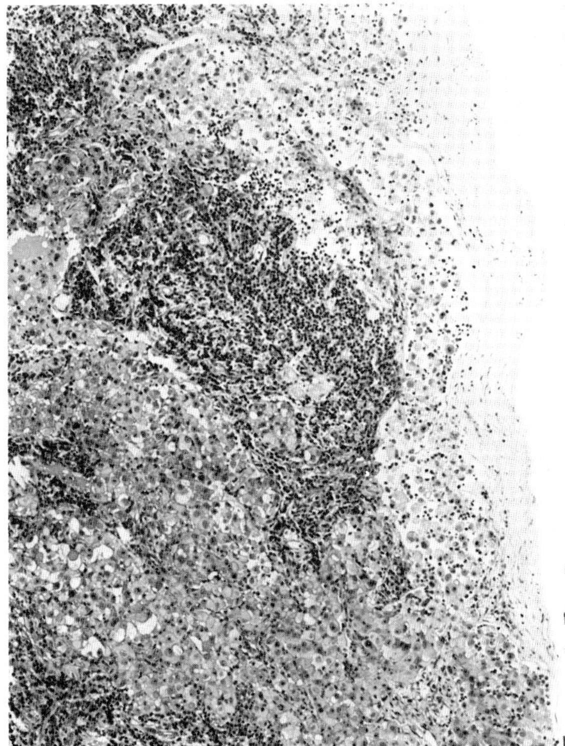

Fig. 15.1 Metastatic carcinoma showing a sinusoidal pattern of infiltration which mimics that of malignant histiocytosis (HE × 60)

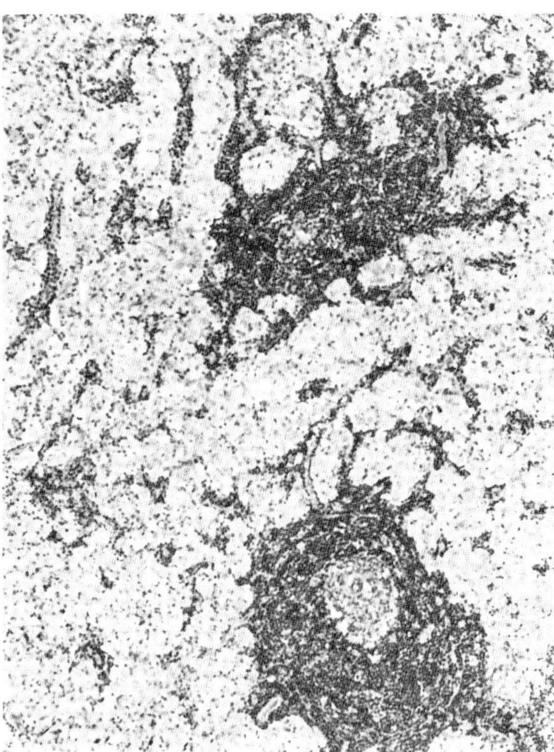

Fig. 15.2 Metastatic nasopharyngeal carcinoma with a quasi-granulomatous pattern of infiltration predominating (HE × 60)

malignant melanoma, a tumour of neuroectodermal derivation, is often intermediate between the above two described patterns (Fig. 15.4). An indeterminate pattern of reticulin may therefore be a useful pointer in the direction of amelanotic malignant melanoma.

Malignant lymphoma has a pattern of invasion of the walls of small veins which, when evident, is virtually specific. This consists of an intimate dissection of the elements of the vessel wall by individual tumour cells to produce a concentric thickening (Fig. 15.5). Staining for reticulin or elastic fibre may be necessary to detect this phenomenon if the tumourous infiltration is heavy. Usually the lumen of the vessel is not occluded although it may be restricted. A solid plug of tumour cells within the lumen of a vessel (Fig. 15.6) argues strongly against a diagnosis of malignant lymphoma although such may sometimes be seen in malignant histiocytosis. This applies also to lymphatic channels in which lymphoid cells remain discrete whilst carcinoma cells tend to form cohesive clusters.

Both primary malignant lymphomas and metastatic carcinomas may display massive or total necrosis of a tumour deposit. Extensive necrosis is, however, more commonly seen in metastatic carcinoma than in lymphomas. Amongst the lymphomas such a feature is not confined to high-grade lymphomas and is quite common in Hodgkin's disease. Under these circumstances a reliable distinction of primary from secondary tumour is often impossible, but it is worth remembering that reticulin staining will probably still show the pattern of fibre. Smaller areas of necrosis within a tumour are not generally a feature of malignant lymphomas other than Hodgkin's disease.

Even though the nature and the source of a metastatic deposit in a lymph node may be perfectly apparent, it is advisable to examine closely

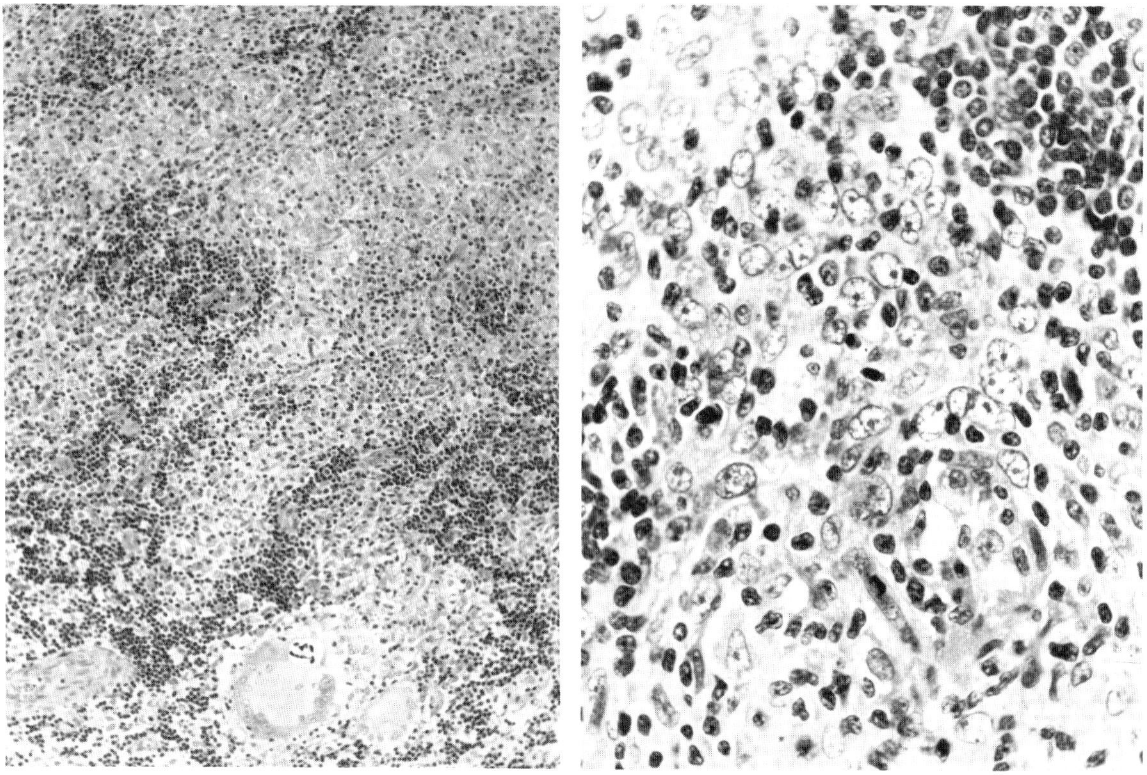

Fig. 15.3 (a) and (b) Metastatic nasopharyngeal carcinoma in a cervical node. (a) at low magnification, the carcinoma is masked by the overlying granulomatous reaction. Note multinucleate macrophages. (b) at a higher magnification, epithelioid cells (top left) mingle with carcinoma cells. (Both HE (a) × 120, (b) × 470)

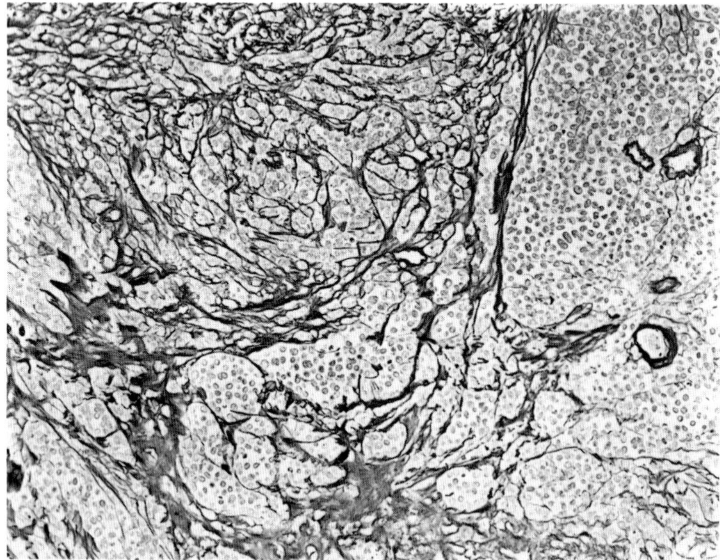

Fig. 15.4 Metastatic malignant melanoma showing a characteristic variation of the reticulin pattern from large cell groups devoid of reticulin to a more intricate pericellular pattern (Gordon and Sweets reticulin × 60)

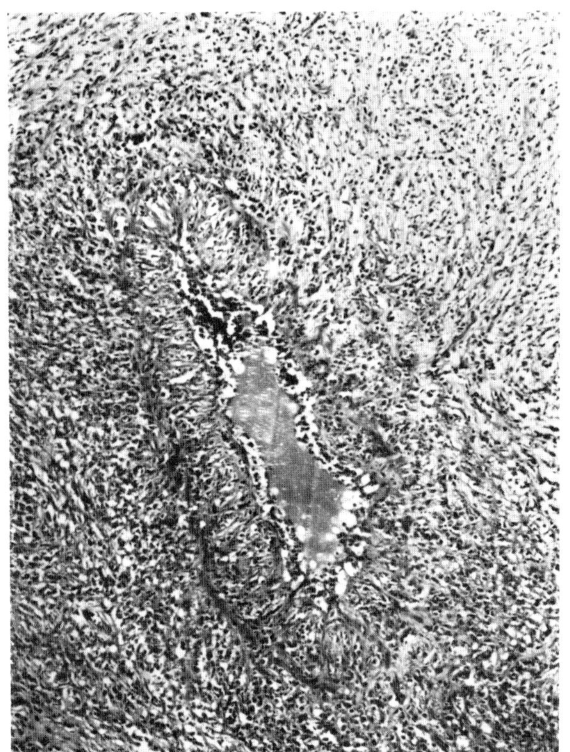

Fig. 15.5 Pattern of vascular invasion characteristic of malignant lymphoma. The lumen of the vein is not occluded. (HE × 60)

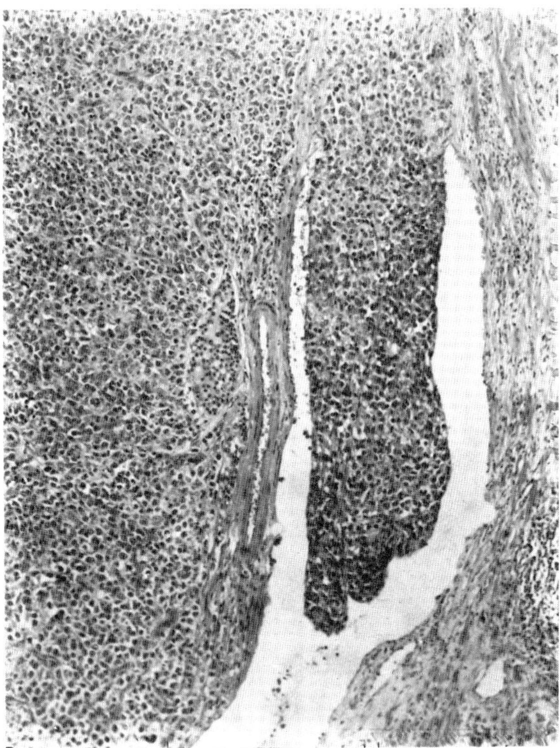

Fig. 15.6 Pattern of vascular invasion typical of epithelial malignancy. A solid core of tumour cells is present in the lumen of the vessel. (HE × 60)

any uninvolved portion of the node. Metastasis may have occurred in a node already involved by lymphoma. There is known to be an increased incidence of various second malignancies in patients who suffer from certain lymphomas such as chronic lymphatic leukaemia.

If fresh unfixed tissue is available, immunohistochemical methods can be employed on imprints or frozen sections as an aid to diagnosis. Today, the final arbiter in distinguishing carcinoma from malignant lymphoma is by the use of monoclonal antisera directed against epithelial antigens (positive in carcinomas but negative in lymphomas) and common leucocyte antigen (positive in lymphomas but negative in carcinomas) (see Ch. 4). Electron microscopy also may be a valuable adjunct. There are characteristic ultrastructural features which may allow the identification of neuroblastoma, rhabdomyosarcoma, malignant melanoma, oat-cell carcinoma, and squamous carcinoma, amongst others.

Although the importance of good fixation for light microscopy of lymph nodes is mentioned elsewhere, the matter will bear repetition and emphasis here. Many of the difficulties which are found in the distinction of primary from secondary neoplasia in nodes are purely a consequence of a poor state of preservation of the tissue with resulting shrinkage of cells.

In the remarks which follow, reference will be made only to those features which may be seen in sections prepared for light microscopy. The ultrastructural features of metastatic malignancies may be found in reference works devoted to electron microscopy.

Metastatic tumours of adults

Malignant melanoma

Malignant melanoma is exceedingly uncommon in childhood but occurs from early adult life onwards. Metastatic tumour may be found in a node at any site and the primary tumour may have been removed years previously, may be small and well hidden at some external or internal location, and may even have undergone spontaneous regression. Malignant melanoma can be completely devoid of melanin pigment or the pigment may be so sparsely distributed that its presence is overlooked. Alternatively, small amounts of melanin may be taken for haemosiderin in the presence of haemorrhage or necrosis. The variability of reticulin pattern (Fig. 15.4) displayed by malignant melanomas has already been mentioned. Because of all these factors malignant melanoma time and again traps the unwary diagnostician. The best safeguard against error is to keep melanoma constantly in mind as being in the differential diagnosis of a very wide range of neoplasms. It could be said that malignant melanoma has a potential for mimicry that is unrivalled by any other neoplasm, and among the tumours with which it is often confused are the malignant lymphomas.

The cells of a malignant melanoma may closely resemble plasma cell precursors at varying stages of maturation. A prominent central eosinophilic nucleolus and margination of nuclear chromatin are characteristic of Hodgkin's cells or immunoblasts, but melanoma may equally well show such an appearance. Eosinophilic cytoplasm, which may be fairly abundant, is shared by plasma cell precursors and malignant melanomas. However, melanoma cells never display quite the degree of pyroninophilia of genuine immunoblasts or plasmacytoid cells. Some of the possible appearances of malignant amelanotic melanoma are illustrated (Figs 15.7, 15.19).

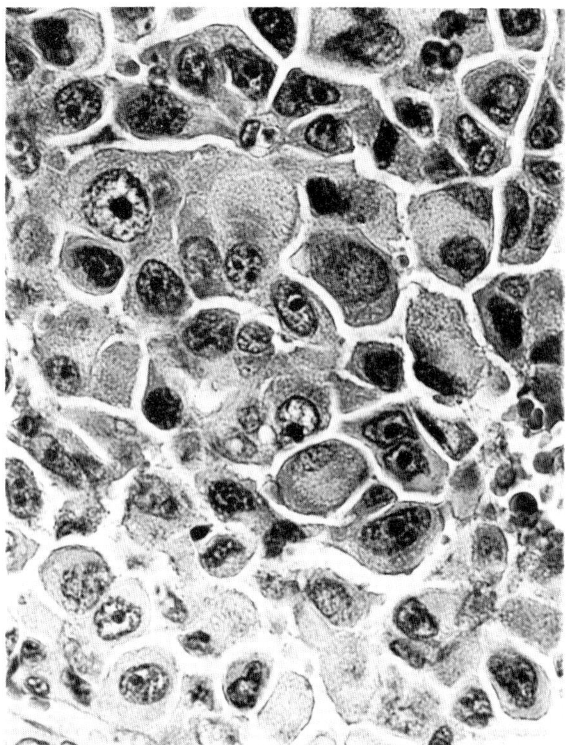

Fig. 15.7 Metastatic malignant melanoma. Eccentric nuclei and abundant eosinophilic cytoplasm mimic the features of the plasma cell series. Note the binucleate spurious 'Sternberg-Reed' cell. (HE × 1000)

Oat cell carcinoma

Oat cell carcinoma is no more than an anaplastic and highly aggressive carcinoid tumour of foregut origin. It shares many of the histological features of carcinoid tumours as a group, which vary in their degree of differentiation and aggressiveness. Although the tumour cells are often arranged in patternless sheets, sometimes a trabecular or a rosette-like pattern is encountered. The reticulin pattern is that of an epithelial malignancy and reticulin staining also serves to display the distinctive vascular pattern. Focal areas of necrosis scattered throughout the tumour also distinguish oat cell carcinoma from malignant lymphoma. Individual tumour cell necrosis with much karyorrhectic debris is another pattern of necrosis, which may be seen in high-grade lymphoma but which is not present to quite the same degree as in oat cell carcinoma. Release of nuclear material from spontaneous dissolution of tumour cells can lead to coating of connective tissue with masses of bare DNA and the haematoxyphil staining which results is very characteristic of oat cell carcinoma. The dense nuclear chromatin pattern of intact tumour cells is unlike that of any lymphoid cell population (Fig. 15.8). Nuclear moulding, whilst it is not exclusive to oat cell carcinoma, is a very useful diagnostic feature which may be displayed in histological material as well as cytological preparations where it is more usually commented upon. Not all oat cell carcinomas are composed of small

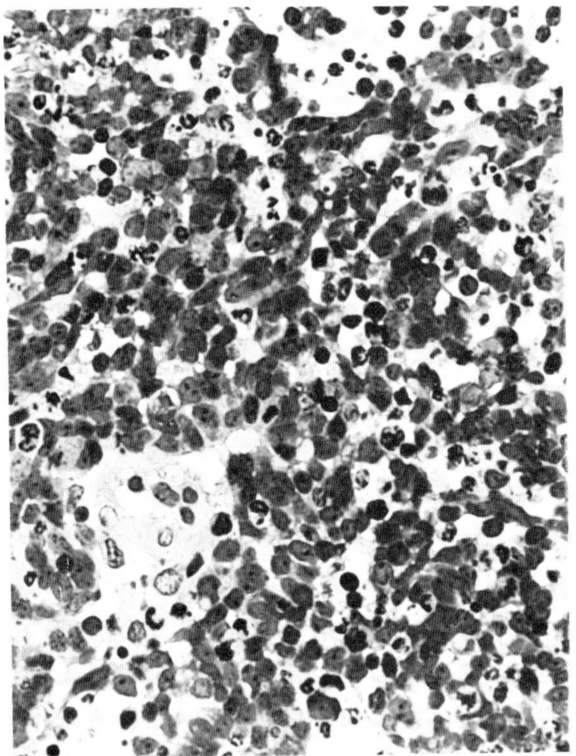

Fig. 15.8 Metastatic oat-cell carcinoma. Nuclear chromatin is dense and finely dispersed. Note the karyorrhectic debris due to individual tumour cell dissolution. (HE × 450)

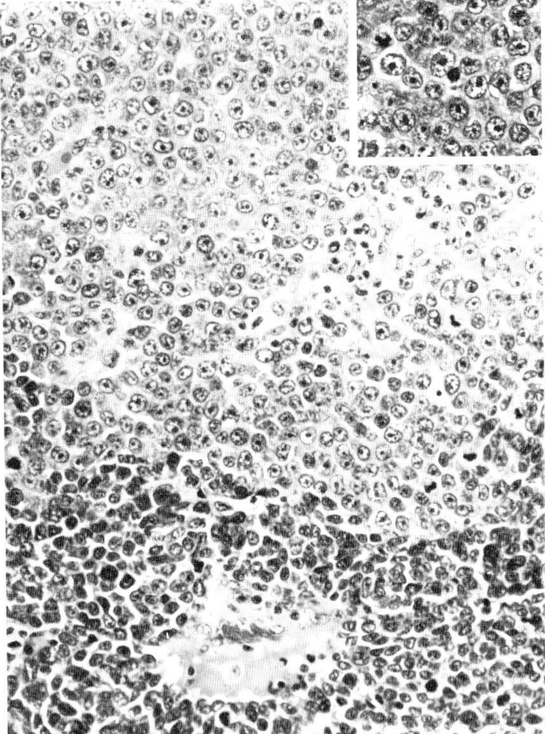

Fig. 15.9 Metastatic oat-cell carcinoma. Much of the tumour shows the typical small cell appearance, but the focus of tumour composed of larger cells (inset) mimics high-grade malignant lymphoma. (HE main fig. × 300, Inset × 900)

cells. An occasional large cell variant may be encountered (Fig. 15.9). Sometimes the sparse neurosecretory granules which all these tumours contain can be demonstrated by an argyrophil staining method.

Metastatic oat cell carcinoma of the bronchus is one of the tumours which is capable of producing a widespread lymphadenopathy. It is also one of the tumours which may have a very small or undetectable primary in the face of wide dissemination. The great majority of oat cell carcinomas arise in bronchial epithelium but the possibility of other primary sites of origin should be recognised. Oat cell carcinoma is recorded as rarely occurring in oesophagus, stomach and pancreas.

Mammary carcinoma

With regard to the differential diagnosis from primary lymph node diseases, there is usually little problem with carcinoma of the breast. For one thing the site of the primary tumour is in most cases obvious from clinical examination. Also, the microscopic appearances of metastatic disease are usually clearly indicative of epithelial malignancy. There is, however, one type of mammary carcinoma which may mimic lymphoma microscopically and which may not produce a definable tumour in the breast. This is infiltrating lobular carcinoma.

Metastatic lobular carcinoma in a lymph node (Fig. 15.10) can closely resemble lymphoma since glandular structures are exceptional and the uniform small rounded cells are arranged in diffuse sheets, sometimes with little or no fibrous reaction. When the malignant cells do excite a fibrous reaction then the diagnosis is immediately obvious. In addition to mimicry of lymphoid neoplasms, mimicry of histiocytic proliferation may result from a sinusoidal pattern of infiltration. Attention

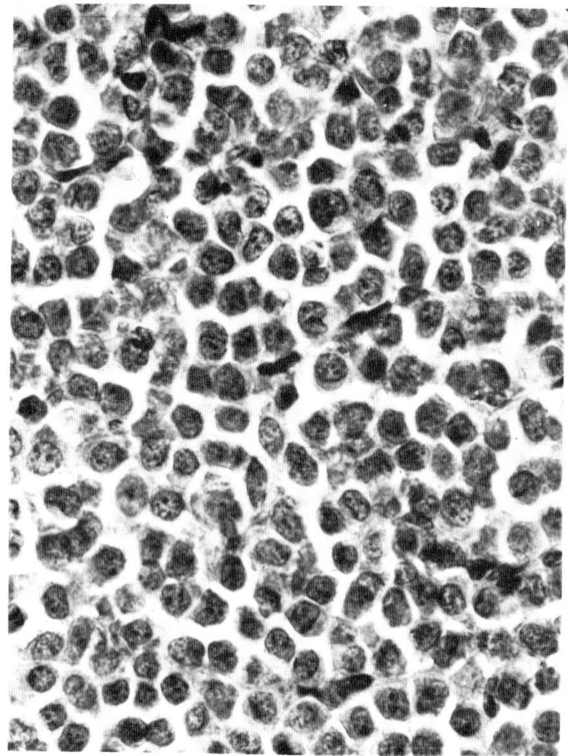

Fig. 15.10 Metastatic carcinoma of the breast. The cells of an infiltrating lobular carcinoma often show very little tendency to cohesion and in this respect are more like the cells of a lymphoid neoplasm. Mucin droplets are not visible in this particular example. (HE × 450)

to cytological detail, particularly nuclear chromatin pattern, and the reticulin pattern should serve to distinguish metastatic lobular mammary carcinoma from lymphoma. An 'indian file' arrangement of cells, typical of infiltrating lobular carcinoma within the breast itself, is not generally seen in metastatic deposits in the pulp of nodes. However, this virtually diagnostic pattern may be apparent in the connective tissue which forms the trabeculae and capsule, and also in connective tissue immediately surrounding the node.

Lobular carcinoma of the breast has a distinctive 'targetoid' or 'bull's-eye' pattern of mucin staining which may be seen both in cytological and histological material (Gad & Azzopardi, 1975; Spriggs & Jerrome, 1975). The basis of this staining pattern is an equally distinctive ultrastructural architecture of the cells which have individual intracytoplasmic lumina with microvillous borders.

Seminoma

The immediate lymphatic drainage of the testis is to para-aortic lymph nodes at the level of the renal arteries. Metastatic seminoma is therefore most often encountered in lymph nodes taken from the abdomen, although occasionally it is found further afield. Inguinal lymph node metastasis implies scrotal involvement and primary tumours as advanced as that are both uncommon in clinical practice and obvious on examination. Massive abdominal lymph node metastasis by seminoma is possible with a small undetected primary tumour in the testis. On rare occasions seminoma (germinoma) arises primarily in an extragonadal site, e.g. mediastinum. Also recorded with seminoma is progressive metastatic tumour with regression of the primary testicular tumour to leave only a fibrous scar.

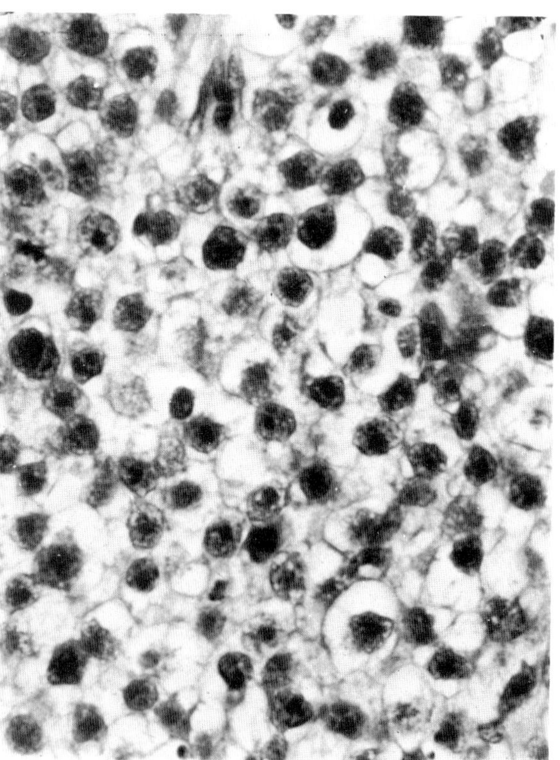

Fig. 15.11 Metastatic seminoma. This example lacks the usual lymphoid stromal infiltrate. The tumour cells have relatively abundant cytoplasm and distinct cell borders. Note the nuclear chromatin pattern. (HE × 450)

Microscopically, seminoma usually has a distinctive lymphoid stroma. Small lymphocytes are present in the delicate connective tissue septa which circumscribe groups of tumour cells. Often the lymphoid component is unevenly distributed, and in some instances it is absent from the entire tumour. Seminoma cells are large — much larger than the cells of most lymphomas — and have a 'clear', slightly granular cytoplasm, which contains abundant glycogen as demonstrated by PAS staining. The cytoplasmic borders are fairly well marked and this is an useful distinguishing feature (Fig. 15.11). Nucleoli are usually prominent but otherwise the nuclear chromatin pattern is unlike that of any lymphoid cell population. Multinucleate giant-cells and granulomatous reaction are sometimes seen in the stroma of seminomas. The reticulin pattern is that of an epithelial tumour.

Merkel cell tumour

Only in the past few years has a distinctive round cell neoplasm of the skin been described which is thought to be derived from Merkel cells. Merkel cells were first described in 1880 by Friedrich Sigmund Merkel, and are now considered to belong to the diffuse neuro-endocrine system. Ultrastructurally they are seen to contain neurosecretory type granules. For the tumours supposedly derived from these cells, the alternative names 'Merkel cell tumour' (Wick et al, 1983) or 'trabecular carcinoma of the skin' (Tang & Toker, 1978) have been proposed.

The microscopic appearances of a typical Merkel cell tumour are illustrated (Fig. 15.12). Tumour cells are medium-sized, polygonal and uniform. The nuclear chromatin is fine and indistinct giving a 'ground glass' or an almost 'empty' look to the nuclei, which are closely apposed to each other because of the very sparse cytoplasm. The cells of a Merkel cell tumour may be arranged in a trabecular formation but often appear as a patternless sheet. This produces a similarity both to malignant lymphoma and to undifferentiated carcinoma.

Clinically the behaviour of these tumours is often less aggressive than the histological appearances might suggest. However, Merkel cell tumours are certainly capable of metastasis to lymph nodes and lymphadenopathy may be the mode of presentation. Metastasis in lymph nodes has therefore to be distinguished from primary nodal lymphoma (and the primary tumour in the skin from primary extranodal lymphoma). The nuclear appearance, which is unlike that of lymphoid cells of any type, should provide a clue to the correct diagnosis. Demonstration of the neurosecretory granules by electron microscopy, or of neuron-specific enolase (NSE) activity by immunostaining provide valuable confirmatory evidence. The reticulin pattern is that of an epithelial tumour.

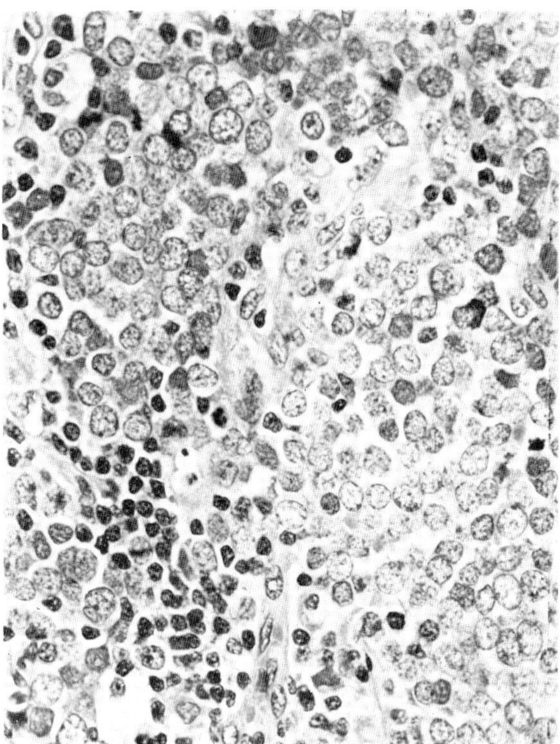

Fig. 15.12 Metastatic Merkel cell tumour. The finely dispersed nuclear chromatin does not resemble that of any lymphoid cell. There are a few remaining lymphocytes present. (HE × 450)

Nasopharyngeal and tonsillar carcinoma of lymphoepitheliomatous type (Schminke tumour)

This distinctive type of carcinoma has a wide range of age incidence. It occurs from childhood to old age and is particularly prevalent in certain populations (Chinese) although by no means confined to them. The tumour commonly presents with enlarged cervical lymph nodes, sometimes bilateral, and the primary tumour may long remain invisible. Even a close inspection of the nasopharynx may fail to reveal the primary. Therefore if a pathologist suspects metastatic nasopharyngeal carcinoma in a cervical node biopsy he would be wise to recommend multiple biopsies of the nasopharynx as an essential part of an ENT examination. Despite the terminology of 'lympho-epithelioma' sometimes applied to this tumour, it is purely epithelial in its genesis. However, it differs from ordinary squamous carcinoma in two respects. First, it is the only known tumour apart from Burkitt's lymphoma which is regularly associated with the Epstein-Barr virus (EBV). Secondly, and perhaps because of this association, the undifferentiated carcinoma cells often show intimate mingling with lymphoid stromal cells, including sometimes plasma cells. It is this feature, which may be seen both in the primary and in nodal metastases, which makes the tumour particularly liable to be mistaken for a malignant lymphoma.

The cells of lymphoepithelioma have these characteristics (Figs 15.3b, 15.13). They are large, with large, almost overlapping, nuclei but with abundant cytoplasm also. The nuclei appear sharply drawn with a crisp nuclear membrane. Nucleoli are usually eosinophilic and are often prominent. The cells display the cohesive character typical of carcinoma cells, at least in some portion of the tumour although this feature tends to be obscured by the lymphoid overlay especially in thick sections. In good quality sections, and particularly in semi-thin (1–2 μm) sections of resin-embedded tissue, the diagnosis becomes much easier. One type of non-Hodgkin's lymphoma which could be confused with metastatic lymphoepithelioma is ML centroblastic/centrocytic (diffuse). On critical examination, however, the very large epithelial cells do not really look like centroblasts and are not strongly pyroninophilic. The small cells in the stroma are lymphocytes and not centrocytes. Reticulin staining is very useful in revealing the epithelial character of this type of metastatic tumour.

Sometimes lymphoepithelioma is mistaken for Hodgkin's disease, which also contains lymphocytes and plasma cells in the stroma. The epithelial cells of metastatic nasopharyngeal carcinoma may have nuclear characteristics very similar to those of Sternberg-Reed cells and Hodgkin's cells. The resemblance to Hodgkin's disease may be heightened by a striking granulomatous reaction which lymphoepithelioma sometimes evokes (see Fig. 15.3a).

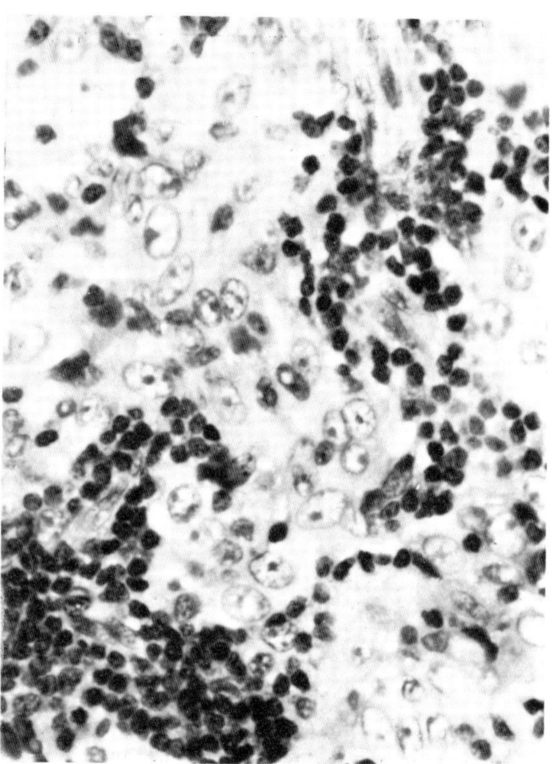

Fig. 15.13 Metastatic nasopharyngeal carcinoma. Poorly differentiated squamous cells show clustering within a lymphoid stroma. Note the nuclear characteristics of the squamous cells. (HE × 450)

Metastatic tumours of children

Neuroblastoma

Neuroblastoma is a malignant tumour very largely confined to childhood. Only exceptionally is it encountered in adult life. This tumour disseminates widely and early and, since the primary tumour is deeply placed in the abdomen or thorax, metastasis in a lymph node at a superficial site may well be the presenting manifestation. In sections of traumatised or poorly-fixed tissue, neuroblastoma may resemble a malignant lymphoma, generally lymphoblastic lymphoma. In this age group it may also be mistaken for metastatic rhabdomyosarcoma or metastatic Ewing's tumour, although the latter seldom presents with lymph node enlargement.

Depending on the degree of maturation of a neuroblastoma, the tumour cells will be of varying size and have a varying amount of cytoplasm which is negative on staining by the PAS method, a useful differentiating feature from Ewing's tumour and rhabdomyosarcoma. At their most primitive, neuroblasts have extremely scanty cytoplasm but then they are most likely to display the neuro-rosette arrangement which is a classical feature of this tumour (Fig. 15.14). Malignant lymphomas and rhabdomyosarcoma do not show rosette formation, but Ewing's tumour may do so occasionally. When slightly more mature, neuroblasts have more abundant cytoplasm and nuclei which begin to approach neuronal nuclei in appearance. The vascular pattern of neuroblastoma is highly distinctive and is observed to best advantage in reticulin stained sections (Fig. 15.15). This pattern is not shared by malignant lymphoma, or by rhabdomyosarcoma or by Ewing's tumour. The fibrillary material, which composes the centres of neuro-rosettes and which is also seen more generally dispersed in those neuroblastomas lacking rosettes, is a useful diagnostic feature when it is noted.

Rhabdomyosarcoma

This is included in the group of small round cell tumours of childhood and the primary site may be undeclared clinically when metastatic disease in lymph nodes becomes apparent. Rhabdomyosarcoma of alveolar type may occur in young adults as well as in children.

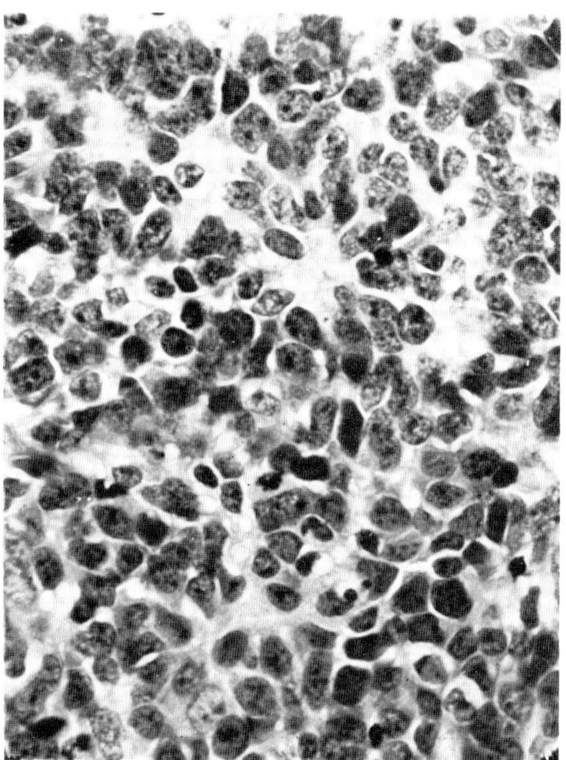

Fig. 15.14 Metastatic neuroblastoma (poorly differentiated). The cells are small with finely dispersed nuclear chromatin and very little cytoplasm. Note the poorly developed rosette formation. (HE × 450)

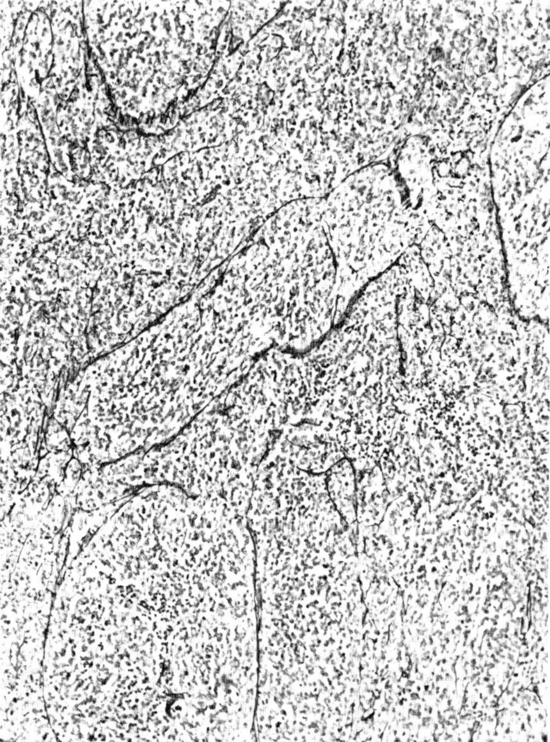

Fig. 15.15 Metastatic neuroblastoma. The tumour cells are arranged in lobules devoid of reticulin fibre. The blood vessels circumscribe the groups of tumour cells. (Gordon and Sweets reticulin × 60)

It is difficult to recognise with certainty completely undifferentiated rhabdomyoblasts since these closely resemble lymphoid cells. Some degree of differentiation may be seen in a proportion of the tumour cells which are larger and display prominently eosinophilic cytoplasm. Such cells often then have an eccentric nucleus after the fashion of plasma cells (Fig. 15.16). A still greater degree of differentiation results in more elongated cells in which striations are demonstrable by appropriate staining methods. It may be that only a few of the cells within the tumour will show striations and a careful search for this diagnostic feature is warranted if the general histological appearances point towards rhabdomyosarcoma. It is worth noting also that rhabdomyoblasts contain glycogen which can be demonstrated by PAS staining although the reaction is generally less intense than that seen in Ewing's tumour. An alveolar pattern in rhabdomyosarcoma is largely an artefact due to imperfect or delayed fixation. The resulting disaggregation of the tumour cells leaves a peripheral rim of cells attached by one pole of their cytoplasm to fibrous connective tissue septa (Fig. 15.17). Observation of this artefact is diagnostically useful since it is characteristic for rhabdomyosarcoma.

Ewing's tumour

Ewing's tumour is a malignant tumour largely but not exclusively encountered in childhood, and usually but not necessarily arising in bone. Its exact histogenesis is unknown. Metastasis to lymph nodes is certainly possible although rare, and rarer still is presentation with metastatic tumour in a lymph node. Despite the infrequency with which Ewing's tumour is found in lymph node biopsies it will be considered here because it enters into the differential diagnosis of the other

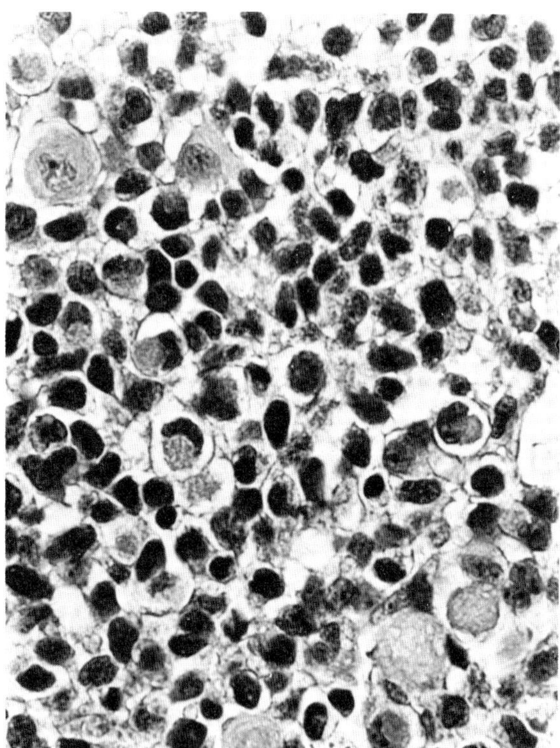

Fig. 15.16 Metastatic rhabdomyosarcoma. Some cells are very primitive with scanty cytoplasm but tend to be ovoid rather than round. Others show more differentiation with abundant eosinophlic cytoplasm. (HE × 450)

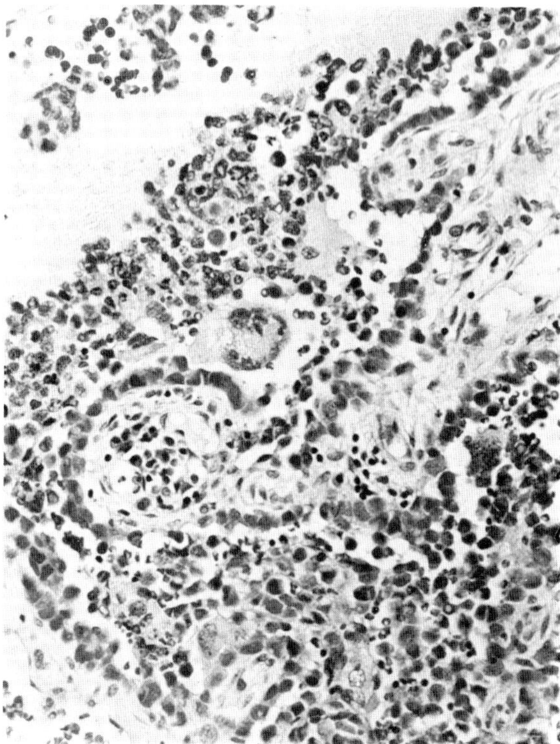

Fig. 15.17 Metastatic rhabdomyosarcoma. Disaggregation of the tumour cells in the centre, leaving a peripheral rim of cells adherent to fibrovascular septa produces the 'alveolar' pattern. (HE × 300)

small round-cell tumours of childhood already mentioned, namely malignant lymphoma, neuroblastoma and rhabdomyosarcoma. Characteristically, the cells of Ewing's tumour contain abundant glycogen which is demonstrable by PAS staining. Rhabdomyosarcomas also often contain glycogen (see above) but seldom in such large amounts as Ewing's tumour. Neuroblastomas are invariably negative when stained for glycogen. Reticulin fibre is very sparse or totally absent within the groups of tumour cells, which explains the often diffluent consistency of the tumour. On rare occasions Ewing's tumour may display rosette-like structures but the usual arrangement is one of patternless sheets of cells.

DETERMINATION OF THE POSSIBLE SITE OF ORIGIN OF METASTASES

In order to assess where a metastasis may have originated a pathologist requires familiarity with the range of possible appearances of tumours at all sites in the body, not excepting even the central nervous system (Wight et al, 1973; Jackson & Graham, 1978). This is clearly too broad a topic to be covered fully here. Not only the histological appearances, but also the vagaries of behaviour of various primary malignancies have to be taken into account when assessing metastatic malignancy in nodes. Both clinicians and pathologists have traditionally enjoyed the game of 'hunt the primary'. In the past the detection of a hidden primary tumour has been largely an academic exercise, pursued for its own interest, rather than a matter of much practical importance for the patient. In recent years, however, advances in chemotherapy and the introduction of more effective forms of treatment for certain types of neoplasm have meant that knowledge of the site of the primary tumour *may* be of much greater consequence than heretofore. The age and the sex of the patient and the site from which a lymph node has been excised are all pieces of highly important information. These must be available if an accurate indication of the likely source of a metastasis is to be given. For example, the probable sites of primary tumours with metastasis in a cervical lymph node in a child are quite different from those metastasising to cervical nodes in an adult, and the differences are obviously greater still if a different region is involved, e.g. inguinal nodes. In general, nodal metastases become clinically apparent within the immediate regional lymphatic drainage of the primary tumour. However, there are many exceptions to this rule, e.g. supraclavicular nodal metastasis from gastric or renal carcinomas. In such instances the regional lymph nodes probably would be affected but this involvement of deep-seated nodes is not readily detectable by clinical examination. It is well to be aware also of the types of primary tumour which may, on occasion, give rise to widespread metastasis, producing generalised lymphadenopathy and a clinical resemblance to primary lymph nodal disease. Examples are neuroblastoma in childhood and oat-cell carcinoma in adults. Certain types of primary malignancy may occasionally regress and disappear in the face of progressive metastatic disease, e.g. malignant melanoma, seminoma.

Some types of tumour have a distinctive histological appearance even in their metastases. Renal tubular carcinoma is often given as a good example. The clear cell appearance in a typical case is very distinctive. It must be borne in mind, however, that not every instance of a given type of primary tumour will conform to a 'classical' pattern. Some renal tubular carcinomas are purely oxyphilic, some are sarcomatoid. Conversely, a particular pattern is not necessarily exclusive to

Table 15.1 Some tumours which may be composed of clear cells

Mucoepidermoid carcinoma of salivary gland
Acinic cell tumour of salivary gland
Follicular carcinoma of thyroid
Squamous carcinoma of lung
Adenocarcinoma of lung
Renal tubular carcinoma
Adrenocortical carcinoma
Hepatocellular carcinoma
Yolk sac tumour
Clear cell (mesonephroid) carcinoma of ovary
Carcinoma of endometrium
Seminoma
Malignant melanoma

one type of malignancy. There are several other tumours besides renal carcinoma, for instance, which may show a clear cell appearance (Table 15.1, Figs 15.18, 15.19).

Tables 15.1–15.4 are provided as brief reminders of some histological features which may

Table 15.2 Some tumours which may have oxyphilic cells

Thyroid follicular carcinoma (Hürthle cell type)
Mammary carcinoma
Renal tubular carcinoma
Hepatocellular carcinoma
Pancreatic carcinoma
Malignant melanoma
Rhabdomyosarcoma

Table 15.3 Some tumours which may contain glycogen

Renal tubular carcinoma*
Seminoma*
Ewing's tumour*
Squamous carcinoma
Hepatocellular carcinoma
Ovarian adenocarcinoma
Thymoma
Rhabdomyosarcoma
Malignant mesothelioma
Malignant melanoma (some examples)

* These particular tumours characteristically contain large amounts of glycogen and give strongly positive staining reactions with the PAS method

Table 15.4 Some tumours with, and some without, intracellular mucin

some tumours with intracellular mucin	some tumours without intracellular mucin
Mucin present	Mucin absent
Adenocarcinomas of:	Carcinomas of:
Gastrointestinal tract	Thyroid
Biliary tract	Kidney
Pancreas	Liver
Lung	Malignant melanoma
Breast	Seminoma
Salivary glands	
Ovary	
Cervix uteri	

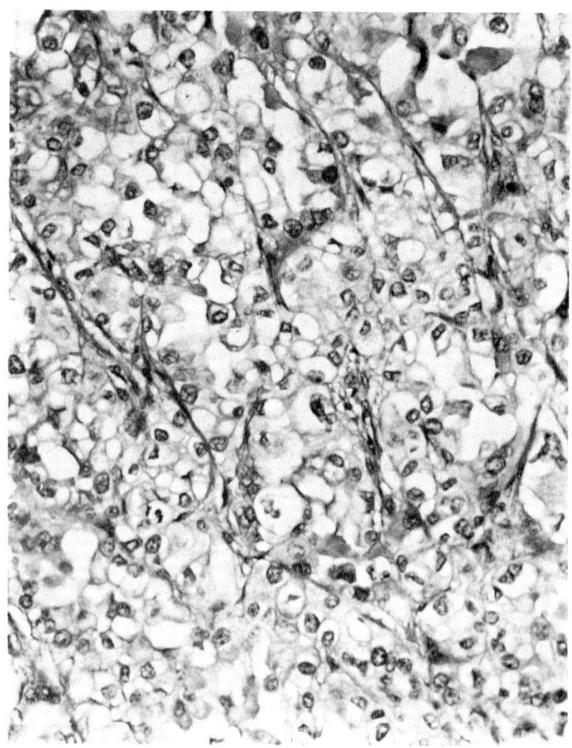

Fig. 15.18 Metastatic clear cell carcinoma of the bronchus. Unlike renal carcinoma the cells of this type of tumour do not contain lipid. (HE × 300)

be relevant to metastatic tumours in lymph nodes. Besides the demonstration of glycogen (PAS staining with and without prior diastase digestion) (Table 15.3), the demonstration of mucin, or the lack of it, may help to determine the primary site of a carcinoma (Table 15.4).

DIFFERENTIATION OF BENIGN LYMPH NODE INCLUSIONS FROM METASTATIC NEOPLASM.

Many benign epithelial inclusions in lymph nodes are infrequent pathological curiosities. A prime requisite for their correct identification is a simple awareness that such conditions exist. Obviously a great deal of anxiety and unnecessary investigation will ensue if benign inclusions are mistaken for metastatic malignancy.

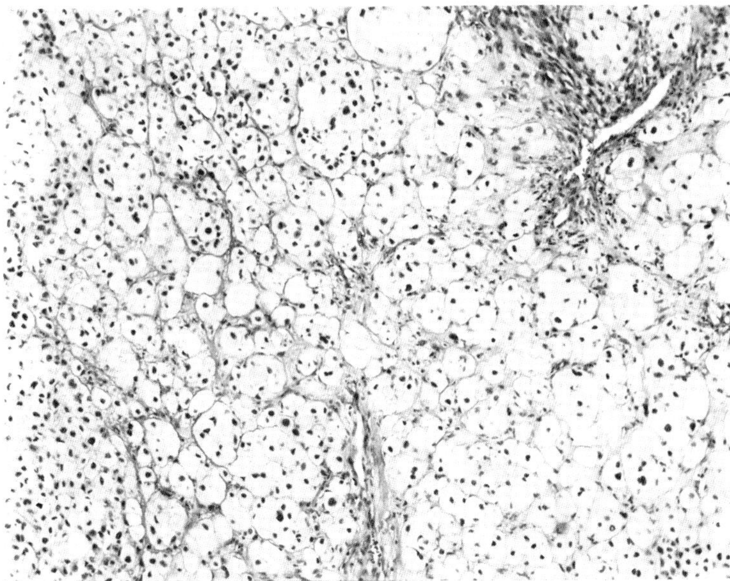

Fig. 15.19 Metastatic clear cell tumour. This is malignant melanoma of the balloon cell variety. The cells contain neither lipid nor glycogen, and in this particular example they are also lacking melanin pigment. (HE × 300)

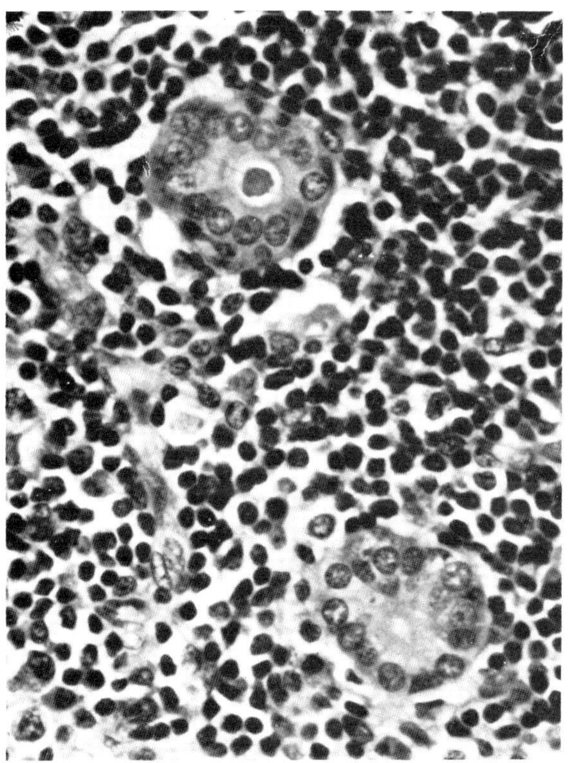

Fig. 15.20 Heterotopic salivary gland tissue in a peri-parotid lymph node. The epithelium lining the small ducts is regular in appearance. (HE × 450)

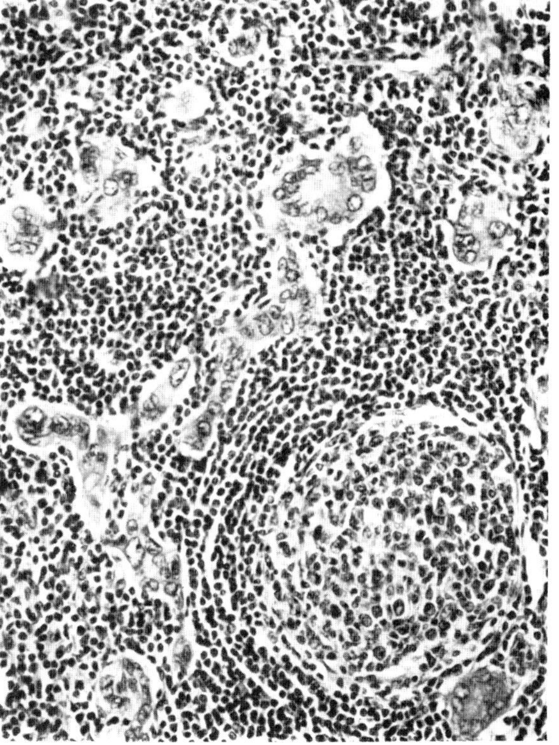

Fig. 15.21 Metastatic gastric carcinoma producing small duct-like structures within a lymph node. Note the pleomorphism of this epithelium in comparison to that of the ducts shown in Fig. 15.20. (HE × 150)

Salivary inclusions

Heterotopic salivary gland tissue in peri-parotid lymph nodes was recognised as a normal feature of foetal and neonatal life as long ago as 1898 (Neisse, quoted by Brown et al, 1953). Persistence of this heterotopic tissue into adult life is extremely common. Small salivary ducts, lined by a double layer of cells (epithelium and myo-epithelium, Fig. 15.20) may be found scattered throughout a lymph node or focally aggregated. Often they are accompanied by salivary acinar tissue. It is conceivable, though unlikely, that the ducts by themselves might be mistaken for metastatic tumour but there can be few pathologists who have not frequently encountered this phenomenon. The uniformity of salivary duct epithelium is not matched even by well-differentiated metastatic adenocarcinoma (cf. Figs 15.20, 15.21).

Breast inclusions

Non-malignant inclusions of breast tissue in axillary lymph nodes are apparently rarely encountered (Turner & Millis, 1980). The usual form that these inclusions take is that of duct-like structures and small cysts (Fig. 15.22). The heterogeneity in size of the ducts and cysts is a feature which distinguishes them from metastatic carcinoma. The lining epithelium lacks any cytological atypia and commonly shows metaplasia to apocrine or squamous type. Squamous metaplasia of the lining is principally seen in the cysts and a granular layer may be discernible. Amorphous eosinophilic material fills the cysts. Like metaplastic apocrine epithelium within the breast as part of benign mammary dysplasia, the apocrine type of epithelium in the lymph node inclusions does not give a positive staining reaction for iron. Normal apocrine sweat gland epithelium from the axilla is positive for iron. For this reason the epithelial inclusions in axillary lymph nodes are thought to be derived in some way from breast tissue rather than from axillary sweat glands (Edlow & Carter, 1973). The duct-like inclusions in axillary lymph nodes often show a double lining (epithelium proper and myo-epithelium), such as is found in normal breast ducts (Garret & Ada, 1957; McDivitt et al, 1968). The lack of associated stroma with epithelial lymph node inclusions at this site suggests that these are not examples of heterotopic breast tissue. The mechanism by which epithelial structures are incorporated into axillary nodes is obscure but may be best explained by postulating lymph transport of benign epithelium from the breasts. It is known that benign sclerosing adenosis in the breast may display invasion of perineural spaces although it is not certain that these perineural spaces represent true lymphatic channels.

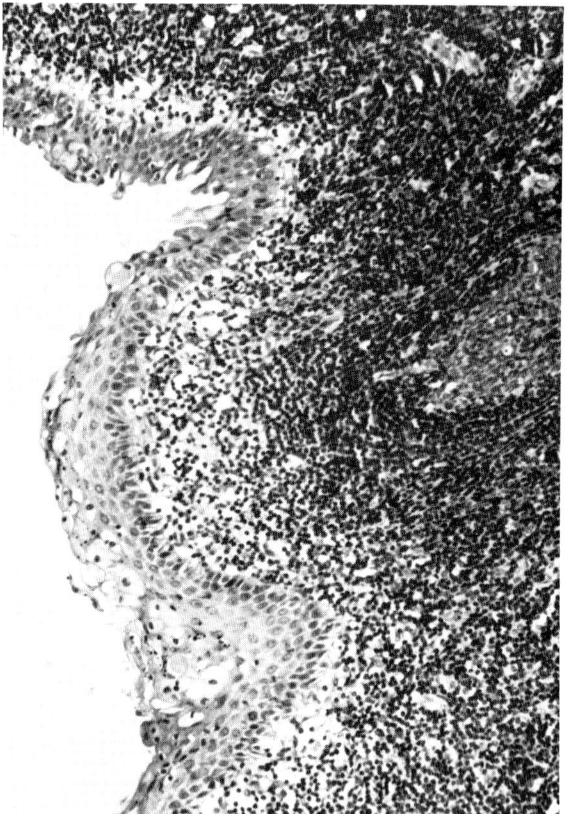

Fig. 15.22 Heterotopic breast tissue in an axillary lymph node. The epithelium lining the cysts of various sizes has undergone extensive squamous metaplasia although there remain some cells with apocrine features. (HE × 150)

Naevus cell inclusions

Naevus cell aggregates are sometimes observed in lymph nodes taken from superficial sites (Ridolfi et al, 1977) and are most commonly found in axillary nodes. They are invariably found enclosed

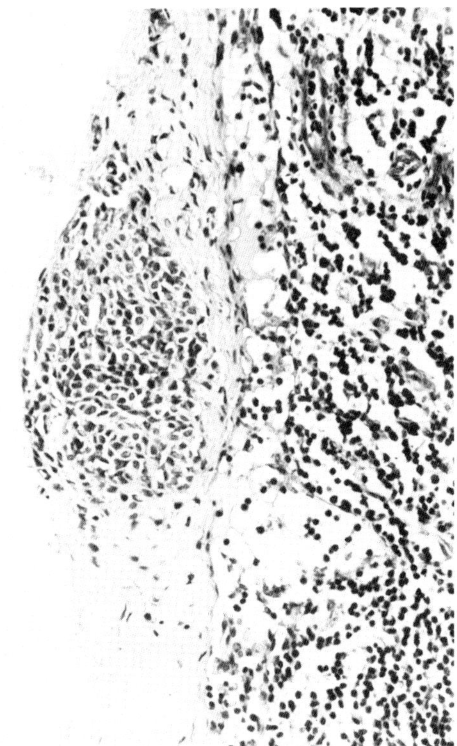

Fig. 15.23 A naevus cell aggregate enclosed in the fibrous tissue of a lymph node capsule. Note the cellular uniformity and the suggestion of an arrangement around small vascular channels. (HE × 150)

within the fibrous tissue which composes the trabeculae or the capsule of the node (Fig. 15.23). The fact that they are not observed within the sinuses argues against their having been transported to the node from benign naevocellular lesions on the skin, quite apart from the absence of any such potential source in many cases. The naevus cells in nodes form clusters similar to those found in benign naevi in the skin. They lack mitotic activity or cellular atypia and can be demonstrated to contain small amounts of melanin pigment sometimes. Probably the best explanation of their origin is an imperfect migration of neural crest derivatives during development. This is exactly similar to the supposed mode of formation of conventional naevi of the skin (Johnson & Helwig, 1969; Hart, 1971).

Some authors believe that the cell clusters referred to here as naevus cell aggregates are glomus cell aggregates rather than being naevocellular in character (Berg et al, 1976). A perivascular arrangement similar to that seen in glomangiomas is admittedly sometimes encountered in these cell clusters. It has not been demonstrated that the clusters are richly endowed with nerve terminals, as true glomangiomas are, however. The exact nature of 'naevus cell aggregates' may be in dispute, but there is no doubt that the differential diagnosis of this uncommon lesion includes metastatic malignant melanoma and metastatic carcinoma of the breast, especially in axillary nodes. The location of the cells, the microscopic size of the lesion, the cellular uniformity and the lack of mitotic activity are features which help to make the distinction. The occasional presence of melanin pigment and the invariable absence of mucin in the cells point away from mammary carcinoma.

Discussion of naevus cells in lymph nodes cannot be left without mention of the special case of the blue naevus. Cellular blue naevi have on several occasions been mistaken for malignant melanomas, even by the experienced. Some cellular blue naevi are associated with 'metastasis' in regional lymph nodes. Doubt has been cast on whether these are true metastases from a progressive and malignant primary tumour or whether they are more in the nature of benign transports — cf. breast inclusions in axillary lymph nodes (Rodriguez & Ackerman, 1968). Primary blue naevus of lymph node capsule has also been described (Azzopardi et al, 1977). This too has to be distinguished from metastatic malignant melanoma.

Thyroid inclusions

Despite some dispute about their frequency and the histological criteria for their diagnosis, there can be no reasonable doubt that benign inclusions of thyroid follicular tissue are occasionally seen in cervical lymph nodes. The mechanism by which benign thyroid follicles find their way into the nodes is as uncertain for this type of inclusion as it is for the other types of epithelial inclusion. The differential diagnosis is, of course, from well differentiated carcinoma metastatic from the thyroid gland. The features which help to distinguish the benign inclusion are its microscopic size (5 to 25 follicles per section), uniformity and small size of the nuclei, exclusively follicular arrangement without any papillary structures, lack of psammoma bodies and of a fibrous stromal reaction, and a location in or adjacent to the lymph node capsule. If an inclusion of thyroid tissue fails to meet any of these criteria then it must be considered to be a metastasis from an occult carcinoma within the thyroid.

Benign thyroid inclusions are possibly more common than is generally realised. They have been discovered in up to 3% of autopsies after careful search (Meyer & Steinberg, 1969). It should be noted that there is also an incidence at autopsy of microscopic foci of carcinoma in the step-sectioned thyroid gland of 5% to over 20% (Fukunaga & Yatani, 1976). However, these are apparently not the same cases as bear the benign lymph node inclusions. Sectioning of the thyroid in those patients will usually fail to disclose a carcinoma. Moreover, the great majority of the microscopic carcinomas found in the thyroid can be dismissed as having no potential for progressive malignant behaviour, i.e. they are mostly 'latent carcinomas'.

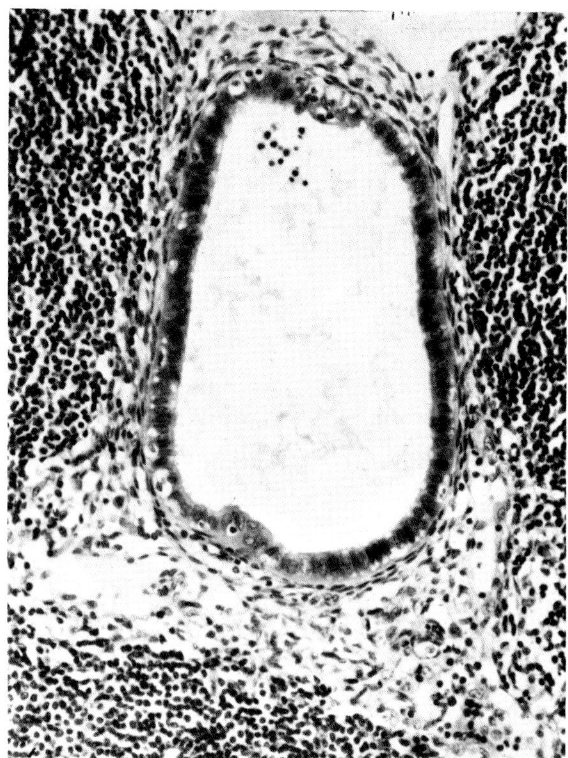

Fig. 15.24 A small focus of endometrial glandular tissue in a mesenteric lymph node taken from a patient with caecal endometriosis. Some endometrial-type stroma surrounds the gland. (HE × 150)

Glandular inclusions in abdominal lymph nodes

Iliac, para-aortic and mesenteric lymph nodes are sometimes found to contain small foci of endometriosis (Karp & Czernobilsky, 1969). The known presence of endometriosis at other sites, the innocent appearance of the epithelium in the glands (Fig. 15.24) and the presence of endometrial stroma around them, all help to distinguish foci of endometriosis from metastatic tumour. The stroma may display a decidual reaction in the appropriate circumstances (Russell, 1945). Sometimes the endometrial stroma is absent around the glands and the explanation of the inclusions in abdominal nodes is said to be from mesothelial rests. This is reminiscent of one previously proposed theory of origin of endometriosis. Tubal epithelium may also be carried to adjacent lymph nodes in cases of salpingitis (Stansfeld, personal observation), and a benign transport mechanism is an alternative theory. As with endometriosis at other sites there is the possibility of the development of endometrial-type carcinoma within a focus of endometriosis. Such an occurrence is only rarely documented (Koss, 1963).

Branchial cysts

Branchial cysts often have an abundance of lymphoid tissue in their walls and may be mistaken for lymph nodes with either benign inclusions or with metastatic malignancy. Close inspection of the lymphoid tissue will generally reveal that it does not have the architectural arrangement of a lymph node, although true lymph nodes are sometimes very closely applied to the walls of branchial cysts. The epithelial elements of a branchial cyst lack the cytological characteristics of malignancy and are usually composed of respiratory-type epithelium with a variable amount of squamous metaplasia. The possibility of malignancy arising primarily in the epithelial component of a branchial cyst has to be admitted and such an event would be difficult to distinguish histologically from metastatic carcinoma in a cervical lymph node. It is most probable, however, that the overwhelming majority of reported cases of carcinoma arising in branchial cysts are in truth cases of metastatic squamous carcinoma in cervical lymph nodes (Batsakis, 1981).

REFERENCES

Azzopardi J G, Ross C M D, Frizzera G 1977 Blue naevi of lymph node capsule. Histopathology 1: 451–461

Batsakis J G 1981 The pathology of head and neck tumours: the occult primary and metastases to the head and neck, part 10. Head and Neck Surgery 3: 409–423

Berg F W R van den, Kaiserling E, Lennert K 1976 Glomus-Zellnester des Lymphknotens. Virchow's Archiv fur pathologische Anatomie und Physiologie A371: 27–34

Brown R B, Gaillard R A, Turner J A 1953 The significance of aberrant or heterotopic parotid gland tissue in lymph nodes. Annals of Surgery 138: 850–856

Edlow D W, Carter D 1973 Heterotopic epithelium in axillary lymph nodes. American Journal of Clinical Pathology 59: 666–673

Fukunaga F H, Yatani R 1975 Geographic pathology of occult thyroid carcinomas. Cancer 36: 1095–1099

Gad A, Azzopardi J G 1975 Lobular carcinoma of the breast: a special variant of mucin-secreting carcinoma. Journal of Clinical Pathology 28: 711–716

Garret R, Ada A E W 1957 Epithelial inclusion cysts in an axillary lymph node. Cancer 10: 173–178

Hart W R 1971 Primary nevus of a lymph node. American Journal of Clinical Pathology 55: 88–92

Ibrahim N B M, Milewski P J, Gillett R, Temple J G 1981 Benign thyroid inclusions within cervical lymph nodes: an alarming incidental finding. Australia and New Zealand Journal of Surgery 51: 188–189

Jackson A M, Graham D I 1978 Remote metastases from intracranial tumours. Journal of Clinical Pathology 31: 794–802

Johnson W T, Helwig E B 1969 Benign naevus cells in the capsule of lymph nodes. Cancer 23: 747–753

Karp L A, Czernobilsky B 1969 Glandular inclusions in pelvic and abdominal lymph nodes. American Journal of Clinical Pathology 52: 212–218

Koss L G 1963 Miniature adenoacanthoma arising in an endometriotic cyst in an obturator lymph node: report of first case. Cancer 16: 1369–1372

Meyer J S, Steinberg L S 1969 Microscopically benign thyroid follicles in cervical lymph nodes. Cancer 24: 302–311

Osborne B M, Butler J J, Mackay B 1980 Sinusoidal large cell (histiocytic) lymphoma. Cancer 46: 2484–2491

Ridolfi R L, Rosen P P, Thaler H 1977 Nevus cell aggregates associated with lymph nodes: estimated frequency and clinical significance. Cancer 39: 164–171

Rodriguez H A, Ackerman L V 1968 Cellular blue naevus: clinicopathologic study of forty-five cases. Cancer 21: 393–405

Russell J B 1945 Decidual reaction of endometrium in abdominal lymph node. Surgery, Gynecology and Obstetrics 81: 218–220

Sidhu G S, Feiner H, Flotte T J, Mullins J D, Schaefler K, Schultenover S J 1980 Merkel cell neoplasms: histology, electron microscopy, biology and histogenesis. American Journal of Dermatopathology 2: 101–119

Spriggs A I, Jerrome D W 1975 Intracellular mucous inclusions: a feature of malignant cells in effusions in the serous cavities, particularly due to carcinoma of the breast. Journal of Clinical Pathology 28: 929–936

Tang C K, Toker C 1978 Trabecular carcinoma of the skin. Cancer 42: 2311–2321

Turner D R, Millis R R 1980 Breast tissue inclusions in axillary lymph nodes. Histopathology 4: 631–636

Wick M R, Goellner J R, Scheithauer B W, Thomas J R, Sanchez N P, Schroeter A L 1983 Primary neuroendocrine carcinomas of the skin (Merkel cell tumours): a clinical, histologic and ultrastructural study of thirteen cases. American Journal of Clinical Pathology 79: 6–13

Wight D G D, Holley K J, Finbow J A H 1973 Metastasizing ependymoma of the cauda equina. Journal of Clinical Pathology 26: 929–935

APPENDIX

The working formulation of non-Hodgkin's lymphomas for clinical usage

In 1975 the National Cancer Institute in Washington sponsored a multi-centre study to compare six classifications of non-Hodgkin's lymphomas. The study was prompted by the earlier failure of pathologists to agree on a classification of these neoplasms at a workshop in Chicago in 1973, and the consequent frustration of clinicians on finding themselves unable to compare results of therapy because of the lack of an agreed classification. Details of the background of the NCI study, its organisation, conduct and results have been subsequently published (National Cancer Institute, 1982).

In summary, the study showed that each of the six classifications that were compared was clinically useful and none was found to be superior to the others in predicting prognosis. At a subsequent meeting of the participating pathologists to discuss these results, a consensus was reached on 'the working formulation of non-Hodgkin's lymphomas for clinical usage', which is set out below. It was agreed at this meeting that the Kiel classification, unlike most of the others, could not be easily equated with the working formulation (WF) and the different categories of the Kiel classification were therefore set out alongside those of the WF.

The 10 categories of the WF are divided into three grades — low, intermediate and high. This division was based on survival data of patients included in the study, not on pathological criteria and the latter were of secondary importance also in determining the 10 individual categories, in which again the prognosis was the primary consideration. For those using the WF, the main heading in each category is 'obligatory', while the sub-headings are 'optional'.

A detailed critique of the NCI study and of the 'working formulation' has been published by Rilke and Lennert (1981), pointing out the major defects of both. Their criticisms will not be repeated here; suffice it to emphasise here that the WF is *not* (nor was it intended to be) a *pathological* classification and the basis of separating the 10 different categories is quite unscientific. Some categories (e.g. category H) quite clearly include a hotch-potch of different entities. Although the WF may prove a useful stop-gap for the comparison of clinical results, it is important that pathologists should not be misled into regarding it as a new pathological classification.

REFERENCES

National Cancer Institute sponsored study of classifications of non-Hodgkin's lymphomas: summary and description of a working formulation for clinical usage 1982 Cancer 49: 2112–2135

Rilke F, Lennert K 1981 A perspective of the Kiel classification in relation to other recent classifications of non-Hodgkin's lymphoma, with special reference to the Working Formulation. In: Lennert K in collaboration with Stein H, Histopathology of non-Hodgkin's Lymphomas (based on the Kiel classification). Springer-Verlag, Berlin p 112–118

A WORKING FORMULATION OF NON-HODGKIN'S LYMPHOMAS FOR CLINICAL USAGE
(equivalent or related terms in the Kiel classification are shown)

Working Formulation	Kiel equivalent or related terms
Low grade	
A. Malignant lymphoma	
Small lymphocytic	
consistent with CLL	ML lymphocytic, CLL
plasmacytoid	ML lymphoplasmacytic/lymphoplasmacytoid
B. Malignant lymphoma, follicular	
Predominantly small cleaved cell	
diffuse areas	
sclerosis	
C. Malignant lymphoma, follicular	ML centroblastic-centrocytic (small), follicular ± diffuse (B and C)
Mixed small cleaved and large cell	
diffuse areas	
sclerosis	
Intermediate Grade	
D. Malignant lymphoma, follicular	
Predominantly large cell	
diffuse areas	
sclerosis	ML centroblastic-centrocytic (large), follicular ± diffuse
E. Malignant lymphoma, diffuse	
Small cleaved cell	
sclerosis	ML centrocytic (small)
F Malignant lymphoma, diffuse	
Mixed, small and large cell	ML centroblastic-centrocytic (small), diffuse
sclerosis	ML lymphoplasmacytic/-cytoid, polymorphic
epithelioid cell component	
G. Malignant lymphoma, diffuse	
Large cell	ML centroblastic-centrocytic (large), diffuse
cleaved cell	ML centrocytic (large)
noncleaved cell	ML centroblastic
sclerosis	
High Grade	
H. Malignant lymphoma	
Large cell, immunoblastic	ML immunoblastic
plasmacytoid	
clear cell	T-zone lymphoma
polymorphous	
epithelioid cell component	Lymphoepithelioid cell lymphoma
I. Malignant lymphoma	
Lymphoblastic	
convoluted cell	ML lymphoblastic, convoluted cell type
nonconvoluted cell	ML lymphoblastic, unclassified
J. Malignant lymphoma	
Small noncleaved cell	
Burkitt's	
follicular areas	ML lymphoblastic, Burkitt type and other B-lymphoblastic
Miscellaneous	
Composite	—
Mycosis fungoides	Mycosis fungoides
Histiocytic	—
Extramedullary plasmacytoma	ML plasmacytic
Unclassifiable	—
Other	—

Index

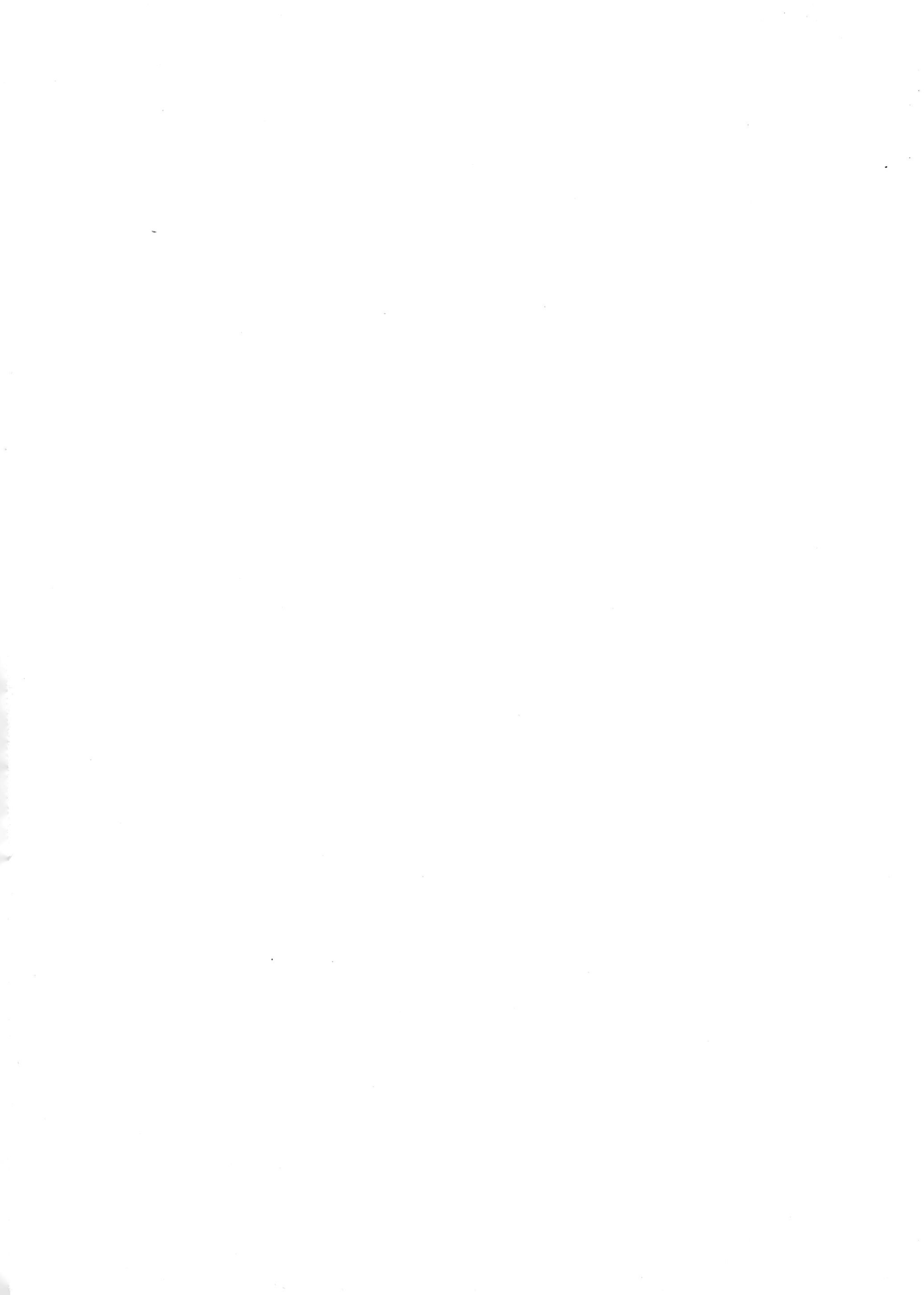